*Embryonic Medicine
and Therapy*

trophoblast, endocrinology, yolk sac, xenobiotics
epidemiology, transgenesis, fetal stem, ultrasound
virology, proliferative disorders, nerve regeneration
oncologists, metabolic diseases, bioethics, cloning
altzheimer's, early pregnancy, diagnostics, paradox
biological warfare defense reproductive technique
embryonic, toxicology, **gene,** yolk sac, virus, therapy
immune-modulatory, **cancer,** cell transplant, I.V.F., fetal
organ transplant, **diabetes,** genetics, cell transplant,
parkinson's **embryonic,** wound healing, endocrinology
transplant, **reproductive,** paradox, organ transplant
detection, **proliferation,** preimplantation factor, I.V.F.
zoology, **endocrinology,** genetics, virology, cloning
gametes, **antiproliferation,** cell biology, early pregnancy
immune, **lupus, bioethics,** oncologists, lupus, teratology
biology, **early detection,** therapy, **gene,** transplant
virology, **trophoblast control,** I.V.F., **metabolic** diseases
cancer, **complex, yolk, fetal stem, teratology,** genetics
diabetes, **detection, paradox, development,** invasion
toxicology, **techniques, cancer, yolk sac,** detection
embryonic, **nerve regeneration, bioethics,** toxicology
proliferation, **early detection, therapy,** embryonical
early pregnancy, **altzheimer's, cloning,** antiproliferation
oncologists, teratology, **cell, biology,** cell transplant, sac
techniques, cancer, yolk sac, xenobiotics, apoptosis
amniotic fluid, cell, oncologists, bioethics, cloning
transgenesis, epidemiology, ultrasound, fetal stem
fetal viability, therapy, integrins, human gametes
marker, proliferation control, in vitro fertilization
endocrinology, yolk sac, xenobiotics, trophoblast

The above graphical rendition is the logo of SIEP, the Society for the Investigation of Early Pregnancy, the not for profit entity, and it has granted inclusion of the logo in this volume. The logo was designed to portray the embryo as a source of understanding and reaching for elements of cure of the representative ailments, disorders, and conditions portrayed therein and depicts typical vehicles used in this medical field.

The logo remains the copyright of the SIEP.

Embryonic Medicine and Therapy

Edited by

ERIC JAUNIAUX
Academic Department of Obstetrics and Gynaecology,
University College London Medical School,

EYTAN R. BARNEA
SIEP (Society for the Investigation of Early Pregnancy),
USA

and

R.G. EDWARDS
Churchill College, Cambridge and
The London Women's Clinic,
London

Oxford   New York   Tokyo
OXFORD UNIVERSITY PRESS
1997

Oxford University Press, Great Clarendon Street, Oxford OX2 6DP

Oxford   New York

Athens   Auckland   Bangkok   Bogota   Bombay
Buenos Aires   Calcutta   Cape Town   Dar es Salaam
Delhi   Florence   Hong Kong   Istanbul   Karachi
Kuala Lumpur   Madras   Madrid   Melbourne
Mexico City   Nairobi   Paris   Singapore
Taipei   Tokyo   Toronto   Warsaw

and associated companies in
Berlin   Ibadan

Oxford is a trade mark of Oxford University Press

Published in the United States
by Oxford University Press Inc., New York

© Oxford University Press, 1997

A catalogue record for this book is available from the British Library

Library of Congress Cataloging in Publication Data
(Data available)

ISBN 0 19 262729 5

Typeset by EXPO Holdings, Malaysia

Printed in Great Britain by
Bookcraft (Bath) Ltd
Midsomer Norton, Avon

Foreword

C.H. Rodeck

Books can be divided into two types: those that fulfil a didactic and aim to represent a summation of knowledge, and those that are exploratory and forward-looking, that aim to define new pathways and to 'change the map'. This book is one of the latter. Its subject matter is early pregnancy and embryonic development in the human, one of the last great areas of ignorance in biology. Paradoxically, the lack of knowledge and understanding is inversely proportional to the crucial importance of the events taking place at this time. They shape and determine the outcome of the pregnancy and the health of both the mother and her offspring. Scientific studies of this area cannot fail to produce information of fundamental importance to biology and have far-reaching consequences for medicine.

How have the editors approached this challenge? They have drawn together a team of outstanding scientists from a variety of fields and disciplines, all relevant to the central theme. There are contributions on the human pre-implantation embryo, on implantation, on the development and biology of the trophoblast and on the disorders of early pregnancy. Results obtained from the use of the most advanced techniques of genetics, cell and molecular biology, sonography and endocrinology are presented. And the implications of transgenesis, gene and stem cell therapy, and ethics are considered. The editors are to be congratulated on their vision and the way in which this book begins to realise it.

Preface

FUTURE DIRECTIONS AND LIMITATIONS

In the past few years, there has been a realization that increased understanding of a major new field of medicine—that of early pregnancy—is now necessary. Firstly, because the field of reproductive medicine, which includes the well advanced assisted reproductive technologies, has reached a point at which greater understanding of implantation if further progress is to be made (the rate-limiting step in reproduction) and the factors contributing to successful pregnancy are essential; and secondly because the medical community has begun to appreciate that the study of this unique period of early pregnancy is having a major impact on a wide variety of disciplines, including transplantation, genetic manipulation, immunology, endocrinology, and control of cell proliferation.

In the preface to their book *Human embryology*, Hamilton and Boyd (1946) recommended that students obtain access to serial sections of mammalian and, if possible, human embryos. Aware of the problem of obtaining intact human embryos, they provided a chapter dedicated to comparative vertebrate embryology. This and their subsequent books continue to be a source, model, and inspiration for the quality of illustrations and original concepts in embryology. Long gone, but not forgotten, are the shy but pioneering attempts made by early workers in the field. Only through their work have we reached where we are today.

In the past 50 years, the advent of *in vitro* fertilization, ultrasound imaging, and progress in biochemistry, cell biology, immunology, molecular biology, pathology, and therapy have revolutionized our understanding of early pregnancy. However, 'modern' embryology textbooks almost totally ignore these extraordinary new developments, and continue to use the same classic descriptive drawings from 50 years ago. Furthermore, embryology remains for students a purely descriptive secondary specialty to anatomy, stimulating nothing but their capability to memorize Latin and Greek-derived terminology.

The growing certainty that recently gained information is becoming applicable to clinical medicine made us realize that a comprehensive and detailed presentation is now needed. At present, there are in fact three main areas of investigation discussed in the literature: *in vitro* embryology and the related techniques of fertilization; developmental molecular biology—an endless source of astonishing discoveries from experiments on animals; and materno-fetal physiology and medicine relating to human life *in utero* and the mechanisms involved in antenatal disorders. There is no doubt that what happens during and around the early phases of pregnancy has an influence not only on the remaining term of pregnancy, from both the fetal and maternal point of view, but also on many pathophysiological conditions of childhood and adult life.

In our view, there is a need to identify and be able to distinguish between correctable/preventable and inevitable early pregnancy disorders; a need to develop, for human use, powerful new investigative tools that are minimally invasive and ethically acceptable; a need to devise specific disease-orientated therapies as elsewhere in medicine, and to move away from empiricism and 'treat-all-or-do-nothing' fatalism; and finally, a need to apply the lessons learned from the study of early pregnancy towards progress in other areas of medicine.

We believe that this novel field of medicine has finally come of age and intend this book to serve as an update on the major basic observations whose translation into clinical practice has not yet fully been explored. Thus we are attempting to link *in vitro* embryology with early human development *in utero*, a subject which has never been presented before. This exciting endeavour has been diligently tackled in an interdisciplinary approach by contributors with a wide spectrum of expertise.

We have divided the book into five sections: Part I deals with the pre-implantation embryo and uterine environment around and immediately after conception; Part II deals with the information of the materno–fetal interface; Part III presents different aspects of embryonic and early fetal life *in utero*; Part IV presents the general medicine of the embryonic and early fetal periods of human pregnancy; and Part V introduces innovative therapeutic techniques for childhood and adult disease along with ethical boundaries for embryonic research in humans.

It is the aim of this treatise to integrate the current knowledge base on post-fertilization reproductive medicine with the medical implications of observations made in early pregnancy. However, caution is in order since the enormous progress expected from implantation enhancement, embryo biopsy, genetic engineering, diagnosis and prevention of early pregnancy disorders, and the use of early pregnancy tissue for medical therapy, raises a spectrum of bioethical questions that, with the advancement of science, will have to be addressed again and again. It is only through an open-minded, judicious approach combined with continuous self- and peer scrutiny that we will progress into the next millennium with this evolving science continuing to play an important role.

London   *E.J.*
New Jersey   *E.R.B.*
London   *R.G.E.*
January 1997

Contents

List of Contributors

A. *Abbas* Harris Birthright Research Centre for Fetal Medicine, King's College Hospital, London SE5, UK

I. *Apaolaza* Academic Unit of Obstetrics, Gynaecology and Reproduction Physiology, St Bartholomew's, *and* The Royal London School of Medicine and Dentistry, Whitechapel, London E1 1BB, UK

E.R. *Barnea* SIEP (Society for the Investigation of Early Pregnancy), 1697 Lark Lane, Cherry Hill, NJ 08003-3157, USA

J.-D. *Barnea* 210 Buxton House, Brown University, Box 2633, Providence, RI 02912, USA

Z. *Blumenfeld* Department of Obstetrics and Gynecology, The Bruce Rappaport Faculty of Medicine, Technion-Israel Institute of Technology, Haifa 31096, Israel

M.*Bronshtein* Department of Obstetrics and Gynecology, The Bruce Rappaport Faculty of Medicine, Technion-Israel Institute of Technology, Haifa 31096, Israel

G.J. *Burton* Department of Anatomy, University of Cambridge, Downing Street, Cambridge CB2 3DY, UK

M. *Bustillo* Mt Sinai Medical Center, 1 Gustave L. Levy Place, Box 1175, New York, NY 10029-6475, USA

T. *Chard* Academic Unit of Obstetrics, Gynaecology and Reproductive Physiology, St Bartholomew's, *and* The Royal London School of Medicine and Dentistry, Whitechapel, London E1 1BB, UK

C.B. *Coulam* Reproductive Immunology, Genetics and IVF Institute, 3020 Javier Road, Fairfax, VA 22031, USA

M. *de Swiet* Institute of Obstetrics and Gynaecology, Queen Charlotte's and Chelsea Hospital, Goldhawk Road, London W6 0XG, UK

J.D.A. *Delhanty* Human Genetics Group, Galton Laboratory, University College London, Wolfson House, 4 Stephenson Way, London NW1 2HE, UK

R.G. Edwards Human Reproduction, Bourn Hall, Bourn, Cambridgeshire CB3 7TR, UK

J.M. Friedman University of British Columbia, Department of Medical Genetics, BC Children's Hospital, 4500 Oak Street, Vancouver, Canada V6H 3N1

O. Genbacev Department of Stomatology, University of California San Francisco, San Francisco, California 94143, USA

J. Goldberg Division of Hematology and Medical Oncology, Department of Medicine, UMDNJ Robert Wood Johnson Medical School, Cooper Hospital/University Medical Center, Camden, NJ 08103, USA

K. Gruboeck Early Pregnancy and Gynaecological Ultrasound Unit, Academic Department of Obstetrics and Gynaecology, King's College School of Medicine and Dentistry, University of London, Denmark Hill, London SE5 8RX, UK

J.G. Grudzinskas Academic Unit of Obstetrics, Gynaecology and Reproductive Physiology, St Bartholomew's *and* The Royal London School of Medicine and Dentistry, Whitechapel, London E1 1BB, UK

B. Gulbis Department of Clinical Chemistry, Hôpital Erasme, Université Libre de Bruxelles, Belgium

A.H. Handyside Department of Obstetrics and Gynaecology, St Thomas' Hospital, Lambeth Palace Road, London SE1 7EH, UK

R. Jaffe Department of Obstetrics and Gynecology, Division of Maternal—Fetal Medicine, University of Rochester, USA

E. Jauniaux Academic Department of Obstetrics and Gynaecology, University College London Medical School, 86–96 Chenies Mews, London WC1E 6HX, UK

C.J.P. Jones Department of Pathological Sciences, University of Manchester, Oxford Road, Manchester M13 9PT, UK

D. Jurkovič Early Pregnancy and Gynaecological Ultrasound Unit, Academic Department of Obstetrics and Gynaecology, King's College School of Medicine and Dentistry, University of London, Denmark Hill, London SE5 8RX, UK

S. Laplace Department of Transplantation and Clinical Immunology, Pavillon P, Hôpital Edouard Herriot, 69437 Lyon cedex 03, France

B.A. Lessey University of North Carolina at Chapel Hill, Department of Obstetrics and Gynecology, Chapel Hill, NC 27599, USA

H.-C. Liu Center for Reproductive Medicine, Cornell University Medical College, Department of Obstetrics and Gynecology, 515 East 71st Street, New York, NY 10021, USA

C. Lockwood Department of Obstetrics and Gynecology, NYU Medical Center/Bellevue Hospital, 550 First Avenue, New York, NY 10016, USA

L.A. Magee Department of Medicine, Mount Sinai Hospital, 600 University Avenue, Suite 428, Toronto, Ontario, M5G 1X5, Canada

D.P. Marazzo Department of Obstetrics, Gynecology, and Reproductive Sciences, Magee Womens Hospital; *and* Department of Genetics, University of Pittsburgh, Pittsburgh, Pennsylvania, USA

T. Mukherjee Mt Sinai Medical Center, 1 Gustave L. Levy Place, Box 1175, New York, NY 10029-6475, USA

K.H. Nicolaides Harris Birthright Research Centre for Fetal Medicine, King's College Hospital, London SE5, UK

M.E. Palmer Department of Anatomy, University of Cambridge, Downing Street, Cambridge CB2 3DY, UK

C. Paul Early Pregnancy and Gynaecological Ultrasound Unit, Academic Department of Obstetrics and Gynaecology, King's College School of Medicine and Dentistry, University of London, Denmark Hill, London SE5 8RX, UK

D. Raudrant Department of Gynaecology, Hôpital de l'Hôtel-Dieu, 69229 Lyon cedex 02, France

M.K. Sanyal Department of Obstetrics and Gynecology, and Comprehensive Cancer Center, Yale University Medical School, 333 Cedar Streets, New Haven, CT, USA

F. Schatz Department of Obstetrics and Gynecology, NYU Medical Center, 550 First Avenue, NY 10016, USA

P.N. Schofield Department of Anatomy, University of Cambridge, Downing Street, Cambridge CB2 3DY, UK

L.B. Schwartz Reproductive Endocrinology, Department of Obstetrics and Gynecology, NYU Medical Center, 550 First Avenue, New York, NY 10016, USA

N.J. Sebire Harris Birthright Centre for Fetal Medicine, King's College Hospital, London SE5, UK

F. Shenfield Fertility Unit, Jules Thorn Building, Middlesex Hospital, Mortimer Street, London W1N 8AA, *and* Academic Department of Obstetrics and Gynaecology, University College London Medical School, 86–96 Chenies Mews, London WC1E 6HX, UK

J.L. Simpson Department of Obstetrics and Gynecology; Department of Molecular and Human Genetics, Baylor College of Medicine, Houston, Texas, USA

C. Sureau Theramex Institute, bioethics, Women's health, and society, 38–40 Avenue de New York, 75116 Paris, France

J.-L. Touraine Department of Transplantation and Clinical Immunology, Pavillon P, Hôpital Edouard Herriot, 69437 Lyon cedex 03, France

A.L. Watson Department of Anatomy, University of Cambridge, Downing Street, Cambridge CB2 3DY, UK

E. Winterhager Institute of Anatomy, Medical School, University of Essen, D-45122 Essen, Germany

List of Abbreviations

α1-AT	α1-antitrypsin
α1-PEG	α1 pregnancy-associated endometrial protein
5-ASA	5-aminosalicylic acid
ACE	angiotension-converting enzyme
aCL	anticardiolipin
ACTH	adrenocorticotrosphic hormone
ADA	adenosine deaminase
ADO	allele dropout
ADP	adenosine diphosphate
AFP	alpha-fetoprotein
AHH	aryl hydrocarbon hydroxylase
ALP	alkaline phosphatase
ALT	alanine aminotransferase
AMP, cAMP	adenosine monophosphate, cyclic AMP
ANA	antinuclear antibody
APS	antiphospholipid antibody syndrome
aPTT	activated partial tromboplastin time
aPL	antiphospholipid
ARMS	amplification refractory system
ART	assisted reproductive technology
ASA	anti-sperm antibody
ASO	allele-specific oligonucleotides
AST	aspartate aminotransferase
AT-III	antithrombin III
ATP	adenosine triphosphate
AVP	arginine vasopressin
AZT	3′-azido-3′-deoxythymidine, zidovudine
BBT	basal body temperature
bFGF	basic fibroblast growth factor
BLG	β-lactoglobulin
BLS	bare lymphocyte syndrome
BM	basement membrane
BP	blood pressure *or* binding protein *or* benzo[a]pyrene
bp	base pairs
bpm	beats per minute
BWS	Beckwith–Wiedemann syndrome

CAH	congenital adrenal hyperplasia
CAM	cell-adhesion molecule
cAMP	cyclic adenosine monophosphate
CAT	chloramphenicol acetyl transferase
CBZ	carbamazepine
CC	choriocarcinoma
CEA	carcinoembryonic antigen
CES	cumulative embryo score
CF	cystic fibrosis
CFU-C, CFU-S	colony forming units, culture; colony forming units, spleen
CG	chorionic gonadotrophin
CHM	complete (or classical) hydatidiform mole
CL	corpus luteum
CML	chronic myelogenous leukaemia
CMV	cytomegalovirus
CNS	central nervous system
COH	controlled ovarian hyperstimulation
CPM	contained placental mosaicism
CRF	corticotropin-releasing factor
CRL	crown–rump length
CRP	cyclic AMP receptor protein *or* C-reactive protein
CSF	colony-stimulating factor
CT, vCT	cytotrophoblast, villous cytotrophoblast
CTD	connective tissue disorders
CVS	chorionic villus sampling
CYP	cytochrome P-450
DCIP	decidual chorionic gonadotrophin-inhibitory protein
DDAVP	desamino-8-arginine vasopressin
DHEA	dehydroepiandrosterone
DIA	differentiation inhibitor activity
DIC	disseminated intravenous coagulation
DD	dihydrodiol dehydrogenase
DM	diabetes mellitus
DMD	Duchenne muscular dystrophy
DMSO	dimethyl sulphoxide
DNA, DNAase	deoxyribonucleic acid, deoxyribonuclease
DNMT	DNA methyltransferase
DRVVT	dilute Russel viper venom time
DVT	deep venous thrombosis
EBV	Epstein–Barr virus
EC cells	embryonal carcinoma cells
ECM	extracellular matrix
EDF	embryo-derived factors

EDPAF	embryo-derived platelet-activating factor
EDTA	ethylene diamine tetra-acetic acid
EGF, EGFR	epidermal growth factor, EGF receptor
EH	epoxide hydrolase
ELISA	enzyme-linked immunosorbent assay
EPF	early pregnancy factor
ERCP	endoscopic retrograde cholangiopathy
ES cells	embryonic stem cells
ESR	erythrocyte sedimentation rate
ET-1	embryo transfer
ET-1	endothelin-1
EVC	extravillous cytotrophoblast
EVT	extravillous trophoblast
FA1, FA2	fetal antigens 1 and 2
FACS	fluorescence–activated cell sorter
FBC	full blood count
FBS	fetal bovine serum
FGF	fibroblast growth factor
FISH	fluorescent *in situ* hybridization
FITC	fluorescein isothiocyanate
FLT	fetal liver transplantation
FSH	follicle-stimulating hormone
FTI	free thyroxine index
FTT	first trimester trophoblast
G_1, G_2	'gap' phases in the cell cycle
GABA	gamma-aminobutyric acid
G-CSF	granulocyte-colony stimulating factor
GDM	gestational diabetes mellitus
GF	growth factor
GGT	gamma glutanyl transferase
GH	growth hormone
GIFT	gamete intrafallopian transfer
GLUT1, GLUT2	glutathion
GM-CSF	granulocyte macrophage-colony stimulating factor
GMP, cGMP	guanosine monophosphate, cyclic guanosine monophosphate
GnRHa	gonadotrophin-releasing hormone agonist
GP215, GP130	glycoproteins of 215 kDa and 130 kDa
GSH-T	glutathione S-epoxide transferase
GST	glutathione *S*-transferase
GvHD	graft-versus-host disease
GvHR	graft-versus-host reaction
hCG	human chorionic gonadotrophin

HELLP	hemolysis, elevated liver enzymes, and low platelets
HGF	hepatocyte growth/scatter factor
HIV	human immunodeficiency virus
HLA	human leucocyte antigen
hPL	human placental lactogen
HPP-CFC	high proliferative potential colony-forming cell
HPRT	hypoxanthine butanine transferase
HSG	hysterosalpingogram
HSPG	heparin sulphate proteoglycan
HSV TK	herpes simplex virus thymidine kinase
5-HT	5-hydroxytryptamine, serotonin
IBD	inflammatory bowel disease
ICAM	cell-adhesion molecule
ICM	inner cell mass
ICSI	intracytoplasmic spermatozoon injection
IDD	immunodeficiency disease
IEM	inborn errors of metabolism
Ig	immunoglobulin
IGF, IGF-BP	insulin-like growth factor, IGF binding protein
IL	interleukin
IRES	internal ribosome entry site
ITP	immune thrombocytopenic purpura
IU, IUGR	intrauterine, intrauterine growth retardation
IV	intravenous
IVF, IVF-ET	*in vitro* fertilization, IVF embryo transfer
IVIg	intravenous immunoglobulin
KCT	kaolin clotting time
LAC	lupus anticoagulant
LAK cell	lymphocyte-activated killer cell
LCR	locus control region
LD_{50}	median lethal dose
LDL-C	low-density lipoprotein cholesterol
LH	luteinizing hormone
LIF	leukaemia inhibitory factor
LP	luteal phase
LPD	luteal phase defect or deficiency
LPI	luteal phase insufficiency
LSP	liver-specific antigens
LTC-IC	long-term culture initiating cell
LTR	long terminal repeat
M, MII	mitosis phase in the cell cycle

M-CSF	macrophage-colony stimulatory factor
MEM	minimal essential medium
MFO	mixed function oxidase
MHC	major histocompatibility complex
MLC	mixed lymphocyte culture
MMP	matrix metalloproteases
MoMulv	Moloney murine leukaemia virus
MPA	medroxyprogesterone acetate
MPF	maturation promoting factor
MRI	magnetic resonance imaging
mRNA	messenger ribonucleic acid
MS-AFP	maternal serum alpha-fetoprotein
αMSH	α-melanocyte-stimulating hormone
MTP	metalloprotease
MUC-1	mucin
MUP	major urinary protein
NAD	nicotinamide–adenine dinucleotide
NADH	nicotinamide–adenine dinucleotide, reduced form
NCAM	neural cell-adhesion molecule
NGF	nerve growth factor
NK cell	natural killer cell
NSAID	non-steroidal anti-inflammatory drug
NTD	neural tube defect
NVP	nausea and/or vomiting of pregnancy
OI	osteogenesis imperfecta
OR	oestrogen receptor
OT	oxytocin
P	progesterone
PA	plasminogen activator
PAF	platelet-activating factor *or* 1-O-alkyl-2-*sn*-glycero-3-phosphocholine
PAH	polycyclic aromatic hydrocarbon
PAI	plasminogen activator inhibitor
PAPP-A	pregnancy-associated plasma protein A
PB	phenobarbital
PBC	primary biliary cirrhosis
PBL	peripheral blood lymphocyte
PCB	polychlorinates biphenyl
PCNA	proliferation cell nuclear antigen
PCO	polycystic ovary
PCR	polymerase chain reaction
PDGF	platelet-derived growth factor

PE	pulmonary embolus
PEG	polyethylene glycol
PEP	primer extension preamplification *or* progestagen-associated endometrial protein *or* progesterone-dependent endometrial protein
PGD	pre-implantation genetic diagnosis
PGE	prostaglandin E
PHM	partial hydatidiform mole
PI	pulsatility index
PIF	pre-implantation factor
PKC	protein kinase C
PKU	phenyketonuria
PL	placental lactogen
POMC	pro-opiomelanocortin
PP	plasma protein *or* placental protein
PR	progesterone receptor
PRL	prolactin
PSTT	placental site trophoblastic tumour
PTT	prothrombine time
PTH, PTHrP	parathyroid hormone, parathyroid, hormone-related protein
PVP	polyvinylpyrrolidone
PZD	partial zona dissection
QR	quinone reductase
RDS	respiratory distress syndrome
RF	radiofrequency
RFLP	restriction fragment length polymorphism
RI	resistive index
RIT	rosette inhibition test
RNA	ribonucleic acid
RTD	residual trophoblastic disease
RU486	antiprogestin
S	synthesis phase of the cell cycle
SCID	severe combined immunodeficiency disease
SCT	stem cell transplant
SDS-PAGE	sodium dodecyl sulphate-polyacrylamide gel electrophoresis
SLE	systemic lupus erythematosus
SP1	placenta-specific glycoprotein 1, schwangerschaft protein 1
SRP	stress response protein
SSCP	single strand conformation polymorphism
ST	syncytiotrophoblast (*or* sulphotransferase)
SUZI	subzonal insemination
SV40	Simian virus 40

SYS	secondary yolk sac
T cell	T lymphocyte, responsible for cell-mediated immunity
T_3, T_4	triiodothyronine, tetraiodothyronine (thyrokine)
TBG	thyroid-binding globulin
TF	tissue factor
TFT	thyroid function test
TGF	transforming growth factor
τGT	τ-glutamyl transferase
TIBC	total iron-binding capacity
TIMP	tissue inhibitor of metalloprotease
TNF	tumour necrosis factor
TRE	trinucleotide repeat expansion
TSH	thyroid-stimulating hormone
TTR	transthyretin
TVS	transvaginal sonography
TVUS	transvaginal ultrasound
UC	ulcerative colitis
UDGAT	uridine diphosphoglucoronie acid transferase
UI	unexplained infertility
UPD	uniparental disomy
US	ultrasound
VEGF	vascular endothelial growth factor
VMA	vanillylmandelic acid
vWD, vWF	von Willebrand's disease, von Willebrand factor
VZIg	varicella zoster immune globulin
YAC	yeast artificial chromosome
ZD	zona drilling
ZP	zona pellucida

I | *Pre-implantation embryo*

1 | *The pre-implantation and implanting human embryo*

R.G. Edwards

Pre-implantation and early post-implantation growth represent a period of rapid growth and differentiation. The embryo differentiates into trophoblast and inner cell mass, the process of implantation is initiated, and the germ layers and early organs are formed. The concepts outlined in this chapter are based on studies in several laboratory mammals and, to a great extent, in lower vertebrates and invertebrates, yet much information is now accruing on the human embryo. Studies on human embryos are closely regulated in many countries, and some types of research are totally restricted in others. Many recent references have been given in a textbook by Edwards and, Brody (1995), and readers are advised to consult it for references up to 1995.

THE CLEAVING EMBRYO AND BLASTOCYST

Migration and growth of embryos in the female reproductive tract

Human fertilization *in vivo* takes place in the oviductal ampulla, and embryos move through the oviducts driven by the ciliary and muscle activity of the Fallopian tube. Their transport may be arrested briefly at the utero-tubal junction. The oviductal lumen offers a suitable and a limited biochemical environment to sustain the embryo as it differentiates under the activity of its own genes and maternal RNA inherited from the oocyte (Dickens *et al.* 1995; Leese 1995). Isolated human oviduct cells cultured *in vitro* produce compounds that improve the development of mouse embryos *in vitro* (Liu *et al.* 1995). Compounds secreted into oviductal fluid may bind to human embryos and exert some sort of role in early embryonic growth. In animals, an oviductal 215 kDa glycoprotein (GP215), 'oviductin' (identical to alpha-fetoprotein), and other polypeptides enter the perivitelline space of eggs and embryos, bind to the zona pellucida, and may attach to blastomeres.

Embryo transport in the oviduct lasts for 24–96 h. The most advanced embryo found in the oviductal lumen had approximately seven cells (Avendano *et al.* 1975). Embryos entered the uterine cavity at eight-cell stage or thereabouts, and six ova and one morula were initially flushed from it on days four and five after ovulation. The first recorded human lastocyst collected from the uterus had 69 mural and 30 polar trophectoderm cells (stage 3–4 of the Carnegie classification) (Hertig 1968). In later studies (Table 1.1), more than one-half of human embryos were abnormal, for they

Table 1.1   Details of human embryos flushed from the
uterus on day 5 post-ovulation (Edwards and Brody 1995)

	Natural cycles	Stimulated cycles
One cell	12	13
Fragmented	13	3
2–18 cells	32	4
Morulae	15	4
Blastocysts	26	11

contained cytoplasmic fragments, arrested or fragmented blastomeres, or advanced signs of degeneration (Edwards and Brody 1995).

The pronucleate egg

Most knowledge on the growth of the pre-implantation human embryo has arisen from studies *in vitro*. Sperm entry into oocytes can occur within 45 min of insemination, and sperm chromatin condenses after one hour due to the replacement of arginine- and cystein-rich protamines by lysine-rich histones. Early stages of growth of the sperm head and movements of the pronuclei occur independently of any control by microfilaments, and the sperm centriole regulates the cleavage spindle (Van Blerkom *et al.* 1995). Sperm centrioles have been isolated and transferred into human oocytes. They are capable of stimulating the enucleation of tubulin and organizing a sperm aster in the recipient oocytes (Van Blerkom and Davis 1995).

The presence of two pronuclei in an egg 15–18 h after insemination provides evidence of normal fertilization, although many fertilized eggs can possess one, three, or more pronuclei. Characteristic nucleoli assemble in the two pronuclei and become active, indicating that ribosomal RNA activity has begun. The pronuclear stage lasts for 20–24 h in human eggs, with typical G_1, S, G_2, and M phases. DNA synthesis begins in male and female pronuclei approximately 12 h after sperm entry and lasts for 3–5 h. The G_2 phase lasts approximately 5 h (Balakier *et al.* 1993). Malfunctions in the sperm centriole can arrest growth at this stage or at syngamy by failing to produce a normal spindle apparatus (Asch *et al.* 1995). Some RNA synthesis may occur during these stages, perhaps to sustain pronucleus formation.

Some human eggs contain a single pronucleus after insemination. This condition may indicate the occurrence of parthenogenesis involving maternal chromosomes, or of androgenesis resulting from a failure of the female pronucleus to form normally. Approximately 5 per cent of fertilized eggs are tripronucleate, rising to 30 per cent under some circumstances. Three pronuclei usually indicate dispermy, which is the primary cause of this condition during *in vitro* fertilization (IVF), or digyny which is its primary cause after the intracytoplasmic injection of a spermatozoon into an oocyte (ICSI) (Edwards and Brody 1995).

Pronuclei enlarge, become closely apposed, then enter syngamy. Their chromosomes condense separately in prophase of the first cleavage division, mingle on the metaphase plate as the spindle forms, and divide at anaphase. One or more pronuclei may fail to decondense, and be expelled from the egg or more entirely into one blastomere of the 2-cell embryo. They may fuse with the blastomere nucleus or continue to develop independently, so producing diploid/triploid and other forms of mosaic embryos. Pronuclei excised from one fertilized egg can be transferred to another using micromanipulation or by applying lasers after the cytoskeleton has been disturbed with colcemid or cytochalasin B.

Syngamy usually lasts for a few hours and is followed by the first cleavage division, which resembles a mitotic division. The embryonic centriole which organizes the spindle during this division is derived from the proximal sperm centriole, which divides to produce two centrioles, located at opposite poles of the cleavage spindle (Van Blerkom *et al.* 1995). Nevertheless, parthenogenetic embryos can undergo cleavage, indicating that centriolar material can form from sources within the oocyte.

The cell-cycle proteins of the mitotic cycle are regulated genetically. They are expressed in embryos, especially during G_1/S phases, and control the mitotic cycle through ionic signals generated via second messenger systems. The successive activities of a series of genes govern the phosphorylation of cell-cycle proteins and their binding to cyclin. Regulatory proteins are transcribed from oncogenes such as *p53*, and are reversibly phosphorylated by cdc2 kinase during the M phase. The cdc2–cyclin B complex and its kinase activity associate to form pre-MPF (maturation promoting factor), and the complex is activated by dephosphorylation to initiate the M phase. Transcripts of the genes c-*mos* and cyclin B1 have been identified in human oocytes and pre-implantation embryos. Level of c-*mos* transcripts are high in mature oocytes and decline sharply after the 6-cell stage, presumably as maternal RNA is degraded. Cyclin B1 transcripts remain at constantly high levels throughout cleavage, presumably associated with the rapid proliferation of cells in the cleaving embryo (Heikenheimo *et al.* 1995).

Cleavage and blastulation

Cleaving embryos increase their cell numbers mitotically. The first cleavage division occurs approximately 24 h after fertilization. One blastomere usually divides before the other, and the cleavage planes like at right angles in the two blastomeres. Blastomeres communicate with each other through spindle midbodies, gap junctions, and microvilli until the 4-stage cell.

Successive closely timed cleavages result in 8- and 16-cell embryos, with each blastomere being round or oval and distinct from the others. These cleavages occur according to a pre-established programme which also regulates 'housekeeping' activities in embryos. Embryos now display 'compaction' as the outer layer of cells adopts a smooth appearance; this phenomenon starts at the 16-cell stage approximately, and results in the formation of the morula as outer and inner cells differentiate at the 8–16-cell stage, many cellular organelles in outside cells become polarized, and outer cells become tightly associated through demosomes and tight junctions. Changes in cytostructure of outer cells include the formation of microvilli and the synthesis of membranal carbohydrates, alkaline phosphatase, and 5′-nucleotidase, and extra-cellular matrix proteins including laminin, fibronectin and collagen (Edwards and Brody 1995).

Embryonic growth and differentiation are regulated genetically. A salient fact about mammalian development concerns the 'totipotency' of blastomere nuclei. This char-acteristic is illustrated by the potential of individual blastomere nuclei of 2- and 4-cell embryos in mice and other species to form an entire fetus when injected into an enu-cleated oocyte. Human blastomeres may display similar properties since the few sur-viving blastomeres of a cryopreserved 8-cell human embryo developed into a normal child (Veiga *et al.* 1987). Totipotency is also shown when a blastomere of a 2-cell embryo develops to full term when the other blastomere is destroyed, or by analyses of the growth of embryos from isolated blastomeres.

Trophectoderm must be produced early in development, since it is essential for implantation to occur. It appears as the blastocyst is formed. Cells may be allocated to inner cell mass and trophectoderm after the first cleavage division has occurred. Outer cells form mural trophectoderm and enclose the blastocoelic cavity; in contrast, polar trophectoderm overlies the inner cells which form the inner cell mass (Fig. 1.1). Membrane proteins such as β_2-microglobulin and antigens form an apical surfaces of differentiating trophectoderm cells as they lose their wide developmental potential. Inner cells remain non-polarized and totipotent (Rosner *et al.* 1990). The distribution of cells to inner cell mass and trophectoderm in animal and human embryos has been assessed by marking blastomeres to identify their fate (Mottla *et al.* 1995). The differ-entiation of these two tissues is partly regulated by the actions of protein kinase C (PKC) and β_4-galactosyl transferase (GalTase).

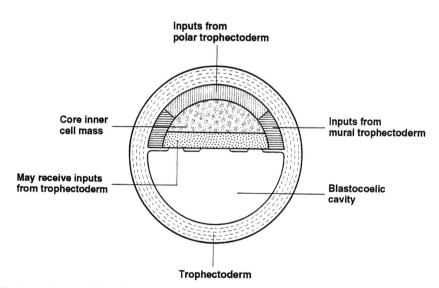

Fig. 1.1   Composition of various cellular zones in the mouse blastocyst (Fleming 1987).

The blastocyst is composed of a distinct inner cell mass placed eccentrically in the blastocoelic cavity, a single-cell layer of enclosing trophectoderm, and a zona pellucida. Some inner cell mass and trophectoderm cells die in these stages of growth, perhaps as part of a programme of cell death. Electrical polarity and apical–basal transcellular currents in outer cells apparently regulate the formation of the blastocoelic cavity, which could be formed via the generation of ATP and large amounts of water. Na^+/K^+ ATPase, a transmembrane enzyme, might utilize ATP to pump Na^+ into intracellular spaces, with water following to form the blastocoelic cavity. Blastocoelic fluid resembles intracellular fluid, and newly synthesized proteins are released into it from the inner cell mass and trophectoderm, including proteins with relative molecular masses of 33 000 and 155 000.

Fully differentiated trophectoderm is associated with the inner cell mass by desmosomes and gap and tight junctions, and there is no basal lamina between them. Trophectoderm resembles an epithelium, and many receptors differentiate on it. Nutrients and other compounds are transported across the trophectoderm. Distinct extracellular matrices containing laminin, fibronectin, and type IV collagen sustain cyto differentiation in the blastocyst.

Metabolism of cleaving embryos and blastocysts

Mammalian embryos display an increasingly active intermediary metabolism as development proceeds. Oocytes contain few nutrient stores, such as glycogen, and the increasing metabolic rate during cleavage is shown by a sharp increase in oxygen consumption, even though mammalian embryos do not tolerate high oxygen concentrations. Pyruvate is a major energy source for cleaving embryos, and lactate is utilized in some species. The tricarboxylic cycle and oxidative phosphorylation are active from 1-cell stage, as shown by the pressure of intermediary metabolites such as citrate, malate, glutarate, aspartate, and alanine in mouse embryos. Glucose metabolism and the glycolytic pathway become active in later cleavage stages, and produce large amounts of CO_2 and lactate. Human blastocysts convert 90 per cent of radiolabelled glucose to lactate (Wales *et al.* 1987), and glucose oxidation accounts for one-half of their oxygen consumption. Glucose is also increasingly metabolized for nucleic acid and lipid synthesis and for oxidation.

Total glucose metabolism in male morulae and blastocyts of cattle on day 7 is twice that in female embryos which have a more active pentose phosphate pathway (Tiffin *et al.* 1991); this difference might explain why male embryos develop more rapidly to blastocysts. Some glucose is converted to glycogen. Its transport is facilitated by GLUT1, a member of the sodium-independent transport system and found in inner cell mass and trophectoderm. GLUT2 appears in trophoblastic membranes facing the blastocoelic cavity (Aghayan *et al.* 1992).

Carrier systems transport amino acids, nucleosides, and purine and pyrimidine bases. Lipid synthesis provides energy sources and membrane precursors. Some maternal proteins are incorporated into embryos by micropinocytotic vesibles, including plasma proteins. Preimplantation embryos may incorporate methionine, a precursor for the universal methylation cofactor *S*-adenosyl methionine (Menezo *et al.* 1989).

REGULATORY ACTIVITY OF MATERNAL AND EMBRYONIC GENES

Maternal and embryonic RNA

Two sources of genetic information exist in early embryos, 'maternal' mRNA inherited from the oocyte, and embryonic mRNA transcribed after fertilization. Maternal poly(A+) mRNA encodes for many factors, including zona glycoproteins, mos protein, products of the oncogene c-*kit*, several enzymes, and connexion, a precursor protein of junctional complexes. Maternal RNA may code for factors acting over several cleavage divisions, such as hypovauthine-guanine transferase (HPRT) activity in mouse embryos, and the genes *oct3* which is the earliest-acting gene containing homeobox sequences which is active in totipotent or undifferentiated embryonic cells, ectoderm, and primordial germ cells.

Regular embryonic transcription begins in 4–8-cell human embryos, that is one cleavage division later than in mouse embryos (Braude *et al.* 1988). Embryonic mRNA codes for embryonic heat-shock proteins, proteins necessary to sustain the second cleavage division, and the activity of some oncogenes during the transition from morula to blastocyst. Embryonic transcription at this time includes genes encoding various enzyme systems which regulate differentiation and distorting growth; it is sensitive to α-amanitin. The first indications of paternal gene expression occur at this time, including the appearance of paternal variants of β_2-microglobulin and other proteins. Human chorionic gonadotrophin β (hCGβ) transcripts in 8-cell human embryos might be coded embryonically (Bonduelle *et al.* 1988), and hCG secretion begins as blastocysts expand on days 7–8 (Fishel *et al.* 1984). The onset and termination of endogenous gene activity in mouse and other embryos can be measured by incorporating reporter gene constructs into specific sites in embryonic DNA, which send a recognizable signal when nearby host genes are activated. The reporter gene is usually *lacZ* with its own promoter removed so that it responds to embryonic promoters.

Genes influence cleavage rates. *Ped* is related to a major histocompatibility complex, and its alleles encode for a surface antigen Qa-2(a) which hastens cleavage. The products of its other alleles can retard cleavage. Growth in mammalian embryos is influenced by their content of sex chromosomes, since human male embryos grow more rapidly than female embryos, a phenomenon previously reported in several species (Pergament *et al.* 1994).

Inactivation of one X chromosome in female embryos

Both X chromosomes are active in female embryos between early cleavage and morulae, when one becomes heteropycnotic. The heteropycnotic X chromosome then becomes genetically inert along much of its length in most cells of female embryos, probably due to the methylation of cytosine in gene promoter sites and in regulatory regions. Paternal alleles on the male X chromosome are transcribed briefly before inactivation occurs, e.g. *pgk1* and *hprt* (Singer-Sam *et al.* 1992). Inactivation begins in trophectoderm, then in inner cell mass, and perhaps finally in embryonic ectoderm.

The paternal X is preferentially inactivated in trophectoderm and primitive endoderm in mice, and in human proximal endoderm and extraembryonic ectoderm.

A few genes on the 'inert' human X apparently escape inactivation (Brown *et al.* 1991). Some of them are located adjacent to the segment pairing with the Y chromosome. These few genes thus remain active in both X chromosomes, i.e. in the Xi (inactive) and the Xa (active) chromosome. A novel gene, *xist* (Xi-specific transcripts), is expressed only from Xi and not from Xa. Located near the X-inactivation centre, it is female specific (Brown *et al.* 1991). These remarkable genetic events in female embryos could be responsible for typical somatic characteristics of XO fetuses and adults. Male embryos may possess rare loci which are active on both the X and the small Y chromosome.

A group of regulatory genes, many of them oncogenes, direct embryonic differentiation. They may contain a highly conserved DNA homeobox sequence of 60 amino acids, i.e. a homeodomain, and some code for proteins or polypeptides which bind to DNA an activate or repress other genes. The genes *oct3*, *oct4*, and *oct6* are transcriptional regulators in human and animal cells. They maintain totipotency or multipotency in embryonic cells, and are transcribed first from maternal RNA and then from embryonic genes in totipotent or multipotent cells (Rosner *et al.* 1990). In human embryos, *oct4* is expressed until approximately the 10-cell stage, and *oct6* thereafter (Abdel Rahman *et al.* 1995). The gene *rig*, with a nuclear location signal and a DNA-binding domain, also regulates transcription in early embryos. The human gene lacks TATA and CAAT boxes but has many CpG islands and multiple copies of a modifier in Sp1, which is a transcription factor. Another regulatory gene codes the protein GAL4, which has 881 amino acids and binds as a dimer to a symmetrical sequence of 17 DNA bases. Like other regulatory genes, it achieves this via a protein containing a residue of 65 amino acids with zinc and cysteine which help to form loops enabling the residue to bind specifically with nucleic acids. GAL4 recognizes a conserved CCG nucleotide triplet at each end of the DNA site (Marmostein *et al.* 1992).

Regulation is also imposed though competition between regulatory proteins and nucleohistones for binding to gene promoter regions in DNA (Felsenfeld 1992), and at the molecular level by RNA splicing or other post-transcriptional modifications. Correct methylation patterns are imposed on some genes in early embryos by demethylation and new methylation, including those carried on the inactive X chromosome. These genes are methylated in the inner cell mass and its derivatives (Singer-Sam *et al.* 1992), but not in trophectoderm and its descendants.

Genes regulate embryonic growth, differentiation, and implantation through the expression of growth factors, cytokines, and substrates. These factors may be derived from adjacent embryonic cells or from the mother, and they are regulated by genes involve in intracellular signalling, such as *Notch* (related to epidermal growth factor, EGF) and *dpp* (related to TGFβ). EGF stimulates protein synthesis, possibly via Na^+/K^+ ATPase and promotes hCG production by syncytiotrophoblasts (Maruo and Mochizuki 1987). Isoforms of TFGβ (β_1, β_2, and β_3) in 4-cell mouse embryos persist in inner cell mass and trophectoderm (Paria *et al.* 1992).

PDGF (platelet-derived growth factor) stimulates the completion of the fourth cell cycle in bovine embryos, and TGFα stimulates blastocyst formation immediately afterwards (Larson *et al.* 1992). Transcripts for insulin, IGF2, and their receptors, are produced in 2-cell mouse embryos, inner cell mass, and trophectoderm. Transcripts for PDGFA chain are present in blastocysts and early stem cells. IGF1 and IGF2 increase cell numbers in blastocysts via a pathway involving imprinted genes. Maternally produced insulin passing through trophectoderm may promote DNA, RNA, and protein synthesis in mouse inner cell mass. A factor known as differentiation inhibitor activity (DIA) may act in inner cell mass to regulate the terminal differentiation of some cell types. DIA has a relative molecular mass (M_r) of 43 000, resembles leukaemia inhibitory factor (LIF) or human interleukin, and its transcription is induced by phorbol esters, EGF, TGF, and cytokines. Many growth factor receptors are expressed on pre-implantation embryos. EGF and possibly FGF (fibroblast growth factor) receptors expressed during morula/blastocyst transition become restricted to trophectoderm.

Genomic imprinting

The activity of some embryonic genes is suppressed as a consequence of earlier inhibitory events occurring in the gonads. This phenomenon, called 'genomic imprinting', is apparently caused by the methylation of these genes in the ovary or testis (Surani *et al.* 1990). Gene expression in early embryos thus depends partly on whether the gene was inherited from mother or father. Many of these effects are reversed in later embryos, although some persist throughout the lifetime. Imprinting may be imposed by the methylation of specific gene sequences, although methylation could be a secondary effect of imprinting. Genes displaying imprinting during early embryogenesis tend to be paternally inherited, especially if they were transmitted through grandfather and father.

Genes can be imprinted for long periods, even permanently. This explains why some genetic diseases seem to be inherited from one parent. Imprinting also causes grandparental effects. A woman afflicted by an active gene inherited from her father may imprint it in her ovaries. The gene is thus inactive in her offspring, which are unaffected. In contrast, her sons transmit an active gene, so grandsons and granddaughters express the gene as in their grandmother. Imprinted genes passing through three or more generations of the same sex might become irreversibly methylated.

Imprinting influences parthenogenetic and androgenetic embryos which inherit their genes from only one parent. Androgenetic embryos, such as the human hydatidiform mole which contain only paternal genes and maternal mitochondria (Surani *et al.* 1990); their trophoblast grows rapidly through paternal imprinting but embryonic linkages develop poorly and are inadequate. Other imprinted genes affecting reproductive processes include mouse IF type 2 and its receptor (IGF2R; IGF, insulin-like growth factor) which is closely linked to the *Tme* locus. The *Igf2* gene is repressed at its maternal locus in mice so that IGF2 is inherited paternally. In some species, the gene for IGF1 receptor (IGF1R) is active only when inherited paternally, whereas *Igf2r* is repressed paternally so the receptor is inherited maternally in mice. These rules do not necessary apply to human embryos and in some species the IGF2 receptor gene is active when inherited from either parent (Barlow *et al.* 1991; Rappolee *et al.* 1992).

Examples of imprinted human genes in adults include neurofibromatosis type 1 (NF1), which is associated with benign tumours, bone defects, and other developmental abnormalities. It is expressed more severely if transmitted maternally, and this sex difference may be due to DNA methylation near the NF1 gene locus. The expression of Huntingdon's disease may be influenced by imprinting. Imprinting takes some highly unusual forms. The human Prader–Willi syndrome involves genetic obesity with mental retardation, and it is often associated with a deletion on chromosome 15 inherited from the father. Some cases (40 per cent) involving maternal uniparental dismay are even more extreme: they possess two maternal chromosomes 15 and no paternal equivalent. Such paternal chromosomes seem to be susceptible to mutation in the testis and are discarded and replaced by a duplicated mutant maternal chromosome in embryos. another human maternal isodisomy involves chromosome 7 and results in a very short stature. Angelman syndrome is exactly the opposite to Prader–Willi syndrome, and arises when inherited on a maternally derived chromosome 15 (Nicholls *et al.* 1989).

THE HUMAN PRE-IMPLANTATION EMBRYO *IN VITRO*

Growth of the human pre-implantation embryos *in vitro*

Approximately 40–50 per cent of embryos develop to blastocysts *in vitro*. Various types of media sustain their growth, such as Earle's medium containing pyruvate and albumin or serum, Whitten's medium, and Ham's 10. MEM (minimal essential medium) also sustain 27 per cent of embryos to blastocysts, and other satisfactory media have been based on human tubal fluid. Omitting glucose, and including EDTA, glutamine, lactate, and pyruvate in the presence of 10 per cent serum may improve growth to blastocysts and result in higher implantation rates per embryo, yet many workers still add serum to the culture medium which negates any prospect of obtaining reliable data in prospective trials.

Growth *in vitro* seems to resemble growth *in vivo*, a fact which questions the role of oviductal secretions as a source of supporting factors. Embryos should be at 2–4-cell stage on days 1–2 post-insemination, and 8–16 cells on days 3–4 (Table 1.2). Many have nucleated or anucleated fragments, an abnormal cytology, cytoplasmic debris, necrosis, uneven-sized blastomeres, or other pathological signs and rare embryos are still pronucleate on day 2. Blastomeres with a single nucleus may produce one-quarter of daughter cells containing multiple nuclei, and a similar proportion of multinucleated cells produce daughter cells which are mononucleate. Such striking events show how many cells in the pre-implantation embryo have a complex history, and are unlikely to be normal genetically (Pickering *et al.* 1995).

Growth *in vitro* is usually measured against a standard by calculating cleavages or cleavage numbers, using log-transformed cell numbers. Yet some embryos with good morphology may arrest at 2 cells by 2.5 days after fertilization (Edwards and Brody 1995), and others may delay at other stages for a day or more. Some arrested human embryos implant and develop into normal babies (Fishel *et al.* 1982), so these delays

Table 1.2   Timing of the growth of human embryos *in vitro*

Mid-stage of development	Hours post-insemination
2 cell	33.2 ± 1.3
4 cell	49.0 ± 1.9
8 cell	64.8 ± 1.8
16 cell	80.7 ± 2.4
Morulae	96.8 ± 1.9
Blastocyst	112.7 ± 2.9
Hatched blastocyst	*c.* 178

could be physiological rather than pathological. Some embryos cleave rapidly and implant when fertilization *in vitro* is delayed, as their cell division apparently catches up with a prearranged timetable. Measurements of uneven blastomeres, fragments, and other anomalies can also be used to assess the growth of human embryos. The timing of morulae or early blastocyst formation on day 4, and the appearance of these embryos, is another guide to human embryonic development *in vitro*. Growth can be assessed in single embryos in 5 μl microdrops by measuring the uptake of metabolites or the secretion of various factors. Assays for other metabolites, such as PAF (platelet-activating factor), may also be helpful.

Blastocysts usually form *in vitro* with 32–64 cells (means 58, range 24–90, 4.6–6.5 cleavages) on day 5 (Steptoe *et al.* 1971; Hardy *et al.* 1989a). More cells are allocated to human inner cell mass than in other species, which also displays more cell death (Hardy *et al.* 1989). The inner cell mass may be prominent or diffuse, with a few associated large cells on the inner cell mass adjacent to the blastocoel. Human blastocysts can form with only five or six cells on day 5 and resemble trophoblastic vesicles. Distinct anomalies include several small blastocoelic cavities, membranous folds or septae traversing the blastocoelic cavity, a diffuse inner cell mass, and localized areas of necrosis. Some blastocysts have two inner cell masses, and others posses a small blastocoelic cavity, no inner cell mass, and display various forms of damage or necrosis.

Chromosomal anomalies in human embryos growing *in vitro*

Up to one-third of all embryos might inherit chromosomal disorders from oocyte or spermatozoon, and this proportion is doubled if fertilization is delayed or many blastomeres are fragmented. These anomalies include monosomies, trisomies, triploidy, tetraploidy, structurally changed chromosomes and other anomalies which distort normal growth (Table 1.3). Even more embryos are apparently chromosomal mosaics. Many of these afflicted embryos can cleave abnormally, and many do not implant or merely give a transient rise in plasma hCGβ at implantation. Some of these disorders *de novo* in the gametes or in early embryos, and others can be inherited from either parent.

Such chromosomal anomalies in embryos arise from anomalous events occurring during meiosis as gamete maturation occurs, or at fertilization. Disperm leads to the formation of fertilized eggs with three pronuclei. Approximately 5–6 per cent of eggs

Table 1.3 Frequency of chromosome imbalance in 391 human oocytes and 261 human spermatozoa: data combined from several studies (Edwards and Brody 1995)

Chromosome complement	Number of oocytes	Number of spermatoza
Total	391	261
Hyperhaploid*	29 (7.5%)	6 (2.3%)
Hypohaploid*	59 (15.5%)	33 (12.6%)
Polyploid	8	–
Structural	15	24
Diploid	34	–

* The incidence of monosomy and trisomy is usually based on hyperhaploids, since chromosome loss during fixing and staining could explain the higher frequency of hypohaploids.

are multipronucleate. Many tripronucleate eggs develop as triploids, but they can form complex haploid mosaics, diploid/triploid mosaics, and complex heteroploids, depending on movements of the three pronuclei at syngamy. One of the pronuclei may be expelled, permitting the other two to form a normal diploid embryo. Mosaicism, haploidy, triploidy (and higher levels of euploidy) stem from parthenogenesis, high-order polyspermy or digyny, and chromosome fragmentation. Most tetraploid embryos probably arise through the suppression of the first or a later cleavage division, or as a consequence of trispermy.

A few embryos contain chromosomes with structural damage or fragmentation, and approximately 8 per cent of chromosome defects in human embryos, including balanced translocations and deletions, are inherited from either parent. Some oocytes (< 2 per cent) are parthenogenotes. In one study, a frequency of 1.6 per cent of them, derived from eggs with one pronucleus, was identified. Many good-quality embryos carry a chromosomal abnormality, and 83 per cent of poor-quality embryos are afflicted (Ederisinghe et al. 1992).

Autosomal trisomies and monosomies, the most frequent anomalies, usually arise during meiotic errors in oocytes, and afflict every autosome pair. Their frequency is correlated with maternal and not paternal age. Chromosome 16 trisomy occurs in 30 per cent of all fetal trisomies, so it must have a high survival rate. Autosomal monosomy and trisomy are responsible for much of the embryonic death before and soon after implantation; one-quarter, perhaps even one-half of fetuses in women over 40 years old, are afflicted (Hassold and Jacobs 1984). More than 5 per cent of births in women of 45 and older are chromosomally imbalanced. Double monosomies and double trisomies, and more complex forms of heteroploidy, share the same fate. Imbalance of the sex chromosomes arises during meiosis in oocytes or spermatocytes.

Mosaic embryos are common, as shown by fluorescent *in situ* hybridization (FISH), and are formed through errors in syngamy or mitotic errors during mitosis in a blastomere. Blastomeres carrying multiple nuclei with differing combinations of sex chromosomes probably arise through mitotic or nuclear irregularities (Munné and Cohen 1993). Some mosaics are diploid/heteroploid mosaics which may arise through nondisjunction during cleavage. Chimeras are rare during preimplantation growth. The division of an oocyte into two halves ('immediate cleavage'), with each half being fertilized, could result in very rare chimeras, since various pronuclear combination have been observed in the two halves.

The introduction of FISH has simplified the identification of many complex mosaics, monosomies, and trisomies. At least four different chromosome pairs were identified in a single nucleus using FISH (Munné *et al.* 1993), which enabled > 90 per cent of the blastomeres to be scored and identified anomalies in 70 per cent of embryos with arrested cleavage. FISH revealed that multiple nuclei within a blastomere arose through a failure of cell division, since they carried the same sex chromosome constitution as mononucleated cells in the same embryo. Other cells with multiple nuclei may form as a syncitium, and could even be precocious syncitiotrophoblast cells. More than five polyploid cells were identified using FISH on 30 per cent of human blastocysts, in tests for chromosomes X, Y, and 18 simultaneously (Benkhalifa *et al.* 1993). FISH also revealed how 30 per cent of morulae and blastocysts had more than five cells which were polyploid for the sex chromosomes and chromosome 18. Similar estimates were obtained using karyotypes.

Many fertilization anomalies are encompassed in the aberrant pregnancy called the hydatidiform mole. Its 'complete' form involves grossly swollen hydatid cysts of trophoblastic villi, composed of trophoblast and endoderm, and evidently nourished by diffusion from maternal blood. The embryos are 46 XX androgenones, arise from a single spermatozoon, and possess paternal chromosomes and maternal mitochondria (Kajii and Ohama 1977). Complete hydatidiform moles apparently arise through anomalies in the second meiotic spindle which cause the entire spindle and its chromosomes to be shed from the oocyte at fertilization (Edwards *et al.* 1992). The sperm chromosomes duplicate during syngamy, resulting in XX or YY androgenic embryos. The YY embryos die, so that only XX embryos are found after implantation (Kajii and Ohama 1977). Partial or incomplete moles arise from diandric triploids, and are often XYY, while some extreme examples have 92, XXXY chromosomes. The risk of a hydatidiform pregnancy increases from 1 in 1000 or more after its first occurrence to less than 1 in 16 after two successive molar pregnancies.

Developmental anomalies in human pre-implantation embryos

Many human embryos appear to develop abnormally *in vitro*, and the same conditions could well arise in those growing *in vivo*. One estimate is that two-thirds of human embryos display some form of anomaly by the 4–8-cell stage (Winston *et al.* 1991). Some blastomeres have a normal ultrastructure yet contain multiple nuclei which incorporate DNA precursors. Others possess extranuclear chromatin with a low precursor uptake, or many pseudonuclei which might be expelled into extracellular spaces. Among 30 embryos examined on day 2, 23 had 2–4 cells but most had multinucleate and anucleate cells and only 10 had a fully satisfactory appearance. On day 3, most embryos were apparently normal, yet many blastomeres were multinucleate or anucleate and only 33 per cent appeared fully normal (Winston *et al.* 1991). Multinucleated nuclei do not necessarily indicate embryo degeneration. Such defects arise through disordered cytokinesis, abnormal spindle mechanics, or 'furrowing' and blebbing during cleavage. Micronuclei or extruded chromatin could result from chromosomal non-disjunction and cause mosaicism and lagging chromosomes.

Embryos growing *in vitro* can also possess fragments or abnormal cells which may be excluded from the inner cell mass. These cells may be extruded into the blasto-coelic cavity, or from trophectoderm to the perivitelline space. Trophectoderm might tolerate binucleate and polyploid nuclei, as it does in later growth as shown by the phenomenon of confined placental mosaicism. The inner cell mass can form despite a modest number of trophectoderm cells, indicating that 'biochemical' pregnancies do not arise through lack of an inner cell mass (Hardy *et al.* 1989). Cryopreserved blas-tocysts with an expanded blastocoel have better chances of implantation (Hartshorne *et al.* 1991) and many with multiple cavities or areas of necrosis will also implant. The blastocoel collapses and expands during culture, apparently as a preliminary to its 'hatching' from the zona pullucida and days 6–7.

Some human embryos can apparently repair such damage and withstand stress. Two-fifths of embryo growing in culture formed blastocysts with between < 10 and > 60 nuclei on day 5, although at best only 13 per cent of all fertilized eggs had devel-oped normally from fertilization (Winston *et al.* 1991). Some of these anomalies could be due to the methods of culture. Reactive oxygen species such as H_2O_2 (hydro-gen peroxide) are synthesized by pre-implantation embryos and may act as second messengers. Hydrogen peroxide levels treble in mouse pronucleate eggs exposed to gas phases containing 20 or 40 per cent oxygen as compared with 5 per cent O_2. Excess light also sharply increases the embryonic production of hydrogen peroxidase, which could invoke excessive lipid and protein peroxidation in high concentrations, affect transcription, spindle assembly, and cell division. Interactions between H_2O_2 and superoxide in the presence of traces of iron or copper can produce highly toxic hydroxyl radicals, which can be prevented by utilizing metal chelators, catalases, or peroxidases to remove H_2O_2. Glutathione peroxidase converts H_2O_2 to H_2O in the presence of reduced glutathione.

Mouse embryos are protected and grow more rapidly when superoxide dismutase, EDTA, or thioredoxin, a protein disulphide reductase, are added to culture medium (Nasr-Esfahani *et al.* 1990). Growing cultures of animal and human embryos under low oxygen status might help, but not sufficiently to overcome the additional effects of transient exposure to light and 20 per cent O_2 in an IVF clinic. Protection is also conferred by removing iron from the medium, and by avoiding excess illumination and high oxygen tension. Cumulus cells could be protective by detoxifying superox-ides or through their high content of reduced glutathione.

Scoring and improving the growth of human embryos *in vitro*

Most embryologist score embryos by their gross appearance; for example grade 1 embryos are normal with no fragments, grades 2–3 display increasing abnormalities, and grade 4 are grossly distorted and fail to implant (Plachot and Mandelbaum 1990). Embryo's 'scores' have been introduced, based on blastomere number and size, anucle-ate fragments, and cleavage rate, or combinations and multiplications of these factors (Fig. 1.2) (Steer *et al.* 1992). Adhesion between blastomeres and zona thickness or

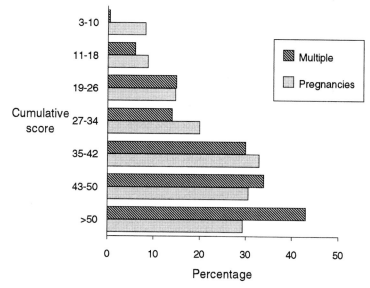

Fig. 1.2   A cumulative embryo score based on the growth rate and quality of human embryos in relation to the establishment of pregnancy (open bars) and the proportion of multiple pregnancies (hatched bars) (Steer *et al.* 1992).

semi-computerized scanning videos may help to indicate good growth (Cohen *et al.* 1989*a*). Blastocyst markers included early cavitation (blastulation), an expanding blastocoel and inner cell mass (grade 1), a transitional phase with multiple and persisting vacuoles with sharp borders and a delay in normal blastocyst formation (grade 2), and foci of degeneration and a collapsed cavity within 24 h (grade 3). Methods of embryo grading do not necessarily discriminate normal embryos or those with better prospects for development.

Biochemical methods have been introduced to score human embryos growing *in vitro* (Edwards and Brody 1995). The uptake or secretion of metabolites into microdrops of medium over a defined interval can be measured at various periods of pre-implantation growth (Leese *et al.* 1986; Hardy *et al.* 1989*a*; Gott *et al.* 1990). Human embryos incorporate pyruvate at rates varying between 36 pmol/embryo/h before fertilization and 27 pmol/embryo/h in morulae. Simultaneous measurements showed how pyruvate uptake rose from 40 pmol/embryo/h on day 2.5 rising to 50 pmol by day 4.5, whereas glucose uptake was < 20 pmol/embryo/h until day 4.5 then 40 pmol on day 5.5. 44 pmol/embryo/h of lactate was released from embryos growing normally in a lactate-free environment on day 2.5, rising to 95 pmol/embryo/h on day 5.5, much more than from arrested embryos (Leese 1995). These three parameters could be combined in a single assay. Metabolic activity can be radically changed by placing embryos *in vitro*, for example with enhanced lactate synthesis. Estimates of ATP and ADP might also identify human embryos with good growth potential. ATP, ADP, and AMP are indices of cell viability, although oxygen consumption has little diagnostic value.

Feeder layers (co-cultures) of various cell types may support the growth of human embryos *in vitro*, by 'conditioning' the medium or absorbing harmful components in it (Bongso *et al.* 1993). The growth of feeder cells must be arrested, e.g. by exposure to X-rays, to prevent them reaching confluence, causing high acidity and exhausting substrates. Feeder cells for human embryos should be human cells since animal cells can introduce harmful viruses and other contaminants, and they should come from one of the embryos' parents, to avoid cross-infection. Cultures of human oviductal epithelium would be the most likely cell type to assist embryos (Liu *et al.* 1995). Some other cell lines produce various products, such as amino acids, growth factors, steroid hormones, proteins, and immunoglobulins (Fig. 1.3). Beneficial effects claimed for co-cultures must be non-specific, since kidney epithelium sustains embryonic growth as effectively as oviductal epithelium. Matrigel has also been investigated as an alternative substrate to culture human pre-implantation embryos (Carnegie *et al.* 1995).

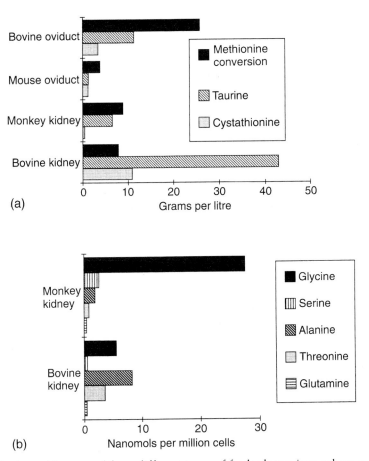

Fig. 1.3 Amino acids secreted from different types of feeder layers into culture medium after 48 h (Edwards and Brody 1995).

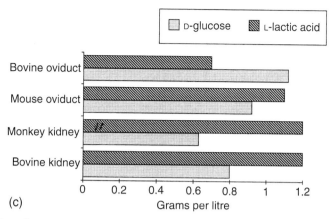

(c)

Fig. 1.3 *continued*

Impressive results with feeder layers still await prospective trials to assess their value. Benefits claimed for co-cultures include less blastomere fragmentation; more blastomeres at transfer; better rates of blastocyst formation, expansion, and hatching; and embryos with higher implantation rates. An equal number of reports contradict the value of feeder layers for human embryos. Many clinics practising co-culture do little more than leaving a few cumulus cells around the embryos.

Improved culture media have been sought in order to overcome the high frequency of anomalies in human embryos growing *in vitro*. These media are based on the composition of oviductal fluid or on analyses of embryonic metabolism. Some novel media might offer unique advantages, for example concentration of 1 g/100 ml protein in T6 medium is similar to that in human tubal fluid (0.4 g/100 ml), which is mostly albumin. Human tubal fluid also contains high levels of potassium, whereas Ham's F10 has high levels of pyruvate and low amounts of calcium and might best be replaced by Ham's F12.

Static droplets of medium may not be optimal for the culture of embryos over a period of 2–3 days, since they fail to reflect dynamic changes in the oviductal and uterine environments. Media may become hypoxic, and mammalian embryos are poorly adapted for anaerobiosis. Culturing several embryos together might help, as they release soluble growth factors which may sustain the growth of adjacent embryos. Two simple media may be all that are needed, one for insemination and the other for embryo growth, but their correct design is still awaited.

Cryopreservation of pre-implantation embryos

Cryostorage is very effective and safe. The only unlikely damage to correctly stored tissues arises from physical processes such as ionizing radiation. The total dose received by a sample over some hundreds of years would hardly impair embryonic growth. The LD_{50} for mutation will ultimately be reached after many years, but this does not seem to be a serious problem even for the most radiosensitive stages in oocytes. All tissue damage accumulated in storage is manifested on thawing, since DNA repair enzymes do not function at such low temperatures (Ashwood-Smith 1992).

The greatest danger of cryopreservation to cells lies in the formation of intracellular ice and its melting on thawing. Large ice crystals damage cells physically, and smaller crystals inflict harm as they expand during thawing. The conditions of cryopreservation must be strictly controlled, since different types of cells have various freezing optima. Such optimal concentrations of cryopreservatives, and their degree of penetration into cells must be assessed. Ice formation is induced at a chosen temperature by 'seeding' samples at –6 to –7 °C, to prevent further supercooling (Ashwood-Smith 1992). Thawing rates are also controlled, and must be balanced with cooling rates for maximum survival.

Success with the cryopreservation of human oocytes is still limited by damage inflicted on cytoplasmic organelles. Recent reports show how 60 per cent of surviving oocytes have a normal spindle (Gook *et al.* 1993). Embryo cryopreservation is much more effective, and enables couples to have two or more successive replacement cycles after a single oocyte collection (Edwards and Brody 1995). Pronucleate and cleaving embryos are usually cultured overnight to ensure that their growth is normal and are replaced after thawing as 2- or 4-cell embryos. Implantation rates approach those obtained with fresh embryos. Propanediol or DMSO are usually used to cryopreserve 1-cell and cleaving embryos, and glycerol for blastocysts. Glycerol has a fusigenic effect on cleaving human embryos. Many embryos tolerate the loss of one or two blastomeres, and three-quarters of blastocysts can survive freezing with glycerol. Hatching human blastocysts survive cryopreservation, some with good post-thaw morphology.

Ultra-rapid methods of cryopreservation and vitrification have not been introduced routinely for human embryos. These methods involve the use of high concentrations or mixtures of cryopreservatives such as DMSO, propanediol, and acetamide with polyethylene glycol or a 1:1 ratio of 3.5 M propanediol and 3.5 M DMSO with sucrose (Ashwood-Smith 1992). These agents are often used in combination with sucrose which extracts some water from cells before freezing begins. Survival rates of 80 per cent or more have been attained with human embryos. Toxicity is avoided because only small amounts of DMSO penetrate into embryos at low equilibrium temperatures and brief exposures.

EXPERIMENTAL INVESTIGATIONS ON PRE-IMPLANTATION EMBRYOS

Micromanipulation of oocytes and embryos

Micromanipulation has been applied to embryos for many years. It may help to avoid the birth of children with inherited disease, by excising one or more blastomeres from cleaving human embryos or small pieces of trophectoderm from them for the diagnosis of inherited disease (pre-implantation diagnosis). The culture of isolated blastomeres to form a clump of several cells for diagnosis may offer an alternative method to excising trophectoderm as a means of obtaining several cells for diagnosis (Geber *et al.* 1995). More unusual, and still experimental approaches, involve methods such as pronucleus excision and transfer, the use of cytoblasts for repairing deficient embryos, injections of DNA into pronuclei, extracting ooplasm to examine mitochondria or for other purposes, destroying one blastomere in a 2-cell embryo or two or three in a 4-cell embryo, fusing embryos together, bisecting morulae or blastocysts, and transferring a donor cell or inner cell mass into a recipient blastocyst.

Inserting gene constructs into eggs, or using spermatozoa as a carrier, to form transgenic animals, has become a most valuable tool in mammalian embryology. Approximately 2 pl of DNA at concentrations of 1 ng/ml are injected, since higher concentrations are toxic. Specific DNA structures, 'fusion gene constructs', are prepared, such as regulatory *cis*-acting genes (i.e. those carried on the same DNA strand as the gene being regulated) linked to foreign genes in order to encourage transgene expression in a desired tissue. For example, the elastase gene directs transgene expression to the pancreas. Regulatory sequences can be incorporated to place transgenes under an external control factor. The metallothionin gene involved in the metabolism of heavy metals as inserted and enables the transgene to be switched on when transfected cells are exposed to heavy metals, glucocorticoid hormones, or zinc (Palmiter *et al.* 1982).

Cloning usually involves the transfer of a donor nucleus to an enucleated oocyte. Constructing identical twins by splitting a 2-cell or later embryo, sometimes called cloning, is different because offspring differ from both parents. Somatic nuclei fuse with oocytes when assisted by viruses, polyethylene glycol, or electroporation. Blastomeres can be excised from 2-cell or later embryos. Excising one cell from an 8-cell embryo is referred to as a 7/8 embryo, and excising two cells results in a cells 6/8 embryo. Many human 3/4 or 7/8 embryos and morulae with 4–5 excised cells grow normally but growth is increasingly jeopardized in 6/8 embryos (Krzyminska *et al.* 1990). Cryopreservation can also breach the zona pellucida and destroy many blastomeres in human embryos. Human embryos may tolerate blastomere excision because more cells are committed to the inner cell mass than in some other species. Tissue can be excised from blastocysts, and embryos may 'collapse' and lose blastocoelic fluid if some mural trophectoderm is excised, but most re-expand *in vitro*.

Chimeric embryos are formed by fusing two embryos or by injecting totipotent cells into the blastocoelic cavity of recipient blastocysts. This work has led to the production of 'knock-out' or 'knock-in' mice. The descendants of a donor cell can differentiate into all cell types in the recipient fetus, including the gonads where they form spermatogonia or oogonia. The chimera produces two types of spermatozoa, derived from the blastocyst and from the donated cell respectively (Gardner 1968). Transgenic animals can be bred in this way, using donor cells with inserted or ablated genes to establish 'humanized' mice and other forms of genetically modified offspring. Knock-out animals are now a regular aspect of research into mammalian embryology and genetics.

More important clinically would be the use of these methods to permit an embryonic cell to be excised, genetically repaired, and then replaced in the blastocyst. The implications of colonizing the germ line would have to be considered carefully.

Pre-implantation diagnosis of human inherited disease

The pre-implantation diagnosis of genetic disease in embryos was introduced in 1968 (Edwards 1993). It relies on on the identification of disease genes in blastomeres or trophectoderm excised from the embryo being diagnosed. It is being applied clinically to relatively simple situations such as sickle-cell anaemia where the mutation involves an A to Y change in codon 6 of the b-globin gene, and to more complex systems such as deletions or *de novo* mutations arising in different exons of the Duchenne and Becker muscular dystrophy genes. As with aminiocentesis and chorionic villous sampling (CVS), knowledge of the exact nature of the genetic risk in a particular family is helpful but not always essential (Table 1.4). Typing embryos for sex using X- or Y-linked markers can avoid the birth of boys afflicted with X-linked mutant genes.

Today's methods mostly involve fluorescent *in-situ* hybridization (FISH), in which radio-, lectin-, or fluorescent-labelled DNA probes of known sequence anneal to complementary sequences in histological sections. DNA methods based on the polymerase chain reaction (PCR) can be used if the nucleotide sequence for the gene is known (Bentley 1993). Specific DNA sequences are amplified greater than 10^6-fold by 30 amplification cycles, to levels easily detectable using routine electrophoresis (Saiki *et al.* 1988). Many different target DNAs can be amplified simultaneously even in a single cell ('multiplexing'). Sensitivity and specificity in PCR are greatly improved by using 'nested primers' for two or more genes. PCR must be carried out in highly clean or sterile conditions, with constant guard against contaminations from external sources.

Other approaches include restriction fragment length polymorphisms (RFLPs) using enzymes to cleave DNA at specific sites and then identifying differing fragment sizes by electrophoresis. Markers can be identified close to a mutant gene. Southern blotting utilizes radiolabelled DNA fragments of known sequences to probe genomic or amplified DNA. An amplification refractory system (ARMS) ensures a matching between the 3′ end of the primer and the mutant gene and so avoids amplifying the

Table 1.4 Value of direct and indirect assays for analysing variations in DNA sequences (Bentley 1993)

Indirect assays	Applied when positive family history of disease exists Informative markers essential Do not require knowledge of the mutant gene Methods include RFLPs and Southern blotting
Direct essays	No need for pedigree analysis The mutation must be known Methods can be applied in all cases PCR methods and its derivatives: e.g. allele-specific oligonucleotide probes (ASO), amplification refractory systems (ARMS), competitive oligonucleotide priming (COP), primer extension preamplification (PEP)

normal allele (Bentley 1993). Fluorescent PCR, in which different electrophoretic bands are stained in a variety of colours, offers a variant of PCR (Findlay *et al.* 1995).

Primer extension preamplification (PEP) involves the amplification of large sequences (78 per cent) of the entire genome of a single cell, such as a spermatozoon. A reaction mixture containing several random primers composed of 15 oligonu-cleotide bases is used initially, followed by the further amplification of specific DNA templates that are now available. More than three-quarters of the whole genomic DNA in a single spermatozoon has been amplified in this way (Zhang *et al.* 1992).

Specific DNA Y primers such as the Y-specific pDP35 can be used to calculate X:Y ratios in human spermatozoa and the frequency of lymphocytes carrying a Y chromo-some (Sarkar 1989). PCR or PEP enable specific X- and Y-linked nucleotide sequences to be identified in a single spermatozoon, and a primer set with a derivative of DXYS1 maps in the distal short arm of the human Y chromosome (Page *et al.* 1989). Human embryos have been sexed using PCR on single excised blastomeres. Several gene pairs have been utilized, including a 149 bp sequence repeated 800–5000 times on the long arm of the Y chromosome and Y sequences on the pseudoautosomal boundary; X-specific repeat sequences including the PERT87-15/BamH1 RFLP; a 130 bp sequence on the X chromosome combined with a 500 bp Page sequence on the Y in a duplex assay; and the two amelogenin alleles present on X and Y chromosomes respectively which were co-amplified with Y-linked DYZ1 receptive elements to detect contamination (Levinson *et al.* 1992). The amelogenin alleles were also identified using fluorescent PCR (Findlay *et al.* 1995). PEP was applied to exon 10 of the cystic fibrosis membrane-conductance gene and repeat sequences on the X chro-mosome of single blastomeres (Xu *et al.* 1993).

These methods are important in the application of ICSI, since Y-chromosome dele-tions are a primary factor in some severe forms of male infertility (Reijo *et al.* 1995). DNA in first polar bodies excised from human oocytes was amplified by PCR to detect the segregation of genes for cystic fibrosis, haemophilia A, β-globulin, and α1 antitrypsin (α1 AT) deficiency in the oocyte (Strom *et al.* 1990). Polar body analysis suffers from the nature of gene segregation in oocytes and polar bodies, and is greatly influenced by the degree of gene cross-over in heterozygotes.

Embryos can be sexed using FISH with specific probes such as pBamX7 to react with a repeat centromeric sequence on the X, and pHY2.1 to react with a repeat sequence on the long arm of the Y (Handyside *et al.* 1989). Up to 90 per cent of blas-tomeres can be labelled. Probes labelled with different fluorochromes distinguish specific chromosomes in addition to the XY, such as 13, 18 and 21. Some repeat sequences may be shared by different chromosomes, e.g. by chromosomes 13 and 21. Identifying these chromosomes is a valuable in averting the birth of trisomies of these types. Triploids, tetraploids, monosomics, and mosaics can also be identified.

As yet, pre-implantation diagnosis has been confined to relatively few clincs. The total number of correctly diagnosed children born cannot exceed 50, and at least three errors in diagnosis have been reported. Alternative approaches are being intro-duced, including the sexing of spermatozoa or the identification of fetal cells in extracts from the lower uterine pole (Briggs *et al.* 1995) or in maternal blood (Lo *et al.* 1990); Bianchi *et al.* 1990).

Embryonic stem cells *in vitro*

Culture lines of embryonic stem cells (ES cells) have proved invaluable in many studies on genetics and differentiation in mammalian embryos. ES cells are usually derived from inner cell mass, and they can be maintained *in vitro* whereupon their properties remain virtually indistinguishable from those of inner cell mass and epiblast.

Many ES cells are totipotent, with a development potential equivalent to inner cell mass/epiblast. Leukaemia inhibitory factor (LIF) maintains their undifferentiated state and could be a regulator of pluripotential embryonic ectoderm. Retinoic acid or transfection by the NF1 gene or the c-*fos* proto-oncogene induces their endodermal differentiation (Toguichida *et al.* 1988; Wagner 1990). Erythropoietin, interleukins 1 and 3 (IL-1, IL-3), M-CSF, and GM-CSF induce them to differentiate into haematopoietic tissue. They colonize all tissues including the germ line in recipient blastocysts. A variant, EC cells derived from trophectoderm, do not have fully totipotent properties.

Genes can be inserted or ablated from ES cells. Gene targeting (i.e. introduced DNA searches for and recombines (with or 'targets' native DNA) is achieved by transfection, electroporation, and other methods. Gene ablation is achieved by introducing an artificial gene construct into the targeted gene site, in order to disrupt its reading frame (Smithies *et al.* 1985; Robertson and Bradley 1986; Thomas and Capecchi 1986). A cloned gene fragment with known intron–exon boundaries and containing inserts for c-*fos* and the gene for neomycin (*neo^r*) is incorporated. Various retroviruses are widely used for targeting, but cellular responses to inserted genes are often weak in the absence of a *cis*-regulating element, or if recipient DNA contains repressors. Transformed cells are then separated by means of positive/negative selection using metabolic markers such as neomycin which has been introduced into the targeted cells by the vector. The position of the inserted or ablated gene is confirmed by vital dyes or DNA methods such as PCR (Robertson and Bradley 1986; Robertson 1991). Many inserted genes are very active but their efficiency is rather low, often less (approximately 1 per cent) than that achieved with DNA injections into pronuclei. No human studies have been reported.

THE HATCHED HUMAN BLASTOCYST

Hatching of the blastocyst

Expanding ('hatching') human blastocysts prepare for implantation by escaping from their enclosing zona pellucida by days 6–7 post-fertilization. *In vivo*, uterine enzymes may have a major role in hatching, by dissolving the zona pellucida. *In vitro*, enzymes digest a hole in the zona pellucida, and blastocysts then escape by a limited series of contractions and expansions—perhaps 5–6 in all. Internal pressure from the blastocysts may assist hatching. The mouse enzyme is strypsin, apparently localized to trophectodermal sites. A similar enzyme in human blastocysts may be secreted over the whole trophectoderm and must be capable of digesting ZP2f and ZP3f formed from

ZP2 and ZP3 after fertilization. A hardened zona pellucida apparently resistant to proteolytic digestion can impair hatching. Trophectoderm blebs through the hole, helped by the periodic contractions and expansions of the blastocyst (Gonzales *et al.* 1995).

Human blastocysts can become semi-constricted during hatching, trapped temporarily half-in and half-out of the slit zona pellucida, and so resemble a figure 8. The empty zona pellucida is seen to be split or punctured after hatching, and it contains living and dead cells and cell debris. These cytoplasmic remnants may be abnormal cells and tissues ejected from the blastocyst during its growth. Embryos failing to hatch perish within zona pellucida *in vitro*, which may be a significant form of embryonic loss *in vivo*. Drilling small incisions in the zona pellucida during cleavage is reported to overcome problems in hatching and improve implantation rates, but no prospective trials have been reported (Cohen *et al.* 1990). Holes 20–30 μm wide can be made in the zona pellucida using an erbium laser (Strohmer *et al.* 1992).

Identical twins might arise from half-hatched figure-8 blastocysts joined in the region of the inner cell mass since inner cell mass and trophectoderm persist in many of the halves (Edwards *et al.* 1986). Identical twins have been born from a thawed human blastocyst with an artificially thinned zona pellucida (Nijs *et al.* 1993). Identical twins may also form if the inner cell mass splits in two.

Differentiation of the germ layers and trophoblast

Hatched human blastocysts double in volume and elongate by 2–3 days after hatching (Edwards and Surani 1978). Their prominent inner cell mass becomes the embryonic disc located in a concave area of surrounding trophectoderm, and further stages of differentiation begin as extra embryonic endoderm differentiates and migrates around the blastocoelic cavity. The primary germ layers form between days 6 and 8 *in vitro* and primitive endoderm forms on days 7–8 (O'Rahilly and Muller 1987). Preparations for implantation at this time exhibit distinct trophoblastic microvilli, large cytotrophoblastic nuclei, intercellular junctions between trophoblast cells, and glycogen synthesis in differentiating endoderm (Edwards 1980). Cytotrophoblast, syncitiotrophoblast and primitive endoderm appear on days 6–7. The co-expression of heparin sulphate proteoglycan (HSPG) and laminin on basement membranes of the trophectodermal surface may initiate the attachment phase and indicate a competence to implant (Carson *et al.* 1993).

Trophoblast expresses inducers, cytokins, and paracine factors including IGF, TGF, FGF and PDGF, TGFα, and IGF2 between 5 and 8 days *in vitro*. Human blastocysts also express receptors for insulin, EGF, PDGF, TGFα, and EGF; IL-1b, IL-1R, and IL-R are also expressed (Simon *et al.* 1995). Trophoblast proliferation and its hormone secretion are stimulated by local EGF receptor ligands (EGF, TGFα). CSF-1, the ligand for the proto-oncogene c-*fms*, has been found in pre-implantation animal embryos (Cullingford and Pollard 1994).

Regulatory factors, substrates, and adhesion molecules confer a considerable liability for paracrine and autocrine functions on differentiating trophoblast. These factors include cytokeratin, placental-type alkaline phosphatase, plasminogen activator (PA) and its inhibitors (PAI-1 and PAI-2), high affinity uPA receptors, HLA class I frame-work antigens, NODG-5 antigen, receptors for integrins and LIF (especially in blast-ocysts), and IGF2 mRNA and protein (Sharkey *et al.* 1995). Heparan sulphate proteoglycan and laminin may be co-expressed on trophectodermal basement mem-branes. Integrins are expressed in human pre-implantation embryos, including a3, a5, av, b1, b3, and b4, together with the E-cadherins, ICAM-1 and NCAM (Fusi *et al.* 1992; Turpeenheim-Hujanan *et al.* 1992; Campbell *et al.* 1995). These include avb3/b5, and the receptors for fibronectin, laminin, and vitronectin. The gene for uPA may confer invasiveness on trophoblasts, as in somatic cells. Receptors for the Steel factor (c-*kit*) may be synthesized in the pre- and post-hatching embryo, and early indication that trophoblast will migrate along genetically defined pathways (Arceci *et al.* 1992).

Paracrinology and endocrinology of the hatched blastocyst

Blastocysts have active endocrine and paracrine roles in implantation. They may signal the uterus to initiate 'true' decidualization. Various types of signal, including hormones, cytokines, and other factors have been considered as potential embryonic signals (Table 1.5).

Most attention is paid to signals such as EDPAF (PAF, 1-O-alkyl-2-*sn*-glycero-3-phosphocholine) released in variable amounts within 48 h of fertilization (O'Neill 1985). Little is known about its structure; it migrates on silica thin-layer chro-matograms with an RF of 0.26. Its endometrial receptors are linked to membranal phospholipase C and calcium ion transport systems. It may activate uterine and sys-temic platelets, raise vascular permeability, and regulate prostaglandin synthetase, provoking thrombocytopenia and reducing circulating blood platelets.

Early pregnancy factor (EPF), another elusive factor, is assayed by complicated and subjective rosette inhibition tests. Its synthesis could depend on the action of EDPAF (Clarke *et al.* 1990). Plasma mononuclear cells from pregnant women each express over 6000 specific EPF receptors. EPF activity is present in the 12-kDa polypeptide thioredoxin, possibly as it interacts with a 68-kDa polypeptide similar to serum albumin (Di Trapani *et al.* 1991). It might be immunosuppressive, inhibit IgG expres-sion in mononuclear and other cells, and modulate the production of superoxides, prostaglandins, and peptide mediators.

Embryos send steroid signals to the mother. Human blastocysts secrete oestradiol, and perhaps progesterone *in vitro*, in amounts correlated with their hCG secretion

Table 1.5 Potential pre-implantation signals from the embryo to the mother (Edwards and Brody 1995)

EDPAF	Pregnancy-specific plasma protein C
EPF	Histamine-releasing factors
Oestradiol 17b	Prostaglandins
Progesterone	Inhibins
hCG	TGFα, IGF2

(Edgar *et al.* 1993). The role of luteal oestrogens during implantation in primates has become a matter of debate (Ghosh and Sengupta 1995).

Human blastocysts secrete HCG, especially after hatching (Fishel *et al.* 1984). *In vivo*, they produce 16 000 mIU daily by day 10 and 160 000 mIU by day 14, more than most blastocysts growing *in vitro* although some can release 19 500 mIU into culture medium (Lopata and Oliva 1993). Weak hCG production could signify the demise of blastocysts, since the corpus luteum may perish or local stimuli to the uterus may be impaired. Insulin, transferrins, and PDGF seem to be involved in initiating hCG secretion from human blastocysts by 7–8 days *in vitro*.

REFERENCES

Abdel-Rahman, B., Fiddler, M., Rappolee, D., and Pergament, E. (1995). Expression of transcription regulating genes in human preimplantation embryos. *Mol. Hum. Reprod.*, 1; see *Human Reproduction*, 10, 2787.

Aghayan, M., Rao, L.V., Smith, R.M. *et al.* (1992). *Development*, 115, 305–12.

Allen, N.D., Norris, M.L., and Surani, M.A. (1990). *Cell*, 61, 853–61.

Arceci, R.J., Pampfer, S., and Pollard, J.W. (1992). Role and expression patterns of CSF-1/c-*fms* and SF/*kit* mRNA during early pre-implantation mouse development. *Developmental Biology*, 151, 1.

Asch, R., Simerly, C., Ord, T., Ord, V.A., and Schatten, G. (1995). The stages at which human fertilization arrests: microtubule and chromosomal configurations which failed to complete development in humans. *Mol. Hum. Reprod.*, 1; see *Human Reproduction*, 10, 1897–906.

Ashwood-Smith, M.J. (1992). The low temperature preservation of fetal cells. In *Fetal tissue transplants in medicine*, (ed. R.G. Edwards), p. 299. Cambridge University Press.

Avendano, S., Croxatto, H.D., Pereda, J., and Croxatto, H.B. (1975). A seven-cell human egg recovered from the oviduct. *Fertility and Sterility*, 26, 1167–72.

Bagshawe, K.D. and Lawler, S.D. (1982). *British Journal of Obstetrics and Gynaecology*, 89, 255–7.

Barlow, D.P., Stöger, R., Hermann, B.G., *et al.* (1991). The mouse insulin-like growth factor type 2 imprinted and closely linked to the Tme locus. *Nature*, 349, 84–6.

Bavister, B.D. (1995). Culture of preimplantation embryos: facts and artefacts. *Human Reproduction Update*, 1, 91–148.

Benkhalifa, M., Janny, L., Vye, P., Malet, P., Boucher, D., and Menezo, Y. (1993). Assessment of polyploidy in human morulae and blastocysts using co-culture and fluorescent *in situ* hybridization. *Human Reproduction*, 8, 895–902.

Bentley, D.R. (1993). The direct diagnosis of genetic defects. In *Preconception and preimplantation diagnosis of human genetic disease*, (ed. R.G. Edwards), p. 183. Cambridge University Press.

Bianchi, D.W., Flint, A.F., Pizzimenti, M.F., *et al.* (1990). *Proceedings of the National Academy of Science (USA)*, 87, 3279–83.

Bonduelle, M.L., Dodd, R., Liebars, I., Van Steirteghem, A., Williamson, R., and Akhurst, T. (1988). Chorionic gonadotrophin-β mRNA, a trophoblast marker, is expressed on human 8-cell embryos derived from tripronucleate zygotes. *Human Reproduction*, 3, 909–14.

Bongso, A., Fong, C.-Y., Ng, S.-C., and Ratnam, S. (1993). The search for improved *in-vitro* systems should not be ignored: embryo co-culture could be one of them. *Human Reproduction*, 8, 1155–60.

Braude, P., Bolton, V., and Moore, S. (1988). Human gene expression first occurs between the four- and eight-cell stages of preimplantation development. *Nature*, **332**, 459–62.

Briggs, J., Miller, D., Bulmer, J.N., Griffiths-Jones, M., Rame, V., and Lilford, R. (1995). Non-syncytial sources of fetal DNA in transcervically recovered cell populations. *Mol. Hum. Reprod.*, **1**; see *Human Reproduction*, **10**, 749–54.

Brown, C.J., Ballabio, A., Rupert, J.L., *et al.* (1991). A gene from the region of the human X-irradiation centre is expressed exclusively from the inactive X chromosome. *Nature*, **347**, 38–44.

Campbell, S., Swann, H.R., Seif, M.W., Kimber, S.J., and Aplin, J.D. (1995). Cell adhesion molecules on the oocyte and preimplantation human embryo. *Mol. Hum. Reprod.*, **1**; see *Human Reproduction*, **10**, 1571–8.

Carnegie, J., Claman, P., Lawrence, C., and Cabaca, O. (1995). Can Matrigel substitute for Vero cells in promoting the *in vitro* development of mouse.

Carson, D.D., Tang, J-P., and Julian, J.A. (1993). Heparan sulfate proteoglycan (perlecan) expression by mouse embryos during acquisition of attachment competence. *Developmental Biology*, **155**, 97–106.

Clarke, F.M., Orozco, C., Perkins, A.V., and Cock, I. (1990). Partial characterization of the PAF-soluble factor which mimics the activity of early pregnancy factor. *Journal of Reproduction and Fertility*, **88**, 459–66.

Cohen, J., Inge, K.L., Suzman, N., and Wright, G. (1989*a*). Videocinematography of fresh and cryopreserved embryos: a retroprospective analysis of embryonic morphology and implantation. *Fertility and Sterility*, **51**, 820–7.

Cohen, J., Elsner, C., Kort, H., Malter, H., Massey, J., Mayer, M.P., and Weimer, K. (1989*b*). Impairment of the hatching process following IVF in the human and improvement of implantation by assisted hatching using micromanipulation. *Human Reproduction*, **5**, 7–13.

Cohen, J., Alikani, M., Trowbridge, J., and Rosenwaks, Z. (1992). Implantation enhancement by selective assisted hatching zona drilling of human embryos with poor prognosis. *Human Reproduction*, **7**, 685–91.

Cullingford, T.E. and Pollard, J.W. (1994). Growth factors as mediators of sex steroid hormone action in the uterus during its preparation for implantation. In *Protooncogenes and growth factors in steroid hormone induced growth and differentiation*, p. 13–29. CRC Press, Boca Raton.

Di Trapani, G., Orosco, C., Perkins, A., and Clarke, F. (1991). *Human Reproduction*, **6**, 450–7.

Dickens, C.J., Maguiness S.D., Cromer, M.T., *et al.* (1995). Human tubal fluid: formation and composition during vascular perfusion of the Fallopian tube. *Human Reproduction*, **10**, 505–8.

Ederisinghe, W.R., Murch, A.R., and Yovich, J.L. (1992). Cytogenetic analysis of human oocytes and embryos in an *in vitro* fertilization programme. *Human Reproduction*, **7**, 230–6.

Edgar, D.H., James, G.B., and Mills, J.A. (1993). Steroid secretion by early human embryos in culture. *Human Reproduction*, **8**, 277–8.

Edwards, R.G. (1980). *Conception in the human female*. Academic Press, London.

Edwards, R.G. (ed.) (1983). *Preconception and preimplantation diagnosis of human genetic disease*. Cambridge University Press.

Edwards, R.G. and Brody, S. (1995). *Principles and practice of assisted human reproduction*. W.B. Saunders, Philadelphia.

Edwards, R.G. and Surani, M.A.H. (1978). The primate blastocyst and its environment. *Uppsala Journal of Medical Science*, **22**, 39–50.

Edwards, R.G., Mettler, L., and Walters, D.E. (1986). Identical twins and *in vitro* fertilization. *Journal of In Vitro Fertilization and Embryo Transfer*, **3**, 114–17.

Edwards, R.G., Morcos, S., Macnamee, M., Balmaceda, J.P., Walters, D.E., and Asch, R. (1991). High fecundity of amenorrhoeic women in embryo-transfer programmes. *Lancet*, **338**, 292–4.

Edwards, R.G., Crow, J., Dale, S., Macnamee, M.C., Hartshorne, G.M., and Brinsden, P. (1992). Pronuclear, cleavage and blastocyst histories in the attempted preimplantation diagnosis of the human hydatidiform mole. *Human Reproduction*, 7, 994–8.

Fehilly, C.B., Cohen, J., Simons, R.F., Fishel, S.B., and Edwards, R.G. (1985). Cryopreservation of cleaving embryos and expanded blastocysts in the human: a comparative study. *Fertility and Sterility*, 44, 638–44.

Felsenfeld, G. (1992). *Nature*, 355, 219–24.

Findlay, I., Urquhart, A., Quirke, P., Sullivan, K., Rutherford, A., and Lilford, R. (1995). Simultaneous DNA fingerprinting, diagnosis of sex and single-gene defect status from single cells. *Mol. Hum. Reprod.*, 1; see *Human Reproduction*, 10, 1609–18.

Fishel, S.B., Edwards, R.G., and Evans, C.J. (1984). Human chorionic gonadotrophin secreted by preimplantation embryos cultured *in vitro*. *Science*, 223, 816–18.

Fleming, T.P. (1987). A quantitative analysis of cell allocation to trophectoderm and inner cell mass in the mouse blastocyst. *Developmental Biology*, 119, 520–6.

Fusi, F.M., Vignalli, M., Busacca, M., and Bronson, R.A. (1992). Evidence for the presence of an integrin on the oolemma of unfertilized human oocytes. *Molecular Reproduction Development*, 31, 215–22.

Gardner, R.L. (1968). Mouse chimaeras obtained by the injection of cells into the blastocyst. *Nature*, 220, 596–7.

Gardner, R.L. (1996). Can developmentally significant spatial palterning of the egg be discounted in mammals? *Human Reproduction Update*, 2, 3–27.

Gardner, R.L. and Edwards, R.G. (1968). Control of the sex ratio in the rabbit at full term by transferring sexed blastocysts. *Nature*, 218, 346–8.

Geber, S., Winston, R.M.L., and Handyside, A.H. (1995). Results of IVF in patients with endometriosis: the severity of the disease does not affect outcome or the incidence of miscarriage. *Human Reproduction*, 10, 1492–6.

Ghosh, D. and Sengupta, J. (1995). Another look at the issue of peri-implantation oestrogen. *Human Reproduction*, 10, 1.

Gonzales, D., Jones, J., Bavister, B.D., and Shapiro, S. (1995). Time-lapse microscopy of the development of the human embryo *in vitro* from the pronuclear stage to the hatching of the blastocyst. *Human Reproduction Update*, 1, No. 2 Item 5, video.

Gook, D.A., Osborn, S.M., and Johnston, W.I.H. (1995). Parthenogenetic activation of human oocytes following cryopreservation using 1,2-propanediol. *Human Reproduction*, 10, 654–8.

Gott, A.L., Hardy, K., Windston, R.M.L., and Leese, H.J. (1990). Non-invasive measurement of pyruvate and glucose update and lactate production by single human preimplantation embryos. *Human Reproduction*, 5, 104–8.

Griffiths-Jones, M.D., Miller, D., Lilford, R.J., Scott, J., and Bulmer, J.N. (1992). Detection of fetal DNA in transcervical swabs from first trimester pregnancies by gene amplification: a new route to prenatal diagnosis. *British Journal of Obstetrics and Gynaecology*, 99, 508–11.

Handyside, A.H., Kontogianni, E.H., Hardy, K., and Winston, R.M.L. (1990). Pregnancies from biopsied human preimplantation embryos sexed by Y-specific DNA amplification. *Nature*, 344, 768–70.

Hardy, K., Handyside, A.H., and Winston, R.M.L. (1989*a*). The human blastocyst cell number, death and allocation during late preimplantation development *in vitro*. *Development*, 107, 597–604.

Hartshorne, G.M., Elder, K., Cros, J., Dyson, H., and Edwards, R.G. (1991). The influence of *in vitro* development upon post-thaw survival and implantation of cryopreserved human blasstocysts. *Human Reproduction*, 6, 136–41.

Hardy, K., Hooper, M.A.K., Handyside, A.H. Rutherford, A.J., Winston, R.M.L., and Leese, H.J. (1989*b*). Non-invasive measurement of glucose and pyruvate uptake by individual human oocyte, and preimplantation embryo. *Human Reproduction*, 2, 188–9.

Hassold, T.J. and Jacobs, P. (1984). Trisomy in man. *Annual Review of Genetics*, **18**, 69–97.

Heikenheimo, O. Lanzendorf, S.E., Baka. S.G., and Gibbons, W.E. (1995). Cell cycle genes c-*mos* and cyclin-B1 are expressed in a specific pattern in human oocytes and preimplantation embryos. *Mol. Hum. Reprod.*, **1**; see *Human Reproduction*, **10**, 699–707.

Henderson, D.J., Bennett, P.R., and Moore, G.E. (1992). Expression of human chorionic gonadotrophin α and β subunits is depressed in trophoblast from pregnancies with early embryonic failure. *Human Reproduction*, **7**, 1474–8.

Hertig, A.T. (1968). *Human trophoblast*. C.C. Thomas, Springfield.

Kajii, T. and Ohama, K. (1977). Androgenetic origin of hydatidiform mole. *Nature*, **268**, 633–4.

Larson, R.C., Ignotz, G.G., and Currie, W.B. (1992). Platelet derived growth factor (PDGF) stimulates development of bovine embryos during the fourth cell cycle. *Development*, 821–6.

Leese, H.J., Hooper, M.A.K., Edwards, R.G., and Ashwood-Smith, M.J. (1986). Update of pyruvate by early human embryos determined by a non-invasive technique. *Human Reproduction*, **1**, 181–2.

Levinson, G., Keyvanfar, K., Wu, J.C., *et al.* (1995). DNA-based X-enriched sperm separation as an adjunct to preimplantation diagnosis testing for the prevention of X-linked disease. *Mol. Hum. Reprod.*, **1**; see *Human Reproduction*, **10**, 979–82.

Li, A., Byllensten, U.B., Cui, X., Saki, R.K., Ehrlich, H.A., and Arnheim, N. (1989). Amplification and analysis of DNA sequences in single human sperm and diploid cells. *Nature*, **335**, 414.

Liu, L.P.S., Chan, S.T.H., Ho, P.C. *et al.* (1995). Human oviductal cells produce high molecular weight factors that improves the development of mouse embryos. *Mol. Hum. Reprod.*, **1**; see *Human Reproduction*, **10**, 2781–2786

Lo, Y. D., Patel, P., Baigent, C.N. *et al.* (1990). Prenatal sex determination fom maternal peripheral blood using the polymerase chain reaction. *Human Genetics*, **90**, 483–8.

Lopata, A. and Oliva, K. (1993). Chorionic gonadotrophin secretion by human blastocysts. *Human Reproduction*, **8**, 932–8.

Marmorstein, R., Carey, M., Ptashne, M., and Harrison, S.C. (1992). *Nature*, **356**, 408–14.

Maruo, T. and Mochizuki, M. (1987). Immunohistochemical localization of epidermal growth factor receptor and *myc* oncogene product in human placenta: implications for trophoblast proliferation and differentiation. *American Journal of Obstetrics and Gynecology*, **156**, 721–7.

Menezo, Y., Nicollet, B., Herbaut, N., and Andre D. (1992). Freezing cocultured human blastocysts. *Fertility and Sterility*, **58**, 977–80.

Mottla, G.L., Adelman, M.R., Hall, J.L., Gindoff, P.R., Stillman, R.J., and Johnson, K.E. (1995). Lineage tracing demonstrates that blastomeres of early cleavage-stage human preembryos contribute to both trophectoderm and inner cell mass. *Human Reproduction*, **10**, 384–91.

Munne, S. and Cohen, J. (1993). Unsuitability of multinucleated human blastomeres for human preimplantation genetic diagnosis. *Human Reproduction*, **8**, 1120–5.

Nasr-Esfahani, M.N., Aitken, J.R., and Johnson, M.H. (1990). Hydrogen peroxide levels in mouse oocytes and early cleavage stage embryos developed in vitro or in vivo. *Development*, **109**, 501–7.

Nicholls, R.D., Knoll, J.H.M., Butler, M.G., *et al.* (1989). Karam, S. and Lalande, M. Genetic imprinting suggest by maternal heterodisomy in non deletion Prader–Willi syndrome. *Nature*, **342**, 281–5.

Novak, E.R. and Woodruff, J.D. (1974). *Novak's gynecological and obstetric pathology*. W.B. Saunders, Philadelphia.

O'Neill, C.J. (1985). *Reproduction and Fertility*, **75**, 375.

O'Rahilly, R. and Muller, F. (1987). *Development stages in human embryos*, Publication 637. Carnegie Institute of Washington.

Palmiter, R.D., Chen, H.Y., and Brinster, R.L. (1983). Metallothionein-human GH fusion genes stimulate growth of mice, **29**, 701–10.

Pergament, E., Fiddler, M., Cho, N., Johnson, D., and Holmgren, W.J. (1994). Sexual differentiation and preimplantation cell growth. *Human Reproduction*, **9**, 1730–2.

Pickering, S., Taylor, A., Johnson, M.H., and Braude, P.R. (1995). An analysis of multinucleated blastomere formation in human embryos. *Mol. Hum. Reprod.*, **1**; see *Human Reproduction*, **10**, 1912–22.

Plachot, M. and Mandelbaum, J. (1990). Oocyte maturation, fertilization and embryonic growth *in vitro*. *British Medicine Bulletin*, **46**, 673–90.

Rall, W.F. and Fahy, G.M. (1985). Ice-free cryopreservation of mouse embryos at –196 degrees C by vitrification. *Nature*, **313**, 573–5.

Rappolee, D.A., Brenner, C.A., Schultz, R. (1988). Wound macrophages express TGF-alpha and other growth factors in vivo: analysis by MRNA phenotyping. *Science*, **241**, 1823–5.

Reijo, R., Lee, T-Y., Salo, P., *et al.* (1995). Diverse spermatogenic defects in humans caused by Y chromosome deletions encompassing a novel RNA-binding protein. *Nature Genetics*, **10**, 383–93.

Robertson, E.J. and Bradley, A. (1986). Production of permanent cell lines from early embryos and their use in studying developmental problems. In *Experimental approaches to mammalian embryonic development*, (ed. J. Rossant and R.A. Pedersen), pp. 475–508. Cambridge University Press.

Rosner, M.H., Vigano, M.A., Ozato, K., *et al.* (1990). A POU-domain transcription factor in early stem cells and germ cells of the mammalian embryo. *Nature*, **345**, 686–92.

Saiki, R.K., Gelfand, D.H., Stoffel, S., *et al.* (1988). Primer-directed enzymatic amplifcations of DNA with a thermostable polymerase. *Science*, **239**, 487–91.

Sarkar, S. (1989). Determining proportions of human X and Y sperm with a recombination deoxyribonucleic acid probe carrying a homologous sequence of sex chromosomes. *Fertility and Sterility*, **51**, 167–9.

Sharkey, A.M., Dellow, K., Blayney, M., Macnamee, M., Charnock-Jones, S., and Smith, S. (1995). Stage-specific expression of cytokine and receptor messenger ribonucleic acids in human preimplantation embryos. *Biology of Reproduction*, **53**, 974–81.

Simon, C., Pellicer, A., and Polan, M.L. (1995). Interleukin-1 cross talk between embryo and endometrium in implantation. In *Regulators of human implantation*, (ed. C. Simon and A. Pellicer). *Human Reproduction* (suppl. 2), 43–54.

Singer-Sam, J., Chapman, V., LeBon, J.M., and Riggs, A.D. (1992). *Proceedings of the National Academy of Science (USA)*, **89**, 10469–73.

Smithies, O., Gregg, R.G., Boggs, S.S., *et al.* (1985). *Nature*, **317**, 230–4.

Steer, C.V., Mills, C.L., Tan, S.L., Campbell, S. and Edward, R.G. (1992). The cumulative embryo score. *Human Reproduction*, **7**, 117–19.

Steptoe, P.C., Edwards, R.G., and Purdy, J.M. (1971). Human blastocysts grown in culture. *Nature*, **229**, 132–3.

Strohmer, H. and Feichtinger, W. (1992). *Fertility and Sterility*, **58**, 212–14.

Strom, C.M., Verlinsky, Y., Milayeva, S., *et al.* (1990). Preimplantation genetic diagnosis for cystic fibrosis by polar body removal and DNA analysis. *Lancet*, **336**, 306–8.

Surani, M.A., Allen, N.D., Barton, S.C., *et al.* (1990). Developmental consequences of imprinting of paternal chromosomes by DNA methylation. *Philosophical Transactions of the Royal Society*, B, **326**, 313–27.

Thomas, K. and Capecchi, M.R. (1986). Introduction of homologous DNA sequences into mammalian cells induces mutations in the cognate gene. *Nature*, **324**, 34–8.

Tiffin, G.J., Rieger, D., Betteridge, K.J., *et al.* (1991). *Journal of Reproduction and Fertility*, **93**, 125–32.

Toguichida, J., Kitshizaki, M., Sasaki, S., *et al.* (1988). *Nature*, **338**, 156–8.

Turpeenheim-Hujanen, T., Ronnberg, L., Kaupila, A., and Puistola, V. (1992). Laminin in human embryo implantation: analogy to the invasion by malignant cells. *Fertility and Sterility*, 58, 105–13.

Van Blerkom, J. and Davis, P. (1995). Evolution of the sperm aster after micromanipulation of isolated human sperm centrioles into meiotically mature human oocytes. *Mol. Hum. Reprod.*, 1; see *Human Reproduction*, 10, 2179–82.

Van Blerkom, J., Davis, P., Merriam, J., and Sinclair, J. (1995). Nuclear and cytoplasmic dynamics of sperm penetration, pronuclear formation and microtubule organization during fertilization and early preimplantation development in the human. *Human Reproduction Update*, 1, 429–61.

Veiga, A., Calderon, G., Barri, P.N., and Coroleu, B. (1987). Pregnancy after the replacement of a frozen-thawed embryo with < 50% intact blastomeres. *Human Reproduction*, 2, 321–3.

Wagner, E.F. (1990). On transferring genes into stem cells of mice. *EMBO Journal*, 9, 3025–92.

Wales, R.G., Whittingham, D.G., Hardy, K., and Craft., I.L. (1987). Metabolism of glucose by human embryos. *Journal of Reproduction and Fertility*, 79, 289–94.

Winston, N.J., Braude, P.R., Pickering, S.J., *et al.* (1991). The incidence of abnormal morphology and nucleocytoplasmic ratios in 2, 3 and 5-day human pre-embryos. *Human Reproduction*, 6, 17–24.

Xu, K.P., Tang, Y.X., Grifo, J., Rosenwaks, Z., and Cohen, J. (1993). Primer extension pre-amplification for detection of multiple genetic loci from single human blastomeres. *Human Reproduction*, 8, 2206–10.

Zhang, L., Cui, X.F., Schmitt, K., Hubert, R., Navidi, W., and Arnheim, N. (1992). Whole genome amplification from a single cell: implications for genetic analysis. *Proceedings of the National Academy of Science (USA)*; 89, 5847–51.

2 | Genetics of human gametes and embryos

Alan H. Handyside and Joy D.A. Delhanty

INTRODUCTION

The incidence of genetic defects at birth is about 2 per cent. Half of these defects are caused by chromosome imbalance and the other half by a combination of genetic contributions to congenital abnormalities and common diseases, and single gene defects, of which around 5000 have now been indentified. Low fecundity rates in fertile women of about 25 per cent per cycle (Wilcox *et al.* 1988) and high pregnancy losses, however, suggest that the incidence earlier in development is likely to be much higher. Spontaneous abortion occurs in 15–20 per cent of clinically recognized pregnancies and about half of these have abnormal karyotypes (Hassold 1986; Burgoyne *et al.* 1991). The development of *in vitro* fertilization (IVF) over the past twenty years for the treatment of infertility and, more recently, pre-implantation genetic diagnosis (PGD) have allowed studies of the genetics of gametogenesis, fertilization, and pre-implantation development. Here we briefly review some of these studies concentrating in particular on chromosomal abnormalities including both conventional karyotyping and more recent molecular cytogenetic studies using fluorescent *in situ* hybridization (FISH). The hybridization of DNA probes *in situ* to metaphase or interphase nuclei and rapid detection by either indirect or direct labelling with various fluorochromes has revolutionized our ability to examine gametes and early embryos and the use of different labels for different probes allows multicolour analysis of several probes simultaneously. Finally we describe recent progress in single-cell genetic analysis for PGD of both chromosomal and single gene defects.

SPERMATOZOA

The tight packaging of chromatin in the nucleus of spermatozoa normally prevents direct karyotype analysis. However, the development of the hamster egg penetration test for male infertility overcomes this problem since human sperm are capable of fusing and penetrating the hamster egg; the nuclei decondense and after a further period in culture, sperm chromosomes condense allowing the karyotype to be ascertained. Analysis of around 16 000 karyotypes accumulated over the past decade has revealed fewer than 200 hyperhaploid sperm, whereas the figure for structural anomalies was tenfold higher (Jacobs 1992). These results of course were limited to sperm capable of fertilization and the extraordinarily high incidence of structural defects suggests these may be a technical artefact.

FISH allows the rapid analysis of large numbers of sperm treated with reducing agents to decondense the chromatin for hybridization. Early studies with single probes to chromosome 1 or the Y chromosome indicated a wide variation in rates of disomy from 0.06–2.7 per cent (Martin *et al.* 1994). Hassold and colleagues used multicolour FISH with two or three probes (X, Y, and 16 or 18) and demonstrated a significant incidence of diploidy 0.2–1 per cent (Williams *et al.* 1993). Interestingly, diploid sperm have never been observed in the hamster egg studies suggesting that they may not be capable of penetrating the egg. The incidence of sex chromosome disomy at meiosis I was 0.09 per cent and, including meiosis II errors, 0.2 per cent. This is 1.5 times the incidence of disomy 16 and twice as common as disomy 18. Since half of 47, XXY individuals are attributable to paternal non-disjunction at meiosis I (Hassold *et al.* 1991), this confirms that the XY bivalent, unlike autosomal bivalents, are particularly prone to failure of disjunction in male meiosis.

More recently, Martin and colleagues have used a similar multicolour FISH strategy to examine the incidence of diploidy and disomy for chromosomes 1, 2, 4, 9, 12, 15, 16, 18, 20, 21, and the sex chromosomes in a large series (in excess of 400 000) of sperm nuclei from a number of chromosomally normal donors (Martin *et al.* 1995; Spriggs *et al.* 1996). The mean frequency of X- and Y-bearing sperm (50.1 and 49.0 per cent) were not significantly different from the expected 50:50 ratio and there was no evidence of a correlation between paternal age and the sperm sex ratio. The mean incidence of diploid sperm was lower than previous studies (0.16 per cent) but ranged between 0.06 and 0.42 per cent. The mean incidence of disomy ranged from 0.08 to 0.29 per cent (chromosomes 2 and 21) for the autosomes and 0.43 per cent for the sex chromosomes. This therefore indicates that both the sex chromosome bivalent and the chromosome 21 bivalent are more susceptible to non-disjunction in male meiosis. Again there was no evidence of a correlation with paternal age for either the incidence of diploidy or disomy.

Most *de novo* mutations causing single gene defects are paternal in origin and there is increasing evidence for an age-related increase (Crow 1993; Drost and Lee 1995). This is thought to be related to differences between spermatogenesis and oogenesis. Before gametogenesis, the numbers of primordial germ cells increase by mitosis as they migrate to the gonads. In the female, this mitotic expansion ceases late in gestation when oogonia enter meiosis and arrest at the dictyate stage of meiosis I until menstrual cycles are initiated at puberty. In the male, by contrast, mitotic division of spermatogonia continues throughout life. Thus the number of mitotic divisions preceeding gametogenesis is much greater in the male, increases with age, and may increase the risk of replication errors.

OOCYTES

The incidence of chromosomal abnormalities in oocytes arrested in metaphase II, mainly after failed fertilization, has been extensively studied by conventional karyotyping. However, in the spreading process chromosomes are easily lost and the contracted morphology of the chromosomes makes them unsuitable for precise banding analysis, limiting the specificity of the information available. Additionally, oocytes remaining unfertilized after exposure to sperm are inevitably aged by at least 40 hours since retrieval and 10–15 per cent, when analysed, turn out to be actually fertilized (see below). These factors combined result in low numbers giving a conclusive answer in each study series, with consequently variable proportions of hyperhaploidy, ranging between 2 and 14.5 per cent in eleven studies (reviewed by Zenzes and Casper 1992). Because it is not possible to distinguish true hypohaploidy from artefactual chromosome loss, total aneuploidy is usually estimated by doubling the figure for hyperhaploidy. Based on the 1120 oocytes in the eleven studies, the reviewers estimated the weighted mean percentage of aneuploidy as about 13 per cent; as expected, this figure is considerably higher than that found in sperm. Almost half of an unselected population of oocytes from cycles in which there was complete failure of fertilization *in vitro* as a result of dysfunctional sperm had chromosome abnormalities by cytogenetic analysis (Almeida and Bolton 1994). However, extrapolating this data to the incidence in oocytes with and without pronuclei following insemination (26.6 and 20.4 per cent, respectively) failed to demonstrate any significant correlation between chromosomal abnormalities and the ability to fertilize.

The karyotyping studies reviewed above suggested that non-disjunction of bivalents is the most common cause of aneuploidy whereas Angell (1991) has reported that hyperhaploid oocytes contain extra copies of single chromatids and not chromosomes indicating that, in particular, trisomy 16 may arise by predivision and abnormal segregation of chromatids rather than non-disjunction of chromosomes. Recent FISH analysis using probes to X, 18, and 13/21 simultaneously of both the first polar body and oocyte have demonstrated that both non-disjunction of bivalents and unbalanced segregation of prematurely divided chromatids can result in aneuploid oocytes (Dailey *et al.* 1996; Cozzi, Winston, and Delhanty, unpublished data). Dailey and co-workers were also able to demonstrate that aneuploidy rates increase with maternal age.

FERTILIZATION

In addition to those arising during gametogenesis, abnormal fertilization also contributes to genetic abnormalities in pre-implantation embryos. A common abnormality which arises with IVF is fertilization by more than one sperm, or polyspermy, which may in part be caused by the relatively high sperm concentrations used to inseminate oocytes. Conversely, some oocytes fail to fertilize and are parthenogenetically activated. Both of these abnormalities are easily detected by removing the cumulus cells which surround the oocytes when they are collected and examining the pronuclei 12–18 hours post-insemination. Fertilization rates for IVF average about 60 per cent with a 5–10 per cent incidence of tripronucleate embryos mainly resulting from dispermic fertilization and a 1 per cent incidence of embryos with one or no pronuclei with a second polar body indicating parthenogenetic activation. Triploid fetuses can develop to advanced stages before aborting and the majority have been shown to result from dispermic fertilization (Jacobs *et al.* 1978). A proportion of three pronucleate embryos develop to the blastocyst stage *in vitro* (Hardy *et al.* 1989). However, in some cases vacuoles can be mistaken for pronuclei so that the embryo may have been normally fertilized (Van Blerkom *et al.* 1987) and in other cases during syngamy a tripolar spindle is formed and the embryo divides into three diploid cells (Kola *et al.* 1987; Sathananthan *et al.* 1991). With tripronucleate embryos resulting from intracytoplasmic sperm injection (ICSI), the origin of the extra pronuleus is thought to be failure to extrude the second polar body (Sultan *et al.* 1995). Zygotes with a single pronucleus and apparently parthenogenetically activated can also undergo cleavage and a minority reach the blastocyst stage. Several studies either using karyotyping or FISH with sex chromosome probes, however, have demonstrated that at least 10 per cent are normally fertilized (Balakier *et al.* 1993; Harper *et al.* 1994; Lim *et al.* 1995). Also, direct analysis of the pronucleus in these zygotes has recently revealed that in some cases both male and female genomes have been combined in true syngamy (Levron *et al.* 1995).

PRE-IMPLANTATION EMBRYOS

The detection of precise chromosomal anomalies in the pre-implantation human embryo is extremely difficult by conventional karyotyping. The usual approach has been to incubate the whole embryo overnight with colchicine to arrest dividing blastomeres at metaphase, followed by attempts to spread the intact embryo. Not surprisingly, this produces poor quality chromosomes, either contracted and difficult to group, or more elongated but overlapping. In these circumstances, complete analysis of a single metaphase is counted as a success and there are few studies with analysis of several cells from individual embryos. Most studies are carried out on 'spare' embryos that are surplus to requirements after those suitable for transfer to the mother have been chosen. A few studies have utilized donated oocytes that are then fertilized specifically for research. In a review of four studies in which a reasonable number of embryos were analysed (30–50), abnormality rates ranging between 23 and 40 per cent were found (Zenzes and Casper 1992). Where sufficient detail was given, mosaicism with normal and aneuploid or polyploid cell lines appeared to be the most common abnormality. In an interesting comparison of the chromosome status of untransferred embryos between two groups of women undergoing IVF treatment, those who became pregnant and those that did not, Zenzes and co-workers analysed one to four mitoses per embryo; overall, 13 per cent of embryos only were normal diploid, 28 per cent aneuploid, and 36 per cent were mosaic (Zenzes *et al.* 1992). They concluded that the proportion of spare embryos that are chromosomally normal is significantly greater in pregnant than in age-matched IVF patients that did not become pregnant and also that detection of chromosomally normal embryos for transfer should improve the success rate in IVF.

Munné and colleagues have used multicolour FISH to analyse chromosome abnormalities in normally developing and arrested cleavage stage embryos (Munné *et al.* 1994*a*,*b*). With probes to X, Y, and chromosome 18, over half of a series of 131 embryos arrested at cleavage stages had nuclei with numerical aberrations and 6.1 per cent were aneuploid (Munné *et al.* 1994*a*). In another study, comparing arrested embryos with those not transferred following pre-implantation diagnosis, 28.8 and 17.1 per cent, respectively, were chromsomally mosaic (Munné *et al.* 1994*a,b*). More recently, 64 normally fertilized embryos were examined with directly labelled probes to X, Y, 18, and 16 (Munné *et al.* 1995). With the four chromosomes tested, 42 and 23 per cent of arrested and normal embryos, respectively, had numerical aberrations. In addition, there were four aneuploid embryos: two monosomies for chromosome 16, one for 18, and a trisomy for 16. We have also observed mosaicism of autosomes and sex chromosomes in morphologically normal, monospermic cleavage stage embryos (Harper *et al.* 1995). With dual analysis of chromosomes 1 and 17, 16 of 35 (46 per cent) had abnormal nuclei. One embryo was triploid, one was monosomic for chromosome 1 and ten were diploid mosaics (three diploid/aneuploid and four diploid/haploid). Four other embryos had different 'chaotic' numbers of the analysed chromosomes in most of the nuclei.

More recently, these observations have been extended by analysing a large series of normal embryos which were not transferred following PGD of sex in X-linked disease (Delhanty *et al.* 1997). In this series triple colour FISH with probes to X, Y, and chromosome 1 were used. Again about half of the embryos in which most nuclei were analysed were abnormal in some way, and around 20 per cent were diploid mosaics. Two-thirds of these were ploidy mosaics, especially diploid/haploid mosaics, and the remainder were diploid/aneuploid mosaics, some due to mitotic non-disjunction. For PGD which is dependent on analysis of single cells biopsied from cleavage stages, it will be important to determine how the haploid nuclei arise since they could cause a misdiagnosis. One possiblity, for example, is that they are supernumerary sperm which did not combine at syngamy. Most strikingly, however, was the recognition that some patients have a high incidence of embryos with chaotic chromosome complements and this was a consistent feature in later cycles. Since these embryos are unlikely to develop much beyond pre-implantation stages, it will be important to understand how they arise in these patients.

Finally, abnormal nuclei also arise during cleavage (Winston *et al.* 1991; Hardy *et al.* 1993). In particular, although most blastomeres have a single nucleus, binucleate blastomeres containing two equal sized nuclei are common and other blastomeres have fragmented nuclei or are anucleate (Hardy *et al.* 1993). Anucleate blastomeres are more frequent in embryos of poor morphology. Careful analysis of the size of binucleate and mononucleate blastomeres at different cleavage stages between days 2 and 4 suggests that they arise by failure of cytokinesis. This could be the result of cleavage arrest *in vitro*, or alternatively, may represent an intermediate stage in the formation of tetraploid and later polyploid cells in the trophectoderm lineage.

PRE-IMPLANTATION GENETIC DIAGNOSIS OF INHERITED DISEASE

The use of assisted reproduction techniques allows pre-implantation genetic diagnosis (PGD) of an inherited disease in early human embryos before implantation. Some genetic defects have even been identified before fertilization by analysis of the first polar body of the oocyte (Verlinsky *et al.* 1990, 1992). By selective transfer of only unaffected embryos, couples at risk of having affected children can avoid the possibility of terminating an affected pregnancy following more conventional diagnostic approaches later in gestation. Clinical experience is still limited but world-wide, approaching 200 hundred cycles have now been reported resulting in 50 pregnancies and over 30 births (Table 2.1) (Harper 1996).

Human embryo biopsy

Human embryos have been successfully biopsied at cleavage stages on day 3 post-insemination, at the 6 to 10-cell stage, and at the blastocyst stage on days 5 or 6 (Dokras *et al.* 1990, 1991; Muggleton Harris *et al.* 1995; Pickering and Muggleton Harris 1995). Blastocyst biopsy has the advantage that a larger number of cells can be removed from the outer trophectoderm layer without affecting the inner cell mass from which the fetus later develops. However, too few embryos reach this stage and implant after transfer to be clinically viable for PGD at the present time. Removal of one or two cells at the equivalent of the 8-cell stage does not appear to affect development to the blastocyst stage *in vitro* (Hardy *et al.* 1990) and has proved to be highly efficient in practise (Ao and Handyside 1995). The procedure involves dissolving a hole in the zona pellucida using acidified Tyrodes (Fig. 2.1) and then aspirating the cells with a second larger micropipette. Also, co-culture of the isolated cells with the biopsied embryo supports limited proliferation and may provide an alternative to the more difficult procedure of blastocyst biopsy (Geber *et al.* 1995). So far there have been no reports of serious abnormalities at birth following cleavage stage biopsy. Human embryos, like other mammalian embryos, appear to be able to regulate their development at these early stages presumably because cells are not yet irreversibly committed to specific fates.

GENETIC ANALYSIS

The genetic analysis of single cells has been made possible by the development of DNA amplification methods involving the polymerase chain reaction (PCR) and FISH for rapid cytogenetic analysis of interphase nuclei. Single cells biopsied at cleavage

Table 2.1 Summary of world clinical experience with pre-implantation genetic diagnosis following IVF and cleavage stage biopsy to February, 1995[a]

	Patients	Cycles	Transfers	Pregnancies	Babies
X-linked (PCR)	41	62	53	14	11
X-lined (FISH)	49	70	56	15	11
Single-gene defects	59	65	62	21	12
Total	149	197	171	50	34

Pregnancy rate: 25 per cent (per cycle); 29 per cent (per ET). Results collated from 14 centres.
[a] Modified from Harper (1996).

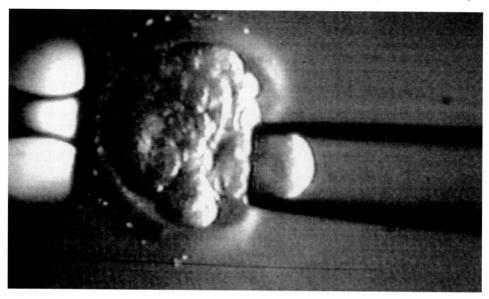

Fig. 2.1 Cleavage stage enbryo biosy. Note the interphase nucleus in the cell being aspirated from this 12-cell embryo early on day 3 post insemination.

stages are therefore prepared for analysis either by carefully placing the cells in lysis buffer in microcentrifuge tubes for PCR or by spreading the nucleus on a microscope slide for FISH.

Single cell analysis by PCR

To amplify sufficient DNA from a single cell for analysis by conventional gel electrophoresis, two rounds of amplification are necessary. 'Nesting' the second pair of oligonucleotide primers, which define the region to be amplified, internally to the first pair has several advantages and provides a safeguard for product contamination carried over into the sample tubes (Fig. 2.2). Theoretically, only a single molecule could be amplified and give an erroneous result. Following amplification, many approaches have been used to identify the presence of different mutations (Table 2.2). Since the aim is to transfer selected embryos on the same day as the biopsy to maximize pregnancy rates, amplification and mutation detection have to be completed in 8–12 h.

Pregnancies and births confirmed to be free of the inherited disease have been established in couples at risk of several common single gene defects including cystic fibrosis (CF) (Handyside *et al.* 1992), Duchenne muscular dystrophy (DMD) (Liu *et al.* 1995), and Tay–Sachs' disease (Gibbons *et al.* 1995). PGD has also been achieved for a specific mutation causing the rare X-linked condition, Lesch–Nyhan syndrome (Hughes, Ray, Winston, and Handyside, unpublished data). With CF and Tay–Sachs' disease, the common 3 base pair (bp) deletion and 4 bp insertion, respectively, were

Table 2.2 Some methods for detecting mutations in amplified fragments for pre-implantation genetic diagnosis

Method	Typical application
Fragment length differences	Distinguishing gene and intronless pseudogene sequences
	Analysis of variable number tandem repeats
Heteroduplex formation	Rapid detection of small insertions or deletions
Restriction digestion	Detection of mutations that eliminate restriction sites
Allele-specific oligonucleotides (ASOs)	Hybridization of normal and mutant ASOs detected by non-radioactive methods
Single strand conformation polymorphism (SSCP)	Detection of majority of mutations anywhere within the amplified fragment
Oligonucleotide ligation	Direct detection of point mutations
Microsequencing	Mutation detection by incorporation of radiolabelled nucleotides—avoids gel electrophoresis

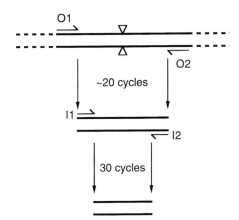

Fig. 2.2 Diagrammatic representation of polymerase chain reaction (PCR) using nested oligonucleotide primers. In the first amplification reaction, an outer pair of primer (O1 and O2) annealing to the sense and antisense strands of the genomic target sequence encompassing the mutation (triangles) is partially amplified. In the second reaction, a second set of 'nested' primers (I1 and I2) annealing to the target sequence internal to that of the outer primers is used to amplify a smaller fragment from an aliquot of the first amplified product. Two rounds of amplification is necessary in most cases to amplify sufficient DNA from single cells for conventional analysis. The use of nested primers reduces non-specific amplification. It is also a safeguard to prevent carry-over contamination of samples tubes with the final amplification product since the outer primers should not anneal to this sequence.

detected by heteroduplex formation (Fig. 2.3). A 3 or 4 bp size difference in the amplified fragment cannot be reliably discriminated by rapid gel electrophoresis. By mixing the amplified DNA from the single cell with DNA previously amplified from homozygous normal or affected individuals, denaturing the double stranded DNA

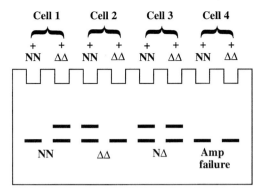

Fig. 2.3 Diagrammatic representation of the use of heteroduplex formation for the rapid detection of, in this example, the common 3 base pair (bp) deletion, ΔF508, causing cystic fibrosis. Amplified product from each of four single cells is mixed with amplified product from either known homozygous normal (NN) or affected (ΔΔ) individuals. The pattern of heteroduplex bands obtained with the two mixtures allows all three possible genotypes as well as amplification failure to be identified on a small polyacrylamide gel run for as little as 30 min.

fragments and allowing the mixtures to cool slowly, heteroduplexes are formed in those cases where both normal length fragments and mutated longer or shorter fragments are present. When these mixtures are then electrophoresed, the heteroduplexes are significantly retarded on the gel and can be interpreted reliably for diagnosing the genotype of the cell biopsied from the embryo.

Single cell analysis by FISH

Dual FISH with X- and Y-specific probes has been used clinically for identifying the sex of embryos in couples at risk of X-linked diseases which only affect boys (Griffin *et al.* 1992, 1993, 1994). This approach has now been further refined using directly labelled probes and an additional autosomal probe to distinguish sex chromosome aneuploidy from abnormal ploidy. Combined with a new spreading procedure involving dissolving the cytoplasm of the single cells and attaching the nuclei to poly-L lysine coated slides, it is now possible to complete the analysis within two hours (Harper *et al.* 1994).

In addition to identifying sex in X-linked disease, FISH analysis is being used for detecting trisomies in couples in which one partner is carrying a reciprocal or Robertsonian translocation or where there is suspected gonadal mosaicism (Conn *et al.* 1995). These couples are often at high risk of trisomic pregnancies and many have repeated miscarriages. These couples are good candidates for PGD since several embryos can be screened in a single cycle. The usual probes specific for repeated sequences in the centromeric region of particular chromosomes may not be suitable and a more distal unique sequence of yeast artificial chromosome (YAC) or cosmid contig probes are being developed. Combinations of probes, specific for the same chromosome, can also be used for accurate detection of particular trisomies, for example, in women believed to be gonadal mosaics (Fig. 2.4). As the majority of aneuploidies arise during maternal meiosis especially meiosis I, first and/or second polar body analysis with combinations of probes detecting X, Y, 21, 18, and 13 are being used to screen embryos in older women undergoing IVF (Verlinsky *et al.* 1995). If sufficient euploid embryos can be identified this may improve pregnancy rates and decrease miscarriage rates in these women.

THE ACCURACY OF PREIMPLANTATION GENETIC DIAGNOSIS

The accuracy of PGD remains to be assessed in clinical practise. The main sources of errors are listed in Table 2.3. Three misdiagnoses have already been reported (Harper and Handyside 1994). However, these involved different diagnostic procedures and probably occurred for different reasons. All five children resulting from a recent series of 18 PGD cycles for the predominant ΔF508 deletion causing CF were confirmed to be homozygous normal (Ao *et al.* 1995). However, analysis of each blastomere from the embryos which were not transferred did reveal some errors, particularly in amplifying both parental alleles in heterozygous carrier cells. Often one parental allele failed to amplify, apparently randomly (allele dropout; ADO), resulting in an incorrect diagnosis as homozygous normal or affected. Further work with single heterozygous lymphocytes has now shown that this phenomenon is partly explained by incomplete denaturation of the genomic template DNA during the initial cycles of PCR (Ray and Handyside 1996). Raising the temperature in the initial cycles improves the efficiency of denaturation and minimizes, but does not eliminate, ADO. Fortunately, in an autosomal recessive condition, ADO cannot cause a serious misdiagnosis leading to the transfer of a homozygous affected embryo (at least in these couples in which both partners were carrying the same mutation). For compound heterozygote detection or

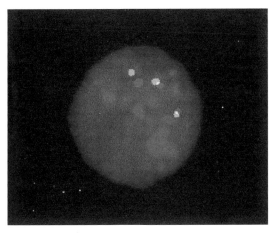

Fig. 2.4 Interphase nucleus from an 8-cell embryo showing three copies of chromosome 21, detected with two specific DNA probes, red, and green.

Table 2.3   Sources of errors in pre-implantation genetic diagnosis

Sources of errors	Potential consequences
PCR failures	
Amplification failure	No diagnosis. Misdiagnosis of deletions
Allele dropout (ADO)	Misdiagnosis of carriers
Preferential amplification	Misdiagnosis of carriers
Non-specific amplification	General misdiagnosis
Carry-over contamination	General misdiagnosis
Extraneous contamination	General misdiagnosis
FISH failures	
Hybridization failure or extraneous signals	Misdiagnosis of sex with single probe. Misdiagnosis as aneuploid
Nuclear abnormalities	
Anucleate blastomeres	No diagnosis. Misdiagnosis of deletions
Binucleate blastomeres	Arise by failure of cytokinesis. No known to cause errors
Multinucleate blastomeres	Mostly fragmenting nuclei. Misdiagnosis likely
Apoptotic or degenerating nuclei	General misdiagnosis
Chromosomal abnormalities	
Haploid	Misdiagnosis of carriers
Triploid	Depending on origin probably not a risk
Tetraploid	Depending on origin probably not a risk
Aneuploid	Only a risk if involving the chromosome with the defect
Chaotic	High risk of misdiagnosis

dominant conditions, however, this could theoretically occur in half the cases of ADO in which the affected allele did not amplify. One way of avoiding these errors for diagnosis of compound heterozygotes is to amplify a single DNA fragment encompassing both mutations. This has recently been demonstrated for β-thalassaemia major diagnosis with single lymphocytes from a boy who is a compound heterozygote for two common Indian mutations of the β-globin gene (Ray *et al.* 1996).

Four general sources of errors have been identified with single blastomere analysis at cleavage stages. However, careful monitoring of FISH or amplification efficiency and contamination levels and reducing ADO by manipulating amplification conditions, together with analysis of two cells from each embryo where possible, should minimize the risk. Estimates of the risk based on analysis of several hundred single blastomeres from the series of PGD cycles for the common ΔF508 mutation causing CF (see above) ranged between 0.1 and 2 per cent depending on the genotype and whether one or two cells are analysed (Ray and Handyside, unpublished data). At the lower end of this range this is probably acceptable though it should be possible to improve on these results and reduce the risk to closer to one in a thousand. In view of the regulative capacity of embryos at these early stages and the possibility that the fetus will be derived from only a subset of cells, however, it may never be possible to exclude errors. For most couples, considerably reducing their risk of an affected pregnancy is sufficient, especially if the *a priori* risk is high.

CONCLUDING REMARKS

The development of techniques for genetic analysis of single cells has given us powerful tools to study early human embryos and understand the contribution of chromosomal and other genetic abnormalities to developmental failure at these early stages. Polar body screening and screening of blastomeres from cleavage stage embryos offer the prospect of improving selection of viable embryos for transfer, which should increase implantation and pregnancy rates in infertile couples following IVF. Progressive improvements in the methods for single-cell analysis should enable the use of PGD for an increasing spectrum of chromosomal and single-gene defects.

REFERENCES

Almeida, P.A. and Bolton, V.N. (1994). The relationship between chromosomal abnormalities in the human oocyte and fertilization *in vitro*. *Human Reproduction*, 9, 343–6.

Angell, R.R. (1991). Predivision in human oocytes at meiosis I: a mechanism for trisomy formation in man. *Human Genetics*, 86, 383–7.

Ao, A. and Handyside, A.H. (1995). Cleavage stage human embryo biopsy. *Human Reproduction Update*, 1, 3.

Ao, A., Ray, P., Lesko, J., Harper, J.C., Handyside, A.H., Hughes, M.R., and Winston, R.M.L. (1995). Clinical experience with preimplantation diagnosis of the ΔF508 deletion causing cystic fibrosis. *Prenatal Diagnosis*, 16, 137–42.

Balakier, H., Squire, J., and Casper, R.F. (1993). Characterization of abnormal one pronuclear human oocytes by morphology, cytogenetics and *in-situ* hybridization. *Human Reproduction*, 8, 402–8.

Burgoyne, P.S., Holland, K., and Stephens, R. (1991). Incidence of numerical chromosome anomalies in human pregnancy estimation from induced and spontaneous abortion data. *Human Reproduction*, 6, 555–65.

Conn, C., Harper, J.C., Winston, R.M.L., and Delhanty, J.D.A. (1995). Preimplantation diagnosis for trisomies 13, 14, 18 and 21 in translocation carriers using multicolour fluorescent *in situ* hybridization. *American Journal of Human Genetics*, 57, (Suppl. A) 1611.

Coonen, E., Harper, J.C., Ramaekers, F.C.S., Delhanty, J.D.A., Hopman, A.H.N., Geraedts, J.P.M., and Handyside, A.H. (1994). Presence of chromosomal mosaicism in abnormal human preimplantation embryos detected by fluorescent *in situ* hybridization (FISH). *Human Genetics*, 54, 609–15.

Crow, J.F. (1993). How much do we know about spontaneous human mutation rates? *Environmental Molecular Mutagens*, 21, 122–9 [erratum p. 389].

Dailey, T., Dale, B., Cohen, J., and Munné, S. (1996). Association between nondisjunction and maternal age in meiosis-II human oocytes. *American Journal of Human Genetics*, 59, 176–84.

Delhanty, J.D.A., Harper, J.C., Ao, A., Handyside, A.H., and Winston, R.M.L. (19967). Multicolour FISH detects frequent chromosomal mosaicism and chaotic division in normal preimplantation embryos from fertile patients. *Human Genetics* (in press).

Dokras, A., Sargent, I.L., Ross, C., Gardner, R.L., and Barlow, D.H. (1990). Trophectoderm biopsy in human blastocysts. *Human Reproduction*, 5, 821–5.

Dokras, A., Sargent, I.L., Gardner, R.L., and Barlow, D.H. (1991). Human trophectoderm biopsy and secretion of chorionic gonadotrophin. *Human Reproduction*, 6, 1453–9.

Drost, J.B. and Lee, W.R. (1995). Biological basis of germline mutation: comparisons of spontaneous germline mutation rates among drosophila, mouse, and human. *Environmental Molecular Mutagens*, 25 (*Suppl.*), 26, 48–64.

Geber, S., Winston, R.M., and Handyside, A.H. (1995). Proliferation of blastomeres from biopsied cleavage stage human embryos *in vitro*: an alternative to blastocyst biopsy for preimplantation diagnosis. *Human Reproduction*, 10, 1492–6.

Gibbons, W.E., Gitlin, S.A., Lanzendorf, S.E., Kaufman, R.A., Slotnick, R.N., and Hodgen, G.D. (1995). Preimplantation genetic diagnosis of Tay–Sachs disease; successful pregnancy after pre-embryo biopsy and gene amplification by polymerase chain reaction. *Fertility and Sterility*, 63, 723–8.

Griffin, D.K., Wilton, L.J., Handyside, A.H., Winston, R.M., and Delhanty, J.D. (1992). Dual fluorescent *in situ* hybridisation for simultaneous detection of X and Y chromosome-specific probes for the sexing of human preimplantation embryonic nuclei. *Human Genetics*, 89, 18–22.

Griffin, D.K., Wilton, L.J., Handyside, A.H., Atkinson, G.H., Winston, R.M., and Delhanty, J.D. (1993). Diagnosis of sex in preimplantation embryos by fluorescent *in situ* hybridisation. *British Medical Journal*, 306, 1382.

Griffin, D.K., Handyside, A.H., Harper, J.C., Wilton, L.J., Atkinson, G., Soussis, I., *et al.* (1994). Clinical experience with preimplantation diagnosis of sex by dual fluorescent *in situ* hybridization. *Journal of Assisted Reproduction Genetics*, 11, 132–43.

Handyside, A.H., Lesko, J.G., Tarin, J.J., Winston, R.M., and Hughes, M.R. (1992). Birth of a normal girl after *in vitro* fertilization and preimplantation diagnostic testing for cystic fibrosis [see comments]. *New England Journal of Medicine*, 327, 905–9.

Hardy, K., Handyside, A.H., and Winston, R.M. (1989). The human blastocyst: cell number, death and allocation during late preimplantation development *in vitro*. *Development*, 107, 597–604.

Hardy, K., Martin, K.L., Leese, H.J., Winston, R.M., and Handyside, A.H. (1990). Human preimplantation development *in vitro* is not adversely affected by biopsy at the 8-cell stage. *Human Reproduction*, 5, 708–14.

Hardy, K., Winston, R.M., and Handyside, A.H. (1993). Binucleate blastomeres in preimplantation human embryos *in vitro*: failure of cytokinesis during early cleavage. *Journal of Reproduction and Fertility*, 98, 549–58.

Harper, J.C. (1996). Preimplantation diagnosis of inherited disease by embryo biopsy. An update of world figures. *Journal Assisted Reproduction Genetics*, 13, 90–5.

Harper, J.C. and Handyside, A.H. (1994). The current status of preimplantation diagnosis. *Current Obstetrics and Gynecology*, 4, 143–9.

Harper, J.C., Coonen, E., Ramaekers, F.C., Delhanty, J.D., Handyside, A.H., Winston, R.M., and Hopman, A.H. (1994). Identification of the sex of human preimplantation embryos in two hours using an improved spreading method and fluorescent *in-situ* hybridization (FISH) using directly labelled probes. *Human Reproduction*, 9, 721–4.

Harper, J.C., Coonen, E., Handyside, A.H., Winston, R.M., Hopman, A.H., and Delhanty, J.D. (1995). Mosaicism of autosomes and sex chromosomes in morphologically normal, monospermic preimplantation human embryos. *Prenatal Diagnosis*, 15, 41–9.

Hassold, T.J. (1986). Chromosome abnormalities in human reproductive wastage. *Trends in Genetics*, 2, 105–10.

Hassold, T.J., Sherman, S.L., Pettay, D., Page, D.C., and Jacobs, P.A. (1991). XY chromosome nondisjunction in man is associated with diminished recombination in the pseudoautosomal region. *American Journal of Human Genetics*, 49, 253–60.

Jacobs, P.A. (1992). The chromosome complement of human gametes. *Oxford Reviews in Reproductive Biology*, **14**, 47–72.

Jacobs, P.A., Angell, R.R., Buchanan, I.M., Hassold, T.J., Matsuyama, A., and Manuel, B. (1978). The origin of triploids. *Annals of Human Genetics*, **44**, 49–57.

Kola, I., Trounson, A., Dawson, G., and Rogers, P. (1987). Tripronuclear human oocytes: altered cleavage patterns and subsequent karyotype analysis of embryos. *Biology of Reproduction*, **37**, 395–401.

Levron, J., Munné, S., Willadsen, S., Rosenwaks, Z., and Cohen, J. (1995). Male and female genomes associated in a single pronucleus in human zygotes. *Biology of Reproduction*, **52**, 653–7.

Lim, A.S., Ho, A.T., and Tsakok, M.F. (1995). Chromosomes of oocytes failing *in-vitro* fertilization. *Human Reproduction*, **10**, 2570–5.

Liu, J., Lissens, W., Van Broeckhoven, C., Lofgren, A., Camus, M., Liebaers, I., and Van Steirteghem, A. (1995). Normal pregnancy after preimplantation DNA diagnosis of a dystrophin gene deletion. *Prenatal Diagnosis*, **15**, 351–8.

Martin, R.H., Chan, K., Ko, E., and Rademaker, A.W. (1994). Detection of aneuploidy in human sperm by fluorescence *in situ* hybridization (FISH): different frequencies in fresh and stored sperm nuclei. *Cytogenetics and Cellular Genetics*, **65**, 95–6.

Martin, R.H., Spriggs, E., Ko, E., and Rademaker, A.W. (1995). The relationship between paternal age, sex ratios, and aneuploidy frequencies in human sperm, as assessed by multicolor FISH. *American Journal of Human Genetics*, **57**, 1395–9.

Muggleton Harris, A.L., Glazier, A.M., Pickering, S., and Wall, M. (1995). Genetic diagnosis using polymerase chain reaction and fluorescent *in-situ* hybridization analysis of biopsied cells from both the cleavage and blastocyst stages of individual cultured human preimplantation embryos. *Human Reproduction*, **10**, 183–92.

Munné, S., Grifo, J., Cohen, J., and Weier, H.U. (1994*a*). Chromosome abnormalities in human arrested preimplantation embryos: a multiple-probe FISH study. *American Journal of Human Genetics*, **55**, 150–9.

Munné, S., Weier, H.U., Grifo, J., and Cohen, J. (1994*b*). Chromosome mosaicism in human embryos. *Biology of Reproduction*, **51**, 373–9.

Munné, S., Sultan, K.M., Weier, H.U., Grifo, J.A., Cohen, J., and Rosenwaks, Z. (1995). Assessment of numeric abnormalities of X, Y, 18, and 16 chromosomes in preimplantation human embryos before transfer. *American Journal of Obstetrics and Gynecology*, **172**, 1191–9.

Pickering, S.J. and Muggleton Harris, A.L. (1995). Reliability and accuracy of polymerase chain reaction amplification of two unique target sequences from biopsies of cleavage-stage and blastocyst-stage human embryos. *Human Reproduction*, **10**, 1021–9.

Ray, P.F. and Handyside, A.H. (1996). Increasing the temperature during the first cycles of amplification reduces allele dropout from single cells for preimplantation genetic diagnosis. *Human Reproduction*, **2**, 213–18.

Ray, P.F., Kaeda, J.S., Bingham, J., Vulliamy, T., Dokal, I., Roberts, I., *et al.* (1996). Preimplantation genetic diagnosis of β-thalassaemia major: accurate detection of mutations in a compound heterozygote following single cell amplification. *Lancet*, **347**, 1696.

Sathananthan, A.H., Kola, I., Osborne, J., Trounson, A., Ng, S.C., Bongso, A., and Ratnam, S.S. (1991). Centrioles in the beginning of human development. *Proceedings of the National Academy of Sciences, USA*, **88**, 4806–10.

Spriggs, E.L., Rademaker, A.W., and Martin, R.H. (1996). Aneuploidy in human sperm: the use of multicolor FISH to test various theories of nondisjunction. *American Journal Human Genetics*, **58**, 356–62.

Sultan, K.M., Munné, S., Palermo, G.D., Alikani, M., and Cohen, J. (1995). Chromosomal status of uni-pronuclear human zygotes following *in-vitro* fertilization and intracytoplasmic sperm injection. *Human Reproduction*, **10**, 132–6.

Van Blerkom, J., Bell, H., and Henry, G.H. (1987). The occurrence, recognition and developmental fate of pseudomultipronuclear eggs after *in vitro* fertilization of human oocytes. *Human Reproduction*, 2, 217–25.

Verlinsky, Y., Ginsberg, N., Lifchez, A., Valle, J., Moise, J., and Strom, C.M. (1990). Analysis of the first polar body: preconception genetic diagnosis. *Human Reproduction*, 5, 826–9.

Verlinsky, Y., Rechitsky, S., Evsikov, S., White, M., Cieslak, J., Lifchez, A., *et al.* (1992). Preconception and preimplantation diagnosis for cystic fibrosis. *Prenatal Diagnosis*, 12, 103–10.

Verlinsky, Y., Cieslak, J., Freidine, M., Ivakhnenko, V., Wolf, G., Kovalinskaya, L., *et al.* (1995). Pregnancies following pre-conception diagnosis of common aneuploidies by fluorescent *in-situ* hybridization. *Human Reproduction*, 10, 1923–7.

Wilcox, A.J., Weinberg, C.R., O'Connor, J.F., Baird, D.D., Schlatterer, J.P., Canfield, R.E., *et al.* (1988). Incidence of early loss of pregnancy. *New England Journal of Medicine*, 319, 189–94.

Williams, B.J., Ballenger, C.A., Malter, H.E., Bishop, F., Tucker, M., Zwingman, T.A., and Hassold, T.J. (1993). Non-disjunction in human sperm: results of fluorescence *in situ* hybridization studies using two and three probes. *Human Molecular Genetics*, 2, 1929–36.

Winston, N.J., Braude, P.R., Pickering, S.J., George, M.A., Cant, A., Currie, J., and Johnson, M.H. (1991). The incidence of abnormal morphology and nucleocytoplasmic ratios in 2-, 3- and 5-day human pre-embryos. *Human Reproduction*, 6, 17–24.

Zenzes, M.T. and Casper, R.F. (1992). Cytogenetics of human oocytes, zygotes, and embryos after *in vitro* fertilization. *Human Genetics*, 88, 367–75.

Zenzes, M.T., Wang, P., and Casper, R.F. (1992). Chromosome status of untransferred (spare) embryos and probability of pregnancy after *in vitro* fertilisation. *Lancet*, 340, 391–4.

3 | *Diagnostic methods for the early embryo*

Tanmoy Mukherjee and María Bustillo

INTRODUCTION

A comprehensive understanding of embryonic growth and differentiation requires promotion of a paradigm which integrates morphologic, metabolic, and genetic elements of pre-implantation development. An integrated model of embryo function will yield many potential benefits, including improved *in vitro* fertilization and embryo transfer (IVF–ET) success rates as well as prevention and treatment of inherited diseases and birth defects. In this chapter we examine morphological, metabolic, and genetic methods of embryonic evaluation and explore clinically relevant correlates.

MORPHOLOGY OF GAMETES AND EMBRYOS

Fertilization failure

In most IVF programmes, the absence of two pronuclei 16–20 post-insemination is taken as evidence of fertilization failure. If the majority of oocytes retrieved in a given cycle of controlled ovarian hyperstimulation (COH) fail to fertilize, it is assumed to be a result of egg or sperm dysfunction, or both. Since the first three cell cycles of the cleaving embryo require oocyte-derived products stored in the cytoplasm (Tesarik *et al.* 1988), and eventual activation of the embryonic genome is dependent on normal genetic contributions from both spermatozoon and oocyte, gamete quality has a direct bearing on embryonic development.

Information correlating developmental potential and gamete morphology was obtained by Van Blerkom and Henry (1994) from an analysis of 373 grossly normal, newly harvested MII oocytes analysed with DNA fluorescence microscopy. (Normality was as defined by the Veeck classification system (Veeck 1986*a*): radiant cumulus, extruded polar body, symmetric/irregular ooplasm, thin matrix/expanded cumulus, large and loosely aggregated granulosa cells.) Approximately 15 per cent of morphologically normal oocytes (Table 3.1) derived from women over 35 years of age, and approximately 11 per cent of normal oocytes from women under 35 (Van Blerkom and Henry 1994) were found to be aneuploid as a result of non-disjunction or single chromatid substitutions arising from precocious centromere division at the

Table 3.1 Estimation of chromosome number by DNA fluorescence microscopy and karyotype in MII-stage human oocytes with normal morphology*

Maternal age	Number of oocytes	Fluorescence microscopy: total aneuploid (%)	Karyotype: total aneuploid (%)
	Newly harvested		
< 35	61	5(11)	4(8)
> 35	312	34(15)	33(15)
Total	373	39(15)	37(14)
	From failed IVF		
	With at least one fertilized in cohort		
< 35	51	3(9)	3(11)
> 35	91	8(14)	10(16)
Total	142	11(12)	14(16)
	With no fertilization in cohort		
< 35	52	3(8)	4(9)
> 35	263	41(25)	40(23)
Total	296	44(22)	44(21)

* Adapted from Van Blerkom and Henry (1994).

first meiosis (Angell *et al.* 1994). Higher rates of aneuploidy (22–53 per cent) were found in oocytes obtained from failed IVF cycles which demonstrated dysmorphic features such as dark granular cytoplasm, clustered organelles, assemblies of smooth endoplasmic reticulum, or intracytoplasmic vesicles (Van Blerkom and Henry 1992). While rates of aneuploidy are positively correlated with worsening oocyte morphology, the high incidence of cytogenetic abnormality suggests that structural and numerical chromosomal disorders may be an important cause of failed fertilization even in the IVF laboratory where morphologically normal oocytes are selected.

While intrinsic defects in egg quality constitute a significant cause of fertilization failure, there is some evidence that poor fertilization may also result from poor oocyte development as a consequence of suboptimal controlled ovarian hyperstimulation (COH) regimens (Van Blerkom and Henry 1992). Some studies have shown that COH after pituitary suppression with gonadotrophin-releasing hormone agonist (GnRHa) results in a higher rate of aneuploidy in human oocytes (De Sutter *et al.* 1992). In addition, Tarín and Pellicer (1990) found more diploid oocytes and a higher incidence of cytoplasmic immaturity in women who produced greater than 11 oocytes when COH with GnRHa was employed. However, the association between GnRHa utilization and higher aneuploidy rates is not a universal finding. Studies by Plachot *et al.* (1988) and Tejada *et al.* (1991) failed to demonstrate a difference in aneuploidy rates as a result of GnRHa treatment. While no clear association exists between gonadotrophin stimulation and aneuploidy rate, the few studies that examine oocytes from unstimulated cycles (Van Blerkom 1991) show a very low rate of aneuploidy, suggesting that hormonal stimulation may be responsible for the rate of aneuploidy observed in IVF oocytes. However, extrapolation of the rate of aneuploidy found in an infertility population to the general population is not appropriate and further study is necessary to assess the impact of gonadotrophins on the rate of chromosomal abnormality in infertile patients.

While poor oocyte quality is responsible for some instances of fertilization failure, the presence of an abnormal semen analysis and/or abnormal Kruger morphology in the setting of fertilization failure is highly suggestive of male factor abnormalities. Because of the morphologic variability inherent in the analysis of human spermatozoa (Kruger *et al.* 1986), strict definitions of biometric and morphologic characteristics of spermatozoa can be utilized to correlate sperm morphology with IVF outcome. Utilizing strict criteria, patients with greater than 14 per cent normal forms demonstrated an *in vitro* fertilization rate of 85 per cent regardless of motility or concentration. Patients with less than 4 per cent normal forms had significantly lower rates of fertilization, implantation, and ongoing pregnancy (Grow *et al.* 1994).

Given the critical role of confirming fertilization failure in the evaluation of the infertile couple, absence of pronuclei should not be pathognomonic for male factor infertility. Defective pronuclei formation may be an underestimated cause of developmental failure, apparently due to the inability to detect such abnormalities by standard light microscopy. Van Blerkom (1989*a*) utilized DNA-specific fluorescent probes in conjunction with epifluoresence microscopy 36 h post-insemination to demonstrate that 15 per cent of oocytes judged to be unfertilized contained sperm nuclear DNA with absent or partial decondensation. Disturbances in sperm pronuclear development may arise from asynchronous maturation of oocyte and follicle as a consequence of non-physiologic conditions resulting from COH, rendering the oocyte unable to facilitate sperm decondensation (Van Blerkom 1989*a*). Alternatively, some patients may have an increased tendency to produce intrinsically defective oocytes. To evaluate this phenomenon a penetration test using zona-free unfertilized human eggs (Tesarik 1989) in conjunction with sperm of proven fertilization potential provides valuable information regarding the capacity of oocyte cytoplasm to support pronuclear formation.

Pronuclear function

The mechanics of gamete fusion in the human and the course of sperm nuclear decondensation and male pronuclear formation have been extensively analysed (Tesarik and Kopecny 1989; Testart and Lassalle 1991). Briefly, stage 1 is characterized by the disappearance of the sperm nuclear envelope, moderate chromatin condensation, and enlargement of the sperm head (Fig. 3.1). In stage 2, the sperm chromatin re-expands, and, in 2–3 h, a dense outline appears around the sperm nucleus heralding pronuclear formation. Stage 3 involves completion of nuclear envelope formation, restructuring of chromatin, assembly of nucleolar precursors, and linear growth of the pronucleus. Finally, stage 4 completes nucleolar precursor development and changes in chromatin distribution. Following syngamy, actual replication of pronuclear DNA is heralded by alterations in nuclear membrane configuration. Knowledge of pre-zygotic development is critical in the evaluation of the early human embryo because normal-appearing concepti may develop after displaying only a single pronucleus or three or more

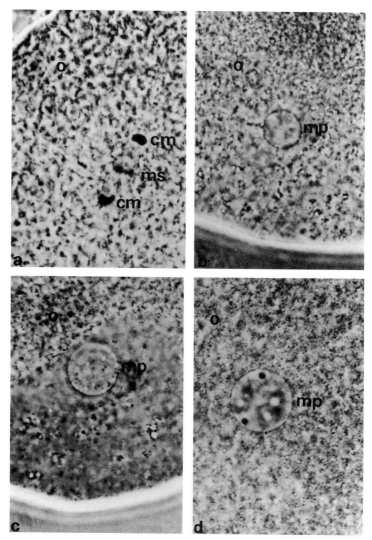

Fig. 3.1 Sequential transformations of human sperm nucleus in human egg. Male pronuclear formation. (a) In the human egg at late anaphase II stage, a condensed sperm head begins to re-expand and a dense outline appeared (120 min after insemination) around the condensed sperm nucleus (b). About 30–60 min after the outline formation, numerous (> 20) dense grains were observed inside the growing male pronucleus (c). (d) A male pronucleus observed after 4 h of culture. Phase contrast ×1000. (From ???, with permission.)

pronuclei. Failing to identify abnormal zygotes could result in transfer of abnormal embryos, and increase the rate of abnormal pregnancies.

Changes in embryonic ultrastructure visible through differential interference optics (DIC) can be correlated with zygotic developmental potential. Alterations in the geometry of the pronuclear membrane observed through DIC microscopy reveal that interdigitation of the pronuclear envelope occurs at the site of juxtaposition as a necessary prerequisite for syngamy (Tesarik 1994). Absence of a conformational alteration in the nuclear membrane envelope is suggestive of incomplete genomic replication and, if present in both nuclei, is suggestive of complete replication failure (Tesarik 1994). Nucleolar distribution is another sign of developmental potential. During the early pronuclear stage the nucleoli are distributed throughout the cytoplasm. Approximately 14 h after insemination, nucleoli migrate to the region of pronuclear juxtaposition and assume an equatorial distribution. The equatorial distribution of nucleoli has been elegantly shown to be an important marker of developmental competence, and has been correlated with normality of cleavage and embryo viability after cryopreservation (Wright *et al.* 1990). Such information is valuable to IVF centres that utilize pronuclear stage embryos for the purposes of cryopreservation and zygote intrafallopian transfer.

Cell stage

The transition from maternal to embryonic developmental control occurs in the early human conceptus between the 4- and 8-cell stages. This hypothesis is supported by induction of an embryonic developmental block in studies examining quantitative patterns of polypeptide synthesis in embryos treated with the transcriptional inhibitor α-amanatin (Braude *et al.* 1988). Prior to embryonic genome activation, protein synthesis is largely unaffected, underscoring the dependence of successful human embryogenesis during the first three cell cycles on stored maternal mRNA. Bolton *et al.* (1988) reported on a series of 317 human embryos which had been cultured for extended periods up to six days, and observed a 50 per cent incidence of developmental failure at the 2- to 4-cell stage (Bolton *et al.* 1988). Although unproven, this high incidence of developmental failure may result from premature exhaustion of oocyte-derived cellular products essential for cell growth.

Post-ovulatory oocytes contain a variety of stored gene products necessary for oocyte development. These consist of different maternal RNAs, enzymes, and DNA synthetic machinery present during a period of development when the embryonic genome is largely quiescent. The cleaving human embryo depletes the storehouse of oocyte-derived products between the 2- and 8-cell stages, including ribosomes, until the embryonic genome is activated. One can speculate that embryonic cells whose ribosome content falls below a critical level would be incapable of performing essential housekeeping functions resulting in cessation of cell development (Tesarik *et al.* 1986), placing oocytes deficient in developmentally relevant molecules at risk for embryogenic arrest following fertilization and early cleavage.

Another striking cytological anomaly evident in the oocyte-dependent portion of embryogenesis is blastomere multinucleation. Multinucleated blastomeres normally appear as a result of endoreduplication during development of trophectoderm, and represent precursors of giant multinucleated trophectoderm cells that develop at the time of implantation. Embryos with multinucleated cells at early cleavage stages have a substantially decreased developmental potential as evidenced by subsequent developmental arrest, chromosomal mosaicism, and extensive cellular fragmentation (Bongso *et al.* 1991). Multinucleation may result from an insufficiency of the microtubular apparatus or as a result of nuclear replication without cytokinesis; either abnormality, in the context of monospermic fertilization, must be considered a defect of oocyte quality (Lopata *et al.* 1983).

As development from pronuclear to cell stage proceeds, a critical transition occurs when control of cellular function is transferred from the maternal to the embryonic genome. A report by Tesarik suggests that up to 29 per cent of human embryos do not successfully activate the embryonic genome (Tesarik *et al.* 1986). Embryonic failure in the human may be due to failure of genome activation in a proportion of blastomeres as suggested by varying embryonic incorporation of uridine into individual blastomeres (Tesarik *et al.* 1986). If all embryonic cells fail to undergo the maternal–embryonic transition, embryo death is inevitable, and while many such embryos arrest at the 4–8-cell stage, some may continue development to the compacted morula stage. However, such embryos cannot form gap junctions and a blastocyst cavity never forms (Tesarik 1988). In the case of maternal–embryonic transition failure in the majority of blastomeres, abnormal tight-junction formation may result in the production of pseudoblastocysts (Tesarik 1988). Such embryos are characterized by a large cavity surrounded by only a few blastomeres. Since routine microscopy will not reveal this detail, appearance of large protruding blastomeres should raise suspicion of developmental compromise. If only a few blastomeres are affected in any given embryo, successful completion of development is possible. The few abnormal cells present undergo fragmentation and are deposited between the trophectoderm and the zona pellucida, and are thus shed during hatching of the blastocyst.

Intrinsic genomic defects may not be the sole aetiology of embryonic activation disorders. While differences in protein synthetic patterns exist between blastomeres within an embryo, data from Artley and Braude (1993) show that blastomeres from a single embryo manifest synchronous genomic activity and demonstrate 'all-or-none' activation of the embryonic genomes. As a result, a subset of developmental abnormalities may result from cytoplasmic anomalies induced by *in vitro* culture conditions. An understanding of the culture requirements of pre-implantation human embryos, and optimizing the conditions required for appropriate genomic activation, should decrease the rates of activation failure in embryos with normal genomes (Fitzgerald and Dimattina 1992).

Embryo grading

Ultrastructural and light microscopy studies in the past ten years have yielded detailed descriptions of morphological factors that serve to predict post-implantation viability of human embryos *in vitro*. Establishing and maintaining accurate embryo grading systems based on such factors are necessary to achieve a maximal pregnancy rate and a minimal multiple gestation rate. To date, most attempts at quantifying morphological parameters have been crude. Factors commonly evaluated for their roles in embryo grading include: visibility of organelles, degree of blastomere symmetry, membrane smoothness, cell to cell adhesion, cellular extrusions, cytoplasmic vacuoles, variation of zona pellucida thickness, presence and degree of extracellular fragmentation, cleavage rates, and the number of abnormal morphologic criteria (Cohen *et al.* 1989). Despite the subjectivity inherent in the utilization of gross morphological features in the cleaving embryo, light microscopic grading is a rapid, easy to perform, and reproducible measure of embryonic developmental potential (Mukherjee *et al.* 1995).

A number of conflicting reports attempt to correlate individual morphologic features with pregnancy outcome. Increased variation in zona pellucida thickness and decreased fragmentation were examined by Cohen and were correlated with increased pregnancy rates (Cohen *et al.* 1989). Studies that specifically examine fragmentation and metabolic rate, however, report dissimilar outcomes. While Staessen *et al.* (1992) and Dor *et al.* (1986) reported decreased pregnancy rates with fragmentation, Claman *et al.* (1987), found no correlation between percentage fragmentation and embryo development. Embryonic metabolic activity has been indirectly assessed by correlating cell number with cleavage rate at various time intervals. In general, the more rapidly cleaving embryos seem to have an increased developmental potential. Testart, however, suggests that extremely rapid cleavage may represent underlying embryo abnormality, i.e. rapidly developing triploid embryos and transfer of rapidly cleaving embryos should be undertaken with caution (Testart 1986). Ultimately the commonly used parameters of embryo quality are simply descriptive, and to date no definite correlation between embryo morphology and developmental competence has been identified. Nevertheless, despite its limitations, embryo grading has been validated as a basis for decision-making in clinical studies.

The Veeck classification system is a widely utilized morphological grading system incorporating blastomere symmetry, fragmentation, and uniform cytoplasmic colour and granularity (Fig. 3.2) (Veeck 1986*b*). However, while such a system has tremendous value in assessing individual embryos, it does not assign an aggregate value to the developmental potential of cohorts of multiple embryos, such as those employed in IVF embryo transfer, and does not take into account embryo cleavage rates. The morphological assessment technique used in our laboratory is the cumulative embryo score (CES) as proposed by Steer *et al.* (1992) which incorporates blastomere symmetry, cytoplasmic fragmentation, and cell number. Grade 4 embryos contain equal sized, symmetrical blastomeres; grade 3 contain uneven blastomeres with < 10 per cent fragmentation; grade 2 contain 10–50 per cent blastomeric fragmentation; and grade 1 contain > 50 per cent blastomeric fragmentation or pronucleate single cell embryos. The morphological grade of the embryo is then multiplied by the number of blastomeres to produce a quality score for each embryo that reflects both morphologic and metabolic activity. The score of all embryos in a given transfer are summed to obtain the cumulative embryo score. In Steer's original report a CES of 42 two days after oocyte retrieval corresponded with a pregnancy rate of 33 per cent per transfer, and further increases in the CES per transfer increased the incidence of multiple gestation rates. A 15.7 per cent multiple pregnancy rate was seen from transfers with CES between 3 and 10, while transfer with CES greater than 50 yielded a multiple pregnancy rate of 43 per cent. Copperman *et al.* (1995) expanded on this model and showed that IVF success could be defined on the basis of cumulative

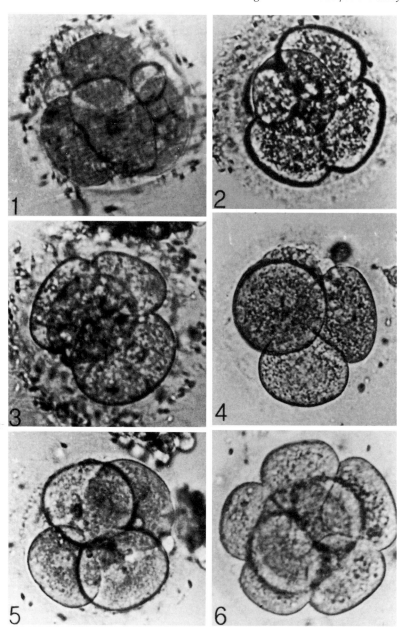

Fig. 3.2 Embryo grading. (1–5) Photographs of various grades of human 4-cell embryos: (1) Grade 5—few or no recognizable blastomeres; major cytoplasmic fragmentation. (2) Grade 4—blastomeres of equal or unequal size; major cytoplasmic fragmentation. (3) Grade 3—blastomeres of unequal size; no cytoplasmic fragments. (4) Grade 2—blastomeres of equal size; minor cytoplasmic fragmentation. (5) Grade 1—blastomeres of equal size; no cytoplasmic fragments. (6) Grade 1—8 cell embryo. (Adapted from Mohr 1983, with permission.)

embryo score. In 60 per cent of women who delivered live-born infants, the CES from all transfers was less than 40, and 95 per cent of all patients achieving a live birth had a cumulative embryo score of less than 280. These kind of data provide valuable prognostic information to infertile couples undergoing successive attempts at *in vitro* fertilization, and may help couples achieve realistic expectations of success. In such a fashion a statistical model for defining IVF failure may provide a sense of closure for couples who have exhausted traditional treatment strategies.

Although embryo classification systems stratify morphological parameters to select embryos capable of achieving high pregnancy rates per transfer, a small percentage of embryos with poor morphological parameters are also able to implant and develop normally. It is important to realize that a significant proportion of embryos (23–29 per cent) with chromsomal abnormalities have an unremarkable morphological appearance (Plachot *et al.* 1988). While limitations such as these clearly exist in the interpretation of any morphological assessment strategy, the utilization of a rapid, easy to perform, and reproducible diagnostic method such as morphological embryo grading is necessary and efficacious and its use will continue to be prevalent until better markers of embryonic implantation and developmental potential are widely available.

METABOLIC ASSESSMENT

Since morphological analysis is often subjective and occasionally unreliable, investigators have attempted to define quantitative parameters of embryo function. Examination of embryonic substrate utilization and metabolism provides another non-invasive means of obtaining information regarding embryo function and may provide useful information relevant to developmental potential. Mammalian oocytes contain few nutrient stores and depend on external substrates for cell metabolism (Biggers and Stern 1973). Although glucose is the primary substrate used by nearly all mammalian cells, Biggers and co-workers demonstrated that pyruvate is the major source of energy for the early cleaving embryo (Biggers *et al.* 1967; Biggers and Stern 1973). In late cleavage stages, glucose metabolism and glycolytic pathways become active, enabling human embryos to convert 90 per cent of radio-labelled glucose to lactate. In 1990, Gott *et al.* observed that increased lactate production could distinguish embryos that developed to the blastocyst stage from those that would subsequently arrest. However, since the difference in lactate levels was small and the overlap in values between normal and arrested embryos considerable, the application of lactate measurement in determining embryonic potential is of limited utility. Similarly, while cleaving blastocysts have a higher rate of pyruvate uptake than arrested blastocysts, pyruvate uptake determination fails to distinguish between embryos which successfully implant from those which fail to implant (Hardy *et al.* 1989). While assessing embryo quality by measuring substrate utilization provides a rapid, non-invasive, and quantitative assessment of the embryo, most existing individual markers cannot be used to assess quality of embryos on the day of transfer.

Current measures of substrate utilization may not be reliable indicators of human embryo development because of a failure to assess directly intracellular substrate utilization. Gardner and Leese (1990) showed that mouse blastocysts cultured *in vitro* demonstrated a decreased level of oxidative metabolism and an increased dependence on less efficient glycolysis in comparison to blastocysts flushed from uteri. A direct measure of oxidative metabolic activity can be obtained in a non-invasive fashion by using NADH fluorimetry to determine the NADH:NAD ratio (Chance *et al.* 1965). Using this technique Hardy *et al.* (1994) demonstrated that increased levels of NADH production were better correlated with developmental potential than morphological grade. Widespread adoption of this technique is clearly hampered by the expense of investing in the equipment and training necessary for accurate embryonic diagnosis.

Growth factors

A number of secretory substances found in the extracellular culture fluid have been reported to correlate either with successful pregnancy after transfer or with development to the blastocyst stage *in vitro*. Levels of human chorionic gonadotrophin (hCG), a product of the syncytiotrophoblast, show a correlation with blastocyst quality. Morphologically poor blastocysts that have a vacuolated appearance and contain extensive degenerative foci often fail to secrete measurable hCG levels and fail to hatch *in vitro* (Dokras *et al.* 1993). Morphologically normal embryos begin secreting hCG from day 7 onwards and increase hCG secretion to a maximum, in culture, by days 10 or 11 and decrease production thereafter. While rapid assays for hCG are available and correlations between hCG and developmental potential exist, the delay of hCG production until day 8 currently makes hCG determination inapplicable within an IVF timeframe.

Platelet-activating factor (PAF) is a phospholipid ubiquitous in body tissues. Investigators have reported a variety of roles for PAF activity in the function of spermatozoa, in the mechanism of ovulation, and in the development of mouse embryos *in vitro* (Pike *et al.* 1992). In 1990, Collier *et al.* found significantly higher levels of platelet activating factor from the medium of human *in vitro* embryos which subsequently produced pregnancies. However, 13 per cent of patients who conceived did so with embryos that failed to secrete measurable quantities of PAF. In addition to a lack of specificity, current PAF measurement is hampered by the tedious, time-consuming, and expensive nature of the assay.

Another non-invasive means of assessing embryo potential explored by several investigators is evaluation of embryo-derived immunosuppressive activity. Reports by Daya *et al.* (1986) and Clark *et al.* (1989) show that 16 per cent and 36 per cent of patients, respectively, who received at least one embryo with an immunosuppressive culture fluid, became pregnant, whereas none of the patients who received embryos that did not demonstrate immunosuppressive activity became pregnant. Other investigators examining immunoactive factors in embryo culture media have also claimed that increased levels of interleukin-1 (IL-1) and increased immunosuppressive activity (Sheth *et al.* 1991) were more likely to be present in culture supernatant obtained from embryos that eventually resulted in a pregnancy. However, subsequent investigators failed to confirm these initials findings. A double blind analysis of the effect of human embryo culture media on lymphocyte proliferation and natural killer activity did not demonstrate a correlation between immunosuppressive activity and pregnancy rate (Armstrong and Chaouat 1993). The complexity of the assay systems may, in part, explain the difficulty in evaluating immunosuppressive activity. The recent identification of monoclonal antibodies to the suppressor factors may standardize experimental protocols and lead to the development of a rapid and reproducible assay system for immunologic factors which mediate embryonic development (Bose *et al.* 1993).

Growth factors such as epidermal growth factor (EGF) and transforming growth factor alpha (TGFα) have been shown to act as mitogens and stimulate differentiation in murine and bovine pre-implantation embryonic development (Harvey *et al.* 1995*a*). Reverse transcriptase PCR (polymerase chain reaction) has been used to examine the expression of growth factors by the embryonic genome and has shown simultaneous expression of EGF, TGFα, and epidermal growth factor receptor (EGFR) in the egg and blastocyst; a pattern of secretion which is unique to the human system and suggests a role for autocrine stimulation in pre-implantation development (Chia *et al.* 1995). Reduced protein levels of EGF, TGFα, and EGFR at later stages of *in vitro* development suggest a switch to paracrine stimulation. Inadequacy of simple culture media to maintain advanced embryo development may reflect insufficient paracrine stimulation of essential developmental pathways.

Growth factor assessment may also yield valuable information regarding implantation potential. Leukaemia inhibitory factor (LIF) is a secreted glycoprotein which triggers blastocyst implantation (Harvey *et al.* 1995*b*). LIF mRNA has been detected in pre-implantation blastocysts as well as in the mid to late stages of development, suggesting several roles in *in vivo* embryonic development (Robertson *et al.* 1993). Preliminary studies by Harvey *et al.* (1995*a,b*) show that addition of LIF to embryonic culture media increases activity of both urokinase-type plasminogen activator and gelatinase B/matrix metalloproteinase; both essential for degradation of the uterine basement membrane and facilitation of implantation.

Determinants of embryo metabolism have great promise in assessing embryo potential. As with morphological indices of embryo potential, no single current method affords completely accurate diagnostic information regarding embryo viability. As metabolic, endocrine, and immunologic pathways are better defined in the early embryo, improved non-invasive methods of embryo analysis will no doubt be developed.

PRE-IMPLANTATION GENETIC ANALYSIS

Pre-implantation genetic diagnosis (PGD) provides a means to diagnose inherited genetic disease by evaluating biopsied embryonic cells. As invasive methods of embryo analysis become more refined, embryonic potential may be determined accurately by direct assessment of the genome. While single blastomere extraction at the 4-cell stage or extraction of greater than 50 per cent of blastomeres at any cell stage has a deleterious effect on embryo development (Roudebush *et al.* 1990), the structural integrity of the 8-cell embryo permits biopsy and eventual embryo replacement in the uterine cavity without affecting developmental potential (Hardy *et al.* 1990).

An alternative to directly extracting blastomeres from the developing embryo is to biopsy the trophectoderm (Dokras *et al.* 1990). As many as 10 to 30 trophectoderm cells from individual blastocysts can be obtained by days 5–6 (Dokras *et al.* 1991). Removal of greater than 10 cells, however, decreases hCG production, and may necessitate exogenous gonadotrophin replacement for luteal support when greater numbers of cells are required (Dokras *et al.* 1991). The ability to perform trophecto-derm biopsy is limited by the fact that only 25–60 per cent of 8-cell embryos reach blastocyst stage *in vitro*.

Trophectoderm cells could also be recovered from blastocysts developed *in vivo*. Flushing devices have been used to recover the pre-implantation blastocyst from the uterine cavity (Sauer *et al.* 1988). The technique may be limited by unsuccessful lavage resulting in retained embryo(s) which cannot be diagnosed, and the theoretical possibility of an ectopic pregnancy resulting from displacement of the blastocyst into the oviduct following lavage. Though the technique of uterine lavage, as first used in humans for oocyte donation, has been replaced by newer methods, the clinical success of trophectoderm biopsy may justify its re-emergence as a technology with potentially useful applications in PGD.

In situ hybridization techniques have been widely used to visualize specific DNA sequences in metaphase chromosomal preparations (Devilee *et al.* 1988; Penketh *et al.* 1989; Griffin *et al.* 1991). Incorporation of a fluorescent reporter molecule such as fluorescein isothiocyanate (FITC) and rhodamine into chromosome-specific probes is termed fluorescent *in situ* hybridization (FISH), and produces striking colour images when viewed through a photomultiplier/confocal microscope assembly or conven-tional fluorescence microscope.

Ploidy assessment of single blastomeres by FISH using a combination of auto-somal and sex chromosome probes is possible in a timeframe compatible with IVF–ET. Munne *et al.* (1993) analysed abnormally developing embryos using FISH probes for chromosomes X, Y, 18, 13, and 21. Successful analysis was achieved in 93 per cent of blastomeres and 70 per cent of embryos were abnormal for one or all of the studied chromosomes. The incidence of chromosomal abnormalities increased to 80 per cent for multinucleated blastomeres. In the same study, normally develop-ing embryos from women greater than 40 years of age were analysed and aneuploidy rates of 43 per cent for chromosomes X, Y, 18, 13 and 21 were calculated. The rate of aneuploidy in women under 40 years of age was 8 per cent (Munné *et al.* 1995). Since aneuploidy may be a major factor in explaining reduced implantation rate in women over 40, the use of FISH to prevent transfer of chromosomally abnormal embryos may increase IVF success in older women if sufficient numbers of embryos are available for selection.

A vast amount of information regarding the morphological, metabolic, and genetic characteristics of the human embryo is available to the practitioner of assisted repro-duction. The appropriate synthesis of relevant data will facilitate reasonable and appropriate clinical decisions regarding the developmental potential of gametes and embryos. While correction of intrinsic genomic defects in gametes and embryos is not an element of current widespread IVF practice, the selection of appropriate stimulation protocols, gametes, and embryos is facilitated by a paradigm of human embryonic development which integrates relevant morphological, metabolic, and genetic correlates of developmental potential.

REFERENCES

Angell, R., Xian, J., Keith, J., Ledger, W., and Baird, D. (1994). First meiotic division abnormalities in human oocytes: mechanism of trisomy formation. *Cytogenetics and Cellular Genetics*, **65**, 194–202.

Armstrong, D. and Chaouat, G. (1993). Immunological aspects of human *in vitro* fertilization and embryo transfer. In *Immunology of pregnancy*, pp. 33–46. CRC Press, Boca Raton.

Artley, J. and Braude, P. (1993). Biochemistry of the preimplantation embryo. *Assisted Reproductive Reviews*, **3**, 13–17.

Biggers, J. and Stern, S. (1973). Metabolism of the preimplantation mammalian embryo. *Advances in Reproductive Physiology*, **6**, 1–59.

Biggers, J., Whittingham, D., and Donahue, R. (1967). The pattern of energy metabolism in the mouse oocyte and zygote. *Proceedings of the National Academy of Science (USA)*, **2**, 560–7.

Bolton, V., Hawes, S., Taylor, C., and Parsons, J. (1988). Development of spare human preimplantation embryos *in vitro*: an analysis of the correlations among gross morphology, cleavage rates and development to the blastocyst. *Journal of In Vitro Fertilization and Embryo Transfer*, **6**, 30–5.

Bongso, A., Ng, S., and Lim, J. (1991). Preimplantation genetics: chromosomes of fragmented human embryos. *Fertility and Sterility*, **56**, 66–70.

Bose, R., Nagy, E., Fleetham, J., Pattinson, H., Berczi, I., and Yang, J. (1993). Production and characterization of monoclonal antibodies to embryo-associated immunosuppressive factor (EASF) produced by human pre-implantation embryos. *Immunology Letters*, **38**, 47–54.

Braude, P., Bolton, V., and Moore, S. (1988). Human gene expression first occurs between the four and eight cell stages of preimplantation development. *Nature*, **332**, 459–61.

Chance, B., Schoener, B., Krejci, K., Russmann, W., Wesemann, W., Schnitger, H., and Bucher, T. (1965). Kinetics of fluorescence and metabolite changes in rat liver during a cycle of ischemia. *Biochemische Zeitschrift*, **341**, 325–33.

Chia, M., Winston, R., and Handyside, A. (1995). EGF, TGF-α, EGFR expression in human preimplantation embryos. *Development*, **121**, 299–307.

Claman, P., Armant, D., Seibel, M., Wang, T., Oskowitz, S., and Taymor, M. (1987). The impact of embryo quality and quantity on implantation and the establishment of viable pregnancies. *Journal of In Vitro Fertilization and Embryo Transfer*, **4**, 218–22.

Clark, D., Lee, S., Fishell, S., Mahadevan, M., Goodall, H., *et al.* (1989). Immunosuppressive activity in human *in vitro* fertilization (IVF) culture supernatants and prediction of the outcome of embryo transfer: a multicenter trial. *Journal of In Vitro Fertilization and Embryo Transfer*, **6**, 51–8.

Cohen, J., Inge, K., Suzman, M., Wiker, S., and Wright, G. (1989). Videocinematography of fresh and cryopreserved embryos: a retrospective analysis of embryonic morphology and implantation. *Fertility and Sterility*, **51**, 820–7.

Collier, M., O'Neill, C., Ammit, A., and Saunders, D. (1990). Measurement of human embryo derived platelet-activating factor (PAF) using a quantitative bioassay of platelet aggregation. *Human Reproduction*, **5**, 323–8.

Copperman, A., Selick, C., Grunfeld, L., Sandler, B., and Bustillo, M. (1995). Cumulative number and morphological score of embryos resulting in success: realistic expectations from *in vitro* fertilization–embryo transfer. *Fertility and Sterility*, **64**, 88–92.

Daya, S., Lee, S., Underwood, J., *et al.* (1986). Prediction of outcome following transfer of *in vitro* fertilized human embryos by measurement of embryo-associated suppressor factor. In *Reproductive immunology*, (ed. D. Clark and B. Croy), pp. 277–85. Elsevier/North Holland, Amsterdam.

De, Sutter, P., Dhont, M., and Vandekerckhove, D. (1992). Hormonal stimulation for *in vitro* fertilization: a comparison of fertilization rates and cytogenetic findings in unfertilized oocytes. *Journal of Assisted Reproduction Genetics*, **9**, 254–8.

Devilee, P., Thierry, R., Kievits, T., Kolluri, R., Hopman, A., Willard, H., *et al.* (1988). Detection of chromosome aneuploidy in interphase nuclei from human primary breast cancer tumors using chromosome-specific repetitive DNA probes. *Cancer Research*, **48**, 5825–30.

Dokras, A., Sargent, I., Ross, C., Gardner, R., and Barlow, D. (1990). Trophectoderm biopsy in human blastocysts. *Human Reproduction*, **5**, 821–5.

Dokras, A., Sargent, I., Ross, C., Gardner, R., and Barlow, D. (1991). Human trophectoderm biopsy and secretion of chorionic gonadotropin. *Human Reproduction*, **6**, 1453–9.

Dokras, A., Sargent, I., and Barlow, D. (1993). Human blastocyst grading: an indicator of developmental potential? *Human Reproduction*, **8**, 2119–27.

Dor, J., Rudak, E., Mashiach, S., Nebel, L., Serr, D., and Goldman, B. (1986). Periovulatory 17 beta-estradiol changes and embryo morphological features in conception and nonconceptional cycles after human *in vitro* fertilization. *Fertility and Sterility*, **45**, 63–8.

Fitzgerald, L. and Dimattina, M. (1992). An improved medium for long-term culture of human embryos overcomes the *in-vitro* developmental block and increases blastocyst formation. *Fertility and Sterility*, **57**, 641–6.

Gardner, D. and Leese, H. (1990). The concentration of nutrients in mouse oviduct fluid and their effects on mouse embryo development and metabolism *in vitro*. *Journal of Reproductive Fertility*, **88**, 361–8.

Gott, A.L., Hardy, K., Winston, R.M.L., and Leese, H.J. (1990). Non-invasive measurement of pyruvate and glucose uptake and lactate production by single human primplantation embryos. *Human Reproduction*, **5**, 104–8.

Griffin, D., Handyside, A., Penketh, R., Winston, R., and Delhanty, J. (1991). Fluorescent *in-situ* hybridization to interphase nuclei of human preimplantation embryos with X and Y chromosome specific probes. *Human Reproduction*, **1**, 101–5.

Grow, D., Oehninger, S., Seltman, H., Toner, J., Swanson, R., Kruger, T., and Mausher, S. (1994). Sperm morphology as diagnosed by strict criteria: probing the impact of teratozoospermia on fertilization rate and pregnancy outcome in a large *in vitro* fertilization population. *Fertility and Sterility*, **62**, 559–67.

Hardy, K., Hooper, M., Handyside, A., Rutherford, A., Winston, R., and Leese, H. (1989). Non-invasive measurement of glucose and pyruvate uptake by individual human oocytes and preimplantation embryos. *Human Reproduction*, **4**, 188–91.

Hardy, K., Martin, K., Leese, H., Winston, R., and Handyside, A. (1990). Human preimplantation development *in vitro* is not adversely affected by biopsy at the 8-cell stage. *Human Reproduction*, **5**, 708–14.

Hardy, R.I., Golan, D.E., and Biggers, J.D. (1994). Metabolic assessment of embryo quality: Correlation between NADH laser fluorimetric measurment and embryo development. From Postgraduate Course VI syllabus. Presented at the 50th meeting of the American Fertility Society 1994, p. 81.

Harvey, M., Leco, K., Arcellana-Panlilio, M., Zhang, X., Edwards, D., and Schultz, G. (1995a). Roles of growth factors during peri-implantation development. *Molecular Human Reproduction*, **10**, 712–18.

Harvey, M., Leco, K., Arcellana-Panlilio, M., Zhang, X., Edwards, D., and Schultz, G. (1995*b*). Roles of growth factors during peri-implantation development. *Human Reproduction* 10, 712–18.

Kruger, T., Lombard, C., and van Zyl, J. (1986). Sperm morphologic features as a prognostic factor in *in vitro* fertilization. *Fertility and Sterility*, 46, 1118–23.

Lopata, A., Kohlman, D., and Johnston, I. (1983). The fine structure of normal and abnormal human embryos developed in culture. In *Fertilization of the human egg in vitro*, (ed. H. Beier and H. Lindner), pp. 189–210. Springer, Berlin. Mohr, (1983).

Mukherjee, T., Copperman, A.B., Lapinski, R., McCaffrey, C., and Obasaju, M. (1995). Interobserver and intraobserver variability of embryo morphology in an IVF program. Presented at the 51st Meeting of the American Society for Reproductive Medicine 1995, Poster 353.

Munné, S., Lee, A., Rosenwaks, Z., Grifo, J., and Cohen, J. (1993). Diagnosis of major chromosome aneuploidies in human preimplantation embryos. *Human Reproduction*, 8, 2185–91.

Munné, S., Alikani, M., Tomkin, G., Grifo, J., and Cohen, J. (1995). Embryo morphology, developmental rates, and maternal age are correlated with chromosome abnormalities. *Fertility and Sterility*, 64, 382–91.

Penketh, R., Delhanty, J., Van de Berghe, J., Finklestone, E., and Handyside, A. (1989). Rapid sexing of human embryos by non-radioactive *in situ*-hybridization: potential for preimplantation diagnosis of X-linked disorders. *Prenatal Diagnosis*, 9, 489–500.

Pike, I., Ammit, A., and O'Neill, C. (1992). Actions of platelet activating factor (PAF) on gametes and embryos: clinical aspects. *Reproductive Fertility Developments*, 4, 399–410.

Plachot, M., Veiga, A., and Montagut, J. (1988). Are clinical and biological IVF parameters correlated with chromosomal disorders in early life? A multicentric study. *Human Reproduction*, 3, 627–35.

Robertson, M., Chambers, I., Rathjen, P., Nichols, J., and Smith, A. (1993). Expression of alternative forms of differentiation inhibiting activity (DIA/LIF) during murine embryogenesis and in neonatal and adult tissue. *Developmental Genetics*, 14, 165–73.

Roudebush, W., Kim, J., and Minhas, B. (1990). The 8 cell pre-embryo is the ideal stage for biopsy in the mouse. *Journal of In Vitro Fertility and Embryo Transfer*, 7, 32–8.

Sauer, M., Bustillo, M., Gorrill, M., Louw, J., Marshall, J., and Buster, J. (1988). An instrument for the recovery of preimplantation human ova. *Obstetrics and Gynecology*, 71, 804–6.

Sheth, K., Roca, G., Al-Sedairy, S., Parhar, R., Hamilton, C., and Jabbar, F. (1991). Prediction of successful embryo implantation by measuring interleukin-1-alpha and immunosuppressive factor(s) in preimplantation embryo culture fluid. *Fertility and Sterility*, 55, 952–7.

Staessen, C., Camus, M., Bollen, N., Devroey, P., and Van Steirteghem, A. (1992). The relationship between embryo quality and the occurrence of multiple pregnancies. *Fertility and Sterility*, 57, 626–30.

Steer, C., Mills, C., Tan, S., Campbell, S., and Edwards, R. (1992). The cumulative embryo score: a predictive embryo scoring technique to select the optimal number of embryos to transfer in an *in vitro* fertilization and embryo transfer programme. *Human Reproduction*, 7, 117–19.

Tarín, J. and Pellicer, A. (1990). Consequences of high ovarian response to gonadotropins: a cytogenetic analysis of unfertilized human oocytes. *Fertility and Sterility*, 54, 665–70.

Tejada, M., Mendoza, R., Corcostegui, B., and Benito, J. (1991). Chromosome studies in human unfertilized oocytes and uncleaved zygotes after treatment with gonadotropin-releasing hormone analogs. *Fertility and Sterility*, 56, 874–80.

Tesarik, J. (1988). Developmental control of human preimplantation embryos: a comparative approach. *Journal of In Vitro Fertility and Embryo Transfer*, 5, 347–62.

Tesarik, J. (1989). The potential diagnostic use of human zona-free eggs prepared from oocytes that failed to fertilize *in-vitro*. *Fertility and Sterility*, **52**, 821–4.

Tesarik, J. (1994). Developmental failure during the preimplantation period of human embryogenesis. In *The biological basis of early human reproductive failure*, (ed. J. Van Blerkom), pp. 327–44. Oxford University Press, New York.

Tesarik, J. and Kopecny, V. (1989). Development of human male pronucleus: ultrastructure and timing. *Gamete Research*, **24**, 135–49.

Tesarik, J., Kopecny, V., Plachot, M., and Mandelbaum, J. (1986). Activation of nucleolar and extranucleolar RNA synthesis and changes in the ribosomal content of human embryos developing *in vitro*. *Journal of Reproductive Fertility*, **2**, 127–36.

Tesarik, J., Kopecny, V., Plachot, M., and Mandelbaum, J. (1988). Early morphological signs of embryonic genome expression in human preimplantation development as revealed by quantitative electron microscopy. *Developmental Biology*, **128**, 15–20.

Testart, J. (1986). Cleavage stage of human embryos two days after fertilization *in vitro* and their developmental ability after transfer into the uterus. *Human Reproduction*, **1**, 29–31.

Testart, J. and Lassalle, B. (1991). Sequential transformations of human sperm nucleus in human egg. *Journal of Reproductive Fertility*, **91**, 393–402.

Van Blerkom, J. (1989a). Developmental failure in human reproduction associated with pre-ovulatory oogenesis and preimplantation embryogenesis. In *Ultrastructure of human gametogenesis and early embryogenesis*, (ed. J. Van Blerkom and P. Motta), pp. 122–80. New York.

Van Blerkom, J. (1989b). The origin and detection of chromosomal abnormalities in meiotically mature human oocytes obtained from stimulated follicles and after failed fertilization *in-vitro*. *Progress in Clinical Biology Research*, **296**, 299–310.

Van Blerkom, J. (1991). Extrinsic and intrinsic influences on human oocyte and early embryo developmental potential. In *Elements of mammalian fertilization. Vol. 2. Practical applications*, (ed. P. Wasserman), pp. 81–109. CRC Press, Boca Raton.

Van Blerkom, J. and Henry, G. (1992). Oocyte dysmorphism and aneuploidy in meiotically-mature human oocytes after ovarian stimulation. *Human Reproduction*, **7**, 379–90.

Van Blerkom, J. and Henry, G. (1994). Cytogenetic, cellular, and developmental consequences of cryopreservation of immature and mature mouse and human oocytes. *Microscopic Research Techniques*, **27**, 165–93.

Veeck, L. (1986a). Human oocytes at the time of follicular harvest. In *Atlas of the human oocyte and early conceptus*, (ed. C. Lynn Brown), pp. 5–132. Williams and Wilkins, Baltimore.

Veeck, L. (1986b). Cleaved human concepti. In *Atlas of the human oocyte and early conceptus*, (ed. C. Lynn Brown), pp. 163–230. Williams and Wilkins, Baltimore.

Wright, G., Wilker, S., and Elsner, C. (1990). Observations on the morphology of pronuclei and nucleoli in human zygotes and implications for cryopreservation. *Human Reproduction*, **5**, 109–15.

4 | *Embryonic signals*

Eytan R. Barnea and Carolyn B. Coulam

INTRODUCTION

This chapter describes the pre-embryonic signals present prior to implantation. The maternal organism recognizes very early that fertilization has taken place, since signals produced by the zygote are already detected in the peripheral circulation by 24 h after ovulation, if conception has occurred (O'Neill 1985a; Roberts *et al.* 1987). None the less, the time from fertilization to implantation *in vivo* (5–7 subsequent days in humans) has remained clinically silent. Most of the data describing the cardinal events leading to successful implantation are derived from experimental animals, due to the limitations on experimentation in humans.

Following sperm penetration of the zona pellucida, egg–sperm fusion at the oolemma or vitelline membrane takes place within the fallopian tubal lumen leading to egg activation. As a result of oocyte activation, cortical granules are released from the ooplasm and meiosis resumes within the nucleus. The incorporated sperm undergoes decondensation to form the male pronucleus. By this time embryonic signals are already detectable. The second polar body is then extruded and the female pronucleus is formed. The sperm's nuclear membrane disintegrates, exposing its chromatin to egg cytoplasm decondensing factors. The chromatin becomes bound by a membrane and syngamy occurs. In the zygote, the first cell division takes place within 12–36 h. Subsequent cell divisions occur more rapidly but are not necessarily symmetrical, leading to an uneven number of cells. The totipotentiality of blastomeres is still evident at the 8-cell stage embryo, but by the 16-cell stage, the embryo undergoes compaction. The inner cell mass leads to the development of the embryo proper, while the outer layer forms the trophoblast. The maternally inherited messenger ribonucleic acid (mRNA) is operative until the activation of the embryonic genome, which takes place at the 2–8-cell stage (Brinster 1973). The timing of this activation is species-specific (Sawicky *et al.* 1978); in humans it probably begins at the 6–8-cell stage.

For implantation to take place, the embryo has to be viable (Hertig *et al.* 1956). Therefore, the expression of various recognition products by the embryo while in contact with the tubal mucosa (during natural conception), or in the endometrial cavity (following *in vitro* fertilization (IVF)) prior to implantation, creates the recognition by the mother and aids in the implantation process. This interaction may contribute to the receptive endometrial environment that is required for the successful start of pregnancy (see Chapter 7).

The following is a description of the various pre-implantation embryonal signals including platelet-activating factor (PAF), early pregnancy factor (EPF), and pre-implantation factor (PIF).

PLATELET-ACTIVATING FACTOR (PAF)

The earliest embryo-derived signal that appears following fertilization and prior to implantation is a transient thrombocytopenia occurring within 8 h of fertilization in women and mice (O'Neill 1985*b*). The component responsible for such an early signal is embryo-derived PAF. PAF is actually a family of acetylated glycerophospholipids that have a significant molecular heterogeneity. One particular form, PAF-acether (1-O-alkyl-2-acetyl-*sn*-glycero-3-phosphocholine) is the compound most frequently studied (Snyder 1989). The presence of PAF appears to be ubiquitous in the organism, and is expressed especially by white cells, platelets, and endothelial cells (Pinckard *et al.* 1979). Effectors of PAF release vary with site as well as pathways of synthesis and release, and are specific for each organ (Braquet *et al.* 1987).

Circulating PAF is rapidly inactivated by an acid-labile factor, acetyl hydrolase (Yasuda *et al.* 1995). In plasma, PAF is converted to lyso-PAF and platelets have also been shown to acetylate PAF to a 2-acyl form (Farr *et al.* 1983). PAF is involved in several reproductive processes and is found in semen, follicular fluid, the endometrium, and in amniotic fluid (Kumar *et al.* 1988; Critser and English 1992). Overall, PAF causes alterations in cell-to-cell interactions, activation of inflammatory processes, changes in vascular permeability, and immunoregulation of graft rejection (Braquet *et al.* 1987; Feurstein and Siren 1988). Conditioned medium from mouse pre-implantation embryos induces a reduction in peripheral platelet count from day one following fertilization in splenectomized mice. This decrease is noticeable until day 7 of pregnancy (Elias *et al.* 1989). In contrast, no such response was obtained by transferring non-fertilized eggs to pseudopregnant mice (O'Neill 1985*b*). PAF can be detected in culture medium where mouse or human embryos have been grown (O'Neill 1985*b*; Collier *et al.* 1988).

Embryo-derived PAF may be important for pregnancy maintenance and tubal transport (Collier *et al.* 1988; Velasquez *et al.* 1995). Human embryos with good morphology secreted higher PAF levels into the culture medium than embryos with poor morphology and, after transfer, embryos that resulted in pregnancy were those that had higher PAF levels.

Using the splenectomized mice model, it appears that the highest expression of PAF is at the 2-cell stage, and it decreases later in the blastocyst phase. It is estimated that the embryo secretes 100 ng/ml of PAF which, when injected to mice, decreases platelet count *in vivo* in a manner which is indistinguishable from that obtained with pure PAF injection (Elias *et al.* 1989). However, because of difficulties in the actual measurement of PAF, this assay is not used clinically at present. The transient thrombocytopenia seen in women following embryo transfer is difficult to document, which is perhaps due to large variations in platelet count among subjects studied (Roberts *et al.* 1987).

Embryo-derived PAF has been suggested to be a facilitator of implantation. Studies in mice, in which the administration of PAF antagonists prior to mating decreased the number of implanted embryos (Spinks *et al.* 1990), support the hypothesis that PAF aids in the synchronization of embryonal/endometrial development. However, other studies have failed to confirm this critical role (Milligan and Finn 1988, 1990). PAF may modify endometrial vascular permeability by acting upon prostaglandins (Smith and Kelly 1988). In humans, PAF is secreted in the endometrium, by stromal but not by epithelial cells, thus a local role may be envisaged as well (Alecozay *et al.* 1989). Overall, PAF of embryonal origin may have a role in the maternal recognition of pregnancy; but at present, the requirements for such a signal and the mechanisms involved are not well defined.

Finally, it has recently been reported (Radonjic-Lazovic and Roudebush 1995) that PAF, when added to mouse embryonal cultures for various time intervals and in a wide range of concentrations, either had no effect, or affected mouse embryonal viability and reduced blastocyst volume. Recent data have questioned whether the embryo-derived substance is actually PAF (Amiel *et al.* 1989; Smal *et al.* 1990). Very sensitive assays using the washed rabbit platelet aggregation assay and a radio-immunoassay with highly sensitive and specific antibody to PAF have failed to confirm the identity of the embryo-derived substance. The use of 10 per cent serum by the aforementioned authors may have contributed to the discrepancies in the results.

A more practical problem is that embryo-derived PAF cannot be distinguished from maternal PAF in serum (Abisogun *et al.* 1989; O'Neill *et al.* 1992). High circulating levels of maternally derived PAF (i.e. fallopian tubes) mask lower concentrations of embryonic-origin PAF, making the measurement of PAF in maternal serum impractical as a pre-implantation marker.

EARLY PREGNANCY FACTOR (EPF)

In the early 1970s, it was recognized that shortly after fertilization an early pregnancy phenomenon called early pregnancy factor (EPF) occurred, also in humans (Morton *et al.* 1977). From its earliest description, the phenomenon has been recognized as reflecting pre-implantation events, but the methodology for its measurement has never reached the stage of allowing a reproducible and systematic study of the phenomenon. EPF is produced within a day after fertilization in several mammalian species including humans, and it is believed mainly to be an immunomodulatory factor (Morton *et al.* 1992a).

The assay used to measure EPF is based on the rosette inhibition test (RIT) (Bach *et al.* 1969). This assay measures the ability of EPF to bind lymphocytes and release genetically restricted suppressor factors (Rolfe *et al.* 1989). These factors affect the activity of Lyt-1+ T cells as demonstrated in the bioassay. Upon the binding of EPF to lymphocytes, two soluble lymphokines are released. The first of these (14 kDa) is related to region I of the major histocompatibility complex (MHC) while the other (55 kDa) is linked to the other major restricting elements of T-cell interactions, i.e. heavy chain immunoglobulins (Rolfe *et al.* 1988). The bioassay is carried out using titre dilutions and the response is a bell-shaped curve in which low and high dilutions are negative.

EPF activity has been detected in both pregnant sera as well as in several other tissues such as sheep placenta, murine ovaries and oviducts, human BeWo choriocarcinoma cells, and ascites fluid (Morton *et al.* 1992b). EPF, of maternal origin, is detected in serum within a day after fertilization. Following implantation, it has been shown that EPF activity is present in embryonic organs and is secreted by first-trimester trophoblast cell cultures (Nahhas and Barnea 1990).

The passive immunization of pregnant mice against EPF causes a loss of embryonic viability (Athanasas-Platsis *et al.* 1989). However, according to recent data, as pregnancy proceeds, EPF levels are not altered, but its inhibitors disappear from circulation soon after implantation (Morton *et al.* 1992*b*). Additionally, PAF injections can induce transient EPF expression in male and female mice (Cavanagh *et al.* 1991) showing that EPF is not specific for pregnancy (Morton *et al.* 1980). Overall, EPF is an interesting biological phenomenon reflecting maternal recognition of the pre-implantation embryo. However, the mechanisms and specific effectors involved still remain unknown after more than twenty years of detailed investigation by several groups (Chard and Grudzinskas 1987).

Whether embryo-derived PAF-acether is the specific effector remains to be established (Cavanagh *et al.* 1991). From a clinical standpoint, the efforts to establish quality control parameters for the RIT suffer from the fact that the assay has been applied mostly to studies on relatively advanced pregnancies. A report by Chen (1985) on embryo transfer is still the only investigation in humans in which EPF was detected in the serum following timed fertilization. In another study, EPF was detected after intercourse in 18/28 cycles, suggesting a fertilization rate of 64 per cent. Early embryonic loss was high (78 per cent), and was detected when EPF disappeared from the circulation before the onset of menses in 14 out of 18 cases (Mesrogli and Maas 1985). In a more recent study, Shahani *et al.* (1992) reported that in cases with missed menses and positive human chorionic gonadotropin (hCG), those that were negative for EPF had an 80 per cent pregnancy failure rate. Similar observations have been made by Gerhard *et al.* (1991). EPF is detected in maternal serum until the third trimester and is associated with viable embryos and fetuses (Clarke 1992). It is also found in fetal sera (Huong and Zhen-Qung 1990).

The identity of EPF has not been yet settled. A report by Mehta *et al.* (1989) identified EPF as being a 21.5-kDa pregnancy serum-derived immunosuppressive protein. More recently, EPF was characterized as being the known platelet-derived low molecular weight heat-shock protein, chaperonin 10 (Cavanagh and Morton 1994). The expression of this class of proteins increases in response to different metabolic insults which represent a universal defence mechanism. The link of EPF to chaperone molecules quite logically suggests that control over early embryonic growth and development may be achieved, in part, by secretion and redirection of chaperonin 10 into the extracellular compartment. Once the identity of EPF is known, it will be necessary to develop a sensitive immunoassay to confirm whether the substance is indeed critical during earliest phases of human or mammalian pregnancy.

EPF-related compounds have been purified from cultured human embryo growth media (Bose *et al.* 1989). Using chromatographic techniques, these authors isolated a number of proteins, the principal of which was a 14.5-kDa molecule containing disulphide bonds. The proteins isolated had immunosuppressive activities as measured by the rosette assay and by their concavalin A-stimulated lymphocyte proliferation. However, not all immunosuppressive activity correlated with that of EPF, suggesting that several immunosuppressors (thus far unrecognized) are secreted by the embryo to aid in creating maternal immunological tolerance.

PRE-IMPLANTATION FACTOR (PIF)

In an attempt to study embryo signalling processes prior to implantation, we have recently described a novel phenomenon of auto-rosette formation between lymphocytes and platelets when treated with serum from pregnant women (Barnea *et al.* 1994). The lymphocyte/platelet binding assay (LPBA) has provided a marker to identify the presence of viable pre-implantation embryos *in vivo* (Coulam *et al.* 1995; Roussev *et al.* 1995). The method is rapid and simple, and requires low volumes of test compounds, test samples, and cell suspensions. However, as with every bioassay, it has some limitations (requiring fresh lymphocytes and platelets, not older than 3–4 h after isolation, and suitable blood donor groups). Of all blood types tested, male O+ donors gave the most distinguishable differences between positive and negative values (Roussev *et al.* 1995). On the other hand, considering that it is a bioassay, it is highly reproducible in blinded testing. When results from two independent observers were compared, a high degree of correlation was found ($r > 0.9$).

A large body of data has been accumulated on PIF. Figure 4.1 shows PIF-positive serum (b) compared with a PIF-negative sample (a). The LPBA was validated for its ability to distinguish between the presence and absence of pregnancy in a large number of samples in prospective studies. To date, more than 200 women have been studied, and in all samples derived from normal pregnancies, PIF-activity has been positive. No correlation with their respective hCGβ levels has been found (Roussev *et al.* 1995). In contrast, no PIF activity has been found in known non-pregnant subjects. The threshold of PIF activity was evaluated prospectively in 67 healthy non-pregnant women and men compared with known pregnant patients. It was established that a result of > 9 per cent of lymphocytes bound to three or more platelets is PIF positive while levels below that are considered PIF negative (Fig. 4.2) (Roussev *et al.* 1995). Table 4.1 shows the sensitivity of the improved assay.

PIF activity has been determined both retrospectively and prospectively, in both cross-sectional and longitudinal studies. In addition, the assay has been carried out in patients who conceived spontaneously and in those subjected to intrauterine insemination or assisted reproductive technologies. The earliest signal for PIF was detected two days after embryo transfer, i.e. 2–3 days prior to implantation (Roussev *et al.*

Table 4.1 Clinical validation of the PIF assay carried out prospectively in 65 patients after embryo transfer following *in vitro* fertilization

Sensitivity	88%
Specificity	97%
Positive predictive value	95%
Negative predictive value	90%

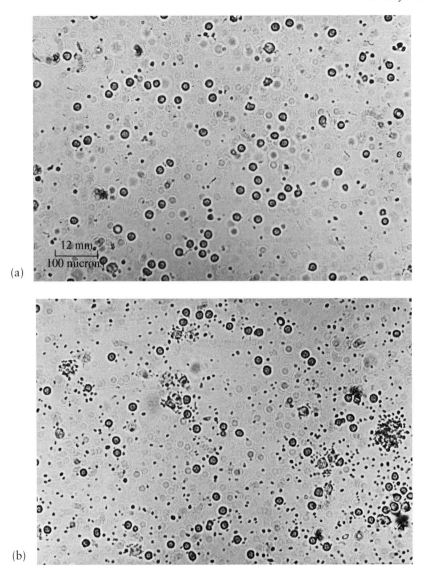

Fig. 4.1 Photographs of the PIF assay from (a) non-pregnant woman (negative control); and (b) pregnant woman (serum from fourth day after embryo transfer that led to a successful pregnancy).

1996). Subsequently, PIF is present in serum all through pregnancy. The following is a brief description of studies carried out to date.

In a prospective study, PIF was measured four days after embryo transfer, and results were compared with hCG levels in serum drawn 11 days after embryo transfer combined with the presence of an intrauterine gestational sac visible on transvaginal

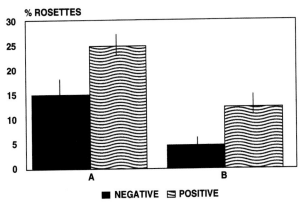

Fig. 4.2 PIF results presented when one or more bound platelets bound to a lymphocyte was considered a rosette (A); and when a minimum of three platelets bound to a lymphocyte was considered a rosette (B). The latter defines a more clear positive threshold.

sonogram using a 7.5 MHz probe three weeks after transfer. Results on 120 serum samples drawn four days after embryo transfer (ET) showed 75 per cent sensitivity, 95 per cent specificity, 94 per cent positive predictive value, and 82 per cent negative predictive value, when compared with pregnant women having > 5 mIU/ml hCG (Roussev *et al.* 1995). In another study, the ability of the PIF assay to detect the presence of viable embryos prior to implantation after ET was examined. Seven out of eight women were PIF positive after ET; four had clinical pregnancies. In the women who did not have clinical pregnancies, PIF activity disappeared 4–13 days after ET. PIF activity continued into the first trimester of pregnancy in those women with clinical pregnancies. In a longitudinal study, samples were tested for PIF in all three trimesters. In all cases, PIF was positive, but the activity in the cord blood was negative.

The value of PIF in predicting early pregnancy loss was also examined (Coulam *et al.* 1995). In 57 women experiencing first trimester losses (46 after IVF–ET and 11 recurrent aborters), PIF was found to be negative at the time of abortion. Of 12 abortuses with normal karyotype, only one woman was initially PIF positive, while the other 11 were all PIF negative. In addition, serial assays were performed in 15 women. Eleven (73 per cent) women were PIF negative four days after ET and remained so until abortion occurred. These patients had a preclinical loss. The other four (27 per cent) were initially PIF positive but became PIF negative a minimum of two weeks prior to demonstration of embryonal demise, while hCG levels remained elevated. These four patients had a clinical loss. Thus, measurement of PIF activity throughout the first trimester of pregnancy predicts not only the presence of a viable pre-implantation embryo, but also the well-being of that embryo and possible subsequent pregnancy loss (Fig. 4.3). In patients who failed to conceive, PIF activity was never detected. Moreover, in patients who conceived but failed to carry to term, PIF activity disappeared prior to appearance of clinical symptoms. Thus PIF activity appears to be required for pregnancy and its disappearance is associated with very poor prognosis.

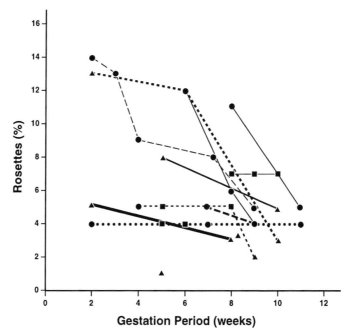

Fig. 4.3 Results of PIF assays from sera of 15 women who had blood drawn serially during their pregnancy prior to experiencing a first-trimester loss. A negative PIF result was considered to be less than 8 per cent rosette formation.

The embryonal origin of PIF

Since PIF can be measured in the sera of women after fertilization but before implantation, the question of determining the source of the measured PIF has become very relevant. To determine whether the embryo was the source of PIF secretion, PIF activity was measured in culture media from 2–8-cell human embryos; each embryo was cultured individually. In all tested human embryo culture media from non-fertilized and fertilized oocytes, PIF activity was negative. However, when the media were concentrated tenfold, PIF activity was detected in all media from 2–8-cell viable embryos, but not in media from unfertilized eggs or atretic embryos. Similar observations were made recently with mouse embryos (Roussev *et al.* 1996).

Thus, a zygote-derived signal(s) is secreted (it is unclear whether PIF activity derives from the paternal or maternal genome which have just barely fused). The potency of the signal is quite impressive, since it derives from only two fused cells and is detected in the circulation; this attests to the force of reproduction. Because of the intensity of the PIF signal, we believe that an amplification process may be operative. Future investigations will be very useful in this respect. Finally, the finding that platelets interact with lymphocytes in the PIF assay may or may not reflect on such an interaction *in vivo*.

In any event, it appears that the recognition process is ingenious, and it is achieved by sensitizing the immune system through lymphocyte activation leading to a generalized maternal immune recognition. Such an early immune recognition may aid in developing endometrial receptivity and synchronization with embryonal development. However, such rapid and widespread recognition may also allow implantation in other unfavourable sites such as the fallopian tubes, ovaries, and within the abdominal cavity. Lack of recognition, on the other hand, may contribute to implantation failure. The specific factors involved and how the signal is transmitted remain unknown at present.

OTHER SECRETORY PRODUCTS

The pre-implantation embryo produces hCG in limited quantities; these levels increase once hatching takes place. It has been shown that at the 6–8-cell stage, hCGβ mRNA expression can already be detected (Bonduelle *et al.* 1988). hCG is recognized to have a major role in the maintenance of the corpus luteum. However, prior to implantation this role may be negligible since no differences are present between the biology of the corpus luteum in fertile and infertile cycles until a few days after implantation. On the other hand, embryo-derived hCG may have other roles as well, and is perhaps involved in maternal recognition processes through action on other target tissues. In fact, Rodway and Rao (1995) have shown that hCG affects lymphocyte proliferation. Moreover, embryonal secretion of hCG may be involved in priming the endometrium through effects on endothelium.

Insulin-like growth factors (IGFs)

The earliest expression of IGF2 is at the 2-cell stage in the mouse, while IGF1 is expressed only after implantation (Schoefield *et al.* 1992). In contrast, in humans the expression of all IGFs occurs only after implantation. This suggests that the pre-implantation embryo is able to develop mainly through autocrine trophic influences. Indeed, when IGF expression was inhibited by using antisense probes to the growth factor, embryonal growth slowed down. However, addition of the two growth factors did not affect pre-implantation mouse embryo development in culture. Whether other growth factors are secreted by the pre-implantation embryos in sufficient quantities to enable maternal recognition is not known at present, and remains an important point for investigation. As discussed earlier, the limitation in all these studies is the lack of a reliable marker that would reflect embryonal signalling to the mother, and which could be monitored in the circulation.

CONCLUDING REMARKS

Embryonic signals are present prior to implantation. Until recently, the detection of those signals was difficult. In the case of EPF this was due to the complexity of the bioassay, and in the case of PAF, to the inability to distinguish between maternally and embryo-derived signals—these signals have not been practical for clinical use.

Our newly developed PIF bioassay and the studies described indicate that PIF is necessary for pregnancy and that viable embryos secrete PIF prior to implantation. The presence of PIF activity suggests that implantation will occur and continued presence of PIF indicates that the pregnancy will be successful. On the other hand, initial presence of PIF but its later disappearance carries, in general, a very poor prognosis for pregnancy outcome. Our data also show that PIF is embryo-derived, is only expressed by viable embryos, and can be detected prior to implantation. Experiments indicate that PIF is a novel phenomenon which is not related to PAF or EPF (Roussev *et al.* 1997). Finally, biochemical evidence shows that PIF is actively secreted by the embryo. Future studies will focus on biochemical characterization and development of an immunoassay for PIF which will be necessary if such an assay is to be widely used clinically.

ACKNOWLEDGEMENTS

We would like to thank Jean-David Barnea for his extensive editorial support in writing this chapter.

REFERENCES

Abisogun, A., Braquet, T., and Tsafriri, A. (1989). The involvement of platelet activating factor in ovulation. *Science*, **234**, 381–3.

Alecozay, A., Calssen, B., and Riehl, R. (1989). Platelet activating factor in human luteal phase endometrium. *Biology of Reproduction*, **41**, 578–86.

Amiel, M., Duquenne, C., Benveniste, J., and Testart, J. (1989). Platelet aggregating activity in human embryo culture media free of PAF acether. *Human Reproduction*, **4**, 327–30.

Athanasas-Platsis, S., Quinn, K.A., Wong, T., Rolfe, B.E., Cavanagh, A.C., and Morton, H. (1989). Passive immunization of pregnant mice against early pregnancy factor (EPF) causes loss of embryonic viability. *Journal of Reproduction and Fertility*, **87**, 495–502.

Bach, J., Dormont, J., Dardenne, M., and Balner, W. (1969). *In vitro* rosette inhibition by anti-human ALS: correlation with skin graft prolongation in primates. *Transplantation*, **8**, 265–80.

Barnea, E.R., Lahijani, K.I., Roussev, R.G., Barnea, J.D., and Coulam, C.B. (1994). Use of lymphocyte/platelet binding assay for detecting a preimplantation factor: a quantitative assay. *American Journal of Reproductive Immunology*, **32**, 133–8.

Bonduelle, M., Dodd, R., Liebaers, I., Streighteghem, A., Williamson, R., and Akhurst, R. (1988). Chorionic gonadotropin β mRNA, a trophoblast marker, is expressed in human 8-cell embryos derived from tripronucleate zygotes. *Human Reproduction*, **3**, 909–19.

Bose, R., Cheng H., Sabbadini, E., McCoshen, J., Mahadevan, M.M., and Fleetman, J. (1989). Purified human early pregnancy factor from preimplantation embryo possess immunosuppressive properties. *American Journal of Obstetrics and Gynecology*, **160**, 954–60.

Braquet, P., Touqui, I., Shen, T., and Vargaftig, B. (1987). Perspectives in platelet-activating factor research. *Pharmacological Reviews*, **39**, 97–115.

Brinster, R. (1973). Parental glucose phosphate isomerase activity in three-day mouse embryos. *Biochemical Genetics*, **9**, 187–93.

Cavanagh, A.C. and Morton, H. (1994). The purification of early pregnancy factor to homogeneity from human platelets and identification as chaperonin 10. *European Journal of Biochemistry*, **222**, 551–60.

Cavanagh, A.C., Rolfe, B.E., Athanasas-Platsis, S., Quinn, K.A., and Morton, H. (1991). The relationship between early pregnancy factor, mouse embryo-conditioned medium and platelet activating factor. *Journal of Reproduction and Fertility*, **93**, 355–44.

Chard, T. and Grudzinskas, J.G. (1987). Early pregnancy factor. *Biological Research of Pregnancy*, **8**, 53–6.

Chen, C. (1985). Early pregnancy factor in an *in vitro* fertilization and embryo transfer programme. In *Early pregnancy factors*, (ed. F. Ellendorf and E. Koch), pp. 215–26. Perinatology Press, Ithaca.

Clarke, F. (1992). Identification of molecules and mechanisms involved in the early pregnancy factor system. *Reproductive Fertility and Development*, **4**, 423–33.

Collier, M., O'Neill, C., Ammit, A., and Saunders, D. (1988). Biochemical and pharmacological characterization of human embryo-derived platelet activating factor. *Human Reproduction*, **3**, 993–8.

Coulam, C.B., Roussev, R.G., Thomasson, E.J., and Barnea, E.R. (1995). Preimplantation factor (PIF) predicts subsequent pregnancy loss. *American Journal of Reproductive Immunology*, **34**, 88–92

Critser, E. and English, J. (1992). The role of platelet-activating factor in reproduction. In *Immunological obstetrics*, (ed. C.B. Coulam, W.P. Faulk, and J.A. McIntyre), pp. 202–15. W.W. Norton, New York.

Elias, K., Das, A., Pardue, D., Coulam, C.B., Critser, J., and Critser, E. (1989). Alteration in platelet count during early pregnancy in the mouse. *American Journal of Reproductive Immunology*, **21**, 82–6.

Farr, R., Wardlow, M., Cox, C., Meng, K., and Greene, D. (1983). Human serum acid labile factor is an acylhydrolase that inactivates platelet activating factor. *Federation Proceedings*, **42**, 3120–2.

Feurstein, G. and Siren, A. (1988). Platelet activating factor and shock. *Progress in Biochemistry and Pharmacology*, **22**, 181–99.

Gerhard, I., Katzer, E., and Runnebaum, B. (1991). The early pregnancy factor in pregnancies of women with habitual abortion. *Early Human Development*, **26**, 83–92.

Hertig, P., Rock, J., and Adams, E. (1956). A description of 34 human ova within the first 17 days of development. *American Journal of Anatomy*, **98**, 435–46.

Huong, W. and Zhen-Qung, Z. (1990). Detection of early pregnancy factor in fetal sera. *American Journal of Reproductive Immunology*, **23**, 69–72.

Kumar, R., Harper, M., and Hanahan, D. (1988). Occurrence of platelet-activating factor in rabbit spermatozoa. *Archives of Biochemistry and Biophysics*, **260**, 497–502.

Mehta, A., Eessaly, T.E., and Aggarwal, B.B. (1989). Purification and characterization of early pregnancy factor from human pregnancy sera. *Journal of Biological Chemistry*, **264**, 2261–71.

Mesrogli, M. and Maas, D.H.A. (1985). EPF as a marker for fertilization and implantation in the human. In *Early pregnancy factors*, (ed. F. Ellendorff and E. Koch), pp. 233–48. Perinatology Press, New York.

Milligan, S. and Finn, C.A. (1988). Failure to demonstrate platelet activating factor involvement in implantation in mice. *Journal of Reproduction and Fertility Abstract Service*, **2**, 29.

Milligan, S. and Finn, C.A. (1990). Failure of platelet-activating factor (PAF-acether) to induce decidualization in mice and failure of antagonists of PAF to inhibit implantation. *Journal of Reproduction and Fertility*, **88**, 105–11.

Morton, H., Rolfe, B.E., Clunie, G., Anderson, M., and Morrison, J. (1977). An early pregnancy factor detected in human sera by the rosette inhibition test. *Lancet*, i, 394–7.

Morton, H., Rolfe, B.E., Neill, L.M., Clarke, P., Clarke, F., and Clunie, G. (1980). Early pregnancy factor: tissues involved in its production in the mouse. *American Journal of Reproductive Immunology*, **2**, 273–77.

74 *Embryonic signals*

Morton, H., Quinn, K.A., Athanasas-Platsis, S., Rolfe, B.E., and Cavanagh, A.C. (1992*a*). Early diagnosis of pregnancy: early pregnancy factor. In *Immunological obstetrics*, (ed. C.B. Coulam, W.P. Faulk, and J.A. McIntyre), pp. 153–66. W.W. Norton, New York.

Morton, H., Rolfe, B.E., and Cavanagh, A.C. (1992*b*). Early pregnancy factor. *Seminars in Reproductive Endocrinology*, 10, 72–82.

Nahhas, F. and Barnea, E.R. (1990). Human embryonic origin early pregnancy factor before and after implantation. *American Journal of Reproductive Immunology*, 22, 105–9.

O'Neill, C. (1985*a*). Partial characterization of the embryo-derived platelet activating factor in mice. *Journal of Reproduction and Fertility*, 75, 375–8.

O'Neill, C. (1985*b*). Thrombocytopenia is an initial maternal response to fertilization in mice. *Journal of Reproduction and Fertility*, 73, 559–66.

O'Neill, C., Ryan, J., Collier, M., Saunders, D., Ammit, A.J., and Pike, I. (1992). Outcome of pregnancies resulting from a trial of supplementing human IVF culture media with platelet activating factor. *Reproductive Fertility and Development*, 4, 109–12.

Pinckard, R., Farr, R., and Hanahan, D. (1979). Physicochemical and functional identity of rabbit platelet activating factor (PAF) released *in vitro* from IgE sensitized basophils. *Journal of Immunology*, 123, 1847–52.

Radonjic-Lazovic, G. and Roudebush, W.E. (1995). The effect of short versus long-term platelet-activating factor exposure on mouse preimplantation embryo development. *Early Pregnancy: Biology and Medicine*, 1, 196–200.

Roberts, T., Adamson, L., Smart, Y., Stanger, J., and Murdoch, R. (1987). An evaluation of peripheral blood platelet enumeration as a monitor of fertilization and early pregnancy. *Fertility and Sterility*, 47, 848–54.

Rodway, M.R. and Rao, Ch.V. (1995). Novel perspectives on the role of human chorionic gonadotropin during pregnancy and in gestational trophoblastic disease. *Early Pregnancy: Biology and Medicine*, 1, 176–87.

Rolfe, B.E., Cavanagh, A.C., Quinn, K.A., and Morton, H. (1988). Identification of two suppressor factors induced by early pregnancy factor. *Clinical and Experimental Immunology*, 73, 219–27.

Rolfe, B., Quinn, K., Athanasas-Platsis, S., Cavanagh, A.C., and Morton, H. (1989). Genetically restricted effector molecules released by human lymphocytes in response to early pregnancy factor. *Immunology and Cell Biology*, 67, 205–9.

Roussev, R.G., Barnea, E.R., Thomasson, E.J., and Coulam, C.B. (1995). A novel bioassay for detection of preimplantation factor. *American Journal of Reproductive Immunology*, 33, 68–73.

Roussev, R.G., Coulam, C.B., Kaider, B.D., Yarkoni, M., Leavis, P.C. and Barnea, E.R. (1996). Embryonic origin of preimplantation factor: biological activity and partial characterization. *Molecular Human Reproduction*, 2, 883–7.

Roussev, R.G., Barnea, E.R., and Coulam, C.B. (1996). Preimplantation factor: the next frontier. Development and validation of an assay for measuring preimplantation factor (PIF) of embrional origin. *American Journal of Reproductive Immunology*, 35, 281–7.

Sawicky, W., Abramczyk, J., and Blaton, O. (1978). DNA synthesis in the second and third cell cycles of mouse preimplantation development. *Experimental Cell Research*, 112, 199–205.

Schoefield, P., Zumkeller, W., Smith, J., Brice, A., Engstrom, W., Morrell, D., *et al.* (1992). Role of growth factors in human development: IGF-II. In *Progress in endocrinology*, (ed. R. Mornex, C. Jaffiol, and J. Leclere), pp. 211–17. Parthenon, Carnforth.

Shahani, S., Monoz, C.L., Chiylange, S., and Meherji, P. (1992). Early pregnancy factor as a marker for the diagnosis of subclinical embryonic loss. *Experimental and Clinical Endocrinology*, 99, 123–8.

Smal, M., Dziadek, M., Cooney, S., Attard, M., and Baldo, A. (1990). Examination for platelet-activating factor production by preimplantation mouse embryos using a specific radioimmunoassay. *Journal of Reproduction and Fertility*, 90, 419–505.

Smith, S. and Kelly, R. (1988). Effect of platelet-activating factor on the release of PGF-2a and PGE-2 by separated cells of human endometrium. *Journal of Reproduction and Fertility*, **82**, 271–6.

Snyder, F. (1989). Biochemistry of platelet activating factor; a unique class of biologically active phospholipids. *Proceedings of the Society of Experimental Biology and Medicine*, **190**, 125–35.

Spinks, N., Ryan, J., and O'Neill, C. (1990). Antagonists of embryo-derived platelet-activating factor act by inhibiting the ability of the mouse embryo to implant. *Journal of Reproduction and Fertility*, **88**, 241–8.

Velasquez, L., Aguilera, J., and Croxatto, H. (1995). Possible role of platelet-activating factor in embryonic signaling during oviductal transport in the hamster. *Biology of Reproduction*, **52**, 1302–7.

Yasuda, K., Takashima, M., and Isamu, S. (1995). Influence of a cigarette-smoke extract on the hormonal regulation of platelet-activating factor acetylhydrolase in rats. *Biology of Reproduction*, **53**, 244–52.

5 | *Embryonic therapy for implantation enhancement*

Hung-Ching Liu

The genetic content, fertilizability, and developmental potential of oocytes are predetermined after ovarian stimulation and retrieval. Genetic abnormalities, failed fertilization, and abnormal embryo development and hatching attribute to implantation failure. Pre-implantation genetic diagnosis, altered embryo culture conditions, assisted fertilization, and assisted hatching are recent advanced technologies in embryonic therapy which will be discussed in this chapter.

PRE-IMPLANTATION GENETIC DIAGNOSIS

Genetic abnormalities constitute as many as 40 per cent of cases of failed implantation. The genetic content is determined by the quality of the oocyte and spermatozoon that participate in the fertilization process. Embryos derived from genetically abnormal spermatozoa and/or oocytes have low frequencies of implantation. By pre-screening for the genetic normality of a single cell biopsied from an embryo, we can eliminate the transfer of genetically abnormal embryos.

Pre-implantation genetic diagnosis involves embryo biopsy using micromanipulation to remove a single blastomere, on which the genetic diagnosis is performed. It has been proved that this embryo, unaffected by biopsy, will continue its normal development and implantation (Handyside *et al.* 1989, 1990; Hardy *et al.* 1990; Cohen *et al.* 1992*a*; Grifo *et al.* 1992). Fluorescence *in situ* hybridization (FISH) (Griffin *et al.* 1992; Munné *et al.* 1993*a*) and polymerase chain reaction (PCR) (Handyside *et al.* 1990; Strom *et al.* 1991*a*; Griffin *et al.* 1992; Grifo *et al.* 1992; Munné *et al.* 1993*a*) are techniques that were developed for genetic diagnosis on a single cell. Although PCR is simple and sensitive, it has the disadvantage of being confused by the amplification of exogenous DNA (Strom *et al.* 1991*b*), unable to distinguish between numerical chromosome abnormalities such as XO, XX, XXX, and inconsistent results between sibling blastomeres. FISH, using fluorochrome-labelled specific probes, after modification became a fast and sophisticated method (Hardy *et al.* 1990) which is able to assess accurately numerical chromosomal abnormalities. Furthermore, the use of multiple probes in FISH provides a method of studying multiple chromosome aneuploidies simultaneously on a single blastomere from pre-implantation human embryos (Benadiva *et al.* 1995; Munné *et al.* 1995). Pre-implantation genetic diagnosis of human embryos using multiple-probe FISH for chromosomes X, Y, 18, 13, and 21 has revealed that aneuploidy for these chromosomes increases significantly with maternal age (Munné *et al.* 1993*b*, 1995; Benadiva *et al.* 1995). Pre-implantation diagnosis is gaining popularity, and has been used to avoid the risk of transmitting X-linked recessive diseases (Handyside *et al.* 1989, 1990; Grifo *et al.* 1992), to eliminate genetically abnormal embryos, and to reduce spontaneous abortions (Benadiva *et al.* 1995).

ALTERING EMBRYO CULTURE CONDITIONS

The implantation potential of normal embryos may be reduced by suboptimal embryo culture conditions. In poor culture conditions, embryo development is inhibited as judged by growth rate and/or formation of abnormalities (Fehilly *et al.* 1985). Conventional *in vitro* human embryo culture systems are suboptimal (Fehilly *et al.* 1985), as indicated by the fact that (1) cell blockage occurs in chemically defined media (Fukui *et al.* 1989; Prichard *et al.* 1992); (2) there are low incidences of formation and hatching of blastocyts *in vitro* (Fehilly *et al.* 1985); and (3) the gamete intrafallopian transfer (GIFT) procedure gives a higher implantation rate than conventional IVF–ET (Yovich *et al.* 1988). Efforts have been made to improve the culture system either by supplementation with specific growth factors or by co-culture with helper cells in order to enhance embryo quality and, ultimately, to enhance implantation (Allen and Wright 1984; Gandolfi *et al.* 1987; Eyestone and First 1989; Wiemer *et al.* 1989; Menezo *et al.* 1990; Bongso *et al.* 1992; Liu 1993).

Recently, co-culture techniques utilizing various types of cell monolayers have exhibited enhanced embryo viability in various species (Wiemer *et al.* 1989; Bongso *et al.* 1992), including humans (Eyestone and First 1989; Bongso *et al.* 1991). Since endometrial cells are physiologically suitable for implantation, they are the ideal cells to use as helper cells in co-culture. There is evidence that endometrial cells significantly improve embryo viability and growth rates when co-cultured with mouse embryos (Liu *et al.* 1994). The major beneficial effects of endometrial cells may be due to the secretion of embryotrophic factors (Liu *et al.* 1994). Embryos exhibited high hatching and outgrowth rates in media supplemented with isolated endometrial secretory proteins (40 μg/ml). This strongly suggests that these secretory proteins are highly specific embryotrophic factors (Liu *et al.* 1994).

Endometrial cells have been shown to synthesize and secrete a large quantity of cytokines and growth factors such as interleukin-1 (IL-1) (De *et al.* 1992; Jacobs and Carson 1993), interleukin-6 (IL-6) (De *et al.* 1992; Jacobs *et al.* 1992; Robertson *et al.* 1992), granulocyte macrophage-colony stimulating factor (GM-CSF) (Robertson *et al.* 1992), tumour necrosis factor α (TNFα) (De *et al.* 1992), epidermal growth factors (EGFs) (Huet-Hudson *et al.* 1990), transforming growth factors (TGFs) (Tamada *et al.* 1990), insulin-like growth factors (IGFs) (Murphy *et al.* 1988; Croze *et al.* 1990), and insulin-like growth factor binding proteins (IGF-BPs) (Croze *et al.* 1990; Bell *et al.* 1991). These cytokines and growth factors are the promoters for both proliferation and differentiation of endometrial and embryonic cells. Growth factor binding proteins are known to modulate the biological activity of their bound growth factors. Therefore, endometrial cells may enhance embryo viability by secreting these cytokines and growth factors.

Co-culture of homologous endometrial cells will eliminate the worry of contamination with HIV and other infectious agents. Jayot *et al.* (1995) evaluated the benefit of co-culturing embryos on homologous endometrial cells in patients with repeated failures of implantation and found that pregnancy rate per transfer significantly increased from 8 per cent to 21 per cent. Co-culture of human embryo and endometrial cells *in vitro* can also be used for investigation into the mechanisms of implantation, in order to increase understanding of the various factors involved in implantation and early embryo development. Identification of these factors and evaluation of their biological functions, using co-culture, may provide a basis for improving embryo culture media.

ASSISTED FERTILIZATION

Failed fertilization is a major problem for male factor infertility patients in conventional IVF–ET. The fertilization rate of these patients is significantly lower than that of patients with other aetiologies such as tubal dysfunction, endometriosis, and idiopathic infertility. However, once the fertilization problem is overcome by whatever means, the pregnancy rate per transfer becomes similar to that of patients with other aetiologies.

Techniques for assisted fertilization such as zona drilling (Gordon *et al.* 1986), partial zona dissection (PZD) (Cohen *et al.* 1988, 1989, 1991; Malter and Cohen 1989), subzonal insemination (SUZI) (Ng *et al.* 1988, 1991; Fishel *et al.* 1990*a,b*, 1992; Cohen *et al.* 1991, 1992*b*; Alikani *et al.* 1992) and intracytoplasmic sperm injection (ICSI) (Lanzendorf *et al.* 1988*a,b*; Palermo *et al.* 1992, 1993) were developed rapidly in the 1980s. When applied to male factor infertility, these techniques not only improved the fertilization rates, but also enhanced implantation rates dramatically. Indeed, these procedures have been considered the greatest advance in IVF–ET since the late 1980s. Hundreds of babies were born to couples who underwent assisted fertilization.

Zona drilling

Gordon and Talansky (1986) performed the very first attempt at zona drilling (ZD) on human embryos using acidified Tyrode's solution and enzymatic digestion. Due to the fact that acid Tyrode's solution was shown to inhibit normal embryo development, the technique of zona drilling was soon abandoned.

Partial zona dissection

In 1989 Cohen *et al.* invented partial zona dissection (PZD) (Malter and Cohen 1989) which is a mechanical technique used to open the zonae. Following dissection, the oocyte was incubated with sperm (100 000 spermatozoa per 50 μl) in microdroplets for fertilization. PZD did improve fertilization rates, resulting in a relatively high pregnancy rate. However, the large opening in the zonae makes the embryo not only vulnerable to attack by leucocytes (Willadsen 1982), but may also cause extrusion of blastomeres through the cut (Payne 1994). In PZD, the presence of biological barriers (vitelline membranes) selects for capacitated and acrosome activated spermatozoa so that only motile spermatozoa can penetrate freely into the zona opening. PZD therefore benefits patients with only moderately severe male internity. High incidences of abnormal fertilization (i.e. polyspermic fertilization) with PZD also reduced the number of embryos for transfer.

Subzonal insemination

Subzonal insemination (SUZI) is the technique of injecting approximately 3 to 5 spermatozoa into the perivitelline space. Ng and colleagues reported the first human pregnancy resulting from subzonal insemination (SUZI) (Ng *et al.* 1988). Two years later, Fishel *et al.* (1990*a*) successfully used a similar procedure which resulted in a set of normal healthy twins and a singleton. Thereafter, SUZI became a popular treatment for human infertility. As with PZD, only capacitated and acrosome activated spermatozoa will fuse with the vitelline membrane, but even those with poor or no motility can be injected into the perivitelline space. With SUZI, normal and abnormal fertilization rates are dependent on the quality and number of spermatozoa injected—injection of too many will dramatically increase polyspermic fertilization. SUZI thus benefits patients with low sperm counts (oligozoospermia), low motility sperm (asteozoospermia), poor morphology sperm (teratozoospermia), or all of these defects (oligoasteoteratozoospermia).

Intracytoplasmic sperm injection

Intracytoplasmic sperm injection (ICSI) involves the direct injection of a single spermatozoon into the cytoplasm. As early as 1962, ICSI was used to investigate the early events of fertilization by injecting homologous or heterogenous spermatozoa directly into the cytoplasm (Hiramoto 1962; Graham 1966; Uehara and Yanagimachi 1976; Thadani 1980; Cohen *et al.* 1994). This micromanipulation technique was widely used in the 1980s to study the fusion between gametes, the activation of oocyte cytoplasm, and the formation of the male and female pronuclei in non-human mammalian species (Gomibuchi *et al.* 1985; Clark and Johnson 1988). Not until the late 1980s was this technology applied clinically to human infertility (Cohen *et al.* 1988, 1989; Lanzendorf *et al.* 1988*a,b*; Ng *et al.* 1988, 1991; Fishel *et al.* 1990*a,b*; Palermo *et al.* 1992, 1993).

Lanzendorf *et al.* (1988*b*) were the first to perform ICSI on a human oocyte to study the formation of the male pronucleus and in 1992, Palermo *et al.* reported the achievement of human pregnancies with ICSI (Palermo *et al.* 1992, 1993). ICSI, which bypasses penetration and membrane fusion, enables any type of spermatozoa to be injected directly into the ooplasm and has been demonstrated to produce decondensation with pronuclear formation after injection of sperm head, immotile sperm, dead sperm, grossly defective sperm, and severely teratozoospermic sperm (Lanzendorf *et al.* 1988*a,b*). ICSI has therefore brought great hope to patients with severe male factor infertility. The efficiency of ICSI is dependent on technique of injection, sperm characteristics, and oocyte maturation. Aspiration of some ooplasm into the pipette before injecting the spermatozoon facilitates the piercing of the oolemma and activates the egg as well. Treatment with polyvinylpyrrolidone (PVP) and immobilizing spermatozoa by damaging the tail significantly increase fertilization rates. Sperm membrane damage is necessary for decondensation to occur (Dozortsev *et al.* 1994) and motile spermatozoa do not fertilize as well as immobilized spermatozoa. Injection should be made in a location which avoids the area where germinal vesicles break down and the first polar body extrudes. Mature oocytes (i.e. metaphase II stage) should be used to ensure fertilization. For successful ICSI, oocyte activation, not acrosome reaction (Lundin *et al.* 1994), is the prerequisite factor. Sperm takes part in the activation and may act as a hormone (Gould and Stephano 1987; Kline *et al.* 1988), or fuse with the oolemma to trigger oocyte activation (Soupart *et al.* 1977), or release a cytoplasmic factor to induce internal calcium release for activation (Swann 1993; Dozortsev *et al.* 1995).

Injection of sperm nucleus or sperm head may lead to nucleus decondensation. The centriole or centrosome, which is located in the mid-section of the spermatozoon (Palermo *et al.* 1994), organizes the embryonic spindle and plays an important role in early embryo cleavage and development. Thus, the sperm head as well as the mid-section are essential for the development of a normal embryo.

The clinical application of PZD, SUZI, and ICSI to male infertility has achieved varying degrees of success. When the outcome among PZD, SUZI, and ICSI groups is compared, ICSI gives the best results followed by SUZI and then PZD. Indeed, ICSI has resulted in the highest fertilization rate, the lowest abnormal fertilization rate, the highest implantation rate, and the highest clinical pregnancy rate. ICSI is now the predominant technique for assisted fertilization world-wide.

ASSISTED HATCHING

The efficiency of IVF is relatively low, the implantation rate being only about 10–30 per cent. A number of embryos may be lost after transfer due to their failure to escape through the zona pellucida (Cohen *et al.* 1990; Khalifa and Tucker 1992). The time of hatching is crucial since late hatching will cause asynchronization between embryo and endometrium and result in failed implantation. Suboptimal follicular stimulation and poor embryo culture conditions may delay embryonic development and the hatching process. A thick and hardened zona pellucida may prevent or inhibit hatching, but the causes of hardened zona pellucida remain unknown. Whether these are dependent on artificial conditions created by follicular stimulation or embryo culture remains to be elucidated. In addition, there may be intrinsic ovarian factors which alter zona glycoprotein synthesis and inhibit the release of proteases, thereby interfering with the hatching process.

Before hatching the zona pellucida undergoes many changes. A thinning zona pellucida is an indication that the embryo is preparing for hatching. Embryos with large variations in the thickness of the zona pellucida (ZP) implant more frequently than those with no variations at all. Thus, cleaved embryos may produce an active component that reduces the thickness of the zona in preparation for hatching (Cohen *et al.* 1989, Wright *et al.* 1990).

Interestingly, microsurgically fertilized mouse and human embryos appear to hatch more frequently and in an accelerated fashion when cultured *in vitro* (Cohen *et al.* 1992*b*, 1994). Therefore, the use of zona drilling on three-day old human embryos was introduced in the hope that it could facilitate the hatching process—called assisted hatching.

Assisted hatching was clinically tested in our centre from 1992 for 330 couples in a randomized fashion (Cohen *et al.* 1992*a*, 1994). In this first trial, the incidence of clinical pregnancy increased significantly ($p < 0.01$) from 37 per cent in the control group to 52 per cent following zona drilling and 27 per cent of zona-drilled embryos implanted compared with 19 per cent of controls ($p < 0.01$). It was found that zona drilling was beneficial for embryos with zonae thicker than 15 μm but was detrimental to embryos with thin zonae (< 12 μm) (Cohen *et al.* 1994). The mean zona thickness was inversely related to maternal age (Cohen *et al.* 1994). For these reasons, selective assisted hatching was incorporated into the IVF procedure for those embryos with thick zonae (corrected for maternal age), slow development, or excessive fragmentation (> 20 per cent) and for all embryos from patients with elevated day 3 FSH (follicle-stimulating hormone) or those over 40 years of age (Cohen *et al.* 1992*a*, 1994).

When we applied assisted hatching to 1834 patients from January 1991 to August 1995, we found that assisted hatching significantly improved both the clinical pregnancy rate per transfer (from 38.2 per cent to 44.9 per cent, $p < 0.0001$) and implantation rates (from 19.9 per cent to 21.9 per cent, $p < 0.01$). The efficiency of assisted hatching is dependent on the size of the opening and the thickness of the zona pellucida, as well as the quality of the embryo. Small openings may cause abnormal hatching such as tripping, twinning, and splitting (Malter and Cohen 1989). Assisted hatching appears to be more successful in younger patients (age < 39) who are able to produce embryos with a high potential for development but with thick zonae. When selective assisted hatching was applied to this group of patients the clinical pregnancy rate per transfer improved from 41.3 per cent to 55 per cent and the implantation rate increased from 21.8 per cent to 26 per cent. On the other hand, assisted hatching provides only minimal benefits for older patients (age > 40) with poor quality embryos. Only marginal changes were observed in the clinical rate per transfer (23 per cent to 30 per cent) and implantation rate (12 per cent to 10.3 per cent) after assisted hatching.

It appears that assisted hatching by zona drilling promotes implantation. The mechanisms involved in this phenomenon remain unclear. The presence of an artificial gap in the zona pellucida may facilitate hatching, allowing for earlier implantation. Therefore, the time of implantation for control and assisted hatching groups was compared. The earliest increase in hCG level in the luteal phase was used to identify the time of implantation (Liu *et al.* 1993). The first increase in hCG occurred no later than day 13 (day 1 = day of oocyte retrieval) in the assisted hatching group. Implantation occurred before luteal day 9 in 75 per cent of pregnant patients in the assisted hatching group and in 53 per cent of pregnancies in the control group ($p < 0.05$) (Liu *et al.* 1993). It appears that assisted hatching promotes accelerated implantation. On average, implantation occurred approximately one day earlier in the assisted hatching group than in the controls. With assisted hatching, not only does implantation take place more frequently within the 'implantation window', but it also allows for earlier embryo–endometrial contact. Early implantation prognosticates viable pregnancy (Liu *et al.* 1988). Delayed implantation, on the other hand, has been associated with high incidences of abortion. Earlier contact may optimize the synchronization between embryo and endometrium, resulting in improved implantation efficiency.

CONCLUDING REMARKS

Embryo viability, endometrial receptivity, and proper synchronization between the embryo and endometrium are essential factors for normal implantation. Both embryo viability and endometrial receptivity are confounded by IVF manipulation. Suboptimal follicular stimulation may generate genetically incompetent eggs and create hormonal imbalances in the luteal phase which may affect endometrial responsiveness and corpus luteum functions.

Ovarian stimulation creates an advanced endometrium within 1–2 days. On the other hand, suboptimal culture conditions inhibit embryo growth by at least 1–2 days. Such asynchronization between the embryo and the endometrium attributes to the big wastage of embryos after IVF–ET.

Enhancing embryo growth and hatching rates can eliminate this synchronization discrepancy. Efforts have been made to improve embryo quality after retrieval. New technologies of alternative culture systems (e.g. co-culture) and assisted hatching have recently been proven to improve embryo implantation by enhancing embryo viability and optimizing synchronization between the embryo and endometrium.

Pre-implantation genetic diagnosis has led to an explosion of research in the areas of genetic and molecular biology, with scientists actively searching for and sequencing all types of human abnormal genes, developing diagnostic methods to screen genetically incompetent embryos, and, where possible, applying gene therapy to embryos with defective genes.

Male factor infertility accounts for the infertility of over 30 per cent of infertile couples. The implementation of assisted fertilization in the IVF treatment of these patients can effectively overcome their fertilization problems by resulting in a higher implantation rate and clinical pregnancy rate PZD, SUZI, and ICSI techniques have all demonstrated the achievement of varying degrees of success. ICSI, which bypasses all the biological barriers and requires only one spermatozoon, has brought great hope to patients with severe male factor infertility. Indeed, ICSI has been used successfully with epididymal and testicular spermatozoa as well. However, though the introduction of grossly defective spermatozoa by ICSI can lead to fertilization and pregnancy, it is highly recommended that patients are checked for chromosomal abnormality by amniocentesis during pregnancy.

REFERENCES

Alikani, M., Adler, A., Reing, A., Malter, H., and Cohen, J. (1992). Subzonal sperm insertion and the frequency of gamete fusion. *Journal of Assisted Reproduction Genetics*, 9, 97–101.

Allen, R. and Wright, R. (1984). *In vitro* development of porcine embryos in coculture with endothelial cell monolayers or cuture supernatants. *Journal of Animal Science*, 59, 1657–61.

Bell, S., Jackson, J., Ashmore, J., Zhu, H., and Tseng, L. (1991). Regulation of insulin-like growth factor binding protein-1 (h1GFBP-1) synthesis and secretion by progestin and relaxin in long term cultures of human endometrial stromal cells. *Journal of Clinical Endocrinology and Metabolism*, 72, 1014–24.

Benadiva, C., Munné, S., and Rosenwaks, Z. (1995). Chromosome 16 aneuploidy increases significantly with maternal age in preimplantation human embryos. (Abstract.) *American Society for Reproductive Medicine*, Annual meeting program supplement, 0–003, S2.

Bongso, A., Ng, S., Fong, C., Mok, H., Ng, P., and Ratnam, S. (1991). Cocultures in human assisted reproduction: support of embryos *in vitro* and their specificity. *Annals of the New York Academy of Science*, 626, 438–44.

Bongso, A., Ng, S.C., Fong, C.Y., Anandakumar, C., Marshall, B., Edirisinghe, R., and Ratnam, S. (1992). Improved pregnancy rate after transfer of embryos grown in human fallopian tube cell coculture. *Fertility and Sterility*, 58, 569–74.

Clark, R.N. and Johnson, L.A. (1988). Factors related to successful sperm microinjection of hamster eggs: the effect of sperm species, technical experience, needle dimensions, and incubation medium on egg viability and sperm deconsensation. *Theriogenology*, 30, 447–60.

Cohen, J., Malter, H., Fehilly, C., Wright, G., Elsner, C., Kort, H., and Massey, J. (1988). Implantation of embryos after partial opening of oocyte zona pellucida to facilitate sperm penetration. *Lancet*, ii, 162.

Cohen, J., Malter, H., Wright, G., Kort, H., Massey, J., and Mitchell, D. (1989). Partial zona dissection of human oocytes when failure of zona pellucida penetration is anticipated. *Human Reproduction*, 4, 435–42.

Cohen, J., Elsner, C., Kort, H., Malter, H., Massey, J., Mayer, M.P., and Wiemer, K. (1990). Impairment of the hatching process following *in vitro* fertilization in the human and improvement of implantation by assisting hatching using micromanipulation. *Human Reproduction*, 5, 7–13.

Cohen, J., Alikani, M., Malter, H.E., Adler, A., Talansky, B.E. and Rosenwaks, Z. (1991). Partial zona dissection or subzonal sperm insertion: microsurgical fertilization alternatives based on evaluation of sperm and embryo morphology. *Fertility and Sterility*, 56, 696–706.

Cohen, J., Alikani, M., Trowbridge, J., and Rosenwaks, Z. (1992a). Implantation enhancement by selective assisted hatching using zona drilling of embryos with poor prognosis. *Human Reproduction*, 7, 685–91.

Cohen, J., Alikani, M., Adler, A., Berkeley, A., Davis, O., Ferrara, *et al.* (1992b). Microsurgical fertilization procedures: the absence of stringent criteria for patient selection. *Journal of Assisted Reproduction Genetics*, 9, 197–206.

Cohen, J., Alikani, M., Liu, H.C., and Rosenwaks, Z. (1994). Rescue of human embryos by micromanipulation. *Bailliere's clinical obstetrics and gynaecology*, Chapter 6: Micromanipulation techniques, (ed. S. Fishel), Vol. 8, pp. 95–116. Bailliere Tindall, Cambridge University Press.

Croze, F., Kennedy, T.G., Schroedter, I.C., Friesen, H.G., and Murphy, L.J. (1990). Expression of insulin-like growth factor-1 and insulin-like growth factor binding protein-1 in the rat uterus during decidualization. *Endocrinology*, 127, 1995–2000.

De, M., Sanford, T.R., and Wood, G.W. (1992). Interleukin-1, interleukin-6 and tumor necrosis factor alpha are produced in the mouse uterus during the estrous cycle and are induced by estrogen and progesterone. *Developmental Biology*, 151, 297–305.

Dozortsev, D., De Sutter, P., and Dhont, M. (1994). Damage of the sperm plasma membrane by touching the sperm tail with the needle prior to intracytoplasmic injection. *Human Reproduction*, 9, (Suppl.), 40.

Dozortsev, D., Rybouchkin, A., De Sutter, P., Qian, C., and Dhont, M. (1995). Human oocyte activation following intracytoplasmic injection: the role of the sperm cell. *Human Reproduction*, 10, 403–7.

Eyestone, W. and First, N. (1989). Co-culture of early cattle embryos to blastocyst stage with oviductal tissue or in conditioned medium. *Journal of Reproduction and Fertility*, 85, 715–20.

Fehilly, C.B., Cohen, J., Simons, R.F., Fishel, S.B., and Edwards, R.G. (1985). Cryopreservation of cleaving embryos and expanded blastocysts in the human: a comparative study. *Fertility and Sterility*, 44, 638–44.

Fishel, S.B., Antinori, S., Jackson, P., Johnson, L., Lisi, F., Chiariello, F., and Versaci, C. (1990a). Twin birth after subzonal insemination. *Lancet*, 335, 8691, 722–3.

Fishel, S.B., Jackson, P., Antinori, S., Johnson, J., Grossi, S., and Versaci, C. (1990b). Subzonal insemination for the alleviation of infertility. *Fertility and Sterility*, 54, 828–35.

Fishel, S.B., Timson, J., Lisi, F., and Rinaldi, L. (1992). The evaluation of 225 patients undergoing subzonal insemination for the procurement of fertilization *in vitro*. *Fertility and Sterility*, 57, 840–9.

Fukui, Y., Urakawa, M., Sasaki, C., Chikamatsu, N., and Ono, H. (1989). Development to the late morula or blastocyst stage following *in vitro* maturation of fertilization of bovine oocytes. *Animal Reproductive Science*, 18, 139–45.

Gandolfi, F., Brezini, J., Richardson, L., Brown, C., and Moor, R. (1987). Characterization of proteins secreted by sheep oviduct epithelial cells and their function in embryonic development. *Development*, 106, 303–12.

Gomibuchi, H., Kayama, F., Sato, K., and Mizuno, M. (1985). Decondensation of sperm head injected into oocyte under micromanipulation. *Acta obstetrica et gynaecologica Japonica*, 37, 2639.

Gordon, J.W. and Talansky, B.E. (1986). Assisted fertilization by zona drilling: a mouse model for correction of oligospermia. *Journal of Experimental Zoology*, 239, 347–54.

Gould, M. and Stephano, J.L. (1987). Electrical responses of egg to acrosomal protein similar to those induced by sperm. *Science*, 235, 1654–6.

Graham, C.F. (1966). The regulation of DNA synthesis and mitosis in multinucleate frog eggs. *Journal of Cell Science*, 1, 363–72.

Griffin, D.K., Wilton, L.J., Handyside, A.H., Winston, R.M.L., and Delhanty, J.D.A. (1992). Dual fluorescent *in situ* hybridization for simultaneous detection of X and Y chromosome-specific probes for the sexing of human preimplantation embryonic nuclei. *Human Genetics*, 89, 18–22.

Grifo, J.A., Tang, Y.X., Cohen, J., Gilbert, F., Sanyal, M.K., and Rosenwaks, Z. (1992). Ongoing pregnancy in a hemophilia carrier by embryo biopsy and simultaneous amplification of X and Y chromosome specific DNA from single blastomeres. *Journal of the American Medical Association*, 6, 727–9.

Handyside, A.H., Pattinson, J.K., Penketh, R.J.A., Delhanty, J.D.A., Winston, R.M.L., and Tuddenhanam, E.G.D. (1989). Biopsy of human preimplantation embryos and sexing by DNA amplification. *Lancet*, i, 347–9.

Handyside, A.H., Kontogianni, E.H., Hardy, K., and Winston, R.M.L. (1990). Pregnancies from biopsied human pre-implantation embryos sexed by Y-specific DNA amplification. *Nature*, 344, 768–70.

Hardy, K., Martin, K.L., Leese, J.H., Winston, R.M.L., and Handyside, A.H. (1990). Human preimplantation development *in vitro* is not adversely affected by biopsy at the 8-cell stage. *Human Reproduction*, 5, 708–14.

Hiramoto, Y. (1962). Microinjection of the live spermatozoa into sea urchin eggs. *Experimental Cell Research*, **27**, 416–26.

Huet-Hudson, Y.M., Chakraborty, C., De, S.K., Suzuki, Y., Andrews, G.K., and Dey, S.K. (1990). Estrogen regulates the synthesis of epidermal growth factor in mouse uterine epithelial cells. *Molecular Endocrinology*, **4**, 510–23.

Jacobs, A.L. and Carson, D.D. (1993). Uterine epithelial cell secretion of interleukin-1α induces prostaglandin E₂ (PGE₂) and PGF₂α secretion by uterine stromal cells *in vitro*. *Endocrinology*, **132**, 300–8.

Jacobs, A.L., Sehgal, P.G., Julian, J., and Carson, D.D. (1992). Secretion and hozmonal regulation of interleukin-6 production by mouse uterine stromal and polarized epithelial cells cultured *in vitro*. *Endocrinology*, **131**, 1037–46.

Jayot, S., Parneix, I., Verdaguer, S., Discamps, G., Audebert, A., and Emperaire, J.C. (1995). Coculture of embryos on homologous endometrial cells in patients with repeated failures of implantation. *Fertilty and Sterility*, **63**, 109–14.

Khalifa, E.M. and Tucker, M.J. (1992). Partial thinning of the zona pellucida for more successful enhancement of blastocyst hatching in the mouse. *Human Reproduction*, **7**, 532–44.

Kline, D., Simoncini, L., Mandel, G., Maue, R.A., Kado, R.T., and Jaffe, L.A. (1988). Fertilization events induced by neurotransmitters after injection of mRNA in Xenopus eggs. *Science*, **241**, 464–7.

Lanzendorf, S.E., Maloney, M., Ackerman, S., Acosta, A., and Hodgen, G. (1988*a*). Fertilizing potential of acrosome-defective sperm following microsurgical injection into eggs. *Gamete Research*, **19**, 329–37.

Lanzendorf, S.E., Maloney, M.K., Veeck, L.L., Slusser, J., Hodgen, G.D., and Rosenwaks, Z. (1988*b*). A preclinical evaluation of pronuclear formation by microinjection of human spermatozoa into human oocytes. *Fertility and Sterility*, **49**, 835–42.

Liu, H.C. (1993). Recent advances to improve human implantation. *Assisted Reproductive Technology Andrology*, **4**, 51–3.

Liu, H.C., Jones, G.S., Jones, H.W., and Rosenwaks, Z. (1988). Mechanisms and factors of early pregnancy wastage in *in vitro* fertilization–embryo transfer patients. *Fertility and Sterility*, **50**, 95–101.

Liu, H.C., Cohen, J., Alikani, M., Noyes, N., and Rosenwaks, Z. (1993). Assisted hatching facilitates earlier implantation. *Fertility and Sterility*, **60**, 871–5.

Liu, H.C., Mele, C., Noyes, N., and Rosenwaks, Z. (1994). Endometrial secretory proteins enhance early embryo development. *Journal of Assisted Reproduction and Genetics*, **11**, 217–24.

Lundin, K., Sjogren, A., Nilsson, L., and Hamberger, L. (1994). Fertilization and pregnancy after intracytoplasmic microinjection of acrosomeless spermatozoa. *Fertility and Sterility*, **62**, 1266–7.

Malter, H.E. and Cohen, J. (1989). Blastocyst formation and hatching *in vitro* following zona drilling of mouse human embryos. *Gamete Research*, **24**, 67–80.

Menezo, Y., Guerin, J., and Czyba, J. (1990). Improvement of human embryo development *in vitro* by coculture on monolayers of Vero cells. *Biology of Reproduction*, **42**, 301–6.

Munné, S., Weier, H.U., Stein, J., Grifo, J., and Cohen, J. (1993*a*). A fast and efficient method for simultaneous X and Y *in situ* hybridization of human blastomers. *Journal of Assisted Reproduction and Genetics*, **10**, 82–90.

Munné, S., Lee, A., Rowenwaks, Z., Grifo, J., and Cohen, J. (1993*b*). Diagnosis of major chromosome aneuploidies in human preimplantation embryos. *Human Reproduction*, **8**, 2185–91.

Munné, S., Benadiva, C., Cohen, J., and Grifo, J. (1995). Preimplantation diagnosis of aneuploidy in women of 40 years or older. (Abstract.) *American Society for Reproductive Medicine* Annual meeting program supplement, 0–076, S37.

Murphy, L.J., Murphy, L.C., and Friesen, H.G. (1988). Estrogen induces insulin-like growth factor expression in the rat uterus. *Molecular Endocrinology*, **1**, 445–50.

Ng, S.C., Bongso, T.A., Ratnam, S.S., Sathananthan, H., Chan, C.L., Wong, P.C., *et al.* (1988). Pregnancy after transfer of multiple sperm under the zona. *Lancet*, **ii**, 8614–790.

Ng, S.C., Bongso, T.A., and Ratnam, S.S. (1991). Micro-injection of human oocytes: the technique for severe oligoasthenoteratozoospermia. *Fertility and Sterility*, **56**, 1117–23.

Palermo, G., Joris, H., Devroey, P., and Van Steirteghem, A.C. (1992). Pregnancies after intracytoplasmic injection of single spermatozoon into an oocyte. *Lancet*, **340**, 17–18.

Palermo, G., Joris, H., Derde, M.P., Camus, M., Devroey, P., and Van Steirteghem, A. (1993). Sperm characteristics and outcome of human assisted fertilization by subzonal insemination and intracytoplasmic sperm injection. *Fertility and Sterility*, **59**, 826–35.

Palermo, G., Munne, S., and Cohen, J. (1994). The human zygote inherits its mitotic potential from the male gamete. *Human Reproduction*, **9**, 1220–5.

Payne, D. (1994). Embryo viability associated with microassisted fertilization. *Baillière's Clinical Obstetrics and Gynaecology*, Chapter 10: Micromanipulation techniques, (ed. S. Fishel), Vol. 8, pp. 157–75. Bailliére Tindall Cambridge University Press.

Prichard, J.F., Thibodeaux, J.K., Pool, S.H., Blakewood, E.G., Menezo, Y., and Godke, R.A. (1992). *In vitro* co-culture of early stage caprine embryos with oviduct and uterine epithelial cells. *Human Reproduction*, **7**, 553–9.

Robertson, S.A., Mayrhofer, G., and Seamark, R.F. (1992). Uterine epithelial cells synthesize granulocyte-macrophage stimulating factor and interleukin-6 in pregnant and nonpregnant mice. *Biology of Reproduction*, **46**, 1069–79.

Soupart, P., Anderson, N.L., and Repp, J.E. (1977). Fusion-induced homogametic activation. *Fertility and Sterility*, **28**, 369–70.

Strom, C.M., Enriquez, G., and Rechitsky, S. (1991*a*). Preimplantation genetic analysis using PCR. In *Preimplantation genetics*, (ed. Y. Verlinsky and A. Kulicy), pp. 131–8. Plenum, New York.

Strom, C.M., Rechitsky, S., and Verlinsky, Y. (1991*b*). Reliability of gender determination using polymerase chain reaction for single cells. *Journal of In Vitro Fertization and Embryo Transfer*, **8**, 225–9.

Swann, K. (1993). The soluble sperm oscillogen hypothesis. *Zygote*, **1**, 273–9.

Tamada, H., McMaster, M.T., Flanders, K.C., Andrews, G.K., and Dey, S.K. (1990). Cell type-specific expression of transforming growth factor-$\beta1$ in mouse uterus during the preimplantation period. *Molecular Endocrinology*, **4**, 965–72.

Thadani, V.M. (1980). A study of hetero-specific sperm–egg interactions in the rat, mouse, and deer mouse using *in vitro* fertilization and sperm injection. *Journal of Experimental Zoology*, **212**, 435–53.

Uehara, T. and Yanagimachi, R. (1976). Microsurgical injection of spermatozoa into hamster eggs with subsequent transformation of sperm nuclei into male pronuclei. *Biology of Reproduction*, **15**, 467–70.

Wiemer, K.E., Cohen, J., Wiker, S., Malter, H.E., Wright, G., and Godke, R.A. (1989). Coculture of human zygotes on fetal bovine uterine fibroblasts: morphology and implantation. *Fertility and Sterility*, **52**, 503–8.

Willadsen, S.M. (1982). Micromanipulation of embryos of the large domestic species. In *Mammalian egg transfer*, (ed. C. Adams), pp. 185–210. CRC Press, Boca Raton, Florida.

Wright, G., Wiker, S., Elsner, C., Kort, H., Massey, J., Mitchell, D., *et al.* (1990). Observations on the morphology of human zygotes, pronuclei and nucleoli and implications for cryopreservation. *Human Reproduction*, **5**, 109–15.

Yovich, J.L., Yovich, J.M., and Edirisinghe, W.R. (1988). The relative chance of pregnancy following tubal or uterine transfer procedures. *Fertility and Sterility*, **49**, 858–64.

6 | *The luteal phase endometrium*

Lisa Barrie Schwartz, Frederick Schatz, and
Charles Lockwood

THE CLINICAL SIGNIFICANCE OF THE LUTEAL PHASE ENDOMETRIUM

Endometrial evaluation for the determination of luteal phase insufficiency (LPI) is an important component of the evaluation of reproductive failure due to infertility or early pregnancy loss. Successful blastocyst implantation requires a receptive luteal phase (LP) endometrium. Hormone-regulated expression of various haemostatic, proteolytic, and vasoactive proteins produced by the endometrium enables the blastocyst to implant, yet promotes menstrual haemorrhage in the absence of implantation. LPI, which can originate from hypothalamic, pituitary, ovarian, or endometrial causes, results in either inadequate progesterone (P) production from the corpus luteum (CL) or impaired P action on the endometrium. Consequently, P-regulated development of the endometrium is insufficient to sustain the implanting embryo. Neither the prevalence of LPI nor its importance as a cause of infertility and early pregnancy loss is clear. Since transient and sporadic LPI has also been documented in women with normal menstrual cycles, there is disagreement as to whether LPI qualifies as a pathological condition. Although there are many modalities with which to evaluate the LP, no universally accepted, thoroughly validated method to diagnose LPI is currently available (Olive 1991).

PHYSIOLOGY OF THE LUTEAL PHASE ENDOMETRIUM

P4 acts on the oestrogen-primed human endometrium to transform stromal cells to decidual cells, initially at perivascular sites, and subsequently throughout the entire endometrium (Noyes *et al.* 1950). Perivascular decidualized endometrial stromal cells are spatially and temporally positioned to regulate menstruation by hormonally controlled expression of haemostatic, proteolytic, and vasoactive proteins. Recent results indicate that *in vitro* decidualization mimics those *in vivo* events in which decidual cells promote haemostasis by enhancing coagulation potential and reducing fibrinolytic activity. The end result is the control of local haemorrhage during trophoblast invasion of the endometrial vasculature. Immunohistochemical studies have shown that both tissue factor (TF), the primary initiator of coagulation, and plasminogen activator inhibitor-1 (PAI-1), the primary inhibitor of fibrinolysis, increase concomitantly with decidualization of human endometrial stromal cells in sections of LP and/or gestational endometrium (Lockwood *et al.* 1993*a*, 1994*a*). Both P and medroxyprogesterone acetate (MPA) enhance the expression of TF and PAI-1 proteins and mRNA in cultured stromal cells derived from predecidualized endometrium (Lockwood *et al.* 1993*b*; Schatz and Lockwood 1993). Although estradiol (E_2) is ineffective alone it enhances progestin actions, which is consistent with the *in vivo* priming action of E_2 to enhance progesterone receptor (PR) levels (Eckert and Katzenellen Bogen 1981; Chan Chereau *et al.* 1992).

Conversely, P withdrawal reduces the expression of TF and PAI-1 while increasing that of urokinase type plasminogen activators (tPA, uPA) and the MMPs (matrix metalloproteinases) (Casslen and Astedt 1981; Gleeson 1994). These changes enhance fibrinolysis, ECM (extracellular matrix) degradation, and ischaemic spiral arterial vascular injury to account for menstrual haemorrhage. Following induction of TF and PAI-1 expression by E_2 and MPA in stromal cell cultures, withdrawal of these steroids from cultured decidual cells results in diminished levels of both TF and PAI-1 proteins and mRNA within seven days (Lockwood *et al.* 1994*b*, 1995), an effect that was produced more rapidly and completely with the antiprogestin RU486 (Lockwood *et al.* 1994*b*, 1995). These *in vitro* findings confirm that steroid withdrawal provokes changes in TF and PAI-1 expression which transforms the haemostatic milieu of the LP endometrium into a haemorrhagic environment characteristic of menstruation.

An inhibition of the expression of ECM degradation proteases, urokinase type plasminogen activators (tPA and uPA), and matrix metalloproteases (MMPs) also accompanies progestin-induced decidualization of oestrogen-primed endometrial stromal cells *in vitro* (Schatz *et al.* 1994). These changes occurring *in vivo* would inhibit fibrinolysis and maintain the structural integrity of the stromal ECM surrounding the blood vessels. Reversed expression of these endpoints following either steroid withdrawal (Schatz *et al.* 1994) or treatment with RU486 (Lockwood *et al.* 1995) promotes fibrinolysis and weakens the ECM. Marked elevations have been found in mRNA levels of stromelysin-1 (MMP-3), interstitial collagenase (MMP-1), and other MMPs in perimenstrual but not early or mid-secretory phase endometrium as assessed by *in situ* hybridization (Rodgers *et al.* 1993). In summary, progressive increases in PA and MMP activity following steroid withdrawal during the late LP enhances degradation of the ECM contributing to enhanced endometrial vascular fragility and menstruation.

Inhibition of endothelin-1 (ET-1) expression also accompanies progestin-induced decidualization of oestrogen-primed endometrial stromal cells (Schatz *et al.* 1994). ET-1 is a potent vasoconstrictor which increases in the perimenstrual period (Casey and McDonald 1992) in association with the intense vasoconstriction with resultant hypoxia immediately preceding menstruation. Enkephalinase, the primary inactivator of ET-1, decreases during this time (Casey and McDonald 1992).

Vasoconstriction and thrombin-induced fibrin plug formation in spiral arterioles located in the basal endometrium restores haemostasis after sloughing of the functional layer. Neovascularization progresses throughout the proliferative-phase endometrium via angiogenesis.

MODALITIES AVAILABLE TO MONITOR THE LUTEAL PHASE
ENDOMETRIUM

Various techniques have been developed to determine whether the LP endometrium is adequate for successful blastocyst implantation. These modalities range from simple, non-invasive recordings of daily basal body temperature (T°) to more invasive blood samplings and endometrial imaging and sampling.

Luteal phase length

Traditionally, basal T° charts have been used to document ovulation via the occurrence of a thermogenic shift, which is thought to reflect P production following ovulation. While a maximal increase in basal T° may occur with P levels greater than 5 ng/ml, changes in basal T° do not accurately monitor circulating P levels. The presence of luteal dysfunction has been linked to a slow rate of basal T° rise following ovulation, and a shortened duration in sustaining this rise (Andrews 1979). The temperature increment alone has not been found to be diagnostic, and is less sensitive than an endometrial biopsy (Downs and Gibson 1983; Olive 1991). However, when correlated with histological changes, i.e. 'out of phase' endometrial biopsies, LP lengths less than 11 days on basal T° indicate a high likelihood of LPI (Downs and Gibson 1983). While basal T° charts fail to time ovulation precisely, they become useful when the defect is severe (Downs and Gibson 1983; Li *et al.* 1987). Urinary LH-predictor kits have been used to detect the LH (luteinizing hormone) surge as a starting point in determining the length of the LP in normal ovulatory women (Lenton *et al.* 1984; Johannisson *et al.* 1987). Lenton *et al.* (1984) reported that 5 per cent of both fertile and infertile women had a shortened LP, with only half of these less than 10 days.

Progesterone and its metabolite

Levels of serum P and its metabolite pregnanediol have been used to evaluate LP function. Initial studies relied on urinary pregnanediol measurements at the mid-LP (Jones 1949). The normal range was established from urine samples of 15 regularly menstruating women of unproven fertility. Abnormally low values were then defined as those levels below the lowest value obtained from normal women, or less than 4 mg per 48 h sample. However, this test diagnosed LPI in an unusually high percentage of cases, 43 per cent of 206 women with unexplained infertility, which indicated a high false-positive rate. Subsequently, LP evaluation relied on serum P measurements in a single mid-LP sample (i.e. day 21) (McNeely and Soules 1988). LPI was defined as a serum P of less than 10–15 ng/ml, or three pooled specimens of less than 15 ng/ml. However, inherent sampling error stemming from frequent and wide fluctuations in serum P levels during the normal LP (Filcori *et al.* 1984) cast doubt on the reliability of single-point serum P4 measurements for LP evaluation (Olive 1991). Instead, integrated values of P secretion, as determined from daily serum P levels throughout the LP, appear to assess hormonal regulation of LP function more accurately (Sherman and Korenman 1974; Landgren *et al.* 1980). Comparisons with mean values from normally menstruating women with unproven fertility (Sherman and Korenman 1974) uncovered a relationship between low daily P sampling and infertility (Lenton *et al.* 1978). A more recently developed, non-invasive modality measures daily salivary P4 during the LP (Li *et al.* 1989). Early–mid-LP daily salivary P levels seem to correlate well with endometrial biopsy results. Despite the obvious potential advantages of both the integrated serum P and salivary levels for LP evaluation, they are not generally used because they are time-consuming and costly and the tests are only in the early stages of development.

Endometrial biopsy

Histological dating

Histological dating of endometrial biopsies by the Noyes' criteria (Noyes *et al.* 1950) is the traditional approach used for LP evaluation. Using Noyes' criteria, the properly timed endometrial biopsy during the late LP (i.e. day 26 of an idealized 28 day cycle) is the method of choice for diagnosing LPI (Wentz 1980). Noyes criteria histologically date the endometrium according to the most advanced portion of the biopsy with the chronological date determined retrospectively by counting backward from the onset of the subsequent menses. Unfortunately, there are numerous flaws with this method, as outlined below. There is inconsistency in both clinical practice and study design as to whether the onset of the next menstrual period is chronologically termed day 28 versus 29 (i.e. day 1 of the subsequent idealized 28 day cycle). The criterion for diagnosing a biopsy 'out of phase' varies from a difference between histological and chronological dating of ≥ 2 days to a lag of ≥ 3 days, and has not been based on controlled studies. An 'out of phase' endometrium occurs in one cycle in up to 20 per cent of women, but the incidence falls to < 3 per cent if two cycles are examined. The number of 'out of phase' biopsies used to diagnose LPI has varied from one to three in both clinical practice and study design. In addition to the inadequate standardization of Noyes' criteria, there is also the inherent problem of inter- and intra-observer variability (Scott *et al.* 1988). Another problem is that the Noyes' criteria were based on endometrial biopsies collected mainly from infertile women. Since endometrial development may be abnormal in such a group of women, it is more valid to base the criteria on biopsies from normal, fertile women. The rate of 'out of phase' biopsies from fertile women was reported to be 31.4–51.4 per cent (Davis *et al.* 1989; Shoupe *et al.* 1989), casting even more doubt on the clinical significance of this finding.

More accurate methods for dating endometrial biopsies were sought. LP dating based prospectively on the LH surge (i.e. counting forward from the day of the LH surge, which is considered cycle day 14) rather than retrospectively on subsequent menses has been promising. Histological and chronological dates correlated well with this method (Koninckx *et al.* 1977). Subsequent studies confirmed that the use of the LH surge for dating is more accurate than subsequent menses in both infertile (Li *et al.* 1987) and fertile (Shoupe *et al.* 1989) patients. An evaluation of integrated serum P levels versus late LP biopsies dated by the Noyes' criteria found that retrospective dating resulted in earlier chronological dates that deviated more from the corresponding histological dates than prospective dating (Johannisson *et al.* 1982). This may be because retrospective dating assumes a fixed 14-day luteal span, whereas, in actuality, there is intrinsic variation in the LP length (Lenton *et al.* 1984). The correlation between integrated serum P levels and endometrial maturation was found to be poor, regardless of the type of chronological dating used (Batista *et al.* 1993). Sixteen per cent of biopsies analysed prospectively from normal, fertile women were interpreted as abnormal (Shoupe *et al.* 1989). Thus, despite the use of a more accurate method for chronological dating, there still remains the need for improved ways to assess the LP endometrium.

Morphometric analysis

The results of morphometric analysis, which is performed by histometric and stereologic methods, lend themselves to regression analysis. Therefore, it is both a more objective procedure than the classic method of dating endometrial biopsies by Noyes' criteria, and more easily validated statistically (Johannisson *et al.* 1982, 1987). Johannison *et al.* (1982, 1987) were the first to relate morphometric analysis of the endometrium to changes in serum steroid levels. They found that changes in glandular diameter were positively correlated with levels of circulating E_2 and P during the proliferative and secretory phase respectively; that the stromal mitotic index correlated negatively with circulating P levels; and that numbers of basal vacuoles were negatively correlated with serum E_2 levels and positively correlated with serum P4 levels during the immediate post-ovulatory phase (Johannisson *et al.* 1982). Endometrial dating by morphometric analysis gave the most significant results from days' –3/–2 LH surge to days' +7/+8 LH surge (Johannisson *et al.* 1982). Thus, endometrial dating is more appropriately related to the time of the LH surge rather than to the 'ideal' 28-day cycle (Johannisson *et al.* 1982; Bjorklund *et al.* 1991). Although these studies used endometria from normal fertile women (Johannisson *et al.* 1982, 1987), a separate study applied morphometric analysis to endometria from infertile women (Bonhuff *et al.* 1990). Li *et al.* (1987, 1988) specifically adapted morphometric analysis to endometrial dating of the LP in fertile women. Of 17 morphometric measurements performed on each endometrial biopsy, only five were required to achieve a highly significant correlation with chronological dating based on the LH surge. (These five measurements were the volume fraction of gland occupied by the gland cell, the amount of predecidual reaction, the amount of secretion in the glandular lumen, the amount of pseudostratification of the gland cell, and the number of mitoses per 1000 gland cells.) This is a significant observation given the labour-intensive nature of morphometric analysis, and the observation that histological dating using morphometric analysis correlated better with chronological dating than did the more conventional Noyes' criteria (Li *et al.* 1988). In summary, the use of morphometric analysis has allowed an objective, more detailed characterization of LP endometrial histology.

Endometrial steroid receptors

As is the case with inadequate steroid production stemming from classic CL insufficiency, defects in endometrial steroid receptors can lead to reproductive failures. Interestingly, the concentration of progesterone receptors (PR) in patients with 'out of phase' endometrial biopsies has been reported to be higher than (Gravanis *et al.* 1984; Saracoglu *et al.* 1985; Spirtos *et al.* 1985), the same as (McRae *et al.* 1984; Jacobs *et al.* 1987), or lower than (Laatikainen *et al.* 1983; Spirtos *et al.* 1985), that of patients with 'in phase' biopsies. Jacobs *et al.* (1987) showed that although there was no difference in PR concentration during the LP in women with LPI, proliferative-phase nuclear PR levels were lower in these women than in normal patients. Thus, a proliferative-phase abnormality may be responsible for the later appearing LPI characterized by an 'out of phase' endometrial biopsy. In contrast to these changes in PR levels, oestrogen receptor (ER) levels were similar in women with LPI compared with normal women (McRae *et al.* 1984). Deserving consideration for future study is the possibility that perhaps only a small subset of patients manifest true endometrial steroid-receptor defects as the underlying cause of LPI.

Progestational responsiveness also depends on PR isoform expression. There are two predominant forms of PR: a high molecular weight form (120 kDa), PRB, and a truncated lower molecular weight form (94 kDa), PRA (Conneely *et al.* 1987; Christensen *et al.* 1991). Transfection studies have demonstrated that the presence of PRA can inhibit PRB-modulated transcription at physiological levels of P (Vegeto *et al.* 1993). Thus, assessing levels of functionally active PR requires ascertaining not only total PR content but also the relative distribution of the isoforms. Future investigation of endometrial PR isoform expression and possible alterations in 'out of phase' endometria is warranted.

Endometrial proteins

Endometrial proteins secreted into the uterine lumen

The endometrium elaborates a wide variety of proteins under the regulatory influence of ovarian-derived E_2 and P (Fay and Grudzinskas 1991), with maximum synthesis occuring during the LP. Secretion of these proteins into the uterine lumen by glandular and luminal epithelial cells and stromal/decidual cells determines the composition of the milieu that the blastocyst encounters during hatching and implantation. Glycoproteins are among the most abundant of the products secreted during the LP. These include large proteins such as the mucins, which are secreted by epithelial cells, and appear to promote blastocyst adhesion. (Aplin 1991; Lindenberg 1991; Mani *et al.* 1992; Rye *et al.* 1993; Kliman *et al.* 1995). Smaller, progestin-regulated glycoprotein products of LP stromal/decidual cells include alpha-1 pregnancy-associated endometrial protein (α1-PEG), and pregnancy-associated plasma protein A (PAPP-A) (Fay and Grudzinskas 1991; Schwartz *et al.* 1993).

The concerted effects of E_2 and P also induce the LP endometrium to synthesize insulin-like growth factor binding protein(s) (IGF-BPs) (Guidice 1994), as well as such hormones as prolactin (Maslar and Ridick 1979) and relaxin. The IGF-BPs and prolactin are also well-studied products of human endometrial stromal cells induced to undergo *in vitro* decidualization by progestins added alone or together with E_2 (see above). The LP endometrium elaborates a wide variety of cytokines, which is the subject of an exhaustive review (Guidice 1994).

Endometrial proteins secreted into peripheral blood

Proteins produced by endometrial glands and stroma during the LP have been detected in the peripheral blood. Measurements of these proteins provide a relatively non-invasive, quantitative modality for assessing the physiological/pathological status of the LP endometrium. One of the most widely studied of these proteins is progesta-gen-associated endometrial protein (PEP), which is also called α2-PEG, and PP-14. PEP is a major secretory product of the endometrial glandular epithelium which appears in serum in the late LP (Joshi *et al.* 1986). Progestational activity of steroids is positively correlated with their ability to stimulate PEP synthesis. Low serum PEP levels on cycle day 28 occurred more frequently in women with LPI than in normal women, which suggests that serum PEP levels reflect the cumulative endometrial effect of P4 secretion during the entire LP (Joshi *et al.* 1986). A second such protein to have been successfully measured in the peripheral blood is stress response protein (SRP)-27, which is maximally expressed by glandular cells at ovulation and in surface epithelium during implantation (Fay and Grudzinskas 1991; Schwartz *et al.* 1993). Circulating levels of SRP-27 are a potential prognosticator of LPI.

Endometrial proteins detected by histology

Immunohistochemical studies have served to delineate the normal secretory pattern of the LP endometrium (Seif *et al.* 1989; Fay and Grudzinskas 1991), and thereby shed light on its functional state (Seif *et al.* 1989). For example, immunohistochemical staining patterns obtained with the monoclonal antibody D9B1, which binds to car-bohydrate epitopes associated with high molecular weight sialoglycoproteins, sug-gested that levels of these moieties may be diagnostic for LPI. Thus, 68 per cent of patients previously diagnosed with LPI by the Noyes' criteria subsequently revealed significantly diminished expression of this epitope, and 92 per cent of endometrial biopsies from infertility patients showed defective production of the D9B1 epitope (Seif *et al.* 1989). Immunohistochemistry has been used to detect progestin-regulated enzymes in the LP endometrium such as carbonic anhydrase and lactoferrin. Predictably, several of the secreted proteins of LP endometria, such as prolactin and IGF-BPs, have been detected in endometrial sections by immunohistochemistry.

Use of immunohistochemistry to identify biochemical markers of normal LP endometrial function may allow for more accurate diagnosis of LPI than that based solely on the histological assessment of a single endometrial biopsy. Since the majority of the secretory products of the endometrium are produced during the early–mid-LP, improved insight into endometrial function may be obtained by performing biopsies for immunohistochemistry during the early, rather than late, LP. Earlier endometrial sampling also allows for LP evaluation at the critical times in the development of endometrial receptivity for blastocyst implantation (Seif *et al.* 1989).

Pelvic ultrasound (US) and magnetic resonance imaging (MRI)

Pelvic imaging allows for less invasive LP endometrial screening than biopsies. Initially, investigators assessed endometrial development throughout the menstrual cycle by measuring the endometrial thickness. This measurement is performed on a single sagittal image of the largest anterior–posterior diameter of the central uterine echo in the most fundal region of the uterus. Endometrial thickness varies throughout the cycle, the endometrium being thin following menstruation and thickening during the follicular phase to approximately 8–15 mm at ovulation and during the LP (Thickman *et al.* 1986; Li *et al.* 1992). A consistent role of endometrial thickness measurements in predicting pregnancy outcome in *in vitro* fertilization (IVF) cycles has not been found. Some investigators found no difference in endometrial thickness between pregnant and non-pregnant cycles (Fleischer *et al.* 1986a; Coulam *et al.* 1994), while others report thicker endometria among subsequently pregnant patients (Rabinowitz *et al.* 1986; Check *et al.* 1991, 1993; Shapiro *et al.* 1993; Check 1994). Cut-off levels have been proposed at which the endometrium is appropriate for implantation: either at ≥ 6 mm (Shapiro *et al.* 1993), ≥ 10 mm (Check *et al.* 1991, 1993; Check 1994), or ≥ 13 mm (Rabinowitz *et al.* 1986).

The application of transvaginal US (TVUS) has enabled endometrial characterization not only in terms of its thickness and growth but also in terms of its echogenicity ('texture') during the cycle (Fleischer *et al.* 1991). The endometrial texture is cyclical, with hypoechogenicity characteristic of the proliferative phase and an echogenic appearance more common in the secretory phase (Fleischer *et al.* 1986b; Randall *et al.* 1989). The early proliferative endometrium appears as a single 'pencil-thin' line representing the endometrial canal. As the follicular phase progresses, a triple-line pattern develops which represents hyperechogenic outer lines (endometrial–myometrial interface) and a central line (uterine cavity) between which there is a hypoechogenic area representing the functional endometrium. After ovulation, the functional layer becomes hyperechogenic and the triple-line sign disappears (Itskovitz *et al.* 1990), which probably represents the development of stromal edema (Fleischer and Kepple 1991). These two distinct US patterns have been confirmed histologically (Forrest *et al.* 1988). Studies of echogenic patterns of the endometrium during IVF cycles suggest that triple or mixed (incomplete) pre-ovulatory patterns can sustain pregnancy, while a homogeneous patterns usually cannot (Check *et al.* 1991; Grunfeld *et al.* 1991; Ueno *et al.* 1991; Coulam *et al.* 1994; Serafini *et al.* 1994).

In summary, TVUS provides promise for the evaluation of the LP endometrium and prediction of pregnancy outcome in IVF endometrial thickness cycles. However, the endometrial thickness and texture on TVUS is not yet standardized or well correlated with other factors to determine the relative clinical importance of these US findings.

The development of the endometrium has also been assessed by magnetic resonance imaging (MRI). The main difference between MRI and TVUS in the normal ovulatory cycle was shown to be at the junctional zone (Mitchell *et al.* 1990). Although the junctional zone was initially promising for the evaluation of the endometrial cycle, since it was thought to represent either the stratum basalis or the vasculature at the endometrial–myometrial junction, subsequently, this anatomic area was histologically identified to be the inner myometrium which corresponds to the low-signal-intensity band that surrounds the bright, central endometrial layer (Scoutt *et al.* 1991). Thus, currently, MRI does not provide any advantage over TVUS in evaluating the LP endometrium.

Doppler waveforms

The evaluation of utero-ovarian perfusion with colour Doppler TVUS has been added to the armamentarium of modalities available to assess ovarian CL and LP endometrial function. The technology of measuring resistive index (RI) and pulsatility index (PI) has been applied to the evaluation of the CL. The RI (systolic peak minus diastolic peak divided by the systolic peak) ranges from 0 to 1.0, with 1.0 representing the highest resistance to forward flow. The PI, another measurement of vascular impedance, is defined as the systolic peak minus the diastolic peak divided by the mean flow velocity (Fleischer 1991). The PI of ovarian blood flow is cyclical. During the follicular phase, the PI is usually high (> 2.0) with a gradual decrease as follicular maturation progresses. With vascularization of the CL, diastolic flow increases (with lower PI values of < 1.0) (Fleischer and Kepple 1991). Taylor *et al.* (1985) demonstrated that high diastolic blood flow and low-impedance Doppler waveforms (low RI and low PI) are present in the ovary containing the active CL. The inactive ovary demonstrates low diastolic flow and high impedance (high RI and high PI).

Colour Doppler TVUS of the uterus examines the uterine artery at the site where it divides into the ascending branch. Colour Doppler signals have also been obtained from the arcuate and radial vessels within the myometrium. It has been reported (Fleischer and Kepple 1991) that uterine artery PI is low and diastolic flow is high during the normal early to mid-secretory phase. Higher PI is characteristic of the late secretory and menstrual phases. Intermediate values are seen during the follicular phase. These changes depend on the formation of a mature dominant follicle and its conversion to a functional CL. Thus, a trend towards decreased PI has been observed in both the uterine and ovarian arteries with the formation of the CL (Fleischer 1991). Increasing uterine perfusion has been shown with rising E_2 levels in the follicular phase, decreasing uterine perfusion with the periovulatory decline in E_2 levels, and a subsequent increase in uterine perfusion (i.e. decreased RI) as P levels rise in the LP (Goswamy and Steptoe 1988; Steer *et al.* 1990). Several studies show that a PI of < 3.3 was more favourable for a positive pregnancy outcome in IVF cycles (Steer *et al.* 1992; Coulam *et al.* 1994).

In summary, Doppler TVUS seems to be of promise for evaluation of normal and abnormal LP utero-ovarian blood flow. A healthy CL seems to be associated with high diastolic blood flow and low impedance in both the ovarian and uterine arteries during the early–mid LP. However, this is not yet well standardized or well correlated with other modalities more traditionally utilized for LP evaluation.

CONCLUDING REMARKS

Despite the recent availability of various morphological and biochemical modalities to evaluate the normal LP endometrium and to distinguish it from LPI, the diagnosis of the abnormal LP still remains elusive and the clinical significance of such a diagnosis is still unclear. Standardization has been lacking, normal ranges have not been well defined, and the clinical relevance (i.e. the association of LPI with infertility) has not been adequately established. Despite these difficulties, the application of technological and biochemical advances to the LP endometrium provide potential new diagnostic modalities that may be useful in conjunction with the more traditional method of dating the endometrial biopsy. The advances of endometrial-derived protein analysis, endometrial imaging, and utero-ovarian blood flow measurements are important steps in the development of more specific and less invasive diagnostic modalities. In the future, these new techniques may serve a functional part of screening tests aimed at preventing unnecessary endometrial biopsies. In this way, the intrinsic problems with the more conventional Noyes' criteria interpretation of the endometrial biopsy for LP evaluation may be circumvented.

REFERENCES

Andrews, W.C. (1979). Luteal phase defects. *Fertility and Sterility*, **32**, 501.

Aplin, J.D. (1991). Glycans as biochemical markers of human endometrial secretory different-iation. *Journal of Reproduction and Fertility*, **92**, 525–41.

Batista, M.C., Cartledge, T.P., Merino, M.J., Axiotis, C., Platia, M.P., Merriam, G.R., et al. (1993). Midluteal phase endometrial biopsy does not accurately predict luteal function. *Fertility and Sterility*, **59**, 294–300.

Bjorklund, T.K., Landgren, B.M., Hamberger, L., and Johannisson, E. (1991). Comparative morphometric study of the endometrium, the fallopian tube, and the corpus luteum during the postovulatory phase in normally menstruating women. *Fertility and Sterility*, **56**, 842–50.

Bonhuff, A., Johannisson, E., and Bohnet, H.G. (1990). Morphometric analysis of the endo-metrium of infertile patients in relation to peripheral hormone levels. *Fertility and Sterility*, **54**, 84–9.

Casey, M.L. and McDonald P.C. (1992). Modulation of endometrial blood flow: Regulation of endothelin-1 biosynthesis and degradation in human endometrium. In *Steroid hormones and uterine bleeding*, (ed. N.J., Alexander, and C. d'Arcangues), p. 209. AAAS Press, Washington, D.C.

Casslen, B. and Astedt, B. (1981). Fibrinolytic activity of human uterine fluid. *Acta Obstetrica Gynecologica Scandinavica*, **60**, 55–8.

Chau Chereau, A., Savouret, J.F., and Milgram, E. (1992). Control of biosynthesis and post-transcriptional modification of progesterone receptor. *Biological Reproduction*, **46**, 174–7.

Check, J.H. (1994). The use of the donor oocyte program to evaluate embryo implantation. *Annals of the New York Academy of Science*, **734**, 198–208.

Check, J.H., Nowroozi, K., Choe, J., and Dietterich, C. (1991). The influence of endometrial thickness and echo patterns on pregnancy rates during *in vitro* fertilization. *Fertility and Sterility*, **56**, 1173–5.

Check, J.H., Nowroozi, K., Choe, J., Lurie, D., and Dietterich, C. (1993). The effect of endometrial thickness and echo pattern on *in vitro* fertilization outcome in donor oocyte–embryo transfer cycle. *Fertility and Sterility*, **59**, 72–5.

Christensen, K., Estes, P.A., and Onate, S.A. (1991). Characterization and functional properties of the A and B forms of the human progesterone receptors synthesized by a baculovirus system. *Molecular Endocrinology*, **5**, 1755–70.

Conneely, O.M., Maxwell, B.Z., Toft, D.O., Schrader, W.T., and O'Malley, B.W. (1987). The A and B forms of the chicken progesterone receptor arise by alternate initiation of translation of a unique mRNA. *Biochemistry and Biophysics Research Communications*, **149**, 493–501.

Coulam, C.B., Bustillo, M., Soenksen, D.M., and Britten, S. (1994). Ultrasonographic predictors of implantation after assisted reproduction. *Fertility and Sterility*, **62**, 1004–10.

Davis, O.K., Berkeley, A.S., Naus, G.J., Cholst, I.N., and Freeman, K.S. (1989). The incidence of luteal phase defect in normal, fertile women determined by serial endometrial biopsies. *Fertility and Sterility*, **51**, 582.

Downs, K.A. and Gibson, M. (1983). Basal body temperature graph and the luteal phase defect. *Fertility and Sterility*, **40**, 466–8.

Eckert, R.L. and Katzenellenbogen, B.S. (1981). Human endometrial cells in primary tissue culture: modulation of the progesterone receptor levels by natural and synthetic *in vitro*. *Journal of Clinical Endocrinology and Metabolism*, **52**, 699–708.

Fay, T.N. and Grudzinskas, J.G. (1991). Human endometrial peptides: a review of their potential role in implantation and placentation. *Human Reproduction*, **9**, 1311–26.

Filcori, M., Butler, J.P., Crowley Jr, W.F. (1984). Neuroendocrine regulation of the corpus luteum in the human: evidence for pulsatile progesterone secretion. *Journal of Clinical Investigation*, **73**, 1638.

Fleischer, A.C. (1991). Ultrasound imaging—2000: assessment of utero-ovarian blood flow with transvaginal color Doppler sonography; potential clinical applications in infertility. *Fertility and Sterility*, **55**, 684–91.

Fleischer, A.C. and Kepple, D.M. (1991). Pelvic anatomy and physiology as depicted by conventional and color doppler transvaginal sonography. *Infertility and Reproduction Clinics of North America*, **2**, 659–72.

Fleischer, A.C., Herbert, C.M., Sacks, G.A., Wentz, A.C., Entman, S.S., and James, Jr, A.E. (1986*a*). Sonography of the endometrium during conception and nonconception cycles on *in vitro* fertilization and embryo transfer. *Fertility and Sterility*, **46**, 442–7.

Fleischer, A.C., Kalemeris, G.C., and Entman, S.S. (1986*b*). Sonographic depiction of the endometrium during normal cycles. *Ultrasound Medicine and Biology*, **12**, 271–7.

Fleischer, A.C., Herbert, C.M., Hill, G.A., Kepple, D.M., and Worrell, J.A. (1991). Transvaginal sonography of the endometrium during induced cycles. *Journal of Ultrasound Medicine*, **10**, 93–5.

Forrest, T.S., Elyaderani, M.K., Muilenburg, M.I., Bewtra, C., Kable, W.T., and Sullivan, P. (1988). Cyclic endometrial changes: US assessment with histologic correlation. *Radiology*, **167**, 233–7.

Gleeson, N.C. (1994). Cyclic changes in endometrial tissue plasminogen activator and plasminogen activator type 1 in women with normal menstruation and essential menorrhagia. *American Journal of Obstetrics and Gynecology*, **171**, 178–83.

Goswamy, R.K. and Steptoe, P.C. (1988). Doppler ultrasound studies of the uterine artery in spontaneous ovarian cycles. *Human Reproduction*, **3**, 721–6.

Gravanis, A., Zorn, J.R., Tanguy, G., Nessman, C., Cedard, L., and Robel, P. (1984). The 'dysharmonic luteal phase' syndrome: endometrial progesterone receptor and estradiol dehydrogenase. *Fertility and Sterility*, **42**, 730.

Grunfeld, L., Walker, B., Bergh, P.A., Sandler, B., Hofmann, G., and Navot, D. (1991). High-resolution endovaginal ultrasonography of the endometrium: a noninvasive test for endometrial adequacy. *Obstetrics and Gynecology*, 200–4.

Guidice, L.C. (1994). Growth factors and growth modulators in human uterine endometrium: their potential relevance to reproductive medicine. *Fertility and Sterility*, **61**, 1–17.

Itskovitz, J., Boldes, R., Levron, J., and Thaler, I. (1990). Transvaginal ultrasonography in the diagnosis and treatment of infertility. *Journal of Clinical Ultrasound*, **18**, 248–56.

Jacobs, M.H., Balasch, J., Gonzalez-Merlo, J.M., Vanrell, J.A., Wheeler, C., Strauss III, J.F., et al. (1987). Endometrial cytosolic and nuclear progesterone receptors in the luteal phase defect. *Journal of Clinical Endocrinology and Metabolism*, **64**, 472–5.

Johannisson, E., Parker, R.A., Landgren, B.M., and Diczfalusy, E. (1982). Morphometric analysis of the human endometrium in relation to peripheral hormone levels. *Fertility and Sterility*, **38**, 564.

Johannisson, E., Landgren, B.M., Rohr, H.P., and Diczfalusy, E. (1987). Endometrial morphology and peripheral hormones levels in women with regular menstrual. *Fertility and Sterility*, **48**, 401–8.

Jones, G.E.S. (1949). Some newer aspects of the management of infertility. *Journal of the American Medical Association*, **141**, 1123.

Joshi, S.G., Rao, R., Henriques, E.E., Raikar, R.S., and Gordon, M. (1986). Luteal phase concentrations of a progestagen-associated endometrial protein (PEP) in the serum of cycling women with adequate or inadequate endometrium. *Journal of Clinical Endocrinology and Metabolism*, **63**, 1247–9.

Kliman, H.J., Feinberg, R.F., Schwartz, L.B., Feinman, M.A., Lavi, E., and Meaddough, E.L. (1995). A human endometrial mucin identified by MAG (mouse ascites golgi) antibodies: menstrual cycle-dependent localization in human endometrium. *American Journal of Pathology*, **146**, 166–81.

Koninckx, P.R., Goddeeris, P.R., Lauweryns, J.M., de Hertogh, R.C., and Brosens, I.A. (1977). Accuracy of endometrial biopsy dating in relation to the midcycle luteinizing hormone peak. *Fertility and Sterility*, **28**, 443.

Laatikainen, T., Andersson, B., Karkkainen, J., and Wahlstrom, T. (1983). Progesterone receptor levels in endometria with delayed or incomplete secretory changes. *Obstetrics and Gynecology*, **62**, 592.

Landgren, B.M., Unden, A.L., and Diczfalusy, E. (1980). Hormonal profile of the cycle in 68 normally menstruating women. *Acta Endocrinologica*, **94**, 89.

Lenton, E.A., Adams, M., and Cooke, I.D. (1978). Plasma steroid and gonadotropin profiles in ovulatory but infertile women. *Clinical Endocrinology*, **8**, 241.

Lenton, E.A., Landgren, B.M., and Sexton, L. (1984). Normal variation in the length of the luteal phase of the menstrual cycle: identification of the short luteal phase. *British Journal of Obstetrics and Gynaecology*, **91**, 685.

Li, T.C., Rogers, A.W., Lenton, E.A., Dockery, P., and Cooke, I.D. (1987). A comparison between two methods of chronological dating of human endometrial biopsies during the luteal phase, and their correlation with histologic dating. *Fertility and Sterility*, **48**, 928.

Li, T.C., Rogers, A.W., Dockery, P., Lenton, E.A., and Cooke, I.D. (1988). A new method of histologic dating of human endometrium in the luteal phase. *Fertility and Sterility*, **50**, 52.

Li, T.C., Lenton, E.A., Dockery, P., Rogers, A.W., and Cooke, I.D. (1989). The relation between daily salivary progesterone profile and endometrial development in the luteal phase of fertile and infertile women. *British Journal of Obstetrics and Gynaecology*, **96**, 445.

Li, T.C., Nuttall, L., Klentzeris, L., and Cooke, I.D. (1992). How well does ultrasonographic measurement of endometrial thickness predict the results of histological dating? *Human Reproduction*, **7**, 1–5.

Lindenberg, S. (1991). Experimental studies on the initial trophoblast endometrial interaction. *Danish Medical Bulletin*, **38**, 371–80.

Lockwood, C.J., Nemerson, Y., Guller, S., *et al.* (1993*a*). Progestational regulation of human endometrial stromal cell tissue factor expression during decidualization. *Journal of Clinical Endocrinology and Metabolism*, **76**, 231–6.

Lockwood, C.J., Nemerson, Y., Krikun, G., *et al.* (1993*b*). Steroid-modulated stromal cell tissue factor expression: a model for the regulation of endometrial hemostasis and menstruation. *Journal of Clinical Endocrinology and Metabolism* **77**, 1014–19.

Lockwood, C.J., Krikun, G., Papp, C., *et al.* (1994*a*). The role of progestationally regulated stromal cell tissue factor and type-1 plasminogen activator inhibitor (PAI-1) in endometrial hemostasis and menstruation. *Annals of the New York Academy of Science*, **734**, 57–79.

Lockwood, C.J., Krikun, G., Papp, C., Aigner, S., Nemerson, Y., and Schatz, F. (1994*b*). Biological mechanisms underlying RU486 clinical effects: inhibition of endometrial stromal cell tissue factor content. *Journal of Clinical Endocrinology and Metabolism*, 79, 786–90.

Lockwood, C.J., Krikun, G., Papp, C., Aigner, S., and Schatz, F. (1995). Biological mechanisms underlying RU486 clinical effects: modulation of endometrial stromal cell plasminogen activator and plasminogen activator inhibitor expression. *Journal of Clinical Endocrinology and Metabolism*, 80, 1100–5.

McNeely, M.J. and Soules, M.R. The diagnosis of luteal phase deficiency: a critical review. *Fertility and Sterility*, 50, 1.

McRae, M.A., Blasco, L., and Lyttle C.R. (1984). Serum hormones and their receptors in women with normal and inadequate corpus luteum function. *Fertility and Sterility*, 42, 58.

Mani, S.K., Carson, D.D., and Glasser, S.R. (1992). Steroid hormones differentially modulate glycoconjugate synthesis and vectoral secretion by polarized human epithelial cells *in vitro*. *Endocrinology*, 130, 240–8.

Maslar, I.A. and Ridick, D.H. (1979). Prolactin production by human endometrium in the normal menstrual cycle. *American Journal of Obstetrics and Gynecology*, 135, 751–4.

Mitchell, D.G., Schonholz, L., Hilpert, P.L., Blum, L., and Rifkin, M.D. (1990). Zones of the uterus: discrepancy between US and MR images. *Radiology*, 174, 827–31.

Noyes, R.W., Hertig, A.T., and Rock, J. (1950). Dating the endometrial biopsy. *Fertility and Sterility*, 1, 3.

Olive, D.L. (1991). The prevalence and epidemiology of luteal phase deficiency in normal and infertile women. *Clinical Obstetrics and Gynecology*, 34, 157–66.

Rabinowitz, R., Laufer, N., Lewin, A., Navot, D., Bar, I., Margalioth, E.J., and Schenker, J.J. (1986). The value of ultrasonographic endometrial measurement in the prediction of pregnancy following *in vitro*, fertilization. *Fertility and Sterility*, 45, 824–8.

Randall, J.M., Fisk, N.M., McTavish, A., and Templeton, A.A. (1989). Transvaginal ultrasonic assessment of endometrial growth in spontaneous and hyperstimulated menstrual cycles. *British Journal of Obstetrics and Gynaecology*, 96, 954–9.

Rodgers, W.H., Matrisian, L.M., Osteen, K.G., and Svitek, C. (1993). Differential expression and cellular localization of matrix metalloproteinases in human endometrial epithelium and stroma during the menstrual cycle. Presented at the 40th Annual Meeting of the Society for Gynecologic Investigation, Toronto, 31st March–3rd April 1993, Abstract #533.

Rye, P.D., Bell, S.C., and Walker, R.A. (1993). Immunohistochemical expression of tumour-associated glycoprotein and polymorphic epithelial mucin in the human endometrium during the menstrual cycle. *Journal of Reproduction and Fertility*, 97, 551–6.

Saracoglu, O.F., Aksel, S., Yeoman, R.R., and Wiebe, R.H. (1985). Endometrial estradiol and progesterone receptors in patients with luteal phase defects and endometriosis. *Fertility*, 43, 851.

Schatz, F. and Lockwood, C.J. (1993). Progestin regulation of plasminogen activator inhibitor type-1 in primary cultures of endometrial stromal and decidual cells. *Journal of Clinical Endocrinology and Metabolism*, 77, 621–5.

Schatz, F., Papp, C., Toth-Pal, E., and Lockwood, C.J. (1994). Ovarian steroid-modulated stromelysin-1 expression in human endometrial stromal and decidual cells. *Journal of Clinical Endocrinology and Metabolism*, 78, 1467–72.

Schwartz, L.B., Laufer, N., and DeCherney, A.H. (1993). The role of the endometrial biopsy and other modalities to evaluate the luteal phase. *Clinical Consultations in Obstetrics and Gynecology*, 5, 188–97.

Scott, R.T., Snyer, R.R., and Strickland, D.M. (1988). The effect of interobserver variation in dating endometrial histology on the diagnosis of luteal phase defects. *Fertility and Sterility*, 50, 888.

Scoutt, L.M., Flynn, S.D., Luthringer, D.J., McCauley, T.R., and McCarthy, S.M. (1991). Junctional zone of the uterus: correlation of M.R. imaging and histologic examination of hysterectomy specimens. *Radiology*, **179**, 403–7.

Seif, M.W., Aplin, J.D., and Buckley, C.H. (1989). Luteal phase defect: the possibility of an immunohistochemical diagnosis. *Fertility and Sterility*, **51**, 273–9.

Serafini, P., Batzofin, J., Nelson, J., and Olive, D. (1994). Sonographic uterine predictors of pregnancy in women undergoing ovulation induction for assisted reproductive treatments. *Fertility and Sterility*, **62**, 815–22.

Shapiro, H., Cowell, C., and Casper, R.F. (1993). The use of vaginal ultrasound for monitoring endometrial preparation in a donor oocyte program. *Fertility and Sterility*, **59**, 1055–8.

Sherman, B.M. and Korenman, S.G. (1974). Measurement of serum L.H., FSH., estradiol, and progesterone in disorders of the human menstrual cycle: the inadequate luteal phase. *Journal of Clinical Endocrinology and Metabolism*, **39**, 145.

Shoupe, D., Mishell, Jr, D.R., Lacarra, M., Lobo, R.A., Horenstein, J., and d'Ablaing, G. (1989). Correlation of endometrial maturation with four methods of estimating day of ovulation. *Obstetrics and Gynecology*, **73**, 88.

Spirtos, N.J., Yurewicz, E.C., Moghissi, K.S., Magyar, D.M., Sundareson, A.S., and Bottoms, S.F. (1985). Pseudocorpus luteum insufficiency: a study of cytosolic progesterone receptors in human endometrium. *Obstetrics and Gynecology*, **65**, 535–40.

Steer, C.B., Campbell, S., Pampiglione, J.S., Kingsland, C.R., Mason, B.A., and Collins, W.P. (1990). Transvaginal color flow imaging of the uterine arteries during the ovarian and menstrual cycles. *Human Reproduction*, **5**, 391–5.

Steer, C.V., Campbell, S., Tan, S.L., Crayford, T., Mills, C., Mason, C., *et al.* (1992). The use of transvaginal color flow imaging after *in vitro* fertilization to identify optimum uterine conditions before embryo transfer. *Fertility and Sterility*, **57**, 372–6.

Taylor, K.J.W., Burns, P.N., Wells, P.N.T., Conway, D.I., and Hull, M.G.R. (1985). Ultrasound Doppler flow studies of the ovarian and uterine arteries. *British Journal of Obstetrics and Gynaecology*, **91**, 240–6.

Thickman, D., Arger, P., Tureck, R., Blasco, L., Mintz, M., and Coleman, B. (1986). Sonographic assessment of the endometrium in patients undergoing *in vitro* fertilization. *Journal of Ultrasound Medicine*, **5**, 197–201.

Ueno, J., Oehninger, S., Brzyski, R.G., Acosta, A.A., Pgilput, C.B., and Muasher S.J. (1991). Ultrasonographic appearance of the endometrium in natural and stimulated *in vitro* fertilization cycles and its correlation with outcome. *Human Reproduction*, **6**, 901–4.

Vegeto, E., Shahbaz, M.M., Wen, D.X., Goldman, M.E., O'Malley, B.W., and McDonnell, D.P. (1993). Human progesterone receptor A form is a cell- and promoter-specific repressor of human progesterone receptor B function. *Moleculor Endocrinology*, **7**, 1244–55.

Wentz, A.C. (1980). Endometrial biopsy in the evaluation of infertility. *Fertility and Sterility*, **33**, 121.

II

From the trophectoderm to the definitive placenta

7 | Integrins and the implantation site

Bruce A. Lessey

INTRODUCTION

Many of us who care for infertile couples share an intense interest in the process of implantation. While much is known about spermatogenesis, folliculogenesis, ovulation, fertilization, and gamete transport, an understanding of the molecular mechanisms of embryo–endometrial interaction has lagged behind. The implantation site is an area of significant cellular activity, including cell attachment and migration, secretion, and degradation of extracellular matrix (ECM) components, chemotaxis, angiogenesis, and apoptosis, orchestrated to a large measure by endocrine, paracrine, and autocrine signalling. The ECM is also involved in cell signalling mediated through integrins, a class of cell-adhesion molecules (CAMs) present on virtually all cells. Further, based on a receptor mediated paradigm of implantation (Yoshinaga 1989), the presence of menstrual cycle-specific changes in integrin expression have been implicated in the initial events of embryo–endometrial interactions (Lessey *et al.* 1992; Tabibzadeh 1992). There is an increasing appreciation of the factors which regulate integrin expression in the endometrium; this aspect of integrin biochemistry is pertinent to the study of factors which favour a receptive endometrium. Thus, the integrins may represent a convergent focus of endocrine, paracrine, and ECM mediators of the implantation process.

As outlined by Psychoyos (1995), uterine receptivity may be the rate limiting event in the implantation of the blastocyst in many species. The endometrium presents a barrier to implantation that must be breached before implantation can occur. The endometrium remains hostile to implantation except for a narrow 'window of implantation' marked by specific, still poorly defined biochemical changes that facilitate embryo–endometrial interactions. The cellular activity surrounding the initial events of implantation has been extensively studied (Enders and Schlafke 1969). The first events occur during *apposition*, when embryonic and endometrial epithelial cells first interact. According to Enders and Schlafke, this is followed by cellular *adhesion*. Early adhesion events are likely to be mediated by specific receptors of the CAM superfamily. So far, only the integrins have been shown to undergo temporal and spatial changes that correlate with the putative window of implantation. Some types of infertility appear to be associated with a loss of certain integrins, suggesting that these glycoproteins may serve as markers for defects in endometrial receptivity. The existence of such defects is of interest for the diagnosis and treatment of infertility and suggests new avenues of research for the development of new contraceptive technologies.

Following initial apposition and adhesion is *penetration* of the luminal epithelium by the embryo. This process involves active protein synthesis and secretion of enzymes capable of degrading the extracellular matrix (ECM) and basement membrane (BM). Contact with ECM results in transduction and gene transcription, again mediated by integrins, leading to this progression from *adhesion* to *penetration* (Werb *et al.* 1990). There also appear to be integrin-mediated events in the decidua which *limit* trophoblast invasion (Irwin *et al.* 1995). While the properties of invading trophoblast have been compared to those of malignant cells, trophoblast invasion appears to be highly regulated. As discussed below, the dynamics of integrin and ECM expression may provide a framework for understanding these events.

The timing of embryo attachment and invasion appears to be critical for successful implantation. Studies performed in the arena of assisted reproductive technologies (ART) using donor embryos transferred into hormonally prepared recipients, documents a 'window of transfer' before which, and after which, implantation will not occur (Navot *et al.* 1991). Studies using statistical evaluation of data based on highly sensitive hCG (human chorionic gonadotrophin) measurements estimate that the window of endometrial receptivity extends from post-ovulatory day 6 to day 10 (cycle day 20 to 24 of an idealized 28 day cycle) (Bergh and Navot 1992). These modern day studies are entirely consistent with the studies of Hertig and colleagues, who searched for and found 34 embryos in hysterectomy samples from pregnant women with known last menstrual periods (Hertig *et al.* 1956). In this seminal work, eight embryos were found to be free floating in the tubes or in the uterine cavity, all prior to cycle day 19 to 20. Of the 26 embryos that were found attached to the uterine lining, all came from uteri obtained at cycle day 21 or beyond. These data imply that initial attachment of the human embryo occurs around cycle day 20, or six days after ovulation. Other 'windows' of receptivity that need to be considered are those of the embryo and corpus luteum. Based on hCG measurements, implantation appears to occur around day 7 post-fertilization, suggesting that the timing of implantation may ordinarily be determined by the embryo (Bergh and Navot 1992). The corpus luteum also appears to have a finite period during which it is responsive to hCG. Late implanting embryos may not be able to effectively rescue the corpus luteum.

Temporal constraints on ovarian, embryonic, and endometrial receptivity may form the basis for the observation that embryo–endometrial synchrony is required for successful implantation. The existence of a defined endometrial window of implantation implies that alterations in the biochemical events which surround this period of endometrial receptivity might predispose to a failure of implantation. In *in vitro* fertilization (IVF), the implantation rate rarely exceeds 25–40 per cent, despite apparent optimization of ovulation induction, fertilization, and embryo manipulation, suggesting the existence of such defects. Luteal phase defect (LPD) caused by a relative deficiency in the serum concentration or action of progesterone, may contribute to infertility and recurrent pregnancy loss. Recently, hydrosalpinges have also been reported to reduce success rates in IVF, presumably due to acquired defects in implantation (Kassabji *et al.* 1994; Strandell *et al.* 1994). Disturbances in endometrial function have also been implicated in unexplained infertility, with numerous examples of alterations in endometrial structure or biochemistry (Graham *et al.* 1990; Li *et al.* 1990; Klentzeris *et al.* 1991; Dockery *et al.* 1993; Lessey *et al.* 1995a), further evidence for occult defects of endometrial receptivity.

INTEGRINS

Integrins are heterodimeric glycoproteins consisting of α and β subunits and comprising a family of CAMs involved in such diverse processes as immunology, wound healing, embryogenesis and development, and the spread of cancer cells (Albelda and Buck 1990). As receptors for the ECM, these molecules are present on virtually all cells and participate in cell–cell and cell–substratum attachment, signal transduction, and interaction with the cytoskeleton. Maintenance of cell shape and polarity may be a primary function of these important molecules and forms the basis for hormone responsiveness and appropriate gene transcription. 'Dynamic reciprocity' was a term coined by Bissell (Bissell and Aggeler 1987) to describe how the ECM made by the cell can subsequently influence cellular phenotype. This vital connection between the outside and inside matrices of the cell has been reviewed by Getzenberg *et al.* (1990).

As shown in Table 7.1, the various integrin subunits pair in predictable ways to form integrins with specific ligand preferences. While some of these 20 known integrins bind only one ECM molecule, others, like $\alpha_3\beta_1$ or $\alpha_v\beta_3$ are promiscuous in their ability to recognize and bind to various ECM proteins. There are additional layers of complexity. Cell membrane composition may alter integrin binding affinity. The availability of certain extracellular components may influence the action of integrins or induce the expression of new integrins. Certain cells, such as platelets, express integrins that must first be activated before they are functional. Topographical distribution of integrins may vary greatly between cell tyes. Certain integrins also rely on other integrins to cooperate in binding to ECM. On balance, these multifaceted molecules are well suited for the diverse functions they serve within the body. It may not be surprising, therefore, that integrins are found to undergo dynamic and complex changes in the endometrium during the menstrual cycle and early pregnancy. Complementary changes are encountered as well as in the pre- and post-implantation embryo and in developing placenta.

INTEGRINS AND THE ENDOMETRIUM

The initial reports of endometrial integrin expression appeared in 1992 (Lessey *et al.* 1992; Tabibzadeh 1992). Based on these early investigations it was immediately apparent that these cell adhesion molecules would be of interest in the study of human implantation. While many integrins were constitutively expressed on both epithelial and stromal cells, it was also noted that at least three integrin subunits (α_1, α_4, and β_3) were regulated during the menstrual cycle. The first two appear at the time of ovulation, and the α_4 subunit 'turns off' at the close of the window of implantation, around cycle day 24 to 25. The latter pairs with the α_v subunit to form the $\alpha_v\beta_3$

Table 7.1   Pairing of individual α and β integrin subunits and ligand preference

	β_1	β_2	β_3	β_4	β_5	β_6	β_7	β_8
α_1	Coll, LM							
α_2	Coll, LM							
α_3	Coll, LM, FN†							
α_4	FN						Peyers patch, FN, VCAM-1, addressin	
α_5	FN†							
α_6	LM			LM				
α_7	LM							
α_8	Tenascin, FN, VN							
α_9	Tenascin							
α_v	FN, VN†		VN, FN, FB, vWF, TSP, OP, BS†		VN†	FN		?
α_x		FB, C3bi						
α_m		FX, FB, C3bi, ICAM-1						
α_L		ICAM-1,2						
α_{IIb}			FB, vWF, FN†					

† recognizes the RGD signal peptide.
Coll = collagen; LM = laminin; FN = fibronectin; VN = vitronectin; FB = fibrinogen; vWF = von Willebrand factor; OP = osteopontin; BSP = bone sialoprotein 1; ICAM-1 and -2 = intercellular adhesion molecules; VCAM = ? cell adhesion molecule; FX = factor X; C3bi = complement component C3bi.

vitronectin receptor, which appears on the endometrial epithelium around cycle day 20, at the same time that Hertig and co-workers had estimated that embryos first attach to the uterine lining. These integrin profiles have subsequently been confirmed by other investigators (Bischof *et al.* 1993; Klentzeris *et al.* 1993; Ruck *et al.* 1994; Taskin *et al.* 1994). Still more complex patterns of cycle-specific integrin changes have recently been reported in glandular (Lessey *et al.* 1994*a*) and luminal (Lessey *et al.* 1995*b*) epithelium and in the decidualized stroma of pregnancy (Lessey *et al.* 1994*a*; Ruck *et al.* 1994). As shown in Table 7.2, the cellular distribution of these molecules in the endometrium is complex and may vary with the time of the cycle and the cell type examined. While not all studies agree on the particular elements of this table, there is general consensus that such changes are important for a better understanding of normal implantation.

The general profile of integrins in human endometrium is similar to that seen in other tissues. As shown in Fig. 7.1, the glandular epithelial cells primarily express receptors for the components of the BM (i.e. laminin, collagen). The pattern of staining for these integrin subunits is also of interest. Note that α_6 and its pairing partner,

Table 7.2 Distribution of integrin subunits in endometrium throughout the menstrual cycle and early pregnancy, shown by degree of immunohistochemical staining

	Coll/LM					FN/VN						Tenascin
	α_1	α_2	α_3	α_6	β_4	α_4	α_5	α_v	β_3	β_5	β_6	α_9
Glandular												
Proliferative	○	●	●	●B	●B	○	○	○	○	*	○	○
Early secretory	●	●	●	●	●	●	○	*	○	●	○	*
Mid secretory	●	●	●	●	●	●	○	●	●	●	○	●
Late secretory	●	●	●	●	●	○	○	●	●	●	○	●
Pregnancy	○	*	●	*	●	○	○	●	●	?	○	?
Stromal												
Proliferative	○	○	○	●	○	○	●	*	*	*	○	○
Early secretory	*	○	○	●	○	○	●	*	*	*	○	○
Mid secretory	*	○	*	*	○	○	●	*	*	●	○	○
Late secretory	●	○	●	*	○	○	●	●	●	●	○	○
Pregnancy	●	○	●	●	○	○	●	●	●	●	○	○
Luminal												
Proliferative	○	*	●	●	●	○	○	○	○	*	*	●
Early secretory	○	*	●	●	●	○	○	○	○	●	*	●
Mid secretory	○	○	●	●	●	○	○	●	●	●	*	●
Late secretory	○	●	●	●	●	○	○	●	●	●	*	●
Pregnancy	○	*	●	*	●	○	○	●	●	?	*	?

B signifies basolateral distribution of staining.
● corresponds to + or ++ staining;
* corresponds to ± staining;
○ corresponds to – staining.

β_4 (panels C and D, respectively) stain the basal pole of the epithelial cells. The $\alpha_2\beta_1$ and $\alpha_3\beta_1$ also localize primarily to the epithelial cells of the endometrium, while the classic fibronectin receptor, $\alpha_5\beta_1$, localizes to stromal cells, in an environment rich in fibronectin. Using panels of antibodies in a blinded study, this pattern was demonstrated convincingly (Lessey *et al.* 1994a). Three cycle-dependent integrins also form a striking pattern of expression, when an index of staining intensity (HSCORE) is plotted against histologic dating criteria. As shown in Fig. 7.2, all three of the integrins $\alpha_1\beta_1$, $\alpha_4\beta_1$ and $\alpha_v\beta_3$ are expressed on endometrial epithelium only during the secretory phase, but each maintains its unique pattern. All three integrins are co-expressed only during the narrow window of implantation, thought to occur on cycle days 20 to 24. As such, these integrins may provide one of the first set of immunohistochemical markers of the time of maximal uterine receptivity.

The endometrial epithelium is not the only cell type that undergoes programmatic changes in integrin expression; the decidua of early pregnancy is also an active site of such changes (Lessey *et al.* 1994a; Ruck *et al.* 1994). With decidualization, the stromal cell invests itself in a pericellular basement membrane, mimicking the epithelial cells of

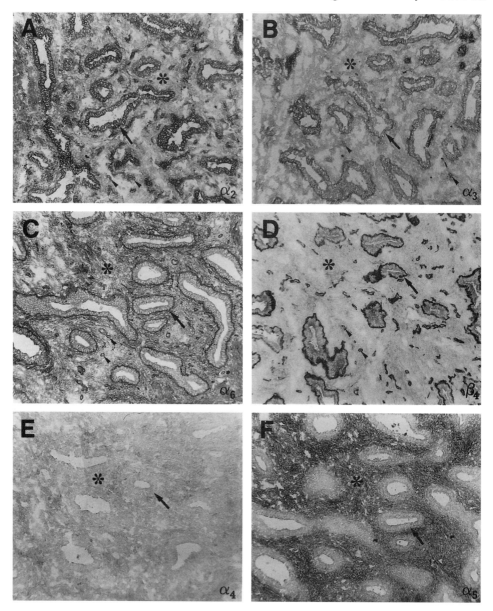

Fig. 7.1 The profile of integrins in normal endometrium in frozen sections. Immuno-histochemical staining of the collagen/laminin receptor subunits α_2 (A), α_3 (B), α_6 (C), and β_4 (D) show prominent staining of epithelium (arrows) and microvessels (arrowheads) without significant stromal staining (asterisks) for α_2, α_3, and β_4. Note basolateral staining for α_3 and α_6, and basal staining for β_4. The immunoreactions (areas of dark staining) were developed by the avidin–biotin–peroxidase complex using diaminobenzidine as a chromogen. For greater sensitivity, no counterstain was applied. Magnification ×125. With permission from the publisher, Rockefeller Press, NY.

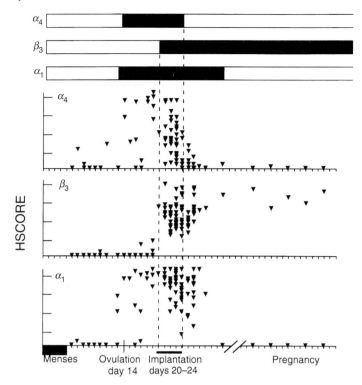

Fig. 7.2 Relative intensity of staining for the epithelial $\alpha4$, $\beta3$ and $\alpha1$ integrin subunits throughout the menstrual cycle and in early pregnancy. Immunohistochemical staining was assessed by a blinded observer using the semi-quantitative HSCORE (ranging from) to 4) and correlated to the estimate of histological dating based on pathologic criteria or by LMP in patients undergoing therapeutic pregnancy termination. The negative staining (open bars) was shown for immunostaining of an average HSCORE ≤ 0.7, for each of the three integrin subunits. Positive staining for all three integrin subunits was seen only during a 4 day interval corresponding to cycle day 20–24, based on histologic dating criteria. This interval of integrin co-expression corresponds to the putative window of implantation. Of the three, only the $\alpha v\beta3$ integrin was seen in the epithelium of pregnant endometrium. Reproduced with permission of the America Society of Reproductive Medicine.

the pre-implantation endometrium. There is a concomitant increase in the BM-specific integrins $\alpha_3\beta_1$ and $\alpha_6\beta_1$; and $\alpha_v\beta_3$. These changes probably serve to both limit trophoblast invasion and initate signal transduction directed towards the embryo. At the same time, the ECM and the associated integrin profile maintains the structural integrity of the decidua, which supports the pregnancy for the length of gestation.

Based on what is presently known, the regulation of integrin expression in the endometrium appears to be quite complex. While the cells of endometrial cancer may lose the ability to express certain integrins, or express inappropriate integrins (Lessey *et al.* 1995c), the pattern observed in the endometrium of normally cycling women is tightly regulated. Evidence for hormonal regulation was first suggested by

Tabibzadeh and Satyaswaroop in 1990, who showed that progesterone would induce the α_1 integrin subunit in explant cultures of proliferative phase endometrium (Tabibzadeh and Satyaswaroop 1990). This phenomenon has also been demonstrated in a well-differentiated endometrial adenocarcinoma cell line (Ishikawa), provided progesterone receptors (PR) are first induced by oestradiol priming (Lessey *et al.* 1995*d*). In normal endometrial epithelium, the loss of PR by cycle days 19 to 20 is associated with the appearance of $\alpha_v\beta_3$. In luteal phase defect, histologic delay is associated with an abnormal persistence of epithelial PR and a lack of $\alpha_v\beta_3$ (Lessey *et al.* 1996*e*). Medical treatment which effectively restores normal histology and epithelial PR results in the appropriate return of the $\alpha_v\beta_3$ integrin. These data suggest that the $\alpha_v\beta_3$ integrin is a progesterone-suppressed protein.

Cytokines and growth factors are also potent inducers and inhibitors of integrins (Lessey and Castelbaum 1995). It is not surprising to find that integrin levels in both stromal and epithelial cells respond to various growth factors and cytokines with either induction or downregulation *in vitro* (Grosskinsky *et al.* 1996; Somkuti *et al.* 1996*a*). Such complexities in integrin regulation probably contribute to the establishment of defects in endometrial receptivity, such as those seen in endometriosis and hydrosalpinx, when a proper endocrine or paracrine milieu is not achieved.

INTEGRINS AND THE EARLY EMBRYO

Placental cells undergo complex developmental patterns of integrin expression that correlate with normal and pathologic conditions (Damsky *et al.* 1994). The ontogeny of integrins in the fertilized ovum suggests a role for both early development and embryo attachment. Clearly, the involvement of integrins in the establishment of embryonic receptivity remains poorly understood. As demonstrated by Damsky and co-workers (Sutherland *et al.* 1993), the mouse embryo expresses two fibronectin receptors ($\alpha_5\beta_1$ and $\alpha_v\beta_3$) on the outer, apical portions of the surface epithelium. The $\alpha_1\beta_1$ collagen receptor is associated with an invasive phenotype and appears only at the time of trophoblast invasion. Others have confirmed these findings in mouse (Schultz and Armant 1995) and human embryo (Campbell *et al.* 1995). Both $\alpha_5\beta_1$ and $\alpha_v\beta_3$ recognize and bind proteins which have the three amino acid sequence Arg–Gly–Asp (RGD). Small peptides with this sequence block embryo attachment and outgrowth *in vitro* (Armant *et al.* 1986).

The $\alpha_4\beta_1$ integrin appears to play a role in implantation as well. Using gene knockout studies, homozygote α_4-deficient mice have early lethal defects involving both placental and cardiac development (Yang *et al.* 1995). The α_4 integrin recognizes the alternatively spliced fetal fibronectin which is elaborated by the embryo and placenta. This material has been toted as embryonic 'glue' that helps embryos adhere to the endometrium (Feinberg *et al.* 1991). This form of fibronectin may interact with endometrial α_4 during the window of implantation to signal the endometrial cells and alter their phenotypic behaviour. It appears that fibronectin may also influence the embryo itself, as was recently reported for hatching rates in cultured embryos exposed to this extracellular component (Turpeenniemi-Hujanen *et al.* 1995).

The presence of $\alpha_v\beta_3$ on the apical surface of the pre-implantation blastocyst and on the luminal surface of receptive endometrium is a fascinating finding. Platelets which maintain the similar integrin, $\alpha_{IIa}\beta_3$, undergo cell–cell attachment through an RGD-containing bridging molecule, fibrinogen. Curiously, the endometrium also synthesizes and secretes a candidate bridging molecule which possesses two RGD sites, named osteopontin (Young *et al.* 1990). Analogous to platelets, embryo–endometrial interaction may be the result of common binding to such a bridging molecule through co-expression of the $\alpha_v\beta_3$ integrin.

MODELS OF IMPLANTATION BASED ON INTEGRINS

The establishment of endometrial receptivity probably involves both the expression of molecules that allow implantation and the removal of barriers to embryo–endometrial interactions. A receptor mediated model of implantation must consider not only the integrins but also members of the cadherin family, immunoglobulin family, and the selectins; models of cell–cell adhesion involving these moieties have been reviewed elsewhere (Hynes 1994). To enable integrins or other small CAMs on the embryo and endometrial luminal epithelium to interact, it appears that certain barriers must first be removed. In the mouse, in which implantation occurs on post-coital days 4 to 5, large bulking molecules known as mucins are expressed by the luminal cells of the pre-receptive endometrium. The study of one of these mucins, MUC-1, reveals that this thick layer of material disappears at the time that implantation normally occurs by post-coital day 4 (Surveyor *et al.* 1993). Mechanisms which block implantation in the human may be similar.

Given what is now known about the patterns of integrin expression during the window of endometrial receptivity, several possible mechanisms of implantation can be proposed. The embryo and endometrium must initially interact through epithelial contacts at their apical surfaces. Three sequential integrin-mediated events that result in successful implantation are summarized in Fig. 7.3. In the initial phase of *apposition* and *adhesion*, endometrial and embryonic surface epithelia recognize and bind to each other. Pinopods are an ultrastructural feature of the peri-implantation endometrium in both rodents and humans (Psychoyos 1995) and are markers of the window of implantation (Nikas *et al.* 1995) It is postulated that these evanescent structures remove extrauterine fluid and bring the embryo into close contact with the surface endometrial epithelium. As shown in Fig. 7.4 A, endometrial pinopods *and* $\alpha_v\beta_3$ expression (Fig. 7.4 C) appear to colocalize to the apical poles of the surface endometrium. The embryo and the invading portions of the early placenta also express this integrin. As shown in Fig. 7.4 B, the distal columns of the human placental cytotrophoblast strongly express this integrin, suggesting that later events of trophoblast/decidua interaction may also involve this receptor. The stroma also expresses $\alpha_v\beta_3$ as early as cycle day 24, in the areas of predecidualization surrounding the arterioles (Fig. 7.4 D). Osteopontin, an RGD-containing peptide made by the glandular epithelium and later by the decidualized stroma, maintains a similar pattern of staining to that of $\alpha_v\beta_3$ (not shown), suggesting that all the elements are present to

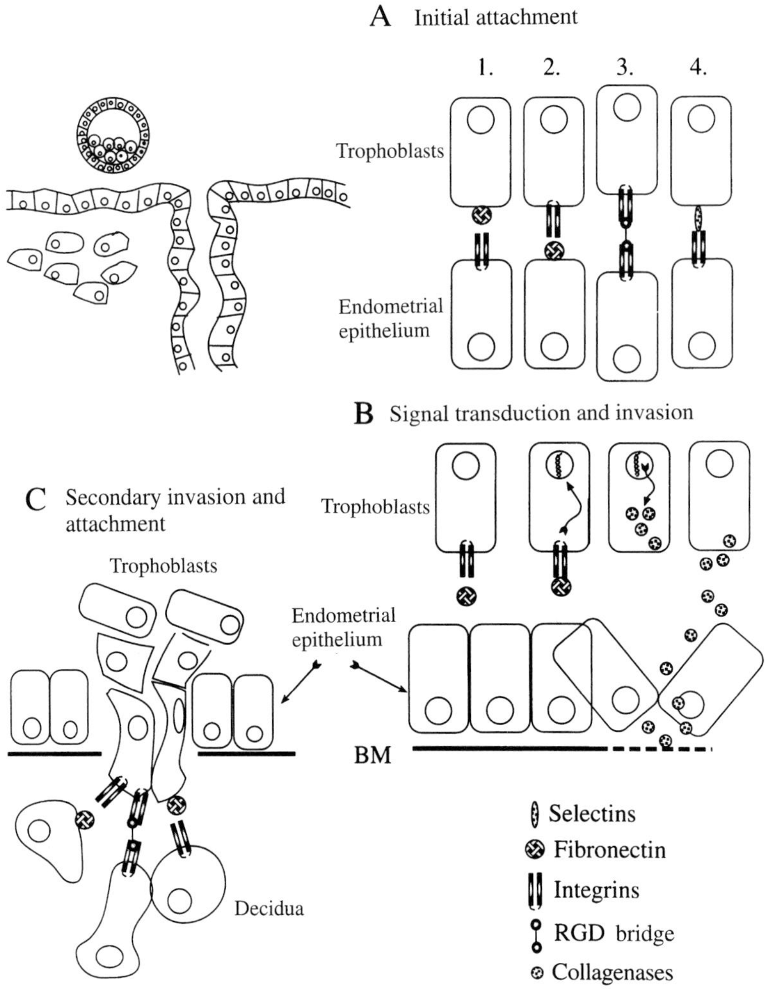

Fig. 7.3 Schematic representation of the early stages of implantation. As illustrated on the upper left, the embryo enters the endometrial cavity between cycle days 16 and 18 prior to implantation. Endometrial–embryonic epithelium must interact as part of the initial adhesion event (A). Models of cell–cell adhesion include integrin interaction with extracellular matrix molecules, like fibronectin, or through homeotypic (integrin–integrin) or heterotypic (integrin–selectin) interactions. Other models are possible (see Hynes 1994). During the phase of invasion through the basement membrane, integrins have been shown to mediate signal transduction leading to the synthesis of matrix metalloproteinases (B). In the secondary invasion and attachment, intruding trophoblast cells interact with the underlying stroma and the fibrinogen-rich extracellular matrix milieu (C). Again, multiple mechanisms of cell–cell adhesion may be postulated. The upregulation of multiple integrins in the human decidua argues for a role of these molecules in this phase of embryo–endometrial interaction.

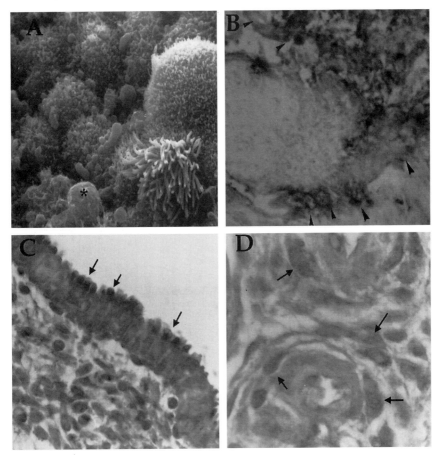

Fig. 7.4 Photomicrographs of endometrial and trophoblast cells. Pinopods are structures that protrude from the apical pole of the endometrial epithelium, demonstrated here using scanning electron microscopy (A; asterisk). These protrusions from the endometrial surface are also the site of intense $\alpha_v\beta_3$ immunostaining (arrowheads; C). The invading columns of cytotrophoblast (arrows) also express large amounts of this integrin (B). The temporal shift from epithelial to stromal attachment is associated with an increase in $\alpha_v\beta_3$ expression by the predecidualized areas in the endometrium (D). These patterns of expression are consistent with a direct role for this integrin in the process of implantation and the cell–cell contact that is observed in the implantation site. (Magnification: A = ×3000; B–D = ×250).

allow embryo–endometrial interaction through the activity of integrins. The possible models of early cell–cell attachment are summarized in Fig. 7.3 A.

As first demonstrated by Werb, placental cells experience signal transduction after engagement with the ECM (Werb *et al.* 1990). Synthesis and secretion of specific matrix metalloprotenases (MMPs) result in the local breakdown of ECM which contributes to the invasive phenotype of trophoblast. Signals may also be transmitted from the embryo to the endometrial cells through elaboration of ECM or by secretion of specific paracrine signals. As an example, cytokines, known to be made by the embryo, such as IL-1 and TNFα have been shown to downregulate the α_6 integrin subunit on both endothelial (Defilippi *et al.* 1992) and decidual cells (Grosskinsky *et al.* 1995) *in vitro*. Loss of $\alpha_6\beta_1$ or $\alpha_6\beta_4$ would result in detachment of epithelial cells from their BM to facilitate access of the MMPs to the underlying ECM. A schematic model of these processes is shown in Fig. 7.3 B.

A secondary phase of invasion and attachment occurs beneath the surface of the luminal epithelium. The decidua is rich in fibronectin, recognized by trophoblast integrins $\alpha_5\beta_1$ and $\alpha_v\beta_3$, which are fibronectin receptors. The distal columns of invading cytotrophoblast cells express large amounts of both these integrins ($\alpha_v\beta_3$ is shown in Fig. 7.4 B). The former has been shown to interact with insulin-like growth factor binding protein 1 (IGF-BP-1), an RGD-containing protein made by the decidua (Irwin *et al.* 1995). The latter binds decidual or embryonic fibronectin, and potentially recognizes decidual osteopontin, bridging between trophoblastic and decidual $\alpha_v\beta_3$. These various models of cell–cell adhesion between invading cytotrophoblast and decidualized stroma are summarized in Fig. 7.3 C. While much remains to be discovered about the molecular events involved in implantation, such theories will form the basis for future experiments in this field using appropriate animal and cell culture models.

DEFECTS IN ENDOMETRIAL RECEPTIVITY

Based on our early studies of the $\alpha_v\beta_3$ integrin, we reasoned that the abrupt increase in expression of this integrin on cycle day 20 of the menstrual cycle could be useful for the study of patients with infertility and luteal phase defect. As a disorder characterized by histologic delay of endometrial maturation, the $\alpha_v\beta_3$ integrin should not be expressed in endometrial biopsies from LPD patients when the biopsy is performed during cycle days 20–24. This was indeed found to be the case (Lessey *et al.* 1992). Abnormally low or absent levels of the $\alpha_v\beta_3$ integrin are also observed in endometrial samples from women without histologic delay, associated with mild forms of endometriosis (Lessey *et al.* 1994*b*). In such cases, the putative defects in endometrial receptivity must be considered *occult*, since these samples would otherwise be considered normal by traditional histologic dating criteria. Other abnormalities of the endometrium have been noted as well in women with endometriosis (Fedele *et al.* 1990) and unexplained infertility (Graham *et al.* 1990; Li *et al.* 1990; Klentzeris *et al.* 1991; Dockery *et al.* 1993; Lessey *et al.* 1995*a*). The lack of $\alpha_v\beta_3$ in these women appears to identify individuals with a profound decrease in cycle fecundity. In follow-up studies of over 50 such patients in the past four years, none conceived with expectant management alone, while over 80 per cent of women with endometriosis and normal $\alpha_v\beta_3$ integrins achieved pregnancy. The cornerstone of the current dogma that minimal or mild endometriosis does not cause infertility resides in this phenomenon of pregnancy with 'expectant management'. The use of specific markers such as the integrins may clarify such controversies and identify modes of therapy that are efficacious in subsets of truly affected individuals.

Using unexplained infertility (UI) in a model population to study for defects in uterine receptivity, we reported that $\alpha_v\beta_3$ was missing in two distinct subsets of patients. The first, which we have named *type I* defects, exhibited endometrium with maturational delay of more than three days, consistent with luteal phase defect. In a second group, women with minimal or mild endometriosis were found who exhibited 'in phase' endometrial biopsies, yet lacked appropriate expression of the epithelial $\alpha_v\beta_3$ integrin. These *type II* defects represent, we believe, an occult endometrial failure, not related to serum progesterone or epithelial PR. While treatment of type I defects with progesterone support restores both histology and integrin status, such treatment in the type II defects is without effect. We postulate that type II defects may reflect an altered paracrine milieu, initiated by endometriotic implants directly, or through the recruitment of activated macrophages in the peritoneal fluid (Lessey *et al.* 1994*b*). Type II defects are also found in some women with hydrosalpinges (Lessey *et al.* 1994*c*). Identification of the substances in the peritoneal or hydrosalpinx fluid which alter integrin expression will be of potential interest for research into contraception targeting the endometruim. The use of oral contraceptives has recently been shown to alter the expression of certain cycle-dependent integrins, effectively arresting the endometrium in a non-receptive state (Somkuti *et al.* 1995). Perhaps other pharmacological strategies will be adopted that shift or eliminate the window of implantation for purposes of contraception.

CONCLUDING REMARKS

Studies of the endometrium and of embryos have provided compelling evidence that the window of implantation is characterized by the expression of certain cell adhesion receptors that could orchestrate the timing and sequence of embryo–endometrial interactions. Due to their sheer complexity and versatility, integrins are good candidate markers of the window of implantation, and perhaps are directly involved in the cascade of molecular events that lead to successful implantation. Future investigations can be divided into three areas. First, by using appropriate research models, we hope to demonstrate the role of integrins and ECM in implantation. Reconstructing the cells of the endometrium *in vitro* has already yielded important clues about the regulation of implantation through signal transduction. Progress is also being made using the mouse as a model for implantation *in vivo*. Similarities between integrins, growth factors, and cytokines suggest this is an excellent model to study.

A second line of research will investigate the utility of integrin expression for the diagnosis and treatment of infertility patients. Current treatment protocols for patients with idiopathic infertility remain largely empiric, and can be expensive and frustrating. Diagnosis of minimal and mild endometriosis through the use of integrins or other endometrial markers may save millions of health care dollars by identifying only those women at risk, who may directly benefit from diagnosis and appropriate therapy.

A third approach will include a search for better and safer forms of contraception. Understanding the mechanisms of implantation will undoubtedly lead to effective methods to block this event by targeting either embryonic or endometrial antigens.

Regulation of integrin expression may also provide a novel pharmacological approach to modulate the window of implantation or embryonic receptivity.

The implantation site is a location of intense cellular activity, mediated by both endocrine and paracrine factors, leading to highly specific interactions of the cells from maternal and embryonic origin. It is, in fact, hard to identify any aspect of this amazing process that does not involve at least one member of the CAM superfamily. The excitement generated by the study of integrins in the endometrium and embryo will probably continue to grow as new discoveries are made. Implantation is, indeed, the last frontier of reproductive biology.

ACKNOWLEDGEMENTS

This work was supported by the National Institutes of Health grants HD-29449 and HD-30476, Bethesa, Maryland, and Berlex Laboratories, Inc. Wayne, New Jersey. The author would like to thank Drs Clayton A. Buck, Art J. Castelbaum, Lynda Wolf, Steve G. Somkuti, and Jinhai Sun for their significant contributions to these studies.

REFERENCES

Albelda, S.M. and Buck, C.A. (1990). Integrins and other cell adhesion molecules. *FASEB Journal*, **4**, 2868–80.

Armant, D.R., Kaplan, H.A., Mover, H., and Lennarz, W.J. (1986). The effect of hexapeptides on attachment and outgrowth of mouse blastocysts cultured *in vitro*: evidence for the involvement of the cell recognition tripeptide Arg-Gly-Asp. *Proceedings of the National Academy of Sciences, USA*, **83**, 6751–5.

Bergh, P.A. and Navot, D. (1992). The impact of embryonic development and endometrial maturity on the timing of implantation. *Fertility and Sterility*, **58**, 537–42.

Bischof, P., Redard, M., Gindre, P., Vassilakos, P., and Campana, A. (1993). Localization of alpha 2, alpha 5 and alpha 6 integrin subunits in human endometrium, decidua and trophoblast. *European Journal of Obstetrics, Gynecology and Reproductive Biology*, **51**, 217–26.

Bissell, M.J. and Aggeler, J. (1987). Dynamic reciprocity: how do extracellular matrix and hormones direct gene expression? In *Mechanisms of signal transduction by hormones and gowth factors*, (ed. J. Smoe), p. 251. Alan R. Liss, New York.

Campbell, S., Swann, H.R., Seif, M.W., Kimber, S.J., and Aplin, J.D. (1995). Cell adhesion molecules on the oocyte and preimplantation human embryo. *Human Reproduction*, **10**, 1571–8.

Damsky, C.H., Librach, C., Lim K-H., Fitzgerald, M.L. , McMaster, M.T., Janatpour, M., *et al.* (1994). Integrin switching regulates normal trophoblast invasion. *Development*, **120**, 3657–66.

Defilippi, P., Silengo, L., and Tarone, G. (1992). $\alpha_6\beta_1$ integrin (laminin receptor) is down-regulated by tumor necrosis factor α and interleukin-1 β in human endothelial cells. *Journal of Biological Chemistry*, **267**, 18303–7.

Dockery, P., Pritchard, K., Taylor, A., Li, T.C., Warren, M.A., and Cooke, I.D. (1993). The fine structure of the human endometrial glandular epithelium in cases of unexplained infertility: a morphometric study. *Human Reproduction*, **8**, 667–73.

Enders, A.C. and Schlafke, S. (1969). Cytological aspects of trophoblast–uterine interactions in early implantation. *American Journal of Anatomy*, 125, 1–30.

Fedele, L., Marchini, M., Bianchi, S., Dorta, M., Arcaini, L., and Fontana, P.E. (1990). Structural and ultrastructural defects in preovulatory endometrium of normo-ovulating infertile women with minimal or mild endometriosis. *Fertility and Sterility*, 53, 989–93.

Feinberg, R.F., Kliman, H.J., and Lockwood, C.J. (1991). Is oncofetal fibronectin a trophoblast glue for human implantation? *American Journal of Pathology*, 138, 537–43.

Getzenberg, R.H., Pienta, K.J., and Coffey, D.S. (1990). The tissue matrix: cell dynamics and hormone action. *Endocrinology Reviews*, 11, 399–417.

Graham, R.A., Seif, M.W., Aplin, J.D., Li, T.C., Cooke, I.D., Rogers, A.W., Dockery, P. (1990). An endometrial factor in unexplained infertility. *British Medical Journal*, 300, 1428–31.

Grosskinsky, C.M., Yowell, C.W., Sun, J., Parise, L., and Lessey, B.A. (1995). Modulation of integrin expression in endometrial stromal cells *in vitro*. *Journal of Endicrinology and Metabolism*, 81, 2047–54.

Hertig, A.T., Rock, J., and Adams, E.C. (1956). A description of 34 human ova within the first 17 days of development. *American Journal of Anatomy*, 98, 435–93.

Hynes, R.O. (1994). The impact of molecular biology on models for cell adhesion. *Bioessays*, 16, 663–9.

Irwin, J.C., Dsupin, B.A., and Giudice, L.C. (1995). Insulin-like growth factor binding protein-1 (IGFBP-1) modulates interaction of isolated placental cytotrophoblasts with fibronectin and endometrial stromal cell cultures. *The Endocrine Society Annual Meeting*, Abst. 1–197, 162.

Kassabji, M., Sims, J.A., Butler, L., and Muasher, S.J. (1994). Reduced pregnancy outcome in patients with unilateral or bilateral hydrosalpinx after *in vitro* fertilization. *European Journal of Obstetrics, Gynecology and Reproductive Biology*, 56, 129–32.

Klentzeris, L.D., Bulmer, J.N., Li, T.C., Morrison, L., Warren, A., and Cooke, I.D. (1991). Lectin binding of endometrium in women with unexplained infertility. *Fertility and Sterility*, 56, 660–7.

Klentzeris, L.D., Bulmer, J.N., Trejdosiewicz, L.K., Morrison, L., and Cooke, I.D. (1993). Beta-1 integrin cell adhesion molecules in the endometrium of fertile and infertile women. *Human Reproduction*, 8, 1223–30.

Lessey, B.A. and Castelbaum, A.J. (1995). Integrins in the endometrium. *Reproductive Medicine Reviews*, 4, 43–58.

Lessey, B.A., Damjanovich, L., Coutifaris, C., Castelbaum, A., Albelda, S.M., and Buck, C.A. (1992). Integrin adhesion molecules in the human endometrium. Correlation with the normal and abnormal menstrual cycle. *Journal of Clinical Investigation*, 90, 188–95.

Lessey, B.A., Castelbaum, A.J., Buck, C.A., Lei, Y., Yowell, C.W., and Sun, J. (1994a). Further characterization of endometrial integrins during the menstrual cycle and in pregnancy. *Fertility and Sterility*, 62, 497–506.

Lessey, B.A., Castelbaum, A.J., Sawin, S.J., Buck, C.A., Schinner, R., Wilkins, B., Strom, B.L. (1994b). Aberrant integrin expression in the endometrium of women with endometriosis. *Journal of Clinical Endocrinology and Metabolism*, 79, 643–9.

Lessey, B.A., Castelbaum, A.J., Riben, M., Howarth, J., Tureck, R., and Meyer, W.R. (1994c). Effect of hydrosalpinges on markers of uterine receptivity and success in IVF. *American Fertility Society Annual Meeting* (Abstract).

Lessey, B.A., Castelbaum, A.J., Sawin, S.J., and Sun, J. (1995a). Integrins as markers of uterine receptivity in women with primary unexplained infertility. *Fertility and Sterility*, 63, 535–42.

Lessey, B.A., Ilesanmi, A.O., Sun, J., Lessey, M.A., Harris, J., and Chwalisz, K. (1995b). Luminal and glandular endometrial epithelium express integrins differentially throughout the menstrual cycle: implications for implantation, contraception, and infertility. *American Journal of Reproductive Immunology*, (In press.)

Lessey, B.A., Albelda, S., Buck, C.A., *et al.* (1995c). Distribution of integrin cell adhesion molecules in endometrial cancer. *American Journal of Pathology*, **146**, 717–26.

Lessey, B.A., Ilesanmi, A., Castelbaum, A.J., Yuan, L.-W., Somkuti, S., and Chwalisz, K. (1995d). Characterization of a functional progesterone receptor in a well-differentiated endometrial adenocarcinoma cell line (Ishikawa). *Journal of Clinical Endocrinology and Metabolism*, (In press.)

Lessey, B.A., Yeh, I.-T., Castelbaum, A.J., Korzeniowski, P., Sun, J., and Chwalisz, K. (1996). Endometrial progesterone receptors and markers of uterine receptivity in the window of implantation. *Fertility and Sterility*, **65**, 477–83.

Li, T.C., Dockery, P., Rogers, A.W., and Cooke, I.D. (1990). A qualitative study of endometrial development in the luteal phase: comparison between women with unexplained infertility and normal fertility. *British Journal of Obstetrics and Gynaecology*, **97**, 576–82.

Navot, D., Bergh, P.A., Williams, M., Garissi, G.J., Guzman, I., Sandler, B. *et al.* (1991). An insight into early reproductive processes through the *in vivo* model of ovum donation. *Journal of Clinical Endocrinology Metabolism*, **72**, 408–14.

Nikas, G., Drakakis, P., Loutradis, D., Mara-Skoufari, C., Koumantakis, E., Michalas, S., and Psychoyos, A. (1995). Uterine pinopodes as markers of the 'nidation window' in cycling women receiving exogenous oestradiol and progesterone. *Human Reproduction*, **10**, 1208–13.

Psychoyos, A. (1995). The implantation window: basic and clinical aspects. In *Frontiers in endocrinology*, (ed. T. Mori, T., Tominaga, T., Aono, and M., Hiroi. p. 57. Ares-Serono Symposia, Tokyo.

Ruck, P., Marzusch, K., Kaiserling, E., Horny, H.-P., Dietl, J., Geiselhart, A. *et al.* (1994). Distribution of cell adhesion molecules in decidua of early human pregnancy: an immunohistochemical study. *Laboratory Investigation*, **71**, 94–101.

Schultz, J.F. and Armant, D.R. (1995). β_1- and β_3-class integrins mediate fibronectin binding activity at the surface of developing mouse peri-implantation blastocysts. Regulation by ligand-induced mobilization of stored receptor. *Journal of Biological Chemistry*, **270**, 11522–31.

Somkuti, S.G., Yowell, C.W., Lei, Y., and Lessey, B.A. (1995). Epidermal growth factor and human uterine receptivity: regulation of the $\alpha_v\beta_3$ integrin vitronectin receptor. *Society of Gynecological Investigation Annual Meeting*, **O120**, 196.

Somkuti, S.G., Yowell, C.W., and Lessey, B.A. (1996). The effect of oral contraceptive pills on markers of endometrial receptivity. *Fertility and Sterility*, **65**, 484–8.

Strandell, A., Waldenström, U., Nilsson, L., and Hamberger, L. (1994). Hydrosalpinx reduces *in-vitro* fertilization/embryo transfer pregnancy rates. *Human Reproduction*, **9**, 861–3.

Surveyor, G.A., Gendler, S.J., Pemberton, L., Spicer, A.P., and Carson, D.D. (1993). Differential expression of Muc-1 at the apical cell surface of mouse uterine epithelial cells. *FASEB Journal*, **7**, 1151a.

Sutherland, A.E., Calarco, P.G., and Damsky, C.H. (1993). Developmental regulation of integrin expression at the time of implantation in the mouse embryo. *Development*, **119**, 1175–86.

Tabibzadeh, S. (1992). Patterns of expression of integrin molecules in human endometrium throughout the menstrual cycle. *Human Reproduction*, **7**, 876–82.

Tabibzadeh, S.S. and Satyaswaroop, P.G. (1990). Progestin-mediated induction of VLA-1 in glandular epithelium of human endometrium *in vitro*. 72nd Annual Meeting of The Endocrine Society, Abstract #700.

Taskin, O., Brown, R.W., Young, D.C., Poindexter, A.N., and Wiehle, R.D. (1994). High doses of oral contraceptives do not alter endometrial α_1 and $\alpha_v\beta_3$ integrins in the late implantation window. *Fertility and Sterility*, **61**, 850–5.

Turpeenniemi-Hujanen, T., Feinberg, R.F., Kauppila, A., and Puistola, U. (1995). Extracellular matrix interactions in early human embryos: implications for normal implantation events. *Fertility and Sterility*, **64**, 132–8.

Werb, Z., Tremble, P., and Damsky, C.H. (1990). Regulation of extracellular matrix degradation by cell–extracellular matrix interactions. *Cellular Differentiation and Development*, **32**, 299–306.

Yang, J.T., Rayburn, H., and Hynes, R.O. (1995). Cell adhesion events mediated by α_4 integrins are essential in placental and cardiac development. *Development*, **121**, 549–60.

Yoshinaga, K. (1989). Receptor concept in implantation research. In *Development of preimplantation embryos and their environment*, (ed. K. Yoshinaga and T. Mori p. 379. Alan Liss, New York.

Young, M.F., Kerr, J.M., Termine, J.D., Wewer, U.M., Wang, M.G., McBride. O.W., and Fischer, L.W. (1990). cDNA cloning, mRNA distribution and heterogeneity, chromosomal location, and RFLP analysis of human osteopontin (OPN). *Genomics*, **7**, 491–502.

8 | *Implantation and trophoblast differentiation*

E. Winterhager and O. Genbacev

INTRODUCTION

Implantation and subsequently placenta formation establish a transient, cooperative physical and biochemical interaction between the fetal and maternal compartments. Contact between fetal and maternal tissue is established by the trophectoderm, the first differentiated and functional embryonic organ which gives rise to the haemochorial placenta.

Several terms for the first steps of feto-maternal interaction have been used which are interchangeable but reflect different aspects of this process. The term 'implantation' emphasizes more the tolerance of uterine tissue to a semi-allograft. 'Nidation' implies a cooperative interaction between blastocyst and endometrium, whereas 'blastocyst invasion' stresses more the aggressive and tumour-like behaviour of the blastocyst. In spite of the fact that the implantation process includes all these different aspects it is a unique phenomenon. The most fascinating aspect is that two genetically different entities, embryo and mother, coexist in close contact for the benefit of the fetus and without harm to the host (mother). The complexity of this interaction and thereby the potential for disturbances is reflected in the high rate (about 50 per cent) of implantation failure. It has been shown recently using site-specific mutagenesis in mouse embryos that a high number of different gene-knockout mice died *in utero* not because of severe embryonic malformation but as a result of an inappropriate differentiation of the trophoblast (for reviews see Cross *et al.* 1994; Copp 1995). These facts confirm that placental development is highly regulated by a coordinated pattern of gene expression and that it is the most critical point for embryonic survival *in utero*. The identification of genes that regulate trophoblast differentiation will give important insights into the causes of embryonic death. To achieve this goal, it is necessary to introduce adequate *in vitro* models that will provide tools to study the regulation of trophoblast gene expression and differentiation under normal and pathological conditions. The focus of this chapter will be on specific markers for trophoblast cell differentiation at the fetal–maternal interface and on *in vitro* models that can be used to study mechanisms for these differentiation processes.

THE PRE- AND PERI-IMPLANTATION TROPHOBLAST

The morphogenesis of the human trophoblast during pre-implantation seems to be, in general, the same as described for other mammals (for a review see Edwards and

Brody 1995). Nearly all investigations on the early human trophoblast during pre-implantation are derived from *in vitro* observations, including *in vitro* fertilization programmes. The trophectoderm represents the trophoblast stem cells and gives rise to the specific epithelial cells unique to the placenta. The first step of differentiation of the trophoblast cell lineage starts with the compaction phase of the 8-cell stage, characterized by the expression of epithelial markers of the outer cells that give rise to the trophectoderm (Edwards and Brody 1995). In human pre-implantation embryos nothing is known about the expression of cell adhesion molecules such as E-cadherin and cell–cell communication via gap junctions, issues that have been investigated extensively in animal models (Magnuson *et al.* 1977; Vestweber *et al.* 1987; Nishi *et al.* 1991). The blastocyst is formed between days 4 and 5 post-fertilization and the expanding blastocyst escapes from the surrounding zona pellucida by hatching out. In *in vitro* experiments, hatching occurs via a small rupture of the zona pellucida through which the trophoblast penetrates, now ready to interact with the uterine epithelium. At this stage the blastocyst starts to produce its first signals, like oestrogen and hCG (Fishel *et al.* 1984; Bonduelle *et al.* 1988; Hay and Lopata 1988) to communicate with the maternal host.

The cell biology of the first steps of implantation in humans remains poorly understood because of very little available data. Most of our knowledge is derived from the Carnegie collection (O'Rahilly 1973) and from studies by Hustin and Franchimont (1992) of early implantation specimens from the collection of the late Professors Boyd and Hamilton (Cambridge, UK). Our understanding of the mechanisms of early implantation events is mainly provided by observations in non-human primates or laboratory animals. The steps common for all species with an invasive implantation modus seem to be blastocyst apposition and adhesion to the uterine epithelium followed by a penetration of the uterine epithelium by the trophoblast cells (Schlafke and Enders 1975). The cell biological mechanisms underlying this unique phenomenon of trophoblast–epithelial interaction are not completely understood either in humans or in animals (for a review see Denker 1993).

A better insight into these early events is of great clinical interest because of high implantation failure rates. A unique *in vitro* approach to study the earliest events of human implantation was made by Lindenberg *et al.* (1986). In these experiments, in which a human blastocyst was co-cultured with endometrium, it was demonstrated that penetration of the epithelium was performed by trophoblast protrusion, followed by establishment of a direct contact between trophoblast and the subepithelial tissue. Additional data about implantation in humans are not forthcoming for ethical reasons. In general, the mechanisms of implantation control in humans are probably less rigid. The fairly frequent occurrence of ectopic implantation in humans points to less tissue-specific embryo–maternal interaction being required than in other mammals.

Differentiation of the trophoblast is initiated during the implantation process, when a subpopulation of cytotrophoblast stem cells differentiates by fusion into the syncytiotrophoblast. These two cell populations, cyto- and syncytiotrophoblast, are characteristic of the prelacunar and lacunar stages of placental development (Boyd and Hamilton 1970; Benirschke and Kaufmann 1990). The ingrowth of mesenchyme into trophoblast sprouts leads to the formation of finger-like primary villi which marks the beginning of the villous stage of placentation (Benirschke and Kaufmann 1990).

POST-IMPLANTATION TROPHOBLAST

Trophoblast differentiation pathways

By branching, the villous tree adapts the growth of the placenta to the growth of the embryo—a process that has been studied and described extensively (Kaufmann *et al.* 1979; Jauniaux *et al.* 1992). In parallel with this process, trophoblast cells differentiate to form several cell subpopulations. Our basic knowledge of trophoblast differentiation is derived from morphological observations of first trimester placental bed biopsy specimens (Boyd and Hamilton 1970; Pijnenborg *et al.* 1980, 1983). The nomenclature for the developing subpopulations of trophoblast are, to a certain degree, confusing. As molecular mechanisms of trophoblast cell differention are still under investigation we propose a slightly modified classification of trophoblast based on their localization at the maternal–fetal interface (Table 8.1). The trophoblast itself can be classified into villous and extravillous cell populations.

The *villous trophoblast* resides in floating and anchoring chorionic villi. The mononuclear trophoblastic stem cells form a monolayer of polarized epithelial cells that are attached to the basal membrane of the chorionic villi that is, the cytotrophoblast, (CT) and are covered by the syncytiotrophoblast (ST). The latter is formed by fusion of the underlying CT, and is responsible for the exchange and transport functions of the placenta.

In the anchoring chorionic villi, CT cells can break through the ST and aggregate into multilayered columns. Cell columns—also referred to as intermediate trophoblast (Kurman *et al.* 1984)—come into contact with the uterine wall and give rise to the extravillous trophoblast. The CT from the distal part of adjacent columns come into close contact and form a continuous layer—the so-called trophoblastic shell. Cell islands are in many respects similar to cell columns, but as they are (in

Table 8.1   Classification of trophoblast cells during placentation based on their localization at the maternal–fetal interface

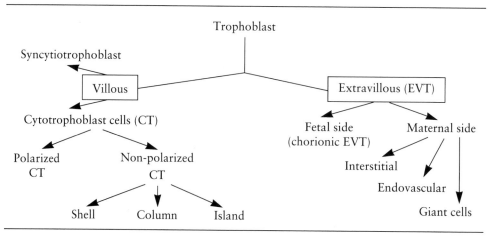

contrast to cell columns) not attached to the uterine wall they can be referred as 'free floating' columns.

Extravillous trophoblast (EVT) differentiates from the proliferating non-polarized CT of the cell column and migrates into the endometrium or ectopic sites of implantation to form interstitial and endovascular EVT cell populations. In addition to extravillous cytotrophoblast mononucleated cells, the placental bed contains multinucleated, non-polarized giant cells that are derived from extravillous cytotrophoblast by fusion and are considered as a final stage of EVT differentiation.

Different approaches have been used to gain more insight into the developmental and functional relationships between these trophoblast cell populations: investigation of specific markers of cell differentiation and function on both mRNA and protein level in specimens *in situ* (placental bed biopsy specimens from different stages of gestation); and use of *in vitro* models to mimic particular stages of post-implantation to study molecular mechanisms of trophoblast differentiation.

SPECIFIC MARKERS OF TROPHOBLAST DIFFERENTIATION

Villous trophoblast

The *syncytiotrophoblast* layer represents the main source of specific placental proteins that are secreted into the maternal circulation. The most extensively studied ones are hCG, the placenta-specific glycoprotein SP1, and human placental lactogen (hPL). Secretion of hCG by the ST is a critical step in maintaining pregnancy because of the signalling by hCG to maintain and develop the corpus luteum gravitates. The hCG α and β chains are regulated by many different factors and are expressed differently during pregnancy (reviewed by Jameson and Hollenberg 1993); hPL is expressed and secreted during pregnancy in increasing amounts, mainly by the ST (for a review see Edwards and Brody 1995). The pregnancy specific β-1-glycoprotein SP1, along with hCG, is one of the earliest proteins secreted by the ST (Bohn and Klaus 1976; Edwards and Brody 1995). The function of both hPL and SP1 during pregnancy is, in spite of many investigations, poorly understood.

The *villous* cytotrophoblastic cells are mitotically active mononucleated trophoblast cells that are organized as a monolayer of polarized cells underneath the ST or as aggregates of non-polarized cells in cell columns and in cell islands. Polarized CTs are characterized by the presence of tight junctions (Metz and Weihe 1980), expression of the integrin adhesion molecule receptor complex ($\alpha_6\beta_4$ integrin) which mediates CT interactions with the basement membrane, and by expression of E-cadherin receptor (Damsky *et al.* 1992).

Identification of the proliferative populations of CTs in the placental bed has been performed immunohistochemically with antibodies directed against different markers of cell proliferation such as Ki67 or PCNA (proliferation cell nuclear antigen). Two populations of mitotically active CTBs were thus identified: polarized CTs that are underlying the ST and non-polarized CTs from the proximal part of cell columns and cell islands. Proliferation of polarized CTs leads to the growth of syncytium, which is assumed to occur by fusion of newly divided cells by a process that has never been documented directly, *in vivo*. The population of proliferative, non-polarized CTs is restricted to the proximal part of the cell column adjacent to the basal lamina (Muehlhauser *et al.* 1991), whereas cells from the distal part of the column, as well as EVT cells, do not express markers of proliferation and are considered to be non-proliferative CTs. Taken together these data suggest that initiation of the different-iation programme within the column coincides with exit from the cell cycle and with cell depolarization. The precise mechanisms involved in the coordination and regu-lation of these processes are still unknown. It is, however, generally accepted that CT proliferation is controlled by complex interactions of growth factors and proto-oncogenes. Proto-oncogenes like c-*myc* and the tumour-suppressor gene products Rb and p53 have been investigated during different phases of gestation. All three gene products were identified in CTs of first trimester placentas and have been shown to decline to different extents during gestation (Roncalli *et al.* 1994; Marzusch *et al.* 1995). Thus these tumour-suppressor genes could be a part of a control mechanism for trophoblast cell proliferation. The role of the epidermal growth factor (EGF) in the regulation of CT proliferation has been studied extens-ively. EGF as well as EGF receptors have been detected in the ST and less so in CTs (Kawagoe *et al.* 1990; Hofmann *et al.* 1992) and were shown to be differentially expressed during gestation.

As already mentioned, the cytotrophoblastic column is the site of CT proliferation as well as of differentiation of EVT cells. Morphologically, the multilayered tro-phoblast cells of the juxtastromal compartment exhibit a close apposition to each other with adherent junctions and numerous desmosomes (Fig. 8.1(a)(b)). With increasing distance from their basal lamina, cell–cell contact is loosening, and cells separate from each other and acquire a more irregular shape. They detach from the cell column and get scattered between the decidual cells. This process is accom-panied by downregulation of the cell adhesion molecule E-cadherin (Damsky *et al.* 1992). Recently we found that the trophoblast cells near to the basal lamina express exclusively connexin40, a gap junction channel protein normally present in endothe-lial cells and heart tissue (Fig. 8.1(c)). Similar to E-cadherin, this connexin is down-regulated towards the distal part of cell islands and cell columns (von Ostau *et al.* 1995).

By analogy with tumour cells, it is believed that a loss of cell adhesion molecules as well as of cell–cell communication is accompanied by cell dedifferentiation and with acquisition of invasiveness (Frixen *et al.* 1991; Yamasaki 1991). In contrast to tumour cells, loss of polarization and of cell–cell contacts is not associated with trophoblast cell dedifferentiation, pointing to some substantial differences between the embryonic and tumour cells in the regulation of both proliferation and differentiation.

Extravillous trophoblast

The fundamental morphological studies of Pijnenborg and co-workers (Pijnenborg *et al.* 1980, 1983) have provided basic information about the organization of tro-phoblast and maternal cells at the maternal–fetal interface. These specimens offer the

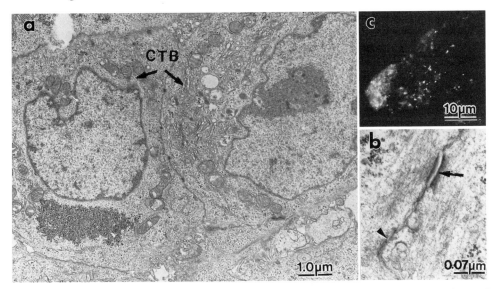

Fig. 8.1 Cytotrophoblast cells (CT) of the proximal part of a cell column from placental anchoring villi of 8–10 weeks of gestation. (a) Electron micrograph of two polygonal shaped CTs in close apposition to each other. (b) Higher magnification reveals desmosomes (arrow) and adherens junction (arrowhead) at the lateral membranes of two adjacent cells. (c) Immunohistochemical staining for connexin-40 demonstrates a punctate reaction typical of gap junction plaques.

unique possibility of visualizing anchoring villi with CTs that are migrating into the maternal tissue giving rise to EVT cells within the placental bed. CT differentiation into EVT cell populations is a complex multistep process that is marked by changes in cell–cell and in cell–matrix interactions, by activation of a cascade of proteolytic enzymes and their inhibitors, and by expression of HLA-G class I molecules.

Placental bed EVT cells that are detached from the cell column and located at the maternal–fetal interface are characterized by a distinctive repertoire of integrins: subunit β_1, but not β_4, has been detected, and the alpha subunit was restricted to the α_1 and α_5 subunits. Thus, the predominant interactions of EVT cells with maternal cell-associated extra cellular matrix (ECM) involves laminin, fibronectin, and type IV collagen (for a review see Damsky *et al.* 1993). These changes in integrin patterns may reflect a greater cell motility due to a different binding capacity to laminin.

Parallel to the switch in the cell programme of cell–cell and cell–matrix interactions the trophoblast cells start to produce different proteases (Polette *et al.* 1994). Proteases, mainly plasminogen activators and metalloproteases, are generally involved in degradation of the ECM by trophoblast cells (for a review see Strickland and Richards 1992; Damsky *et al.* 1993). Using an *in vitro* Matrigel assay to study cytotrophoblast invasion and differentiation it was shown by Librach *et al.* (1991) that the 92 kDa type IV collagenase seems to be more responsible for trophoblast invasion than the plasminogen activations PA1 and PA2.

An additional 72 kDa type IV collagenase is secreted predominantly by the first trimester placenta in all types of trophoblast cells, giving a hint that both metallo-proteases are involved in the invasion process (Fernandez *et al.* 1992). Trophoblast invasiveness seems to be controlled by the uterine microenvironment, by production of the tissue inhibitor of metalloproteases, TIMP-1 and TIMP-2 (Graham and Lala 1992; Polette *et al.* 1994).

The transforming growth factor, TGFβ, produced by the decidua has a dual effect: it induces TIMP-1 secretion by trophoblast and decidua and also stimulates the inter-stitial trophoblast to form non-invasive multinucleated giant cells (for a review see Graham and Lala 1992). The stimuli involved, autocrine and/or paracrine, that are responsible for inducing the switch in gene expression from non-invasive to invasive trophoblast are still under investigation.

The observation that human CTs can express an unusual MHC class Ib molecule, HLA-G, is probably of great importance (Kovats *et al.* 1990; McMaster *et al.* 1995) because the expression of this class of molecule may protect these cells from destruc-tion by natural killer-like cells (Burt *et al.* 1991). At least this unusual expression of an MHC class I antigen in the trophoblast population seems to support this unrecog-nized invasion process. A subpopulation of the EVT cells colonize maternal arterial blood vessels by penetrating the arterial walls and replacing the endothelium. During this event the muscular layer of the arterial wall is replaced by fibrinoid material and the lumen of the spiral arteries becomes plugged by EVT cell aggregates (Wells and Bulmer 1988). Almost nothing is known about the cell biological mechanisms of endothelial replacement, reorganization of the blood vessels, and the fate of endo-vascular EVT plugs. The physiological significance of these changes is an increase in blood vessel diameter and in restistance to vasoconstrictive signals, resulting in an increase of blood flow in the placental bed. It has been suggested that EVT cells may contribute to the increase in vascularization of the implantation site by production of angiogenic factors by the EVT cells (Sharkey *et al.* 1993; Jackson *et al.* 1994). This hypothesis, however, awaits further experimental confirmation.

IN VITRO MODELS FOR DIFFERENTIATION OF THE POST-IMPLANTATION TROPHOBLAST

Explant culture of first trimester villi

Intact first trimester villi maintained on a matrix similar to either decidual ECM or basal lamina (Matrigel) can replicate many of the characteristics observed *in vivo* (Genbacev *et al.* 1992, 1993*a*,*b* 1994; Genbacev and Miller 1993). By 6–12 weeks of gestation the fetal portion of the placenta recovered from abortus material consists of both floating and anchoring chorionic villi and cell islands (Fig. 8.2(a),(b)). Anchoring villi that are detached from uterine decidua after abortion retain on their tips rem-nants of cell columns (Fig. 8.2(d)) that are *in vivo* sites of differentiation of EVTs. Therefore it is possible, by culturing the intact anchoring villi under appropriate con-ditions, to study the factors that are involved in the regulation of differentiation of EVT cell populations. In addition to cell columns, cell islands cultured on Matrigel

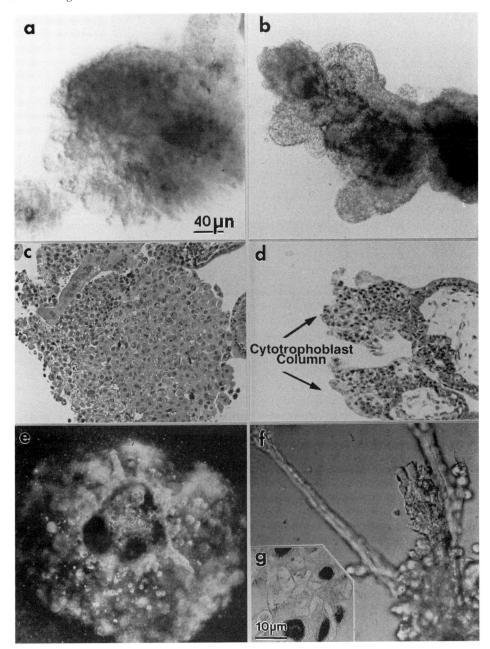

Fig. 8.2 Cell islands (a) and placental anchoring villi (b) of 8–10 weeks' gestation. Histological examination reveals that both cell islands (c) and columns (d) are formed from aggregates of non-polarized CTs. Cell islands (e) and villous explants (f) cultured on Matrigel show tremendous outgrowth. (a)–(f) are at the same magnification; at higher magnification (g) is an outgrowth generated by proliferation of CTs immunostained with antibodies against a proliferation cell nuclear antigen (PCNA).

(Fig. 8.2(c)) also give rise to EVT-like cells (Fig. 8.2(e),(f)). CTs from cell columns (Fig. 8.2(g)) and cell islands continue to proliferate *in vitro*, as demonstrated by their ability to incorporate bromodesoxyuridine or by expression of markers of cell proliferation such as PCNA and Ki67 (Genbacev *et al.* 1992, 1994). Newly formed CTs from the distal zone of anchoring villi (Genbacev *et al.* 1992) and from cell islands (Genbacev *et al.* 1996) lose their polarization and intercellular membrane contacts and switch their integrin expression to follow that characteristic for the distal zone of cell columns from the placental bed of the first trimester of pregnancy (Damsky *et al.* 1992; Fisher and Damsky 1993). Furthermore, CT cells stream out of the column, penetrate into the matrix by producing a zone of lysis (Genbacev *et al.* 1992), express markers of EVTs, and some of them form giant cells after 4–6 days in culture.

As this *in vitro* system replicates many of the *in vivo* characteristics of CT differentiation, it can be used to address different issues related to the regulation of this process. One of the factors involved in the regulation of trophoblast differentiation is the oxygen partial pressure, p_{O2}. Morphological studies of the placental bed have shown that the growing embryo is separated from the maternal circulation by the trophoblast shell at 12 weeks' gestation, when endovascular trophoblastic plugs are dislocated, and direct communication between maternal blood vessels and intervillous space becomes possible (Hustin and Franchimont 1992). The absence of intervillous space during the first trimester of pregnancy was further confirmed by angiography in first trimester hysterectomy specimens (Hustin and Schaaps 1987) and by colour Doppler imaging *in vivo* (Jaffe and Woods 1993). That this physical barrier affects oxygen supply to the tissue at the maternal–fetal interface was demonstrated directly by Rodesch *et al.* (1992) who showed that to p_{O2} in the intervillous space before 12 weeks of pregnancy is much lower (18 mmHg or 2.4 kPa) than later during the second and third trimester (40 mmHg or 5.3 kPa) of pregnancy.

By exposing villous explants or CTs to p_{O2} that are equal, lower, or higher than the p_{O2} of the intervillus space during the first trimester of pregnancy, we have demonstrated that oxygen is one of the factors regulating trophoblast differentiation along the invasive pathway (Genbacev *et al.* 1996). In the hypoxic environment (18 mmHg) the trophoblast cells progress only through the initial stages of the EVT differentiation programme. They upregulate DNA synthesis and express an integrin pattern characteristic for trophoblast cells from the proximal part of the columns, failing to switch their integrin pattern to $\alpha_1\beta_1$, that normally required for the acquisiton of an invasive phenotype. This failure in the differentiation programme is associated with the reduced ability of CTs to invade both Matrigel and decidual tissue explants (Genbacev *et al.* 1996). These *in vitro* data suggest that the balance between CT cell proliferation and differentiation can be modulated by oxygen tension and that, under *in vivo* conditions, p_{O2} at the maternal–fetal interface may regulate the shift of trophoblast gene expression.

The fact that many *in vivo* characteristics of trophoblast differentiation can be mimicked *in vitro* in the absence of endometrium supports the view that the early stages of placentation are not dependent on decidual signals (Fox 1992). As trophoblast differentiation along the invasive pathway in vitro does not occur in the absence of matrix proteins and is triggered by CT–ECM interactions (Genbacev *et al.*

1992), we hypothesize that similar mechanisms are operating *in vivo*, both at intrauterine as well as ectopic sites of implantation.

The pattern of EVT cells' differentiation from villous explants co-cultured with decidua on collagen type I (Vicovac *et al.* 1995) is very similar to the pattern described in explants maintained on ECM alone. However, its is difficult to compare quantitatively trophoblast invasion into matrix versus decidual fragments and to assess the role of maternal tissue in the regulation of EVT cell invasion.

In addition to supporting CT differentiation into EVT cells, ECM also supports the synthesis and secretion of placental hormones by syncytiotrophoblast. The production rate of both hCG and progesterone by villous explants cultured on Matrigel or collagen type I can be maintained at a constant rate for at least six days, along with a morphologically well preserved ST (Genbacev *et al.* 1992).

Various explant culture techniques have been used to study differentiation of the ST. They include both static (Cemerikic and Genbacev 1989; Castellucci *et al.* 1990; Maruo *et al.* 1992) and dynamic (by superfusion) (Barnea *et al.* 1991) culture systems. Since during the first 12 weeks of gestation materno–placental circulation is not yet established, the static culture system in which the villous explants are immersed seems to mimic more accurately the intervillous space environment. The factors regulating ST hormone and protein expression are discussed elsewhere (see Chapter 10).

Cell culture of first trimester cytotrophoblast

Trophoblast cells isolated from placentas obtained from first trimester abortions comprise a mixture of villous CTs containing CTs that are underlying ST and CTs derived from cell columns and cell islands. *In vitro* models have been developed in which isolated human cytotrophoblasts were plated on Matrigel or matrix components. Those cells from first trimester placentas are capable of degrading this matrix rapidly and penetrating it (Fisher *et al.* 1989; Librach *et al.* 1991; Fisher and Damsky 1993). They resemble, in many aspects, non-polarized CTs from the cell columns and differentiate *in vitro* into invasive subpopulations of EVT cells.

Isolated CT cells express three classes of molecules that are characteristic for interstitial and endovascular EVT cell populations *in vivo*: integrins (Damsky *et al.* 1993), metalloproteases (Fisher *et al.* 1989; Librach *et al.* 1991), and the unusual MHC-1 antigen (McMaster *et al.* 1995). The CT cultures have been also used to identify factors that regulate CT differentiation pathways through paracrine/autocrine mechanisms. For example, isolated CTs express EGF receptor mRNA and do not express transcripts for EGF and TGFα. Of five growth factors (TGFβ, PDGF-AA, PDGF-BB, EGF, and TNFα) tested, only EGF treatment led to an impressive increase in trophoblast invasiveness (Bass *et al.* 1994). Similar to results with explant cultures, isolated trophoblast cells cultured in hypoxic conditions for three days are not able to switch their integrin expression, nor can they invade Matrigel or penetrate decidual explants (Genbacev *et al.* 1996). Isolated CTs are therefore a unique model that can be used to study molecular mechanisms involved in the differentiation of villous tissue cytotrophoblast stem cells and assess CT invasiveness.

CONCLUDING REMARKS

Substantial progress has been made in our understanding of early peri-implantation stages of human trophoblast development. A rapidly growing list of cell and differentiation stage-specific markers has provided a better insight into trophoblast differentiation programmes under both *in vivo* and *in vitro* conditions. Mechanisms of cytotrophoblast invasion, as well as changes in cell–cell and cell–matrix interactions have been unravelled. However, many important aspects of implantation and trophoblast differentiation remain poorly understood. Signals responsible for the establishment of feto-maternal cooperation, an important characteristic of implantation, as well as factors that control trophoblast differentiation, are almost unknown. Based on some experimental evidence it is interesting to speculate that trophoblast cells may, by producing their own angiogenic factors, control microvascularization of the implantation site needed for subsequent vascular invasion, an essential step for the establishment of the feto-maternal circulation. Establishment of the feto-maternal circulation marks the end of the peri-implantation stage of trophoblast differentiation. As trophoblast stem cells during first trimester of pregnancy are exposed to a lower p_{O2} than later in gestation, the role of oxygen in the regulation of CT differentiation has been investigated recently and it has been shown that oxygen plays a role in regulating the balance between CT cell proliferation and differentiation programmes.

In contrast to the secretory products of the syncytiotrophoblast that are released into the maternal circulation, the identification of local factors produced by different trophoblast cell populations is much more difficult. Development and better characterization of *in vitro* models that can be used to mimic different stages of trophoblast development have provided new dynamic approaches which can be used to study the regulation of these differentiation programmes. It can be expected that by combining different organ, cell culture, and co-culture systems, it will become possible to identify and characterize both maternal and fetal signals. This information is essential for the future medical treatment of implantation failures and of some diseases of pregnancy.

ACKNOWLEDGEMENT

We would like to thank Dr Rebecca Beaconsfield, SCIP, University of London, UK, for critical reading and editing of this manuscript.

REFERENCES

Barnea, E.R., Feldmann, D., and Kaplan, M. (1991). Gestational age dependent, rapid and delayed effect of EGF upon hCG secretion by the first trimester explants. *Trophoblast Research*, **6**, 173–87.

Bass, K.E., Morrish, D., Roth, I., Bhardwaj, D., Taylor, R., Zhou, Y., and Fisher S.J. (1994). Human cytotrophoblast invasion is up-regulated by epidermal growth factor: evidence that paracrine factors modify this process. *Developmental Biology*, **164**, 550–61.

Benirschke, K. and Kaufmann, P. (1990). Nonvillous parts of the placenta. In *Pathology of the human placenta*, (ed. K. Bernirschke and P. Kaufmann), pp. 244–305. Springer, New York.

Bohn, H. and Klaus, W. (1976). Isolierung und Charakterisierung des Plazentaproteins PP1. *Archiv der Gyneokologie*, 221, 165–75.

Bonduelle, M.-L., Dodd, R., Liebaers, I., Van Steirteghem, A., Williamson, R., and Akhuers, R. (1988). Chorionic gonadotrophin-β mRNA, a trophoblast marker is expressed in human 8-cell embryo derived from trinucleate zygotes. *Human Reproduction*, 3, 909–14.

Boyd, J.D. and Hamilton, W.J. (ed.) (1970). *The human placenta*. W. Heffer and Son, Cambridge.

Burt, D., Johnston, D., Rinke de Wit, T., Van den Elsen, P., and Stern, P.L. (1991). Cellular immune recognition of HLA-G-expressing choriocarcinoma cell line Jeg-3. *International Journal of Cancer*, (Suppl.), 6, 117–22.

Castellucci, M., Kaufmann, P., and Bischof P. (1990). Extracellular matrix influences hormone and protein production by human chorionic villi. *Cell and Tissue Research*, 262, 135–42.

Cemerikic, B. and Genbacev, O. (1989). Tissue explant technique in the study of human chorionic gonadotrophin (hCG) production *in vitro*. In *Placenta as a model and source*, (ed. O. Genbacev, A. Klopper, and R. Beaconsfield), pp. 93–102. Plenum, New York.

Copp, A.J. (1995). Death before birth clues from gene knockouts and mutations. *Trends in Genetics*, 11, 87–93.

Cross, J.C., Werb, Z., and Fisher, S.J. (1994). Implantation and the placenta. *Science*, 266, 1508–18.

Damsky, C.H., Fitzgerald, M.L., and Fisher, S.J. (1992). Distribution pattern of extracellular matrix components and adhesion receptors are intricately modulated during first trimester cytotrophoblast differentiation along the invasion pathway, *in vivo*. *Journal of Clinical Investigations*, 89, 210–22.

Damsky, C.H., Sutherland, A., and Fisher, S.J. (1993). Extracellular matrix 5: adhesive interactions in early mammalian embryogenesis, implantation, and placentation. *FASEB Journal*, 7, 1320–9.

Denker, H.-W. (1993). Implantation: a cell biological paradox. *Journal of Experimental Zoology*, 266, 541–58.

Edwards, R.G. and Brody, S.A. (ed.) (1995). *Principles and practice of assisted human reproduction*. W.B. Saunders, Philadelphia.

Fernandez, P.L., Merino, M.J., Nogales, F.F., Charonis, A.S., Stetler-Stevenson, W., and Liotta, L. (1992). Immunohistochemical profile of basement membrane proteins and 72 kilodalton type IV collagenase in the implantation placental site. *Laboratory Investigations*, 66, 572–9.

Fishel, S.B., Edwards, R.G., and Evans, C.J. (1984). Human chorionic gonadotrophin secreted by pre-implantation embryos cultured *in vitro*. *Science*, 223, 816–18.

Fisher, S.J. and Damsky C.H. (1993). Human cytotrophoblast invasion. *Seminars in Cell Biology*, 4, 183–8.

Fisher, S.J., Cui, T.Y., Zhang, L., Hartman, L., Grahl, K., Zhang, G.Y., et al. (1989). Adhesive and degradative properties of human placental cytotrophoblast cells *in vitro*. *Journal of Cell Biology*, 109, 891–902.

Fox, H. (1992). Ectopic sites of implantation. Early human placenta morphology. In *The first twelve weeks of gestation*, (ed. E.R. Barnea, J. Hustin, and E. Jauniaux), pp. 297–309. Springer, New York.

Frixen, U., Behrens, J., Sachs, M., Eberle, G., Voss, B., Warda, A., et al. (1991). E-cadherin-mediated cell–cell adhesion prevents invasiveness of human carcinoma cells. *Journal of Cell Biology*, 113, 173–85.

Genbacev, O. and Miller R.K. (1993). Three-dimensional culture of placental villous—an *in vitro* model for peri-implantation. *Methods in Toxicology*, 3, 205–44.

Genbacev, O., Cemerikic, B., Vicovac, L., Vuckovic, M., and Sulovic, V. (1992). Long term tissue culture of first trimester villous trophoblast in collagen gel—evaluation of its possible use as a model system. *Trophoblast Research*, 6, 163–72.

Genbacev, O., de Mesy Jensen, K., Schubach Powlin S., and Miller R.K. (1993*a*). *In vitro* differentiation and ultrastructure of human extravillous trophoblast (EVT) cells. *Placenta*, 14, 463–75.

Genbacev, O., White T., Gavin, C., and Miller, R.K. (1993*b*). Human trophoblast in cultures: models for implantation and peri-implantation toxicology. *Reproductive Toxicology*, 7, 75–94.

Genbacev, O., Powlin, S., and Miller, R.K. (1994). Regulation of human extravillus tro-phoblast (EVT) cell differentiation and proliferation *in vitro*—role of epidermal growth factor (EGF). *Trophoblast Research*, 8, 427–42.

Genbacev, O., Joslin, R.J., Damsky, C.H., Polliotti, B.M., and Fisher, S.J. (1996). Hypoxia alters early gestation human cytotrophoblast differentiation invasion *in vitro* and models the placental defects that occur in preeclampsia. *Journal of Clinical Investigations*, 97, 540–50.

Graham, C.H. and Lala, P.K. (1992). Mechanisms of placental invasion of the uterus and their control. *Biochemistry and Cell Biology*, 70, 867–74.

Hay, D.L. and Lopata, A. (1988). Chorionic gonadotrophin secretion by human embryos *in vitro*. *Journal of Clinical Endocrinology and Metabolism*, 67, 1322–4.

Hofmann, G.E., Drews, M.R., Scott Jr, R.T., Navot, D., Heller, D., and Degligdisch, L. (1992). Epidermal growth factor and its receptor in human implantation trophoblast: immunohisto-chemical evidence for autocrine/paracrine function. *Journal of Clinical Endocrinology and Metabolism*, 74, 981–8.

Hustin, J. and Franchimont, P. (1992). The endometrium and implantation. In *The first twelve weeks of gestation*, (ed. E.R. Barnea, J. Hustin, and E. Jauniaux), pp. 26–42. Springer, New York.

Hustin, J. and Schaaps, J.P. (1987). Echographic and anatomic studies of the maternotro-phoblastic border during the first trimester of pregnancy. *American Journal of Obstetrics and Gynecology*, 157, 162–8.

Jackson, M.R., Carney, E.W., Lye, S.J., and Ritchie, J.W. (1994). Localization of two angio-genic growth factors (PDECGF and VEGF) in human placenta throughout gestation. *Placenta*, 15, 341–53.

Jaffe, R. and Woods, J.R. (1993). Color Doppler imaging and *in vivo* assessment of the anatomy and physiology of the early uteroplacental circulation. *Fertility and Sterility*, 60, 293–7.

Jameson, J.L. and Hollenberg, A.N. (1993). Regulation of chorionic gonadotropin gene expres-sion. *Endocrine Reviews*, 14, 203–21.

Jauniaux, E., Burton, G.J., and Jones C.J.P. (1992). Early human placenta morphology. In *The first twelve weeks of gestation*, (ed. E.R. Barnea, J. Hustin, and E. Jauniaux), pp. 45–64. Springer, New York.

Kaufmann, P., Sen, D., and Schweikhart, G. (1979). Classification of human placental villi. I. Histology. *Cell and Tissue Research*, 200, 409–23.

Kawagoe, K., Akiyama, J., Kawamoto, T., Morishita, Y., and Mori, S. (1990). Immuno-histochemical demonstration of epidermal growth factor (EGF) receptors in normal human placental villi. *Placenta*, 11, 7–15.

Kovats, S., Main, E.K., Librach, C., Stubblebine, M., Fisher, S.J., and DeMars, R. (1990). A class I antigen, HLA-G, expressed in human trophoblasts. *Science*, 248, 220–3.

Kurman, R.J., Main, C.S., and Chen, H.C. (1984). Intermediate trophoblast: a distinctive form of trophoblast with specific morphological, biochemical and functional features. *Placenta*, 5, 349–69.

Librach, C.L., Werb, Z., Fitzgerald, M.L., Chiu, K., Corwin, N.M., Esteves, R.A., *et al.* (1991). 92-kD type IV collagenase mediates invasion of human cytotrophoblast. *Journal of Cell Biology*, **113**, 437–49.

Lindenberg, S., Hyttel, P., Lenz, S., and Holmes, P.V. (1986). Ultrastructure of the early human implantation *in vitro*. *Human Reproduction*, **1**, 533–8.

McMaster, M.T., Librach, C.L., Zhou, Y., Lim, K.-H., Janatpour, M.J., DeMars, R., *et al.* (1995). Human placental HLA-G expression is restricted to differentiated cytotrophoblasts. *The Journal of Immunology*, **154**, 3771–8.

Magnuson, T., Anthony, D., and Stackpole, C.W. (1977). Characterization of intercellular junctions in the preimplantation mouse embryo by freeze-fracture and thin section electron microscopy. *Developmental Biology*, **61**, 252–61.

Maruo, T., Matsuo, H., Murata, K., and Mochizuki, M. (1992). Gestational age-dependent dual action of epidermal growth factor on human placenta early in gestation. *Journal of Clinical Endocrinology and Metabolism*, **75**, 1362–7.

Marzusch, K., Ruck, P., Horny, H.-P., Dietl, J., and Kaiserling, E. (1995). Expression of p53 tumor suppressor gene in human placenta: an immunohistochemical study. *Placenta*, **16**, 101–4.

Metz, J. and Weihe, E. (1980). Intercellular junctions in the full term human placenta. II Cytotrophoblast cells and blood vessels. *Anatomy and Embryology*, **158**, 167–78.

Muehlhauser, J., Crescimanno, C., Kaufmann, P., Hoefler, H., Zaccheo, D., and Castellucci, M. (1991). Differentiation and proliferation patterns in human trophoblast revealed by c-erB-2 oncogene product and EGF-R. The *Journal of Histochemistry and Cytochemistry*, **41**, 165–73.

Nishi, M., Kumar, N.M., and Gilula, N.B. (1991). Developmental regulation of gap junction gene expression during mouse embryonic development. *Developmental Biology*, **146**, 117–30.

O'Rahilly, R. (1973). *Development stages in human embryos. Part A: embryos of the first three weeks gestation (stages 1 to 9)*. Carnegie Institute of Washington Publication, Washington DC.

Pijnenborg, R., Dixon, G., Robertson, W.B., and Brosens, I. (1980). Trophoblast invasion of human decidua from 8 to 18 weeks of pregnancy. *Placenta*, **1**, 3–19.

Pijnenborg, R., Bland, J.M., Robertson, W.B., and Brosens, I. (1983). Uteroplacental arterial changes related to interstitial trophoblast migration in early human pregnancy. *Placenta*, **4**, 397–414.

Polette, M., Nawrocki, B., Pintiaux, A., Massenat, C., Maquoi, E., Volders, L., *et al.* (1994). Expression of gelatinase A and B and their tissue inhibitors by cells of early and term human placenta and gestational endometrium. *Laboratory Investigations*, **71**, 838–46.

Rodesch, F., Simon, P., Donner, C., and Jauniaux, E. (1992). Oxygen measurements in endometrial and trophoblastic tissues during early pregnancy. *Obstretics and Gynecology*, **80**, 283–5.

Roncalli, M., Bulfamante, G., Viale, G., Springall, D.R., Alfano, R., Comi, A., *et al.* (1994). C-myc and tumor suppressor gene product expression in developing and term human trophoblast. *Placenta*, **15**, 399–409.

Schlafke, S. and Enders, A.C. (1975). Cellular basis of interaction between trophoblast and uterus at implantation. *Biology of Reproduction*, **12**, 41–65.

Sharkey, A.M., Charnock-Jones, D.S., Boocock, C.A., Brown, K.D., and Smith, S.K. (1993). Expression of mRNA for vascular endothelial growth factor in human placenta. *Journal of Reproduction and Fertility*, **99**, 609–15.

Stickland, S. and Richards, W.G. (1992). Invasion of the trophoblast. *Cell*, **71**, 355–7.

Vestweber, D., Gossler, A., Boller, K., and Kemler, R. (1987). Expression and distribution of the cell adhesion molecule uvomorulin in mouse pre-implantation embryos. *Developmental Biology*, **124**, 451–6.

Vicovac, L., Jones, C.J., and Aplin, J.D. (1995). Trophoblast differentiation during formation of anchoring villi in a model of the early placenta *in vitro*. *Placenta*, **16**, 41–56.

von Ostau, C., Gruemmer, R., Kohnen, G., Kaufmann, P., and Winterhager, E. (1995). Expression verschiedener Connexine waehrend der Entwicklung der humanen Placenta. *Anatomischer Anzeiger*, **177**, 102.

Wells, M. and Bulmer, J.N. (1988). The human placental bed: histology, immunohistochemistry and pathology. *Histopathology*, **13**, 483–98.

Yamasaki, H. (1991). Aberrant expression and function of gap junctions during carcinogenesis. *Environmental Health Perspectives*, **93**, 191–7.

9 | *Formation of the trophoblastic barrier*

G.J. Burton, M.E. Palmer, and A.L. Watson

INTRODUCTION

The trophoblastic covering of the placental villous tree plays a variety of essential roles during pregnancy. Amongst these are the facilitation and modulation of placental transport, the synthesis of essential steroid and protein hormones, and the concealment of fetal antigens from the maternal immune system. Normal development and differentiation of the trophoblastic covering of the placental villous tree are of key importance in a healthy pregnancy. Recent advances in molecular biology are beginning to elucidate some of the cytokine networks which may regulate these processes. Many of the data are based on experiments conducted *in vitro* and the question of how closely these equate with the situation *in vivo* remains to be resolved. None the less, an array of possible regulatory factors as diverse as parental chromosomal imprinting and the uterine oxygen tension have been identified. By influencing levels of cytokine expression, the number of receptors, or transduction activities these factors may ensure that under normal circumstances trophoblast development is responsive to the uterine milieu and to fetal requirements. At present the picture is far from clear, but it is almost certain that ultimately it will prove to be the balance of a variety of stimulatory and inhibitory influences that is of critical importance. It is with the formation and maintenance of this villous covering that the present chapter is concerned.

ESTABLISHMENT OF THE TROPHECTODERM LINEAGE

The origin of the trophoblast can be traced back to the very earliest stages of development, and the introduction of *in vitro* fertilization techniques has provided the opportunity to examine these stages in great detail. How closely the timings correspond to those *in vivo* remains uncertain, however. Even at the 2-cell stage it has been reported that morphological differences can be observed between different parts of the blastomere surface at the ultrastructural level. The free surface bears microvilli and displays evidence of endocytic activity, whereas those areas in mutual contact show a tendency to develop focal submembrane densities and cell junctions (Tesarík 1989). These differences become more marked over the next two cell divisions during the formation of the morula, although each cell remains totipotential. Late on day 3 following *in vitro* fertilization the morula undergoes the process of compaction, during which the intercellular contacts and junctional complexes become more extensive. As a result the cells become polarized, with inner and outer domains, and this crucial change allows for asymmetrical cell division. Consequently two distinct cell lineages are established. The deeper portions of the cells give rise to the inner cell mass (ICM) from which the embryo develops, whereas the superficial parts become trophectoderm (TE) cells which will contribute to the formation of the extra-embryonic membranes.

Accumulation of fluid in the intercellular spaces leads to blastulation occurring on day 5 or 6. Estimates indicate that TE cells are more numerous than those of the ICM throughout this period. Discounting degenerating cells, which are commonly observed, there are approximately six cells allocated to the ICM and 10 to the TE at the 16-cell stage. By day 7 these figures have increased to approximately 46 and 81 cells in the ICM and TE shell respectively (Hardy *et al.* 1989). Again, how closely the numbers reflect the situation *in vivo* is difficult to judge. The divergence of these two cell lineages is of fundamental importance for embryogenesis. That it should occur so early in development and at a time of rapid cell division may explain why karyotypic differences can exist between the TE cells and those of the fetus. Although cell death may provide a mechanism for the removal of mitotic errors, placental mosaicism must be considered when interpreting genetic analyses based on chorionic villus sampling (Gosden 1993).

By day 7 the blastocyst has hatched from the zona pellucida and will soon undergo implantation. The trophectodermal shell of such an *in vitro* fertilized blastocyst was described in detail by Mohr and Trounson (1982). The cells possessed long microvilli on their apical surface and numerous vesicles and mitochondria were present within the cytoplasm. Extensive junctional complexes consisting of tight junctions and desmosome-like junctions closed the apical ends of the intercellular spaces. Along their lateral cell boundaries adjacent cells appeared to communicate via gap junctions. Physical contacts were also made with the cells of the ICM by way of desmosomes, and notably the authors make no reference to a trophoblastic basal lamina. They do, however, comment that the polar trophoblast cells are less attenuated than their mural counterparts, and of course it is the former that will be involved in the process of implantation.

Very little is known about the process of implantation in the human. The earliest specimens available for study were described by Hertig *et al.* (1956), but in even the youngest of these (estimated to be day 7 post conception) the blastocyst is almost completely embedded within the endometrium. Attempts have been made to explore the events taking place using *in vitro* fertilized blastocysts and monolayer cultures of endometrial epithelial cells (Lindenberg *et al.* 1986). Such model systems suffer through the lack of an endometrial stroma, and inevitably there is a loss of polarization of the epithelial cells. However, within their limitations they have produced some valuable insights. The polar trophectoderm cells establish the initial contact and send out long protrusions which penetrate between the endometrial cells. No cell contacts are made between the two cell types and neither is there any evidence of cell degeneration. The endometrial cells simply become displaced, forming stacks 3–4 cells high at the margins.

In the centre of these implantation sites the trophoblast cells make contact with the culture dish and then undergo a remarkable transformation. A true multinucleated syncytium is formed, and from now on the trophoblastic covering can be divided into two layers, the outer syncytiotrophoblast and the inner cytotrophoblast. This transformation takes place less than 24 h after adhesion in the *in vitro* system (Lindenberg *et al.* 1986). In the earliest *in vivo* specimen examined, estimated to be at day 7 post-conception (Hertig *et al.* 1956), an extensive mantle of syncytiotrophoblast is seen abutting the endometrial stroma. This mantle becomes more complete as the blastocyst embeds further into the uterine wall over the next few days.

At the same time a series of isolated, fluid filled vacuoles develop within the syncytiotrophoblastic mass. These coalesce to form larger lacunae which are the precursors of the intervillous space. Separating them initially are sheets or trabeculae of syncytiotrophoblast, but beginning on day 12 post-conception, cytotrophoblast cells penetrate into the sheets, reaching their distal segments by day 14. Shortly after, the cytotrophoblast cells are followed by extraembryonic mesoderm, and proliferation of these tissues results in the formation of the earliest villi (Kaufmann and Burton 1994).

THE RELATIONSHIP BETWEEN CYTOTROPHOBLAST AND SYNCYTIOTROPHOBLAST

The syncytiotrophoblast forms the outer covering of the villi and so is bathed directly by the maternal blood circulating in the intervillous space. This is a true multinucleated syncytium which extends uninterrupted over the entire villous tree (Figs 9.1 and 9.2). Vertical cell membranes dividing it into a series of subunits are extremely rare and most probably represent the result of repair mechanisms (see below). The structure of the syncytiotrophoblast has recently been reviewed at length by Benirschke and Kaufmann (1990) and Jones and Fox (1991).

Syncytial nuclei display varying chromatin patterns but generally as gestation advances, dense aggregates of chromatin develop beneath the nuclear membrane. These appearances are somewhat similar to those seen in apoptosis. It is notable that neither mitotic figures nor the incorporation of tritiated thymidine has ever been observed in the syncytiotrophoblastic nuclei. Transcription also seems to be suppressed or reduced to barely detectable levels (Benirschke and Kaufmann 1990). The overwhelming picture is that the syncytiotrophoblast is a terminally differentiated tissue which depends on the continual recruitment of its progenitor cells, the cytotrophoblasts, for both its generation and maintenance.

The cytotrophoblast cells lie below the syncytiotrophoblast on the trophoblastic basal lamina (Fig. 9.1). For much of the first trimester they form a complete layer of cells but towards term they are seen less frequently in sectioned material. Traditionally this has been interpreted as indicating that the number of cytotrophoblast cells declines as pregnancy advances. Recent stereological analyses have challenged this view, however, revealing that the absolute number of these cells continues to increase throughout pregnancy (Simpson *et al.* 1992). This apparent paradox may be explained on the basis that the surface area of the villous tree

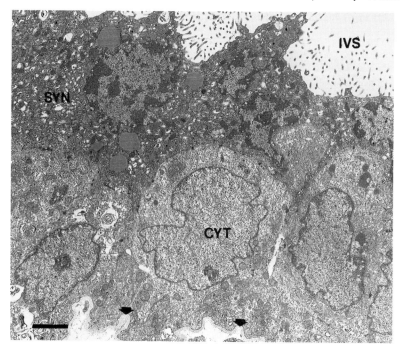

Fig. 9.1 A transmission electron micrographs of first trimester placental tissue illustrating the two layers of the trophoblast present at this stage of gestation. The outer layer facing the inter-villous space (IVS) is the multinucleated syncytiotrophoblast (SYN), which carries numerous microvilli on its free surface. This layer is generated from the underlying population of cyto-trophoblast cells (CYT), resting on the basal lamina (arrowed). Scale bar = 2 μm.

increases dramatically during the third trimester and so the cytotrophoblast cells inevitably become more dispersed. The quantitative analyses further indicate that a consistent ratio between the number of villous syncytiotrophoblastic and cyto-trophoblastic nuclei is maintained throughout pregnancy, in the region of 9:1.

Such analyses cannot take into account the number of syncytiotrophoblastic nuclei which are continually being lost through the shedding of syncytial knots or sprouts into the maternal circulation. None the less they demonstrate that trophoblast pro-liferation would appear to be under tight control. The number of cytotrophoblast cells present at any time will depend on various factors, but principally on the rate at which the cells undergo division, the length of the cell cycle, and the rate at which daughter cells fuse with the syncytiotrophoblast. Autoradiographic studies based on first trimester tissue indicate a cell cycle time of approximately 15 h, with an S phase of 5–6 h (Gerbie *et al.* 1968). As gestation advances the cycle time increases, but the proliferative rate of the cytotrophoblast cells remains constant (Arnholdt *et al.* 1991). It may change under pathological conditions, however, and for example appears to be increased in pregnancies complicated by pre-eclamptic toxaemia (Arnholdt *et al.* 1991).

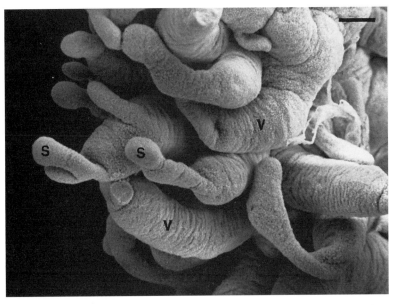

Fig. 9.2   A scanning electron micrograph of first trimester tissue demonstrating that the covering of microvilli extends over the entire surface of the villi (V). Numerous sprouts (S) composed wholly of syncytiotrophoblast are present at this stage of gestation, and the tips of these may break away and be deported through the maternal venous system. Scale bar = 50 μm.

An excessive number of villous cytotrophoblast cells has been associated with a variety of pathological conditions, many of which are associated with intrauterine hypoxia (Fox 1978; Benirschke and Kaufmann 1990). This has led to the suggestion that the prevailing oxygen tension may play a pivotal role in regulating cytotrophoblastic cell function. Estimating the oxygen tension at the placental interface *in vivo* is extremely difficult, but one situation in which it is unquestionably reduced is during pregnancy at high altitude. Morphometric data obtained from normal term placentas indicate that the percentage volume of the terminal villi occupied by cytotrophoblast cells increases from 1.2 per cent at sea level to 2.6 per cent at 2800 m ($t = 2.93$, $p > 0.01$) (Reshetnikova and Burton, unpublished observations). This change is not due to an alteration in mean cell volume but appears to be the result of a real increase in the number of cells, with a shift in the ratio of syncytiotrophoblastic to cytotrophoblastic nuclei (Ali and Burton, unpublished observations).

Under normal conditions villous cytotrophoblast cells do not appear to be continuously cycling. How their proliferation and subsequent differentiation is regulated at the cellular level is largely unknown, but an increasing number of candidates are being identified. Some of these factors may be of maternal origin and so present in the fluids within the intervillous space bathing the trophoblastic surface. Others are derived from the cells of the mesenchymal villous core and whose expression may be responsive to the fetal milieu or to changes in the uterine environment.

CONTROL OF CYTOTROPHOBLASTIC PROLIFERATION

Control of cell proliferation can be exerted at several levels, through differential expression of growth factors, their receptors, or the regulation of transcriptional processes.

   1. *Epidermal growth factor (EGF).* During the first 4–5 weeks of gestation EGF and its receptor (encoded by the c-*erb-B* proto-oncogene) are primarily localized to the cytotrophoblast cells, whereas later in pregnancy a switch occurs and they become predominantly associated with the syncytiotrophoblast (Ladines-Llave *et al.* 1991; Mühlhauser *et al.* 1993). Administration of exogenous EGF to villous explant cultures at 4–5 weeks of development leads to increased proliferation of the cytotrophoblast cells within 12 h as quantified by the marker Ki-67, but older tissue, 6–12 weeks gestational age, did not respond in this manner (Maruo *et al.* 1992). Placental trophoblast is capable of secreting EGF during *in vitro* culture, and this is enhanced by the addition of thyroid hormone to the medium (Matsuo *et al.* 1993). The possibility for an autocrine/paracrine control system therefore exists. In the earliest stages of pregnancy this may regulate proliferation, but as gestation advances it appears that EGF exerts more of a role in stimulating the release of human chorionic gonadotrophin and placental lactogen from the syncytiotrophoblast (Morrish *et al.* 1987; Maruo *et al.* 1992).

   2. *Insulin-like growth factors (IGFs).* Considerable evidence exists suggesting that IGF2 may play a major role in regulating trophoblast growth, and it has been selectively localized to the cytotrophoblast layer of first trimester villi by *in situ* hybridization (Ohlsson *et al.* 1989). These cells coexpress the IGFI and IGFII receptors, suggesting that short range signalling may be important. Binding to the IGFI receptor is thought to mediate proliferation in other cell lines, and so may be the most relevant in this context (Czech 1989). However, mice deficient in a functional IGFII gene notably display a considerably smaller placenta (DeChiara *et al.* 1990). In the mouse the IGF2 gene is known to be parentally imprinted, being expressed on the paternally inherited chromosome 7 (Ferguson-Smith *et al.* 1991). There may therefore be some connection between overexpression of the gene and the excessive proliferation of trophoblast that occurs in complete hydatidiform moles. In this condition both sets of chromosomes are paternally derived.

   3. *Platelet-derived growth factor (PDGF).* PDGF may exist as either a homodimer (AA or BB chains) or as the heterodimer (AB). The c-*sis* proto-oncogene encodes the B chain and the distribution of this has been localized within first trimester placental tissue by *in situ* hybridization. The gene product is expressed in a subset of proliferative cytotrophoblast cells, principally within the cytotrophoblastic shell but also to a lesser extent within the villi (Goustin *et al.* 1985). Cultured cytotrophoblast cells express high affinity receptors for PDGF and addition of the factor to such cultures induces DNA synthesis. Again, there is a strong possibility that autocrine control of trophoblastic growth could be operative.

4. *Hepatocyte growth/scatter factor (HGF)*. HGF is generally believed to be an important modulator of mesenchymal–epithelial interactions since it is expressed by mesenchymal cells whilst its receptor c-*met* is found on nearby epithelial cells. Recent work on mice lacking HGF has revealed severe impairment of placental development, and in particular a marked reduction in the number of trophoblast cells (Schmidt *et al.* 1995; Uehara *et al.* 1995). Both HGF protein and mRNA have been detected in the mesenchymal cells of the villous core of human placental villi, but are absent from the trophoblast layers (Saito *et al.* 1995). By contrast, c-*met* protein is expressed by cytotrophoblast cells but not by the syncytiotrophoblast. Administration of HGF to cytotrophoblast cells grown in serum-free medium causes enhanced DNA synthesis but does not influence hormone secretion. There is evidence to suggest therefore that HGF may act as a promoter of cytotrophoblast proliferation but not of differentiation.

5. *Vascular endothelial growth factor* (VEGF). This factor is a potent mitogen for endothelial cells, and being freely diffusible is found throughout the villous stroma. Intriguingly, the receptor *flt* has been localized on villous cytotrophoblast cells, although its actions are at present unknown (Charnock-Jones *et al.* 1994).

A number of other growth factors, such as colony stimulating factor 1 (CSF1), do not appear to stimulate cytotrophoblast proliferation but may play important roles in promoting subsequent differentiation into syncytiotrophoblast (see later).

The binding of growth factors to their respective receptors can lead to the activation of proto-oncogenes and the stimulation of cell proliferation (reviewed by Ohlsson *et al.* 1993). For example, addition of PDGF to cytotrophoblast cells in culture leads to a 10-fold increase in c-*myc* mRNA content per cell within 2 h (Goustin *et al.* 1985). Within 24 h over 90 per cent of the cells moved through the S phase of the cell cycle. A similar correlation between c-*myc* expression and cell proliferation was made in intact first trimester villi by comparing the number and distribution of cells staining positively for c-*myc* RNA by *in situ* hybridization with those incorporating tritiated thymidine (Pfeifer-Ohlsson *et al.* 1984). An equivalent pattern is observed when the gene product is detected using immunohistochemistry (Maruo and Mochizuki 1987). This congruence is strongly suggestive that the products of the c-*myc* gene are directly or indirectly involved in control of cytotrophoblast proliferation. By comparison, the roles of other proto-oncogenes such as c-*fos* and c-*ras* in trophoblast development are unclear, but they are expressed at maximal levels in term placentas.

Regulation of trophoblastic growth could also occur at the transcriptional level but little is known regarding this possibility in the human. Work on the mouse has demonstrated that the product of the *Mash-2* gene may be a lineage-specific factor essential for the development of the trophoblast (Guillemot *et al.* 1994). *Mash-2* is not required for the generation of the trophectoderm at the blastocyst stage, but appears to be essential at post-implantation stages for the development of differentiated trophoblast cell types.

THE PROCESS OF CYTOTROPHOBLASTIC DIFFERENTIATION

Cytotrophoblast cells vary in their appearance and a spectrum can be observed within normal villi. At one extreme are cuboidal cells displaying a large rounded nucleus with evenly dispersed chromatin. The cytoplasm contains few organelles and secretory droplets are infrequent. Such cells are considered to represent the resting or undifferentiated state (Benirschke and Kaufmann 1990; Jones and Fox 1991; Kaufmann and Burton 1994). At the opposite extreme are more flattened cells whose cytoplasm closely resembles that of the syncytiotrophoblast. Mitochondria are more numerous and rough endoplasmic reticulum and Golgi bodies are conspicuous. The nucleus is often irregularly shaped and aggregations of chromatin beneath the nuclear membrane are characteristic. These are referred to as intermediate cells, and the fact that some are occasionally seen in the process of fusing with the syncytiotrophoblast indicates that they are a highly differentiated form of cytotrophoblast.

Evidence supporting this view may be drawn from studies which have followed the endocrine activity of cytotrophoblast cells. For example, human chorionic gonadotropin (hCG) has been localized to the cisternae of rough endoplasmic reticulum and perinuclear spaces of intermediate cells. It has also been demonstrated by *in situ* hybridization that the messenger RNAs for the alpha and beta subunits of hCG are present in only a few villous cytotrophoblast cells *in vivo* (Hoshina *et al.* 1985). Hence it has been concluded that the *genes* responsible for the synthesis of the hormone are activated late in the differentiation pathway. Commensurate with this change in endocrine activity is an increase in aerobic and anaerobic glycolysis as evidenced by a rise in the cells' level of the enzyme lactate dehydrogenase (Benirschke and Kaufmann 1990). Full activation of endocrine activity may not take place until fusion with the syncytiotrophoblast since messenger RNA for the hormone human placental lactogen (hPL) has not been detected in cytotrophoblast cells (Hoshina *et al.* 1985).

FUSION OF CYTOTROPHOBLAST CELLS WITH THE
SYNCYTIOTROPHOBLAST

Undifferentiated and differentiating cytotrophoblast cells are linked to the overlying syncytiotrophoblast by numerous desmosomes, and the respective cell membranes are clearly visible separated by a narrow intercellular cleft. The normal fate for a cytotrophoblast cell is to fuse with the syncytiotrophoblast, and isolated fragments of cell membranes and desmosomes within the syncytioplasm bear witness to this phenomenon (Fig. 9.3). Two contrasting but not necessarily mutually incompatible mechanisms have been put forward as mediators of this process.

Firstly, it has been claimed that the formation of gap junctions is an essential prerequisite. Gap junctions have been observed between the syncytiotrophoblastic and cytotrophoblastic layers of the human placenta by freeze-fracture replication (de Virgillis *et al.* 1982). A marked increase in their formation has also been shown to immediately precede fusion of cytotrophoblast cells to form syncytial plaques *in vitro* (Cronier *et al.* 1994). These junctions will permit the exchange of second messengers

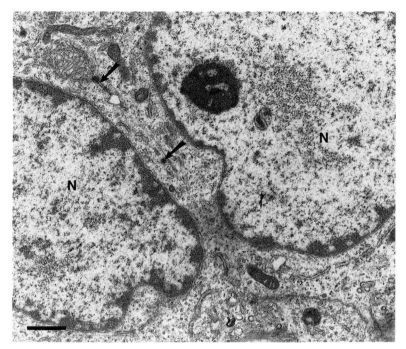

Fig. 9.3   A transmission electron micrograph showing two cytotrophoblast cells that have recently fused. Only isolated fragments of the cell membranes (arrowed) are visible between the two nuclei (N). Scale bar = 1 μm.

between the cell types and so may play an important role in coordinating the final events leading up to cell fusion. From evidence based on the guinea-pig it has been suggested that the junctions themselves may act as the foci for fusion (Firth *et al.* 1980).

Secondly, endogenous retroviral proteins are known to be expressed by the trophoblast and have been implicated in fusion processes in other cell lines (Lyden *et al.* 1994*a*). Budding of type C retroviral particles from the deep surface of the syncytiotrophoblast can be seen in most placentas if sufficient sections are examined, and particles have been isolated and characterized at the ultrastructural level (Lyden *et al.* 1994*b*). In marmosets this budding is particularly pronounced at the time of implantation when, of course, the cytotrophoblast is at its most proliferative (Smith and Moore 1988). Whether differentiation related expression of retroviral envelope proteins is responsible for mediating syncytial transformation in the human placenta remains to be tested, however.

CONTROL OF CYTOTROPHOBLAST CELL DIFFERENTIATION

Differentiation of purified cytotrophoblast cells into syncytiotrophoblastic masses can occur *in vitro*, allowing for the investigation of its control. As with the case of proliferation an increasing number of cytokines are being identified as potential regulators of this process. Several possible autocrine, paracrine, and endocrine pathways have been proposed.

1. *EGF*. Addition of EGF to such cultures established from term placentas induces syncytial formation and raises the level of secretion of hCG into the medium (Morrish *et al.* 1987). The formation of syncytial aggregates is associated with a twofold increase in the number of high affinity EGF binding sites, and with a significant rise in EGFR-kinase activity. Higher levels of EGFR gene expression in syncytiotrophoblast compared with cytotrophoblast cells indicate that the increase in EGF receptors is due to a change in the rate of their synthesis (Alsat *et al.* 1993*a*). Evidence that this cytokine may play a significant role *in vivo* is provided by the recent finding of aberrant receptor function in cases of intrauterine growth retardation compared with controls (Fondacci *et al.* 1994). In some cases the number of high affinity binding sites for EGF on the syncytiotrophoblastic microvillous surface was reduced, whereas in others there was abnormal transduction of the EGF-induced signal.

2. *Parathyroid hormone (PTH)*. Administration of PTH, and also of parathyroid hormone-related protein (PTHrP), at physiological levels to *in vitro* cultures results in an elevation of EGFR mRNA levels (Alsat *et al.* 1993*b*). This effect is accompanied by a rise in EGF binding, suggesting that these factors which are found in the uterine environment may be able to modulate trophoblastic development.

3. *Transforming growth factor β_1*. By contrast, the stimulatory action of EGF on cytotrophoblast differentiation can be blocked by the administration TGFβ_1, indicating that this factor may play an inhibitory role (Morrish *et al.* 1991). Whether this is acting through downregulation of EGF receptors is not known. However, since TGFβ_1 mRNA has been localized to the syncytiotrophoblast but not to villous cytotrophoblast cells, the possibility of paracrine control exists (Lysiak *et al.* 1995).

4. *Colony-stimulating factor (CSF)*. Administration of macrophage CSF will stimulate first trimester cytotrophoblast cells grown in serum-free medium to fuse and secrete both hCG and hPL (Saito *et al.* 1993). Both CSF$_1$ and granulocyte-macrophage CSF have been immunolocalised to villous cytotrophoblast cells and to mesenchymal cells in the villous core *in vivo* during the first and second trimester (Daiter *et al.* 1992; GarciaLloret *et al.* 1994). The production of these factors from stromal fibroblasts *in vitro* can be upregulated by the trophoblast-derived cytokines interleukin 1 and tumour necrosis factor alpha. Cytokine regulated interactions could therefore be taking place between the trophoblast and the villous core. Whereas cytotrophoblast cells express low levels of the receptor for CSF$_1$, high levels are seen in the syncytiotrophoblast, suggesting that CSF is more involved in the regulation of trophoblast differentiation than proliferation (Pampfer *et al.* 1992; Jokhi *et al.* 1993).

5. *hCG*. The addition of hCG itself has been shown to promote the syncytial trans- formation of cytotrophoblast cells in culture, and to increase the levels of mRNAs for the hCG subunits (Shi *et al.* 1993; Rodway and Rao 1995). These effects are medi- ated via the cAMP–protein kinase A system. Exogenous hCG also stimulates the formation of gap junctions between cytotrophoblast cells, lending confirmatory support of the importance of these communications to the fusion process (Cronier *et al.* 1994).

6. *Leukaemia inhibitory factor (LIF)*. LIF can inhibit differentiation commitment in pluripotential embryonic stem cells and so could be of importance in trophoblast development. Using Northern blotting, expression of the LIF receptor gene has been detected in both first trimester and term villous tissue (Kojima *et al.* 1995). It is not yet known whether the receptor itself is expressed and if so, on which cell populations within the villi. Addition of LIF to cytotrophoblast cells grown *in vitro* has been reported to promote differentiation into syncytiotrophoblast (Sawai *et al.* 1995). This effect can be blocked by anti-hCG antibodies, and so it is thought that in this situa- tion LIF exerts its effect by stimulating hCG secretion rather than by acting on the cytotrophoblast cells directly.

THE INTEGRITY OF THE TROPHOBLASTIC COVERING

Most epithelial surfaces suffer injury during their lifespan and the villous tro- phoblastic covering appears to be no exception. One well-documented cause of discrete superficial lesions is rupture of points of syncytial fusion between neigh- bouring villi (Burton 1986). Uterine contractions or fetal movements that cause displacement of the villi in relation to each other may be sufficient to break these delicate connections, leaving a defect in the syncytiotrophoblastic surface approxi- mately 20–40 μm in diameter. Such defects have been observed in first trimester placental material but are more frequently seen during the third trimester when the increasing complexity of villous branching predisposes to a greater number of physical interactions. More extensive and deeper lesions may well be caused by vig- orous actions of the fetus, some of which are forceful enough to cause placental abruption and antepartum haemorrhage (Eden 1987). Tears of the villous covering which penetrate below the trophoblastic layer will expose stromal cells bearing fetal histocompatability antigens to the maternal immune system. These antigens are not expressed by either the syncytiotrophoblast or cytotrophoblast cells, and so under normal circumstances the placenta presents an antigenically inert surface. Deep tears may also result in rupture of fetal capillaries and transplacental blood exchange. Either circumstance could lead to maternal sensitization to fetal anti- gens, and this occurs in 3–10 per cent of women in their first pregnancy before 20 weeks, rising to 15 per cent at term (Regan and Braude 1987). The question then arises as to how effective repair mechanisms are in reinstating the trophoblastic covering.

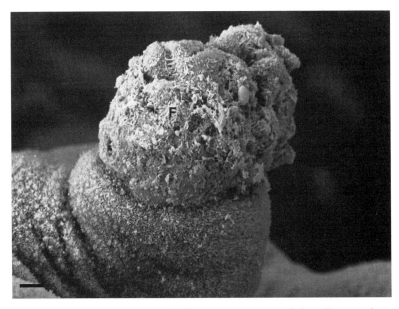

Fig. 9.4   A scanning electron micrograph illustrating an area of the villous surface where the trophoblastic surface is deficient and is replaced by a fibrin clot (F). Activated platelets and cells can be seen entrapped within the fibrin. Since the trophoblastic covering is breached, such areas may represent sites of paracellular materno-fetal transfer. Scale bar = 10 μm.

The microvillous border of the syncytiotrophoblast displays strong platelet-aggregation inhibiting activity (Iioka *et al.* 1994), and as soon as this is disrupted platelet adhesion and activation takes place (Figs 9.4 and 9.5). A fibrin plug will result, in which maternal leucocytes and platelet fragments become enmeshed. This plug not only provides a temporary seal but has the potential to modulate local cytotrophoblastic activity. A comparison of cytotrophoblast cells cultured on a variety of substrates has shown that a fibrin matrix can switch the cells away from the secretion of specific products such as hCG towards a more repair orientated phenotype (Farmer and Nelson 1992). This is evidenced by their ability to form a bilayer consisting of a well-differentiated syncytiotrophoblast with occasional mononucleated cytotrophoblast cells beneath. The latter secrete laminin, an important component of the trophoblastic basal lamina. Elevated levels of $TGF\beta_1$ have been identified at the sites of villous injury *in vitro*, and by inhibiting cytotrophoblast cell differentiation this could also facilitate coverage of the plaque (Watson *et al.* 1996).

In delivered placentas, perivillous fibrin plaques account for approximately 7 per cent of the villous surface (Nelson *et al.* 1990). They display a variety of appearances. Examples such as that illustrated in Fig. 9.4 show evidence of continuing platelet activation. At the margins, however, tongues of syncytiotrophoblast, sometimes in

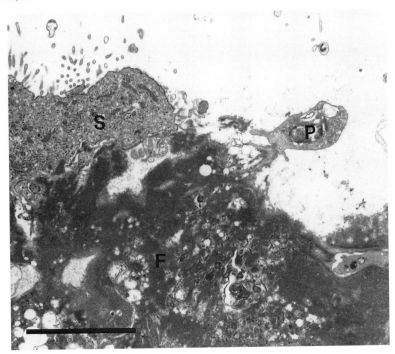

Fig. 9.5 A transmission electron micrograph of a similar region to that illustrated in Fig. 9.4 showing the heterogenous nature of the fibrin clot (F). The accumulation of cell debris, derived in part from maternal platelets (P), and extracellular matrix proteins has led to these deposits being termed perivillous fibrinoid. A healthy layer of syncytiotrophoblast (S) can be seen apparently migrating over the surface of the deposit. Scale bar = 5 μm.

conjunction with cytotrophoblast cells, may be observed apparently migrating over the surface (Fig. 9.5). Others are completely re-epithelialized (Fig. 9.6). This spectrum suggests that the trophoblastic surface can be repaired *in vivo*, although the time course of the process is unknown. It is notable that the extracellular matrix protein tenascin is expressed at high levels in the immediate vicinity of perivillous fibrin deposits (Castellucci *et al.* 1991). This protein is known to be involved in wound healing in other systems, where it is thought to facilitate cell migration. Indeed, the secretion of a number of other proteins into the original fibrin clot has led to the use of the term fibrinoid to denote the more established deposits (Frank *et al.* 1994).

During the time that the fibrinoid deposits are exposed to the contents of the inter-villous space they may act as paracellular routes of placental transport. Perfusion studies *in vitro* have demonstrated that horseradish peroxidase (48 000 Da; 3.0 nm molecular radius) can penetrate these areas and reach the stromal core (Edwards *et al.* 1993). The possibility exists, therefore, that solutes and even pathogens could cross the trophoblastic covering in a similar non-selective fashion.

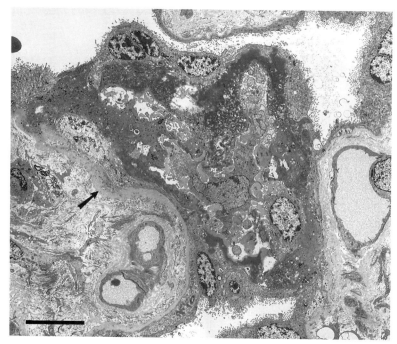

Fig. 9.6   A more extensive and most likely older deposit of fibrinoid which links two villi and has a complete covering of syncytiotrophoblast. Note that the trophoblastic basal lamina (arrowed) is thickened beneath the deposit. Scale bar = 10 μm.

REFERENCES

Alsat, E., Haziza, J., and Evainbrion, D. (1993*a*). Increase in epidermal growth-factor receptor and its messenger-ribonucleic-acid levels with differentiation of human trophoblast cells in culture. *Journal of Cellular Physiology*, **154**, 122–8.

Alsat, E., Haziza, J., Scippo, M.L., Frankenne, F., and Evainbrion, D. (1993*b*). Increase in epidermal growth-factor receptor and its messenger-RNA levels by parathyroid-hormone (1–34) and parathyroid hormone-related protein (1–34) during differentiation of human trophoblast cells in culture. *Journal of Cellular Biochemistry*, **53**, 32–42.

Arnholdt, H., Meisel, F., Fandrey, K., and Löhrs, U. (1991). Proliferation of villous trophoblast of the human placenta in normal and abnormal pregnancies. *Virchows Archiv B Cell Pathology*, **60**, 365–72.

Benirschke, K. and Kaufmann, P. (1990). *The pathology of the human placenta*. Springer, Heidelberg.

Burton, G.J. (1986). Scanning electron microscopy of intervillous bridges in the human placenta. *Journal of Anatomy*, **147**, 245–54.

Castellucci, M., Classen-Linke, I., Mühlhauser, J., Kaufmann, P., Zardi, L., and Chiquet-Ehrismann, R. (1991). The human placenta: a model for tenascin expression. *Histochemistry*, **95**, 449–58.

Charnock-Jones, D.S., Sharkey, A.M., Boocock, C.A., Ahmed, A., Plevin, R., Ferrara, N., *et al.* (1994). Vascular endothelial growth factor localisation and activation in human trophoblast and choriocarcinoma cells. *Biology of Reproduction*, **51**, 524–30.

Cronier, L., Bastide, B., Hervé, J.C., Délèze, J., and Malassiné, A. (1994). Gap junctional communication during human trophoblast differentiation: influence of human chorionic gonadotropin. *Endocrinology*, **135**, 402–8.

Czech, M.P. (1989). Signal transmission by the insulin-like growth factors. *Cell*, **59**, 235–8.

Daiter, E., Pampfer, S., Yeung, Y.G., Barad, D., Stanley, E.R., and Pollard, J.W. (1992). Expression of colony-stimulating factor-1 in the human uterus and placenta. *Journal of Clinical Endocrinology and Metabolism*, **74**, 850–8.

DeChiara, T.M., Efstratiadis, A., and Robertson, E.J. (1990). A growth deficiency phenotype in heterozygous mice carrying an insulin-like growth factor II gene disruption by targeted mutagenesis. *Nature*, **345**, 78–80.

Eden, J.A. (1987). Fetal-induced trauma as a cause of antepartum hemorrhage. *American Journal of Obstetrics and Gynecology*, **157**, 830–1.

Edwards, D., Jones, C.J.P., Sibley, C.P., and Nelson, D.M. (1993). Paracellular permeability pathways in the human placenta: a quantitative study of maternal–fetal transfer of horseradish peroxidase. *Placenta*, **14**, 63–73.

Farmer, D.A. and Nelson, D.M. (1992). A fibrin matrix modulates the proliferation, hormone secretion and morphologic differentiation of cultured human placental trophoblast. *Placenta*, **13**, 163–77.

Ferguson-Smith, A.C., Cattanach, B.M., Barton, S.C., Beechey, C.V., and Surani, M.A. (1991). Embryological and molecular investigations of parental imprinting on mouse chromosome 7. *Nature*, **351**, 667–70.

Firth, J.A., Farr, A., and Bauman, K. (1980). The role of gap junctions in trophoblastic cell fusion in the guinea-pig placenta. *Cell and Tissue Research*, **205**, 311–18.

Fondacci, C., Alsat, E., Gabriel, R., Blot, P., Nessmann, C., and Evainbrion, D. (1994). Alterations of human placental epidermal growth-factor receptor in intrauterine growth retardation. *Journal of Clinical Investigation*, **93**, 1149–55.

Fox, H. (1978). *Pathology of the placenta*. Saunders, London.

Frank H.-G., Malekzadeh F., Kertschanska S., Crescimanno C., Castellucci M., Lang I., et al. (1994). Immunohistochemistry of two different types of placental fibrinoid. *Acta Anatomica*, **150**, 55–68.

GarciaLloret, M.I., Morrish, D.W., Wegmann, T.G., Honore, L., Turner, A.R., and Guilbert, L.J. (1994). Demonstration of functional cytokine-placental interactions: CSF-1 and GM-CSF stimulate human cytotrophoblast differentiation and peptide hormone secretion. *Experimental Cell Research*, **214**, 46–54.

Gerbie, A.B., Hathaway, H.H., and Brewer, J.I. (1968). Autoradiographic analysis of normal trophoblastic proliferation. *American Journal of Obstetrics and Gynecology*, **100**, 640–8.

Gosden, C. (1993). Genetic diagnosis, chorionic villous biopsy and placental mosaicism. In *The human placenta*, (ed. C.W.G. Redman, I.L. Sargent, and P.M. Starkey), pp. 113–54. Blackwell Scientific Publications, Oxford.

Goustin, A.S., Betsholtz, C., Pfeifer-Ohlsson, S., Persson, H., Rydnert, J., Bywater, M., et al. (1985). Coexpression of the *sis* and *myc* proto-oncogenes in developing human placenta suggests autocrine control of trophoblast growth. *Cell*, **41**, 301–12.

Guillemot, F., Nagy, A., Auerbach, A., Rossant, J., and Joyner, A.L. (1994). Essential role of *Mash-2* in extraembryonic development. *Nature*, **371**, 333–6.

Hardy, K., Handyside, A.H., and Winston, R.M.L. (1989). The human blastocyst: cell number, death and allocation during late preimplantation development *in vitro*. *Development*, **107**, 597–604.

Hertig, A.T., Rock, J., and Adams, E.C. (1956). A description of 34 human ova within the first 17 days of development. *American Journal of Anatomy*, **98**, 435–91.

Hoshina, M., Boothby, M., Hussa, R., Pattillo, R., Camel, H.M., and Boime, I. (1985). Linkage of human chorionic gonadotropin and placental lactogen biosynthesis to trophoblast differentiation and tumorigenesis. *Placenta*, **6**, 163–72.

Iioka, H., Akada, S., Shimamoto, T., Yamada, Y., Sakamoto, Y., Yoshida, T., *et al.* (1994). Platelet-aggregation inhibiting activity of human placental chorioepithelial brush border membrane vesicles and basal membrane vesicles. *Trophoblast Research*, **8**, 383–92.

Johki, P.P., Chumbley, G., King, A., Gardner, L., and Loke, Y.W. (1993). Expression of the colony stimulating factor-1 receptor (*c-fms* product) by cells at the human uteroplacental interface. *Laboratory Investigation*, **68**, 308–20.

Jones, C.J.P. and Fox, H. (1991). Ultrastructure of the normal human placenta. *Electron Microscopy Reviews*, **4**, 129–78.

Kaufmann, P. and Burton, G.J. (1994). Anatomy and genesis of the placenta. In: *The physiology of reproduction*, (ed. E. Knobil and J.D. Neill), pp. 441–84. Raven, New York.

Kojima, K., Kanzaki, H., Iwai, M., Hatayama, H., Fujimoto, M., Narukawa, S., *et al.* (1995). Expression of leukaemia inhibitory factor (LIF) receptor in human placenta: a possible role for LIF in the growth and differentiation of trophoblasts. *Human Reproduction*, **10**, 1907–11.

Ladines-Llave, C.A., Maruo, T., Manalo, A.S., and Mochizuki, M. (1991). Cytologic localization of epidermal growth factor and its receptor in developing human placenta varies over the course of pregnancy. *American Journal of Obstetrics and Gynecology*, **165**, 1377–82.

Lindenberg, S., Hyttel, P., Lenz, S., and Holmes, P.V. (1986). Ultrastructure of the early human implantation *in vitro*. *Human Reproduction*, **1**, 533–8.

Lyden, T.W., Johnson, P.M., Mwenda, J., and Rote, N.S. (1994*a*). Anti-HIV monoclonal antibodies cross-react with normal human trophoblast. *Trophoblast Research*, **8**, 19–32.

Lyden, T.W., Johnson, P.M., Mwenda, J.M., and Rote, N.S. (1994*b*). Ultrastructural characterisation of endogenous retroviral particles isolated from normal human placentas. *Biology of Reproduction*, **51**, 152–7.

Lysiak, J.J., Hunt, J., Pringle, G.A., and Lala, P.K. (1995). Localization of transforming growth factor β and its natural inhibitor decorin in the human placenta and decidua throughout gestation. *Placenta*, **16**, 221–31.

Maruo, T. and Mochizuki, M. (1987). Immunohistochemical localization of epidermal growth factor receptor and *myc* oncogene product in human placenta: implication for trophoblast proliferation and differentiation. *American Journal of Obstetrics and Gynecology*, **156**, 721–7.

Maruo, T., Matsuo, H., Murata, K., and Mochizuki, M. (1992). Gestational age-dependent dual action of epidermal growth factor on human placenta early in gestation. *Journal of Clinical Endocrinology and Metabolism*, **75**, 1362–7.

Matsuo, H., Maruo, T., Murata, K., and Mochizuki, M. (1993). Human early placental trophoblasts produce an epidermal growth factor-like substance in synergy with thyroid hormone. *Acta Endocrinologica*, **128**, 225–9.

Mohr, L.R. and Trounson, A.O. (1982). Comparative ultrastructure of hatched human, mouse and bovine blastocysts. *Journal of Reproduction and Fertility*, **66**, 499–504.

Morrish, D.W., Bhardwaj, D., Dabbagh, L.K., Marusyk, H., and Siy, O. (1987). Epidermal growth factor induces differentiation and secretion of human chorionic gonadotropin and placental lactogen in normal human placenta. *Journal of Clinical Endocrinology and Metabolism*, **65**, 1282–90.

Morrish, D.W., Bhardwaj, D., and Paras, M.T. (1991). Transforming growth factor $\beta 1$ inhibits placental differentiation and human chorionic gonadotropin and human placental lactogen secretion. *Endocrinology*, **129**, 22–6.

Mühlhauser, J., Crescimanno, C., Kaufmann, P., Höfler, H., Zaccheo, D., and Castellucci, M. (1993). Differentiation and proliferation patterns in human trophoblast revealed by c-*erbB-2* oncogene product and EGF-R. *The Journal of Histochemistry and Cytochemistry*, **41**, 165–73.

Nelson, D.M., Crouch, E.C., Curran, E.M., and Farmer, D.R. (1990). Trophoblast interaction with fibrin matrix. Epithelialization of perivillous fibrin deposits as a mechanism for villous repair in the human placenta. *American Journal of Pathology*, **136**, 855–65.

Ohlsson, R., Holmgren, L., Glaser, A., Szpecht, A., and Pfeifer-Ohlsson, S. (1989). Insulin-like growth factor 2 and short-range stimulatory loops in the control of human placental growth. *EMBO Journal*, **8**, 1995–9.

Ohlsson, R., Glaser, A., Holmgren, L., and Franklin, G. (1993). The molecular biology of placental development. In *The human placenta*, (ed. C.W.G. Redman, I.L. Sargent, and P.M. Starkey), pp. 33–81. Blackwell Scientific Publications, Oxford.

Pampfer, S., Daiter, E., Barad, D., and Pollard, J.W. (1992). Expression of the colony stimulating factor-1 receptor (c-*fms* proto-oncogene product) in the human uterus and placenta. *Biology of Reproduction*, **46**, 48–57.

Pfeifer-Ohlsson, S., Goustin, A.S., Rydnert, J., Wahlström, T., Bjersing, L., Stehelin, D., *et al.* (1984). Spatial and temporal pattern of cellular *myc* oncogene expression in developing human placenta: implications for embryonic cell proliferation. *Cell*, **38**, 585–96.

Regan, L. and Braude, P.R. (1987). Is antipaternal cytotoxic antibody a valid marker in the management of recurrent abortion? *Lancet*, **ii**, 1280.

Rodway, M.R. and Rao, Ch. V. (1995). A novel perspective on the role of human chorionic gonadotropin during pregnancy and in gestational trophoblastic disease. *Early Pregnancy: Biology and Medicine*, **1**, 176–87.

Saito, S., Saito, M., Enomoto, M., Ito, A., Motoyoshi, K., Nakagawa, T., *et al.* (1993). Human macrophage-colony-stimulating factor induces the differentiation of trophoblast. *Growth Factors*, **9**, 11–19.

Saito, S., Sakakura, S., Enomoto, M., Ichijo, M., Matsumoto, K., Nakamura, T., *et al.* (1995). Hepatocyte growth factor promotes the growth of cytotrophoblasts by the paracrine mechanism. *Journal of Biochemistry*, **117**, 671–6.

Sawai, K., Azuma, C., Koyama, M., Ito, S.I., Hashimoto, K., Kimura, T., *et al.* (1995). Leukemia inhibitory factor (LIF) enhances trophoblast differentiation mediated by human chorionic gonadotropin (hCG). *Biochemical and Biophysical Research Communications*, **211**, 137–43.

Schmidt, C., Bladt, F., Goedecke, S., Brinkman, V., Zschlesche, W., Sharpe, M., *et al.* (1995). Scatter factor/hepatocyte growth factor is essential for liver development. *Nature*, **373**, 699–702.

Shi, Q.J., Lei, Z.M., Rao, Ch. V., and Lin, J. (1993). Novel role of human chorionic gonadotropin in differentiation of human cytotrophoblasts. *Endocrinology*, **132**, 1387–95.

Simpson, R.A., Mayhew, T.M., and Barnes, P.R. (1992). From 13 weeks to term, the trophoblast of human placenta grows by the continuous recruitment of new proliferative units: a study of nuclear number using the disector. *Placenta*, **13**, 501–12.

Smith, C.A. and Moore, H.D.M. (1988). Expression of C-type viral particles at implantation in the marmoset monkey. *Human Reproduction*, **3**, 395–8.

Tesarík, J. (1989). Involvement of oocyte-coded message in cell differentiation control of human embryos. *Development*, **105**, 317–22.

Uehara, Y., Minowa, O., Morl, C., Shlota, K., Kuno, J., Noda, T., *et al.* (1995). Placental defect and embryonic lethality in mice lacking hepatocyte growth factor/scatter factor. *Nature*, **373**, 702–5.

de Virgillis, G., Sideri, M., Fumagalli, G., and Remotti, G. (1982). The junctional pattern of the human villous trophoblast: a freeze fracture study. *Gynecological and Obstetrical Investigation*, **14**, 263–72.

Watson, A.L., Palmer, M.E., and Burton, G.J. (1996). An *in vitro* model for the study of wound healing in first trimester human placenta. *Cell and Tissue Research*, (in press).

10 | *The trophoblast* in vitro *and* in vivo

Eytan R. Barnea

INTRODUCTION

The separation of the conceptus into extraembryonic structures including the tro-phoblast and the embryoblast occurs around implantation, when cell proliferation begins to accelerate. Around implantation, the trophoblast starts to differentiate from the cytotrophoblast (CT) into the syncytiotrophoblast (ST). There are three main forces that are operative during implantation and the first few weeks thereafter. The first involves recognition and immunological allowance, and is due to embryo-derived recognition factors and endometrial receptivity (see Chapters 4 and 7). The second is the attachment and invasion of the trophoblast through the action of proteolytic enzymes (principally metalloproteases), through a system of checks and balances involving local cell regulators, i.e. integrins and growth factors (see Chapter 8). The third is the migration and penetration of CT cells into decidual blood vessels, thereby becoming extravillous and changing their biochemical and secretory properties. By invading the endothelium and lining endothelial surfaces, these cells lower blood flow to the trophoblastic cast, and serve, among other roles, as a shield and anchor for the conceptus.

The properties of extravillous trophoblastic cells, as shown by several studies, are different from those of villous trophoblastic cells (e.g. lack of human chorionic gonadotrophin (hCG), expression of alkaline phosphatase and other markers) (see Chapter 8) and will not be further discussed here.

TROPHOBLASTIC DEVELOPMENT AND CONTROL

Knowledge of the trophoblast during the pre-embryonic period (before five weeks) is rather limited (see Chapter 1). While the trophoblast undergoes rapid growth, the growth of the embryoblast is slow in comparison. Strategically, the embryoblast is located behind the trophoblast where it is shielded both physically and metabolically from the maternal environment (see Chapter 23). According to Maruo *et al.* (1992), at 4–5 weeks of gestation hCG is only present in the CT; in contrast, immunohisto-chemical studies show that its expression shifts to the ST by the sixth week. Moreover, epidermal growth factor (EGF), a known hCG stimulator, and its receptor are also found in the CT at 4–5 weeks of gestation and then shift to the ST. Together, such data point to an autocrine control of hCG (and perhaps also of human placental lactogen (hPL)) secretion in very early pregnancy. This shift in location also points to the lack of the need in very early gestation for trophoblast differentiation in order to express hCG, and subsequently hPL, which is clearly the case later in gestation.

This suggests that the placenta undergoes several distinct stages of development which are brought about by the shifting needs of the embryo/fetus. Recent observation supports the view that placental function and regulation change substantially during gestation (e.g. hCG secretion). Once the pre-embryonal stage of the trophoblast is completed, a major increase in hCG secretion is noted which is coupled with very rapid embryonic development. The signals responsible for such a massive start of cell proliferation are not clear at present. However, it is clear that both genetic and epigenetic factors play a role.

Prior to 1980, the first trimester trophoblast (FTT) was rarely investigated. More recent studies have revealed that the placenta is a dynamic organ whose function and regulation change dramatically across gestation requiring longitudinal comparative studies as we and others have carried out (Kato and Braunstein 1990). These studies show changes in morphologic features, metabolism, immunology, proliferation, and invasivity. Currently, the FTT is under intensive investigation because of the view that insight into the subject will have implications that are far beyond the understanding of that period (see later for examples).

During embryogenesis, the regulation of the FTT becomes responsive to hormonal control through the effect of several paracrine factors (Table 10.1) deriving from the decidua (leukaemia-inhibitory factor (LIF)), autocrine influences (gonadotrophin-releasing hormone (GnRH), interleukin-6 (IL-6), EGF, and insulin-like growth factors (IGFs)), and endocrine factors deriving from the corpus luteum (progesterone, oxytocin (OT), arginine vasopressin (AVP), and relaxin) and the embryo itself (Barnea *et al.* 1989*a*); and the list continues to grow. Decidual cells are a rich source for hormonal and regulatory agents; among others, EGF, somatostatin, prolactin (PRL), activin, inhibin, plasma proteins 12 and 14 (PP12, PP14), and prorenin. On the other hand, tumor necrosis factor alpha (TNFα), LIF, interleukin-1 (IL-1), and IGF binding protein-I (IGF-BP-I) were described to be produced locally (Barnea and Shurtz-Swirski 1992). Some of these agents were shown to modulate placental hormonal function

Table 10.1 Sources of influences of placental hormone secretion according to gestational age

| Source | Gestational age (weeks) | | | |
	1–2	3–5	6–9	10–40
Maternal pituitary	+	=	=	=
Maternal ovary	+	++	+	=
Decidua	+	++	+	=
Embryo/amniotic fluid	=	+	++	+
Trophoblast	+	++	++	+++

= no effect; + low effect; ++ moderate effect; +++ large effect.

(see later). More recently, a decidual factor was isolated; this 10 kDa protein (decidual chorionic gonadotrophin-inhibitory protein (DCIP)) inhibits hCG secretion in a time- and dose-dependent manner (Ren and Braunstein 1994; see also Chapter 6).

The distinction among different types and relative contributions of various factors is difficult to make since there are several which are expressed at the same time in the FTT, decidua, and perhaps elsewhere. An illustrative example is progesterone, which is initially secreted by the corpus luteum, but consequently produced by the FTT. With respect to function, this steroid has several roles including a trophic effect on the endometrium and decidua, a complex role in inducing immune tolerance, and a complex effect on hCG secretion (p. 10).

During embryogenesis, embryo-derived factors may begin to play a regulatory role as well. The potential role of embryo-derived factors in hCG and progesterone regulation has been described (Barnea *et al.* 1989*a*; Shurtz-Swirski *et al.* 1991), and summarized (Barnea 1994*a*). Briefly, several visceral and neural organs contain low size proteinaceous compounds which have a time-, dose-, and gestational age-dependent effect on both hCG and progesterone secretion by placental explants in static and dynamic cultures. This was evidenced, in general, by an inhibitory effect on hCG secretion by fractions prior to nine weeks, but an opposite effect later in the first trimester (see also Chapter 15).

As embryonal size and complexity grow, the link between the embryo and the FTT very quickly becomes of endocrine nature, mainly through the umbilical cord (although exchange of regulatory compounds through the amniotic fluid is not excluded). The functional dependence between the embryo and FTT is supported by the finding that the end of the embryonic period coincides with a plateau and subsequent decline in hCG secretion. Following embryogenesis, a shift towards the formation of ST cells from CT cells, the development of functional blood vessels, and mesenchymal proliferation (Hustin 1992) lead to the formation of the placenta itself.

Thus, the development of the FTT may be divided functionally into the autonomous period, the embryonic period, and the fetal period, with additional subdivisions which may or may not be needed (Table 10.2). Many of the aforesaid statements are supported by *in vitro* findings and some are also supported by *in vivo* observations.

Table 10.2 Proposed evolution of the trophoblast during gestation, based on morphologic and functional parameters (see text for details)

Developmental stages	Period	Invasivity	Vascular stroma	hCG secretion
Zygote	1–4 days	N/A	N/A	No
Pre-implantation	5–16 days	High	No	Minimal
Embryonal (< 6 weeks)	2–6 weeks	High	No	Exponential
Embryonal (> 6 weeks)	6–9 weeks	High	Minimal	Slows down
hCG plateau	9–10 weeks	High	Moderate	Plateau
Fetal period	11–36 weeks	Low	High	Decrease
Senescent	36–40 weeks	Low	Low	Low

HORMONES OF THE FTT

Human chorionic gonadotropin (hCG)

hCG is the prime functional marker of the FTT. This glycoprotein (approximately 36 000 Da) is composed of two dissimilar subunits, α and β, which are joined non-covalently. Both hCG and the pituitary glycoprotein hormones (follicle-stimulating hormone, FSH; thyroid-stimulating hormone, TSH; and luteinizing hormone, LH share a similar α subunit; it is their specific β subunit which dictates their function. The specificity of hCG β is due to a 24 amino acid extension on its carboxyl terminal. The tertiary structure of the subunits is achieved through internal disulphide bonds and carbohydrate moieties. Much of the micro-heterogeneity of the hormone is due to variation in carbohydrate structures and the degree of sialylation (Ren and Braunstein 1992).

Biochemical and morphological results suggest that formation of the ST from the CT is the principal event leading to hCG biosynthesis after six weeks (Maruo *et al.* 1992). The α and β subunits are encoded for on different chromosomes (6 and 19, respectively); there are six β genes, of which only three are functional. After formation of the protein core, the hCG subunits are glycosylated and then combine (Hoshina *et al.* 1982).

Immunohistochemical studies have demonstrated that hCG is found within the trophoblast surface, in the microvilli and cisterns of the rough endoplasmic reticulum, but not in the Golgi apparatus. Newly synthesized hCG is rapidly secreted by the trophoblast which involves its attachment to the plasma membrane. Storage of hCG by secretory granules in the trophoblast has also been demonstrated in the first trimester, but not at term (Morrish *et al.* 1987). Several studies have been carried out regarding the precise regulation of hCG formation and secretion. Despite all efforts, however, there is no consensus on the identity of the real regulators, although several important modulatory factors have been identified. Evidently, *in vitro* observations show only part of the picture and *in vivo* data on the subject remain limited.

Human placental lactogen (hPL)

hPL is a 190-amino acid, single-chain polypeptide which is cross-linked with two disulphide bonds (cystine bridges). The polypeptide, a 22 308 Da-molecule, has 85 per cent homology to human growth hormone, and is similar to PRL (64 per cent). In circulation, a small quantity exists in a dimeric form, and a large precursor molecule (25 kDa) may exist. At term, hPL secretion accounts for 10 per cent of all placental secretions, and is four-fold higher than in the FTT, due to increased transcription. hPL acts by binding to lactogenic receptors (growth hormone, GH, and PRL), since there are no specific receptors for hPL. Since the ST is the site for hPL production and secretion, its increase in the circulation is mainly seen after the first trimester. There are five genes for hPL, all located on chromosome 17.

Little is known about the regulation or post-binding action of the polypeptide. Opioid peptides, angiotensin II, cyclic adenosine monophosphate (cAMP), insulin, and IGF2 have been shown to exert a stimulatory effect, while prostaglandins E_2 and $F_{2\alpha}$ and somatostatin (a hormone of CT origin) may also act as negative regulators of hPL since somatostatin secretion decreases with advancing gestation (Handwerger *et al.* 1994). The involvement of hPL in fetal growth may be exerted through an increase in somatomedins. However, hPL may not be necessary for pregnancy since in some placentae the polypeptide is not detected (Hubert *et al.* 1983).

Moreover, while the role of hPL in other species has been established, the hormone's function in humans remains poorly defined. Overall, as compared to hCG, placental hPL is insensitive to the effects of several hormonal factors, but it is sensitive to metabolic factors, such as the addition of high-density lipoprotein *in vitro*, and fasting *in vivo* (Handwerger and Brar 1992). Circulating apolipoproteins, even in a delipidated form, increase hPL secretion by cells, acting through adenylate cyclase and phosphoinositide hydrolysis pathways. Placenta-derived GH is detected in the ST from the ninth week onwards (Falcone and Little 1994*a*). Its regulation is not known and the secretion is not stimulated by the GH-releasing factor.

Opioid peptides

Pro-opiomelanocortin (POMC) is a 31-kDa precursor for several opioid peptides (including β-lipotropin, adrenocorticotrophic hormone (ACTH), β-endorphin, and α-melanocyte-stimulating hormone (αMSH) in the placenta (Odagiri *et al.* 1979). In early pregnancy, significant levels of opioid peptides are found in amniotic fluid and are thought to be derived from the FTT. Both β-endorphin and dynorphin have significant, but opposing, specific effects on hCG secretion in static and dynamic FTT cultures (Barnea *et al.* 1991 *a,b*). Their effect is time-, dose-, and receptor-dependent, and is not mimicked by inactive analogues. The use of naloxone, an opioid antagonist, has revealed that endogenous opioid peptides exert a negative effect on basal hCG secretion.

The opioid peptides tested so far are known to exert their effect through receptors which are different from those described at term (k receptors). Therefore, in order to determine the sites of action of β-endorphin and dynorphin, we conducted preliminary experiments which show that other receptors are present in the FTT as well (Barnea and Sarne, unpublished data). The post-receptor events of opioid peptide action in the FTT have not been studied, but our data on dynorphin 1–13 fragment suggest its involvement in suppressing the entry of calcium ions to cells or in blocking adenylate cyclase (see the positive effect of cAMP in this context on hCG secretion, p. 166). The positive effect on hCG secretion may also be exerted by inhibiting local progesterone secretion (Barnea *et al.* 1991*c*). Finally, several other derivatives of POMC have effects on hCG and sex steroid secretion in the FTT. With respect to corticotrophin-releasing factor (CRF), its expression in the FTT is low, and is localized in the ST (Mochizuki *et al.* 1994).

Steroids

The FTT progressively takes over steroid production. The earliest steroid produced is oestradiol, which is already present by the sixth week of gestation since it requires the presence of local androgens. This is followed by progesterone around 7–8 weeks following regression of the corpus luteum. The third and final steroid production to be taken over by the placenta is that of corticosteroids.

The production of sex steroids involves the attachment of low-density lipoprotein cholesterol (LDL-C), which is the main source for local steroid production. The binding of LDL-C to specific receptors ('coated pits') on the microvilli leads to endocytosis; when these are internalized, they fuse with acid lipase, leading to the hydrolysis of cholesterol esters. Expression of LDL-C receptors is highest in the FTT (Furuhashi *et al.* 1989). These receptors are expressed from the sixth week, reaching a peak in the FTT. The production of progesterone occurs by breakdown of maternal LDL-C, while oestrogens are derived from maternal or fetal dehydroepiandrosterone (DHEA). In the case of hypobetalipoproteinaemia, progesterone, 17 β-oestradiol, and oestriol secretion are much below normal, illustrating the need for maternal precursors for placental steroid secretion (Parker *et al.* 1986).

The placental enzymes responsible for steroid synthesis belong to the P-450 cytochrome family. The classical description of the feto-placental unit with respect to steroid metabolism and its control may not be applicable for the first trimester. The trophoblast has intracellular oestrogen and progesterone receptors that are localized in the nucleus, suggesting the presence of an autocrine mode of control. Regulation of placental progesterone secretion is complex, and limited data are available on its regulation in the FTT. Overall, β-adrenergic agents have a stimulatory effect, while dynorphin 1–13 and GnRH have an inhibitory effect (Barnea *et al.* 1992*a*). Progesterone, in addition to its effect on hCG (discussed below, p. 164), also decreases CRF secretion. Data from *in vitro* studies show that the addition of RU486, a specific progesterone antagonist, decreases hPL and as well as progesterone secretion.

Inhibin and related compounds

Transforming growth factor β (TGFβ) and inhibin are members of a family of growth factors which share structural, but not functional similarities. Activin is a homodimer of the β subunit of inhibin (Qu *et al.* 1992). Two forms of inhibin have been described, A and B. The expression, and possibly the function, of inhibin changes with gestation. Minami *et al.* (1995) examined the expression of inhibin in the FTT using immunohistochemical techniques (Falcone and Little 1994*a*). The results show that the inhibin αA and βA subunits are expressed in the ST; in contrast, the staining for the βB subunit is faint in the FTT. No changes in the intensity of staining have been found during the first trimester (Table 10.3). It is of note that in capillaries, erythroblastic cells stained for the βB subunit, indicating that perhaps the growth factor may be involved in haemopoiesis. With respect to inhibin function, Mersol-Berg *et al.* (1990) have shown that inhibin suppresses hCG secretion at term but not in the FTT.

Prorenin

Prorenin is a precursor peptide whose active form, renin, is a powerful peptide involved in blood pressure regulation by the kidney. The placenta contains both

Table 10.3   Inhibin-related compounds in the FTT

Compounds	mRNA	Localization
Inhibin α	High	CT
Inhibin βA	High	CT/ST
Inhibin βB	Low	ST
Activin	No	CT

CT, cytotrophoblast; ST, syncytiotrophoblast.

prorenin and renin; but the FTT has higher prorenin and renin levels than at term. In contrast, the decidual content does not change with gestation (Downing *et al.* 1995). Moreover, we have preliminary data showing that prorenin is detected in the effluent of superfused placental explants and that the secretion is episodic and is stimulated by GnRH (Barnea and Poisner, personal communication). It was shown by Szilágyi *et al.* (1995) that prorenin secretion in static cultures of FTT is modulated by sex steroids. This information, coupled with earlier findings that activity of both angiotensins I and II is present in the placenta and that high levels of prorenin are found in the amniotic fluid during the first trimester, raises intriguing questions regarding this hormone's function. One intriguing possibility is that it is involved in promoting angiogenesis locally.

USE OF THE FTT AS AN EXPERIMENTAL MODEL

The scope of this section is not to describe in detail the large body of data accumulated in the field of early pregnancy investigation *in vitro*, but instead to emphasize the need for a thorough investigation of this critical period of gestation. This emphasis is necessary since animal models, although very useful, are not suitable for investigating hCG regulation; what is lost by using *in vitro* investigations is gained by obtaining specific information on humans. On the other hand, animal models provide information on intact subjects. However, only primates, with their chorionic gonadotrophin (CG) production, are capable of mimicking conditions in humans, and it is recognized that this source is limited in access, and is very expensive.

Models used

The FTT was, until recently, studied using static-cell, tissue-explant, or spheroid cultures. The use of choriocarcinoma or immortalized cell lines in this context will not be discussed further because their regulation, particularly with respect to hCG, appears to be quite different (Licht *et al.* 1994; Rodway and Rao 1995). Dynamic culture systems to study the FTT have also been developed, attempting to mimic the conditions present *in vivo*, which at best is only partial (Barnea 1994*b*). When static cultures are compared with dynamic cultures, important information regarding hormones, patterns of secretion, and their control is acquired, but information on FTT morphology, proliferation, and metabolism is limited. Moreover, the release of hCG in long-term static cultures may not correlate with the viability of the tissues (Watson *et al.* 1995).

Cell cultures are viewed as important for FTT investigation, but it is now recognized that cell to cell contact and interaction may be particularly important in the FTT and are required for maintaining spontaneous episodic hormonal secretion, an important aspect of trophoblast function *in vivo* and *in vitro* (Owens *et al.* 1981; Barnea and Kaplan 1989; Barnea *et al.* 1992*b*). Other investigations have utilized cell cultures since only in that manner can cell differentiation and invasivity be examined and the regulatory factors involved be determined (see Chapter 8). On the other hand, cells isolated in the preparation of cultures are mostly CT and white cells, while the ST layer is lost during cell isolation procedures. Therefore, functional links between CT and ST elements are not present, requiring *de novo* differentiation of the CT *in vitro* to ST, which is limited in the first trimester. Overall, it has to be recognized that any experimental model is only valuable if the questions asked are appropriate and if their limitations are recognized beforehand, so that conclusions drawn from the data are not overstated.

Comparison of static and dynamic cultures

The specifics of the superfusion models available have been discussed (Barnea 1994*b*). In static cultures, exposure to test agents is continuous (hours, days) and collection of medium is infrequent; this is clearly different from the situation *in vivo* where the placental environment is continuously changing (Merz *et al.* 1991) through the introduction and elimination of elements through the circulation, the presence of the decidua, bathing in the amniotic fluid, and links to the embryo. On the other hand, dynamic cultures (superfusion) provide the tissue with a continuous flow of fresh nutritive medium while constantly eliminating secretory products and waste materials, apparently creating a quasi-optimal surrounding for the trophoblast. This is especially important since it is not possible to conduct placental perfusion experiments (a very valuable model at term) in the first trimester due to the lack of functional blood vessels in the FTT. In addition, since the transport of nutrients and oxygen from the mother to the FTT is primarily achieved through diffusion and not through the vascular system which evolves later, use of the superfusion model adds a new dimension to trophoblast investigation (Barnea 1994*b*). Using this model, evidence has been provided to show that hormonal secretions are episodic, resembling patterns present *in vivo* (Barnea 1993*b*). As Fig. 10.1 shows, the patterns of episodic hCG and progesterone secretion, measured simultaneously in superfused FTT explants, appear to be different since the peaks rarely correlate.

Moreover, the spontaneous pulsatility of hCG is protein-synthesis dependent since it is blocked by addition of cycloheximide (Barnea *et al.* 1992*b*). As experiments with tritiated leucine have shown, newly formed proteins (as shown by incorporated leucine) also have a spontaneous pulsatile pattern which is different from that of hCG measured simultaneously. The pattern of hCG secretion is very consistent, both in explants from the same placenta and in different placentas.

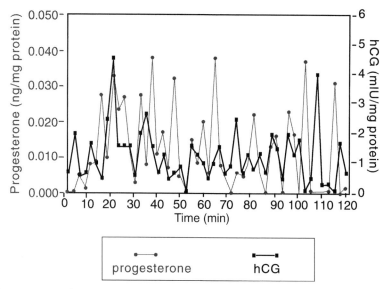

Fig. 10.1 Patterns of spontaneous episodic hCG and progesterone secretion by superfused FTT explants determined in the same placenta. There is a low concordance between the two hormone peaks.

Secretion profiles change with gestational age (Kaplan *et al.* 1991) and factors which control spontaneous episodic hormone secretion (mostly hCG) have been investigated (Table 10.4). The superfusion model provides valuable additional parameters by which the patterns of FTT secretory products can be examined. In addition to increases or decreases in secretion, changes in pulse frequency, amplitude, and the area under the curve can be measured, and trend analyses can be carried out. The

Table 10.4 Compounds that were shown to have an effect on superfused placental explants following *in vivo* and *in vitro* exposure

In vivo	
Maternal exposure	Neuroleptics, xenobiotics, cigarette smoking
In vitro	
Peptides	GnRH, GnRH agonist and antagonists, dynorphin 1-13, dynorphin 2-13, naloxone
Growth factors	EGF, human parathyroid hormone 1-34, insulin
Cytokines	IL-1β
Xenobiotics	Benzo(a)pyrene, cadmium, mercury, benzodiazepines
Steroids	Progesterone, RU486
Embryonal tissues and extracts	Brain, spinal cord, lung, adrenal, kidney
Miscellaneous	Calcium, EDTA, cAMP, cycloheximide, GABA, GABA inhibitor

effect of test compounds on any or all of these parameters can be determined in a quantitative manner. A given test compound could affect one or more parameters and its effects could change with gestational age, supporting the view that placental function is not static but adjusts to particular needs at various stages of gestation.

Overall, in the superfusion model, the effects noted are specific, and are achieved at low concentrations (physiological range). The intermittent administration of test compounds is much more advantageous than continuous exposure. In addition, the effects of single factors can be determined while minimizing the interference of the FTT itself by its own secretory products, which may be the case in static cultures. When comparing basal hormonal secretion in static and superfusion models, the total hCG secretion in dynamic cultures for the same period has been found to be higher (Merz *et al.* 1991; Barnea 1994*b*). This illustrates that under more favourable conditions, the FTT is better at expressing its secretory products. Furthermore, the superfusion model enables comparison of patterns of different hormonal secretion, both under basal and experimental conditions, determination of receptor dependence, distinction between the effects of hormone agonists and antagonists, and establishing whether the effect is positive or negative on hormone secretion (Barnea *et al.* 1991*d*).

The superfusion model also enables testing of environmental pollutants, such as cigarette smoke and its constituents, showing specific, non-toxic effects, making it a valuable tool in non-invasive toxicological studies as well (Boadi *et al.* 1992; Shurtz-Swirski *et al.* 1992*a*; Barnea 1994*b*). In addition, the superfusion model has been used to determine unidirectional paracrine interactions between embryonal tissues, showing that potent secretory products are produced by the embryo, which modulate placental hCG and progesterone secretion (see Chapter 15).

Overall, the exact rationale for episodic secretion by the FTT is not known at present, but we hypothesize that it may be advantageous for several reasons:

(1)   it saves energy for the cell;

(2)   it enables the cell to maintain high circulating hormone levels;

(3)   it prevents downregulation of receptors both locally and at a distance; and

(4)   it creates both a tonic and clonic mode of secretion, which may have different but complementary functions.

CONTROL OF PLACENTAL HORMONE SECRETION *IN VITRO*

Hormonal secretion by the FTT is responsive to several internal and external influences. These factors are secreted by the pituitary, ovary, and decidua in the mother, by products derived from the embryo and perhaps extraembryonic structures, and by local regulatory pathways (Table 10.1). The relative importance of these factors frequently changes with advancing gestation. The complex and far-from-being-elucidated interplay among the internal and external influences described determines overall hormone secretion. The simple loops of endocrine control seen in the central nervous system (i.e. hypothalamus, pituitary, and gonads) do not appear to be applicable to the placenta in which feedback loops are much more complex.

Figure 10.2 describes the various factors that have been shown to affect hCG secretion (the glycoprotein which is most commonly investigated) *in vitro*. It is clear that there is a redundancy in the control systems and that several factors may play only a permissive role while others may be critical for production/secretion of hCG. Since it is recognized that without production/secretion of hCG there can be no viable pregnancy (contrary to hPL), hCG itself must have a pivotal role.

The effect produced, whether stimulatory or inhibitory, depends on the experimental conditions used. Spontaneous episodic hCG secretion requires cell-to-cell contact or interaction (present in explants), since this pattern was not observed in viable isolated cells (Barnea *et al.* 1992*b*). hCG is stored in specific secretory granules and its secretion is protein-synthesis dependent, as are other placental proteins (Morrish *et al.* 1987). Spontaneous hCG episodic secretion is modulated by secondary messengers, calcium ions, and cAMP, and spontaneous hCG pulsatility can be up- or downregulated in a reversible manner (Barnea and Check 1992*a*; Barnea 1994*b*).

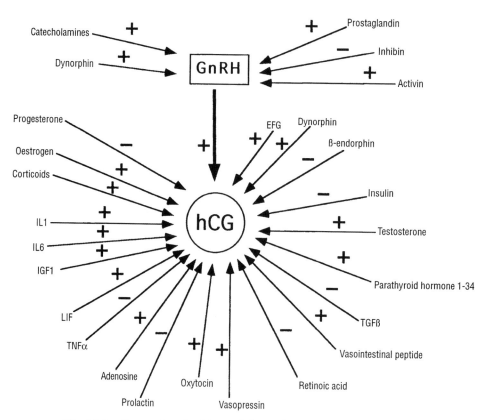

Fig. 10.2   Factors involved in modulating hCG secretion by the FTT.

Several novel functions of hCG have been described, beyond its being a controller of corpus luteum secretion in early pregnancy (Rodway and Rao 1995); hCG may also have autocrine effects exerted through local receptors. However, hCG secretion is not decreased by having the glycoprotein itself added to cell cultures of FTT, an observation similar to that seen in choriocarcinoma cells but different from that seen at term (Licht *et al.* 1993). Therefore, a fresh look at the subject is required.

The role of gonadotrophin-releasing hormone (GnRH)

This locally secreted decapeptide is regarded as an important positive regulator of hCG secretion/production in the FTT but not at term (Siler-Khodr *et al.* 1991; Barnea *et al.* 1992*c*). Placental GnRH is similar but not identical to the pituitary decapeptide (Gautron *et al.* 1989). Both GnRH and its precursor are produced by the placenta, and GnRH secretion is controlled by several agents (i.e. insulin and adrenaline) at term (Petraglia *et al.* 1989); whether the regulation is similar in the FTT is not known. GnRH has a major stimulatory effect on hCG production and secretion in the FTT; the effect is potent, and is time- and dose-dependent (Currie *et al.* 1993). The effect is specific, and is exerted through binding to high-affinity sites on the membrane (Barnea, unpublished data). In superfusion, short pulses of a GnRH analogue had a markedly higher effect (4–5 orders of magnitude) than that seen by adding the decapeptide to static cultures (Barnea and Check 1992*b*). The effect exerted is calcium-dependent (Mathialgan and Rao 1989); it is mimicked by calcium (Barnea 1994*b*) and blocked by calcium-channel blockers.

Immunohistological studies have reported the presence of GnRH-like material in the CT, but recent data show that messenger ribonucleic acid (mRNA) for GnRH is also present in the ST. In an earlier study using *in situ* hybridization assays, no differences in the presence of GnRH mRNA were found throughout gestation. Very recently, however, it was reported that the level of GnRH-receptor mRNA changes in proportion to that of hCG. The expression of the receptor mRNA is present by six weeks, becomes maximal at nine weeks, and declines to non-detectable levels at term, further supporting the role of GnRH in hCG regulation (Lin *et al.* 1995). Spontaneous episodic hCG secretion is also, in part, regulated by endogenous GnRH, since addition of a GnRH antagonist decreases both basal secretion and peak amplitude of spontaneous episodic hCG secretion (Barnea *et al.* 1991*d*; Tables 10.5, 10.6).

Table 10.5 GnRH in the FTT and term placenta

	FTT	Term placenta
Concentration	High	Low
Effect on hCG in superfusion	Marked	None
Effect on hCG in static culture	Mild	Only in high doses
High-affinity receptor	Present	Present
Receptor mRNA	Present	Absent

Table 10.6   The effect of GnRH and GnRH-agonist on hCG in the FTT

Stimulation of hCG biosynthesis
Rapid genome-independent stimulatory effect
Highly effective stimulation with short pulses
Time- and dose-dependent stimulation
Effectivity in the K_M range of the high-affinity receptor
100:1 effectiveness of GnRH-agonist:GnRH
Up- and downregulation of basal hCG pulsatility
Effect blocked by specific GnRH antagonist
Neutralization of effect by coadministration with progesterone

The role of steroids

Progesterone is involved in controlling hCG secretion; the steroid exerts differing effects on patterns of spontaneous pulsatile hCG secretion under basal and stimulated conditions. The effect of short progesterone pulses in low doses is profoundly inhibitory and decreases hCG pulse frequency (Barnea and Kaplan 1989; Barnea *et al.* 1991*c*). Furthermore, when both hormone levels are determined in superfusion, a complex pattern of interaction emerges: progesterone secretion is episodic and corre-lates with spontaneous hCG pulse frequency, but the peaks of the two hormones rarely coincide. Moreover, pulses of GnRH and dynorphin increase hCG secretion while lowering progesterone secretion (Barnea, unpublished data), confirming earlier observations (Wilson and Jawad 1980). Maruo *et al.* (1986) have shown that in static cultures, adding progesterone for 48 h decreases hCG secretion by lowering the levels of the mRNAs of both the α and β subunits of hCG.

The antagonism between the effects of GnRH and progesterone has been demon-strated by giving both agents together in short pulses during superfusion, without effect (Barnea 1994*b*). The specificity of progesterone action was also shown by adding RU486, a specific progesterone-receptor blocker, which abolished the progesterone-induced effect (Szilágyi *et al.* 1993). Overall, the effect of progesterone can be exerted on hCG biosynthesis (genome-dependent), but the steroid may also act by preventing the release of hCG storage granules through action on the cell surface, an effect which is produced within minutes. Recently, genome-independent effects of progesterone action were described elsewhere (xenopus oocyte). The steroid's negative effect on hCG secretion may also be exerted through action on corticoid receptors, as these steroids have been shown to stimulate hCG secretion as well. The stimulatory effect of low dose 17β-oestradiol and cortisol on hCG secretion by the FTT was also reported (Barnea *et al.* 1991*c*). In addition, the androgen DHEA has a stimulatory effect, while testosterone exerted an inhibitory effect on hCG secretion in four-day cultures (Ahmed and Murphy 1988).

The role of cytokines

A GnRH-independent pathway of hCG regulation has been described in isolated cell cultures (Matsuzaki *et al.* 1994): it involves a complex cascade of positive and negative regulation by cytokines. According to the model, IL-1 and TNFα stimulate IL-6 secretion which, in turn, through receptor binding, releases hCG. On the other hand, TGFβ blocks IL-1 and IL-6 action, thereby blocking hCG secretion. Very recently, soluble IL-6 receptors were found to be present in the sera of pregnant women. These receptors were shown to form complexes with IL-6 and thereby stimulate the secretion of hCG by the FTT. As inhibition experiments show, this effect may be exerted by homodimerization of glycoprotein 130 (GP 130) and activation of the JAK family of tyrosine kinases in the FTT (Matsuzaki *et al.* 1995). The stimulatory role of locally produced LIF on hCG secretion has also been described (Sawai *et al.* 1995).

Experiments using tyrosine kinase antagonists have revealed that its effect is exerted through tyrosine-kinase dependent GP130 activation. Evidence for the location of IL-1 in the endometrium during early pregnancy has also been provided, suggesting that the cytokine may have a paracrine role (Yang *et al.* 1995).

The role of growth factors

Early pregnancy is characterized by a massive growth of the FTT. The involvement of growth factors in this process has been investigated. Table 10.7 shows the growth factors that have been found in the FTT; the function of many of them is unclear. This is due to several factors, including the presence of several species of binding proteins for IGFs which may limit or enhance their function, the putative sites of action, and their differential expression during gestation.

The growth factor which has received most attention is EGF, which causes phosphorylation of membrane proteins and acts as a mitogen by increasing deoxyribonucleic acid (DNA) and ribonucleic acid (RNA) synthesis; it may have also a direct

Table 10.7 Presence of growth factors and their binding sites in the FTT

Growth factor	Presence	Binding site
Epidermal growth factor (EGF)	+	+
Insulin	+/−	+
Insulin-like growth factor 1 (IGF1)	+	+
Insulin-like growth factor 2 (IGF2)	+	+
Interleukin-1 (IL-1)	+	+
Interleukin-6 (IL-6)	+	+
Parathyroid hormone 1-34 (PTH 1-34)	?	+
Macrophage colony-stimulating factor (M-CSF)	+	+
Granulocyte colony-stimulating factor (G-CSF)	+	+
Transforming growth factor α (TGFα)	+	+
Transforming growth factor $β_{1,2}$ (TGF$β_{1,2}$)	+	+
Interferon α,β (INFα,β)	+	+
Tumour necrosis factor α (TNFα)	+	+
Platelet-derived growth factor (PDGF)	+	+
Amphiregulin	+	?
Nerve growth factor (NGF)	+	?
Basic fibroblast growth factor (bFGF)	+	+

effect on nuclear receptors (Maruo *et al.* 1987). In the FTT, its effect is stimulatory on hCG secretion in both static and dynamic cultures. The effects noted are specific, time- and dose-dependent, and appear to be exerted on both secretion and production. In addition, EGF changes both the amplitude and frequency of spontaneous pulsatile hCG secretion in superfusion (Barnea *et al.* 1990; Barnea and Shurtz-Swirski 1992). However, the effect is gestational-age dependent since it changes after the hCG plateau and becomes inhibitory. Overall, the effect is independent of GnRH action since a specific GnRH antagonist was unable to block the EGF-induced effect. The local production of EGF and its receptor in the FTT has been demonstrated (Maruo *et al.* 1987). Additionally, a cytological change is noted in the FTT; both the ligand and its receptor are located in the CT prior to six weeks' gestation, while thereafter they are localized in the ST (Maruo *et al.* 1992).

Transforming growth factor α (TGFα) and EGF have similar structures and bind to a common receptor. The placenta contains an active receptor and TGFα mRNA is expressed throughout gestation (Falcone and Little 1994*a*). Very recent data suggest that amphiregulin, a glycoprotein which has a significant amino acid homology to the members of the EGF family, is expressed by the first-trimester ST. Its effect on hCG secretion, however, remains unknown (Lysiak *et al.* 1995).

Several other factors have been found to affect hCG secretion in the FTT. These include parathyroid hormone (PTH) and insulin, both of whose effects are also gestational-age dependent. Parathyroid hormone also increases the expression of EGF receptors in isolated cells. The effect of the hormone is unclear, but it may be adenylate-cyclase dependent, while that of EGF is mediated through tyrosine kinase (discussed by Shurtz-Swirski *et al.* 1993). Insulin is also a major hormone responsible for glucose regulation. Specific receptors for the hormone have been reported to be present in the brush-border membrane of the ST. Our data show that insulin has both a rapid and delayed effect on hCG secretion in the FTT, which is inhibitory and time-, dose-, and gestational-age dependent. The effect obtained may have been produced by a decrease in hCGβ subunit secretion (as measured by a specific radioimmunoassay) (Barnea *et al.* 1993*a*).

It is hypothesized that the effect noted, since it was obtained at very low concentrations, is exerted by binding to a high-affinity receptor and not an IGF receptor whose affinity is much lower for the ligand. In addition, IGF1 has no effect on static cultures of explants. Others have, however, found a positive effect on hCG secretion at higher concentrations (Maruo *et al.* 1995). As for IGF2, its effect on hCG secretion is not known. Its expression increases with gestation in the placenta while that of IGF 1 appears to follow an opposite course. According to our data, basic fibroblast growth factor (bFGF) does not affect hCG secretion *in vitro* (Barnea *et al.* 1993*a*).

The role of cellular mediators

We have investigated the effect of calcium and cAMP on hCG secretion. In both cases, the effect is stimulatory and achieved with 1 min pulses in superfusion. The effect of calcium chloride was blocked by a calcium chelator, ethylenediaminetetraacetic acid (EDTA) (Barnea and Check 1992*a*; Barnea *et al.* 1992*b*). This strongly suggests that the rapid release noted is due to exocytosis of stored hCG. The effect of cAMP appears to be exerted through a protein kinase. The activation of adenylate cyclase and the resulting elevation of cAMP is a common initial response of many cells to hormones that bind to surface receptors. In addition, cyclic guanosine monophosphate (cGMP) was shown to have a stimulatory effect on early tissues (Hilf and Merz 1985). There is an additional suggestion that protein kinase C is involved in the release of hCG (Iwashita *et al.* 1988).

The FTT is a source for prostaglandin production, including prostaglandin E (PGE). It has been shown that both hCG and GnRH participate in the regulation of PGE production in the FTT (North *et al.* 1991; Siler-Khodr *et al.* 1991). There is also evidence that IL-1, a major cytokine, is also involved in secretion of PGE in the FTT. The effect is attenuated by the addition of TGFβ_1 (Shimonovitz *et al.* 1995).

The roles of other factors

Several neuropeptides have a significant effect on hCG secretion in static and dynamic cultures. The effect of oxytocin (OT) is stimulatory and is exerted through a specific binding site since it is blocked by the addition of a specific receptor blocker, CAP-450 (Tal *et al.* 1991). AVP stimulates hCG secretion in both models used. On the other hand, the effect of PRL was in general inhibitory. Gamma-aminobutyric acid (GABA) stimulates hCG secretion when added in superfusion by binding to specific receptors (Merz *et al.* 1991). We have presented preliminary evidence that benzodiazepines have a similar stimulatory effect on hCG secretion in both static and dynamic cultures, which is apparently exerted through binding to specific sites present in the FTT cell membrane (Barnea *et al.* 1989*a*, 1992*d*). More recently, we reported that retinoic acid, which is known to accumulate in the FTT (Sartre *et al.* 1992), exerts a negative regulatory effect on hCG secretion in a time-dependent manner, the effect being biphasic and gestational-age dependent (Barnea *et al.* 1993*b*). Thus, retinoic acid and its teratogenic derivatives have similar negative effects prior to the hCG peak, an effect which is not noted after that stage.

Overall, these studies strongly suggest that several and diverse factors have a role in controlling hCG secretion and production. The rationale for each of them may be different; for example, OT and AVP are nonapeptides that are derived from the corpus luteum and may have a role in placental maintenance (discussed by Tal *et al.* 1991), while PRL is a hormone which is secreted during stressful situations and may cause adverse effects, and is also produced by the decidua and present in the amniotic fluid. Finally, retinoic acid, which operates through specific receptors, may, by promoting cell differentiation, cause a decrease in hCG secretion in a paracrine manner.

In this context, the role of triiodothyronine (T$_3$), which belongs to the same family of hormones as retinoic acid, is of interest. Its addition to explants stimulates hCG secretion by increasing the production rate of the two hCG subunits, as well as increasing secretion of sex steroids, an effect which is not noted at term (Maruo *et al.* 1991, 1994). The effect produced by low T$_3$ concentrations appears to be exerted through binding to the thyroid hormone receptor present in the nucleus, whose expression is highest in the FTT. This may explain the high rate of pregnancy loss that takes place in hypothyroidism, which is correctable and preventable by thyroid hormone replacement (Maruo *et al.* 1994).

PLACENTAL SECRETORY PRODUCTS *IN VIVO*

The value of placental index measurements under normal and pathological conditions has been widely discussed for the past twenty years, where the major impetus has been the development of sensitive radio-and immunoassay methods. Table 10.8 lists the hormones, cytokines, and other agents that are known to be of trophoblastic origin and which are used clinically for pregnancy monitoring. In some instances, controversy still exists regarding the origin of the compound (e.g. pregnancy-associated plasma protein A (PAPP-A), which is produced and secreted by the FTT (Barnea *et al.* 1986*a*), but may also be present in the decidua. The number of secretory products of the placenta are numerous; those that are easy to detect and are present in large concentrations have been investigated in detail (i.e. hCG, progesterone, hPL), while there is very limited information about others (i.e. inhibin, SP_1) (Table 10.8).

As *in vitro* data reveal, the placenta is a rich source of secretory products, many of which may never be detected in the circulation because their concentration is very low (i.e. agents which have autocrine functions, such as cytokines). The present description deals mainly with peripheral levels of specific placental products. The reader is referred to Chapter 13 for descriptions of the amniotic and coelomic fluid contents and dynamics.

With respect to the origin of circulating products, many are secreted by several reproductive and non-reproductive organs (p. 153). For example, there is evidence that hCG is detected in the plasma of non-pregnant women where it is presumably of CNS origin (Odell and Griffin 1987). In addition, embryonal organs have been shown to produce some hCG (McGregor *et al.* 1983). However, hCG that is measured in the periphery is clearly of FTT origin. On the other hand, no such distinctions are possible for oestradiol, progesterone, prorenin, or inhibin, just to mention a few which are also produced by the ovary in early gestation.

Table 10.8   Placental markers measurable in maternal circulation in early pregnancy

Proteins	Human chorionic gonadotrophin (hCG), free hCGα, free hCGβ human placental lactogen (hPL), schwangerschaftsprotein (SP1), pregnancy-associated plasma protein A (PAPP-A), alkaline phosphatase, inhibin, prorenin, prolactin, corticotrophin-releasing hormone, leucine aminopeptidase, relaxin, C-reactive protein, gonadotrophin-releasing hormone (GnRH)
Steroids	Progesterone, 17-hydroxyprogesterone, oestrone, oestradiol, oestriol, androgens, deoxycorticosterone (DOC)

Another point is that the metabolic clearance rate of each secretory product actually reflects the net result of its rate of production, secretion, binding to binding proteins, half-life in circulation, metabolism, and excretion (for a detailed description on these topics, the reader may consult an excellent review on the subject by Falcone and Little (1994*a*,*b*)); obviously, the longer the half-life, the higher the hormone level will be. Therefore, episodic secretion appears to be advantageous and is noted for hCG and progesterone in the periphery (Nakajima *et al.* 1990). This is not surprising, since for control of the corpus luteum, episodic LH secretion is a necessity, and the profile of progesterone secretion by the corpus luteum is episodic as well, closely following that of LH. Although it is recognized that monitoring the placental secretory pattern *in vivo* would be ideal, it has its limitations because it is impractical to perform frequent measurements on a given individual.

The following is a brief description of the dynamics of several placental products in the FTT and their use in a clinical setting.

Dynamics of hCG

The use of trophoblastic markers such as hCG has led to major progress in monitoring pregnancies at risk (Grudzinskas and Chard 1992). It was recognized rather early that single measurements of potential markers may not be accurate and of prognostic value, and therefore repetitive measurements were sought to provide a better index. In the early 1980s, evidence was presented that, for example, the secretion of hCG *in vivo* is episodic, although the pulses noted are infrequent (Owens *et al.* 1981; Nakajima *et al.* 1990). However, later studies have shown that there is also a rapid pattern of pulsatility, although in order to identify it, frequent serial measurements have to be made (Cvetkovic and Genbacev 1992).

With respect to trends, the concept of 'doubling time' has been advocated by Kadar *et al.* (1981), in which the failure of observing such a pattern strongly suggests that the pregnancy is abnormal and is most likely in an ectopic location, especially if a gestational sac is not seen in the uterus by ultrasound. More recent data suggest that simultaneous measurement of progesterone might increase the diagnostic accuracy (Barnea *et al.* 1986*b*; Choe *et al.* 1992). Indeed, it has been suggested that a single measurement of progesterone in early pregnancy may be as useful in predicting early pregnancy pathology as serial hCG measurements (Daily *et al.* 1994; Isaacs *et al.* 1994).

Other markers for diagnosing ectopic pregnancy, including PAPP-A, SP_1, hPL, 17-hydroxy progesterone, and free hCG α, have been tried, but their clinical value is limited (Barnea and DeCherney 1986; Barnea *et al.* 1986*b*; Gargosky *et al.* 1990; Chard and Grudzinskas 1992; Ren and Braunstein 1994). Therefore, as of 1996, the diagnosis of abnormal pregnancies is mostly based on progesterone, the rate of change of hCG, and advanced transvaginal ultrasound. Other early pregnancy pathologies (such as threatened abortion or habitual abortion), are discussed in Chapter 21. In addition, trophoblastic markers for diagnosing chromosomal abnormalities are discussed elsewhere (Chapter 13/19).

What have we learned from measuring placental indices *in vivo*? First, that the organ changes its secretion pattern throughout gestation in a rather unique manner

(Fig. 10.3). hCG is already secreted by the pre-implantation embryo in culture. This secretion increases dramatically once the embryos hatch in culture (Copperman and Bustillo 1995). hCG becomes detectable in the peripheral circulation within a few days after implantation (within 10 days of conception), which is related to trophoblastic mass, combined with access to blood vessels. During this early period, the increase is not linear and only reaches 200 mIU/ml (Lenton *et al.* 1982). Subsequently, a quasi-linear increase in hCG levels takes place, up to 5000–6000 mIU/ml. Here, a doubling time of 1.4–2 days is observed (Kadar *et al.* 1981). Subsequently, the hCG increase slowly diminishes, reaching a plateau around 40 000–80 000 mIU/ml, around nine weeks of gestation. Following this, levels decline to a nadir (15 000–20 000 mIU/ml) around 17 weeks, and thereafter hCG levels only fluctuate mildly until term.

Free hCG subunits have been detected in pregnant sera. These forms are native molecules rather than products of hCG dissociation. The free β subunit is the same size as the dissociated component of hCG and is readily associated with free α subunit to form hCG, but the free α subunits are somewhat larger than those dissociated from the dimer (24 kDa v. 22 kDa). This difference is based on size, charge, and inability to combine with the β subunit (Chen *et al.* 1986).

Levels of the free α and β hCG subunits undergo major changes during gestation. At first, the free subunits are rather abundant, but subsequently their levels decline as that of hCG rises. After hCG peaks, free hCG β levels become very low while those of hCG α rise with advancing gestation, reflecting placental mass. This indicates that the rate-limiting factor in hCG secretion is the hCG β subunit (Ren and Braunstein 1992). However, hybridization studies reveal that mRNA expression of both subunits is greater in the first trimester than at term. This occurs because the steady-state levels of hCG α mRNA decrease eightfold. The ability of hCG α to combine changes as gestation advances, secondary to changes in the glyco portion of the molecule (Ren

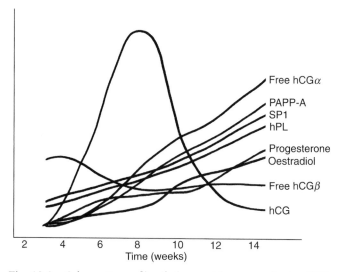

Fig. 10.3 Schematic profile of placental hormones in the FTT.

and Braunstein 1994). It has also been shown that except for being eliminated in intact form in urine, a certain degree of metabolism of the hCG molecule takes place. This is carried out through the formation of the β-core fragment (Cole and Birken 1988) and hCG β nicking (positions 44–45 and 47–48) which increases with advancing gestation (Cole *et al.* 1991). The metabolic clearance of hCG is 10- and 30-fold slower than the β and α subunits, respectively (Falcone and Little 1994*a*).

Important lessons on the nature of the trophoblast can be learned from the rate of hCG increase in the serum. Obviously, in multiple gestations, the absolute levels and the rate of rising are different from those noted in singleton pregnancies. On the other hand, if the rise and the absolute levels are very high, it strongly suggests the presence of a trophoblastic neoplasm (Maruo and Mochizuki 1994). Beyond the ready information reflecting hCG and its subunits' secretion, it has been shown that this marker may have a role in diagnosing several high-risk conditions such as diabetes mellitus, toxaemia, and intrauterine growth retardation later in pregnancy (Ren and Braunstein 1994). Thus, not only immediate prognostic value but also future occurrences can be derived from these observations. Except for hCG and its β subunit, all other secretory products appear to increase with advancing gestation (Fig. 10.3).

Regulation of hCG

The large body of data available on regulation of placental hormone secretion *in vitro* is contrasted by the paucity of information on its regulation *in vivo*. Most of the information available suggests that peripheral hCG levels in the first trimester can be modulated *in vivo*. Administration of progesterone has been shown to cause an increase in hCG secretion (Yosef *et al.* 1984); this may not be through direct action of the steroid but may act by supporting the decidua. On the other hand, it was shown that the antiprogestin RU486 lowers hCG as well as other hormone secretion, presumably by interfering with decidual function, thus creating a retro-placental clot. However, a direct effect can not be excluded (Szilágyi *et al.* 1993).

Another regulatory agent is GnRH which, *in vitro*, has a clear paracrine stimulatory role supported by several observations (p. 164). Exposure to GnRH agonists *in vivo* in early pregnancy apparently does not interfere with gestation; but data from primates with higher doses have shown that they can interfere (Siler-Khodr *et al.* 1991). Clearly, *in vivo* exposure is complex and has to take into account several factors, such as half-life and the concentration that reaches the placenta, while *in vitro* the exposure is direct. Moreover, the effect produced may also be indirect (i.e. through the decidua). Therefore, direct evidence for placental hormonal regulation *in vivo* is hard to obtain and is hard to document. However, an *ex vivo* model serves as a compromise.

We have used this approach to document the effects of toxins on placental hormonal secretion and embryo–placental interaction (see Table 10.4). Indeed, spontaneous placental hCG pulsatility was affected in a significant manner *in vitro* when the subject was exposed to cigarette smoke or neuroleptic drugs *in vivo* prior to the collection of the placenta, documenting *in vivo*-induced effects in a quantifiable manner (Shurtz-Swirski *et al.* 1992*b*). Since hCG and progesterone hormonal secretions are episodic *in vivo*, it would be advantageous to carry out frequent hormone measurements for diagnosing early pregnancy pathology, in the authors' view. This would not only document absolute levels, which change continuously, but may also add further parameters as we have documented *in vitro* and others have *in vivo*, with respect to pulse frequency, amplitude, and area under the curve (p. 00). A similar approach was suggested in a non-pregnant state when evaluating corpus luteum function.

Other placental glycoproteins

SP1 is a major placental product; several human SP1 members have been identified which share over 90 per cent sequence homology and 80 per cent amino-acid homology. The major form has a molecular weight of 64 kDa. Its antigens are similar to those of carcinoembryonic antigen (CEA), a major tumour marker (Chou and Plouzek 1992). In serum, it is detected shortly after implantation and its levels double every 2.4 days rising to very high levels at term. SP1 mRNA expression remains unchanged with gestation, but we have shown that its spontaneous pulsatility increases with gestation, which may help to create the high levels seen at term (Kaplan *et al.* 1991). SP1 is produced by the ST and the three major forms of SP1 mRNA were identified to be 2.3, 2.2, and 1.7 kb in length. However, the expression of mRNA from different gestational ages varies. The longer half-life at term, due to glycosylation, may contribute to the higher circulating levels.

The secretion of PAPP-A has been reported in the FTT in both explants and cells. This large (800 kDa) molecule may have an important role in immunomodulation and increases with gestational age (Bischof 1992). PAPP-A secretion appears to be protein-synthesis dependent (Barnea *et al.* 1986*a*).

CONCLUDING REMARKS

Placental hormone dynamics are complex; in some cases, hormone secretion is episodic and its regulation changes during early gestation. Hormone regulation is clearly multifactorial and also changes with gestational age. Observations *in vitro* are valuable and add significantly to our understanding, specifically of paracrine, autocrine, or short endocrine loops (i.e. ovarian, embryonal, and decidual influences). Placental products such as hCG and PAPP-A have major clinical utility, and identification of other specific secretory products should be actively pursued. The use of the *ex vivo* model as a study method of the FTT should also be pursued since it provides information on aspects of placental function and dysfunction which is not achievable by other means. Finally, as novel methods of pregnancy evaluation develop, such as advanced ultrasound, Doppler, and magnetic resonance imaging (MRI), the future of the value of placental markers in conjunction with other means will be better defined.

Insight into the secretory products of the FTT and their regulation continues to provide a fertile field of investigation with important implications for early pregnancy and well beyond. In the future, identification of specific conceptus-derived products will provide effective tools for diagnosis and treatment. The FTT, while once simply regarded as a young placenta, has become an entity in itself with unique characteristics and far-reaching ramifications.

ACKNOWLEDGEMENTS

I would like to thank Jean-David Barnea for his extensive editorial input into this chapter.

REFERENCES

Ahmed, N.A. and Murphy, B.E. (1988). The effects of various hormones on human chorionic gonadotropin production by early and late placental explant cultures. *American Journal of Obstetrics and Gynecology*, **159**, 1207–20.

Barnea, E.R. (1993). Placental dynamic cultures: workshop report. In *Trophoblast research*, Vol. 7, (ed. H. Schneider, P. Bischof, and R. Leiser), pp. 265–9. University of Rochester Press.

Barnea, E.R. (1994*a*). Dual effects of embryo-derived factors on hCG secretion by placental explants. In *Implantation and early pregnancy in humans*, (ed. E.R. Barnea, J.H. Check, J.G. Grudzinskas, and T. Maruo), pp. 271–82. Parthenon, Carnforth.

Barnea, E.R. (1994*b*). Placental dynamic cultures: the state of the art. In *Implantation and early pregnancy in humans*, (ed. E.R. Barnea, J.H. Check, J.G. Grudzinskas, and T. Maruo), pp. 201–27. Parthenon, Carnforth.

Barnea, E.R. and Check, J.H. (1992*a*). Comparative effects of GnRH and cAMP on hCG secretion by placental explants in dynamic and static cultures. *Assisted Reproductive Technology and Andrology*, **4**, 55–60.

Barnea, E.R. and Check, J.H. (1992*b*). Comparative role of GnRH in pituitary and placental gonadotropin secretion. *Assisted Reproductive Technology and Andrology*, **3**, 385–96.

Barnea, E.R. and DeCherney, A.H. (1986). β-HCG and other chemical parameters of ectopic pregnancy. In *Ectopic pregnancy*, (ed. A.H. DeCherney), pp. 65–81. Aspen Press, Baltimore.

Barnea, E.R. and Kaplan, M. (1989). Spontaneous, gonadotropin-releasing hormone-induced, and progesterone-inhibited pulsatile secretion of human chorionic gonadotropin in the first trimester placenta *in vitro*. *The Journal of Clinical Endocrinology and Metabolism*, **69**, 215–17.

Barnea, E.R. and Shurtz-Swirski, R. (1992). Endocrinology of the placental and embryo-placental interaction. In *The first twelve weeks of gestation*, (ed. E.R. Barnea, J. Hustin, and E. Jauniaux), pp. 128–53. Springer, Berlin.

Barnea, E.R., Sanyal, M.K., Brami, C., and Bischof, P. (1986*a*). *In vitro* production of pregnancy-associated plasma protein-A (PAPP-A) by trophoblastic cells. *Archives of Gynecology*, **237**, 187–90.

Barnea, E.R., Oelsner, G., Benveniste, R., Romero, R., and DeCherney, A.H. (1986*b*). Progesterone, estradiol, and alpha-human chorionic gonadotropin secretion in patients with ectopic pregnancy. *The Journal of Clinical Endocrinology and Metabolism*, **62**, 529–31.

Barnea, E.R., Simon, R.J., and Kol, S. (1989*a*). Human embryonal extracts modulate placental function in the first trimester: effects of visceral tissues upon chorionic gonadotropin and progesterone secretion. *Placenta*, **10**, 331–4.

Barnea, E.R., Fares, F., and Gavish, M. (1989*b*). Modulatory action of benzodiazepines on human term placental steroidogenesis *in vitro*. *Molecular and Cellular Endocrinology*, **64**, 155–9.

Barnea, E.R., Feldman, D., Kaplan, M., and Morrish, D.W. (1990). Dual effect of epidermal growth factor upon human chorionic gonadotropin secretion by the first trimester placenta *in vitro. The Journal of Clinical Endocrinology and Metabolism*, **71**, 923–8.

Barnea, E.R., Ashkenazi, R., and Sarne, Y. (1991a). Effect of dynorphin upon placental pulsatile human chorionic gonadotropin secretion *in vitro. The Journal of Clinical Endocrinology and Metabolism*, **73**, 1093–8.

Barnea, E.R., Ashkenazi, R., Tal, Y., Kol, S., and Sarne, Y. (1991b). Effect of beta-endorphin on human chorionic gonadotropin secretion by placental explants. *Human Reproduction*, **6**, 1327–31.

Barnea, E.R., Feldman, D., and Kaplan, M. (1991c). The effect of progesterone upon first trimester trophoblastic cell differentiation and human chorionic gonadotropin secretion. *Human Reproduction*, **6**, 905–9.

Barnea, E.R., Kaplan, M., and Naor, Z. (1991d). Comparative stimulatory effect of gonadotropin releasing hormone (GnRH) and GnRH agonist upon pulsatile human chorionic gonadotropin secretion in superfused placental explants: reversible inhibition by a GnRH antagonist. *Human Reproduction*, **6**, 1063–9.

Barnea, E.R., Check, J.H., Ashkenazi, R., and Sarne, Y. (1992a). Evidence for a paracrine interaction between progesterone and hCG secretion in the first trimester placenta. *Society for Gynecologic Investigation 39th Annual Meeting*, San Antonio.

Barnea, E.R., Shurtz-Swirski, R., and Kaplan, M. (1992b). Factors controlling spontaneous human chorionic gonadotrophin (hCG) pulsatility in superfused first trimester placental explants. *Human Reproduction*, **7**, 1022–6.

Barnea, E.R., Check, J.H., Levi, Y., and Sharoni, Y. (1992c). Gestational dependent effect of GnRH in the placenta. *Ninth International Congress of Endocrinology, Satellite Symposium on Gonadotropins, GnRH, GnRH Analogs, and Gonadal Peptides*, Paris.

Barnea, E.R., Amiri, Z., Fares, F., Gavish, M., and Check, J.H. (1992d). Evidence that benzodiazepine ligands bind to peripheral binding sites of first trimester placenta, and embryonal organs and subsequent effect on hormonal secretion. *12th Rochester Trophoblast Conference*, Rochester.

Barnea, E.R., Neubrun, D., and Shurtz-Swirski, R. (1993a). Effect of insulin on human chorionic gonadotropin secretion by placental explants. *Human Reproduction*, **8**, 858–62.

Barnea, E.R., Diamant, M., Maruo, T., and Shurtz-Swirski, R. (1993b). Gestational age-dependent effects of retinoids on hCG secretion by placental explants. *Human Reproduction*, **9**, 1166–9.

Bischof, P. (1992). Pregnancy-associated plasma protein-A. *Seminars in Reproductive Endocrinology*, **10**, 127–35.

Boadi, W.Y., Shurtz-Swirski, R., Barnea, E.R., Urbach, Y., Brandes, J.M., Philo, E., *et al.* (1992). Secretion of human chorionic gonadotropin in superfused young placental tissue exposed to cadmium. *Archives of Toxicology*, **66**, 95–9.

Chard, T. and Grudzinskas, J.G. (1992). Pregnancy protein secretion. *Seminars in Reproductive Endocrinology*, **10**, 61–71.

Chen, R., Barnea, E.R., and Benveniste, R. (1986). Characterization of glycoprotein hormone free alpha-subunit from human pituitary and placental extracts. *Hormone Research*, **23**, 38–49.

Choe, J.K., Check, J.H., Nowroozi, K., Benveniste, R., and Barnea, E.R. (1992). Serum progesterone and 17-hydroxyprogesterone in the diagnosis of ectopic pregnancies and the value of progesterone replacement in intrauterine pregnancies when serum progesterone levels are low. *Gynecological and Obstetrical Investigation*, **34**, 133–8.

Chou, J.Y. and Plouzek, C.A. (1992). Pregnancy-specific β_1-glycoprotein. *Seminars in Reproductive Endocrinology*, **10**, 116–26.

Cole, L.A. and Birken, S. (1988). Origin and occurrence of human chorionic gonadotropin β-subunit core fragment. *Molecular Endocrinology*, **2**, 825–30.

Cole, L.A., Kardana, A., Andrade-Gordon, P., Gawinowicz, M.-A., Morris, J.C., Bergert, E.R., *et al.* (1991). The heterogeneity of human chorionic gonadotropin (hCG). III. The occurrence of biological and immunological activities of nicked hCG. *Endocrinology*, **129**, 1559–67.

Copperman, A.B. and Bustillo, M. (1995). Biochemical and sonographic evaluation of the very early intrauterine pregnancy. *Early Pregnancy: Biology and Medicine*, **1**, 1–13.

Currie, W.D., Steele, G.L., Yuen, B.H., Kordon, C., Gautron, J.P., and Leung, P.C. (1993). LHRH and hydroxyproline 9-LHRH-stimulated human chorionic gonadotropin secretion from perfused first trimester placental cells. *Endocrinology*, **130**, 2871–6.

Cvetkovic, M. and Genbacev, O. (1992). Pulsatile secretion of hCG in early pregnancy. *Placenta*, **13**, A.11.

Daily, C.A., Laurent, S.L., and Nunley, W.C. (1994). The prognostic value of serum P and quantitative beta human chorionic gonadotropin in early human pregnancy. *American Journal of Obstetrics and Gynecology*, **171**, 380–4.

Downing, J., Poisner, A.M., and Barnea, E.R. (1995). First trimester villous placenta has high prorenin and active renin concentrations. *American Journal of Obstetrics and Gynecology*, **172**, 864–7.

Falcone, T. and Little, A.B. (1994*a*). Placental polypeptides. In *Maternal–fetal endocrinology*, 2nd edn, (ed. D. Tulchinsky and A.B. Little), pp. 15–32. W.B. Saunders, Philadelphia.

Falcone, T. and Little, A.B. (1994*b*). Placental synthesis of steroid hormones. In *Maternal–fetal endocrinology*, 2nd edn, (ed. D. Tulchinsky and A.B. Little), pp. 10–14. W.B. Saunders, Philadelphia.

Furuhashi, M., Seo, H., Mizutani, S., Narita, O., Tomoda, Y., and Matsui, N. (1989). Expression of low density lipoprotein receptor gene in human placenta during pregnancy. *Molecular Endocrinology*, **3**, 1252–6.

Gargosky, S.E., Moyse, K.J., Walton, P.E., Owens, J.A., Wallacw, J.C., Robinson, J.S., and Owens, P.C. (1990). Circulating levels of insulin-like growth factors increase and molecular forms of their serum binding proteins change with human pregnancy. *Biochemical and Biophysical Research Communications*, **170**, 1157–63.

Gautron, J.P., Pattou, E., Bauer, K., Rotten, D., and Kordon, C. (1989). LHRH-like immuno-reactivity in the human placenta is not identical to LHRH. *Placenta*, **10**, 19–32.

Grudzinskas, J.G. and Chard, T. (1992). Diagnosis of abnormalities of early pregnancy by measurement of fetoplacental products in biological fluids. In *The first twelve weeks of gestation*, (ed. E.R. Barnea, J. Hustin, and E. Jauniaux), pp. 347–57. Springer, Berlin.

Handwerger, S. and Brar, A. (1992). Placental lactogen, placental growth hormone, and de-cidual prolactin. *Seminars in Reproductive Endocrinology*, **10**, 106–15.

Handwerger, S., Richards, R.G., and Myers, S.E. (1994). Novel regulation of the synthesis and release of human placental lactogen by high density lipoproteins—a review. In *Trophoblast research*, Vol. 8, (ed. R.K. Miller and H.A. Thiede), pp. 339–54. University of Rochester Press.

Hilf, G. and Merz, W.E. (1985). Influence of cyclic nucleotides on receptor binding, and micro-heterogeneity of human chorionic gonadotropin synthesized in placental tissue culture. *Molecular and Cellular Endocrinology*, **39**, 151–9.

Hoshina, M., Boothby, M., and Boime, I. (1982). Cytological localization of chorionic gonadotropin α and placental lactogen mRNAs during development of the human placenta. *Journal of Cell Biology*, **93**, 190–8.

Hubert, C., Descombey, D., Mondon, F., and Daffos, F. (1983). Plasma human chorionic somatomammotropin deficiency in a normal pregnancy is the consequence of low concentra-tion of messenger RNA coding for human chorionic somatomammotropin. *American Journal of Obstetrics and Gynecology*, **147**, 676–8.

Hustin, J. (1992). The maternotrophoblastic interface: uteroplacental blood flow. In *The first twelve weeks of gestation*, (ed. E.R. Barnea, J. Hustin, and E. Jauniaux), pp. 97–110. Springer, Berlin.

Isaacs, J.D., Whitworth, N.S., and Cowan, B.D. (1994). Relative operating characteristic analysis in reproductive medicine: comparison of P and human chorionic gonadotropin doubling time as predictors of early gestational normalcy. *Fertility and Sterility*, 62, 452–5.

Iwashita, M., Watanabe, M., Adachi, T., Shinozaki, Y., Takeda, Y., and Sakamoto, S. (1988). The effect of diacylglycerol on hCG release by trophoblast cells: comparison with GnRH. In *Placental protein hormones*, (ed. M. Mochizuki and R. Hussa), p. 287. Excerpta Medica, Amsterdam.

Kadar, N., Caldwell, B.U., and Romero, R. (1981). A method of screening for ectopic pregnancy. *Obstetrics and Gynaecology*, 58, 162–6.

Kaplan, M., Barnea, E.R., and Bersinger, N. (1991). Patterns of spontaneous pulsatile secretion of human chorionic gonadotropin and pregnancy specific beta-1 glycoprotein by superfused placental explants in first and last trimester: lack of episodic human placental lactogen secretion. *Acta Endocrinologica*, 124, 331–7.

Kato, Y. and Braunstein, G.D. (1990). Purified first and third trimester placental trophoblasts differ in *in vitro* hormone secretion. *The Journal of Clinical Endocrinology and Metabolism*, 70, 1187–92.

Lenton, E.A., Neal, L.M., and Sulaiman, R. (1982). Plasma concentrations of human chorionic gonadotropin from the time of implantation until the second week of pregnancy. *Fertility and Sterility*, 37, 773–8.

Licht, P., Cao, H., Lei, Z.M., Rao, Ch. V., and Merz, W.M. (1993). Novel self-regulation of human chorionic gonadotropin biosynthesis in term pregnancy human placenta. *Endocrinology*, 133, 3014–25.

Licht, P., Cao, H., Zuo, J., Lei, Z.M., Rao, Ch. V., Merz, W.E., *et al.* (1994). Lack of self-regulation of human chorionic gonadotropin biosynthesis in human choriocarcinoma cells. *The Journal of Clinical Endocrinology and Metabolism*, 78, 1188–94.

Lin, L.S., Roberts, V.J., and Yen, S.S. (1995). Expression of human gonadotropin-releasing hormone receptor gene in the placenta and its functional relationship to human chorionic gonadotropin secretion. *The Journal of Clinical Endocrinology and Metabolism*, 80, 580–5.

Lysiak, J.J., Johnson, G.R., and Lala, P.K. (1995). Localization of amphiregulin in the human placenta and decidua throughout gestation: role in trophoblast growth. *Placenta*, 16, 359–66.

McGregor, W.G., Kuhn, R.W., and Jaffe, R.B. (1983). Biologically active chorionic gonadotropin: synthesis by the human fetus. *Science*, 220, 306–8.

Maruo, T. and Mochizuki, M. (1994). Molecular endocrine aspects in the diagnosis of gestational trophoblastic diseases. In *Implantation and early pregnancy in humans*, (ed. E.R. Barnea, J.H. Check, J.G. Grudzinskas, and T. Maruo), pp. 485–504. Parthenon, Carnforth.

Maruo, T., Matsuo, H., Ohtani, T., Hoshina, M.H., and Mochizuki, M. (1986). Differential modulation of chorionic gonadotropin (CG) subunit messengers ribonucleic acid levels and CG secretion by progesterone in human placenta in normal placenta and choriocarcinoma cultured *in vitro*. *Endocrinology*, 119, 855–64.

Maruo, T., Matsuo, H., Hayashi, M., Nishino, R., and Mochizuki, M. (1987). Induction of differentiated trophoblast function by epidermal growth factor: relation of immunohistochemically detected cellular epidermal growth factor receptor levels. *The Journal of Clinical Endocrinology and Metabolism*, 64, 744–9.

Maruo, T., Matsuo, H., and Mochizuki, M. (1991). Thyroid hormone as a biological amplifier of differentiated trophoblast function in early pregnancy. *Acta Endocrinologica*, 125, 58–66.

Maruo, T., Ladines-Llave, C.A., Matsuo, H., Manalo, A.S., and Mochizuki, M. (1992). A novel change in cytologic localization of human chorionic gonadotropin and human placental lactogen in first trimester placenta in the course of gestation. *American Journal of Obstetrics and Gynecology*, 167, 217–22.

Maruo, T., Matsuo, H., Katayama, K., Hayashi, M., and Mochizuki, M. (1994). The role of thyroid hormone during the functional shift from corpus luteum to placenta in maintaining early gestation. In *Implantation and early pregnancy in humans*, (ed. E.R. Barnea, J.H. Check, J.G. Grudzinskas, and T. Maruo), pp. 177–94. Parthenon, Carnforth.

Maruo, T., Murata, K., Matsuo, H., Samoto, T., and Mochizuki, M. (1995). Insulin-like growth factor-I as a local regulator of proliferation and differentiated function of the human trophoblast in early pregnancy. *Early Pregnancy: Biology and Medicine*, 1, 54–61.

Mathialgan, N. and Rao, A.J. (1989). A role for calcium in gonadotropin releasing hormone (GnRH) stimulated secretion of chorionic gonadotropin by first trimester placental minces *in vitro*. *Placenta*, 10, 61–70.

Matsuzaki, N., Shimoya, K., Taniguchi, T., Neki, R., Okada, T., Saji, F., *et al.* (1994). Paracrine effect of trophoblast-derived cytokines on placental hCG secretion. In *Implantation and early pregnancy in humans*, (ed. E.R. Barnea, J.H. Check, J.G. Grudzinskas, and T. Maruo), pp. 229–34. Parthenon, Carnforth.

Matsuzaki, N., Neki, R., Sawai, K., Shimoya, K., Okada, T., Sakata, M., *et al.* (1995). Soluble interleukin-6 (IL-6) receptor in the sera of pregnant women forms a complex with IL-6 and augments human chorionic gonadotropin production by normal human trophoblasts through binding to the IL-6 signal transducer. *The Journal of Clinical Endocrinology and Metabolism*, 80, 2912–17.

Mersol-Berg, M.S., Miller, K.F., Choi, C.M., Lee, A.C., and Kim, M.H. (1990). Inhibin suppresses human chorionic gonadotropin secretion at term, but not first trimester, placenta. *The Journal of Clinical Endocrinology and Metabolism*, 71, 1294–8.

Merz, W.E., Erlewein, C., Licht, P., and Harbarth, P. (1991). The secretion of hCG as well as the α and β-messenger ribonucleic levels are stimulated by exogenous gonadoliberin pulses applied to first trimester placenta in a superfusion culture system. *The Journal of Clinical Endocrinology and Metabolism*, 73, 84–92.

Minami, S., Yamoto, M., and Nakano, R. (1995). Sources of inhibin in early pregnancy. *Early Pregnancy: Biology and Medicine*, 1, 62–6.

Mochizuki, M., Kitagawa, M., Otani, T., and Maruo, T. (1994). Gene expression of placental corticoprotein releasing hormone and its clinical relevance. In *Implantation and early pregnancy in humans*, (ed. E.R. Barnea, J.H. Check, J.G. Grudzinskas, and T. Maruo), pp. 283–94. Parthenon, Carnforth.

Morrish, D.W., Marusyk, H., and Siy, O. (1987). Demonstration of specific secretory granules for human chorionic gonadotropin in placenta. *Journal of Histochemistry and Cytochemistry*, 35, 93–101.

Nakajima, S.T., McAuliffe, T., and Gibson, M. (1990). The 24 hour profile of the levels of serum progesterone and immunoreactive human chorionic gonadotropin in normal early pregnancy. *The Journal of Clinical Endocrinology and Metabolism*, 71, 345–53.

North, R.A., Whitehead, R., and Larkins, R.G. (1991). Stimulation by human chorionic gonadotropins of prostaglandin synthesis by early human placental tissue. *The Journal of Clinical Endocrinology and Metabolism*, 73, 60–70.

Odagiri, E., Sherrill, B.J., Mount, C.D., Nicholson, W.E., and Orth, D.N. (1979). Human placental immunoreactive corticotropin, lipotropin, and β-endorphin: evidence for a common precursor. *Proceedings of the National Academy of Sciences, USA*, 16, 2027–38.

Odell, W.D. and Griffin, J. (1987). Pulsatile secretion of human chorionic gonadotropin in normal adults. *The New England Journal of Medicine*, 317, 1688.

Owens, O.M., Ryan, K.J., and Tulchinsky, D. (1981). Episodic secretion of human chorionic gonadotropin in early pregnancy. *The Journal of Clinical Endocrinology and Metabolism*, 53, 1307–10.

Parker Jr, C.R., Illingworth, D.R., Bissonnette, J., and Carr, B.R. (1986). Endocrinology of pregnancy in abetalipoproteinemia: studies in a patient with homozygous familial hypobetalipoproteinemia. *The New England Journal of Medicine*, 314, 557–60.

Petraglia, F., Sutton, S., Vale, W. (1989). Inhibin and activin modulate the release of GnRH, hCG, and progestrone from cultured human placental cells. *Proceedings of the National Academy of Sciences (USA)*, **86**, 5144–22.

Qu, J., Ying, S.Y., and Thomas, K. (1992). Inhibin production and secretion in human placental cells cultured *in vitro*. *Obstetrics and Gynaecology*, **79**, 705–12.

Ren, S.G. and Braunstein, G.D. (1992). Human chorionic gonadotropin. *Seminars in Reproductive Endocrinology*, **10**, 95–105.

Ren, S.G. and Braunstein, G.D. (1994). Comparison of *in vivo* and *in vitro* trophoblast hormone production at different stages of pregnancy. In *Implantation and early pregnancy in humans*, (ed. E.R. Barnea, J.H. Check, J.G. Grudzinskas, and T. Maruo), pp. 247–70. Parthenon, Carnforth.

Rodway, M.R. and Rao, Ch. V. (1995). A novel perspective on the role of human chorionic gonadotropin during pregnancy and in gestational trophoblastic disease. *Early Pregnancy: Biology and Medicine*, **1**, 176–87.

Sartre, M.A., Ugen, K.E., and Kochlar, D.M. (1992). Developmental changes in endogenous retinoids during pregnancy and embryogenesis in the mouse. *Biology of Reproduction*, **46**, 802–10.

Sawai, K., Matsuzaki, N., Kameda, T., Hashimoto, K., Okada, T., Shimoya, K., *et al.* (1995). Leukemia inhibitory factor produced at the fetomaternal interface stimulates chorionic gonadotropin production: its possible implication during pregnancy, including implantation period. *The Journal of Clinical Endocrinology and Metabolism*, **80**, 1449–56.

Shimonovitz, S., Yagel, S., Anteby, E., Finci-Yeheskiel, Z., Adashi, E.Y., Mayer, M., *et al.* (1995). Interleukin-1 stimulates prostaglandin Embryo production by human trophoblast cells from first and third trimester. *The Journal of Clinical Endocrinology and Metabolism*, **80**, 1641–6.

Shurtz-Swirski, R., Simon, R.J., Cohen, Y., and Barnea, E.R. (1991). Human embryo modulates placental function in the first trimester: effects of neural tissues upon chorionic gonadotropin and progesterone secretion. *Placenta*, **12**, 521–31.

Shurtz-Swirski, R., Barnea, E.R., Korenblum, R., and Check, J.H. (1992*a*). Effect of maternal cigarette smoking upon placental hCG secretion *in vitro*. *Assisted Reproductive Technology and Andrology*, **3**, 397–403.

Shurtz-Swirski, R., Cohen, Y., and Barnea, E.R. (1992*b*). Patterns of secretion of human chorionic gonadotropin by superfused placental explants and the embryo–placental relationship following maternal use of medications. *Human Reproduction*, **7**, 300–4.

Shurtz-Swirski, R., Check, J.H., and Barnea, E.R. (1993). Effect of 1–34 human parathyroid hormone upon first trimester placental human chorionic gonadotrophin secretion *in vitro*: potentiation by epidermal growth factor. *Human Reproduction*, **8**, 107–11.

Siler-Khodr, T.M., Kang, I.A., and Khodr, G.S. (1991). Current topic: symposium on placental endocrinology; 1. Effects of chorionic GnRH on intrauterine tissues and pregnancy. *Placenta*, **12**, 91–103.

Szilágyi, A., Benz, R., and Rossmanith, W.G. (1993). Human chorionic gonadotropin secretion from the early human placenta: *in vitro* regulation by progesterone and its antagonist. *Gynecological Endocrinology*, **7**, 241–50.

Szilágyi, A., Mukhopadhyay, A.K., Werling, J., and Szabó, I. (1995). Regulation of placental prorenin secretion from the early human placenta *in vitro*. *Early Pregnancy: Biology and Medicine*, **1**, 119–23.

Tal, J., Kaplan, M., Sharf, M., and Barnea, E.R. (1991). Stress-related hormones affect human chorionic gonadotropin secretion from the early human placenta *in vitro*. *Human Reproduction*, **6**, 766–9.

Watson, A.L., Palmer, M.E., and Burton, G. (1995). Human chorionic gonadotrophin release and tissue viability in placental organ culture. *Human Reproduction*, **10**, 2159–64.

Wilson, E.A. and Jawad, M.J. (1980). Luteinizing hormone-releasing hormone suppression of human placental progesterone secretion. *Fertility and Sterility*, **33**, 91–4.

Wilson, E.A. and Jawad, M.J. (1982). Stimulation of human chorionic gonadotropin secretion by glucocorticoids. *American Journal of Obstetrics and Gynecology*, **142**, 344–8.

Yang, E.M., Chen, D.B., Lee, S.P., and Harper, M.J.K., (1995). Interleukin-1 α in the rabbit uterus during early pregnancy. *Early Pregnancy: Biology and Medicine*, **1**, 201–6.

Yosef, S.M., Nesher, R., Navot, D., Hadani, P.E., and Anteby, S.O. (1984). Effect of administration of progesterone on beta hCG blood level in early pregnancy. *Gynecological and Obstetrical Investigation*, **18**, 113–15.

11 | *The life and death of the embryonic yolk sac*

Carolyn J.P. Jones

INTRODUCTION

The human yolk sac is an extraordinary structure. During its short life it performs a multitude of functions, including absorption, secretion, fetal nutrition, haemato-poiesis, and germ cell production, before slowly degenerating after about the eighth week of gestation. Delicate and fragile, at the peak of its development it floats in the exocoelomic cavity like a miniature balloon. Its honeycombed surface is almost translucent, yet this belies the intense activity within its walls, rendering it essential to the well-being and growth of the embryo to which it is attached.

In this chapter, a brief description of the development and microscopic anatomy of the yolk sac is followed by a review of its ultrastructure, illustrated with examples of yolk sacs between 6 and 10 weeks of gestation, and a discussion of the biological significance of its main characteristics.

DEVELOPMENT OF THE SECONDARY YOLK SAC

During the first week of life, the blastocyst consists of an inner cell mass and outer trophoblast. At the beginning of the second week, an outer layer differentiates on the surface of the inner cell mass, which becomes the hypoblast or primary endoderm, and splits appear between this and the remaining epiblast or primary ectoderm (Moore 1988; Larsen 1993). Over the next few days, a wave of new endodermal cells migrates out from the hypoblast to line the blastocyst cavity, transforming it into the primary yolk sac or exocoelomic cavity. There are conflicting theories about the formation of the definitive, or secondary yolk sac (Gonzalez-Crussi 1979; Larsen 1993), which have been discussed by Vögler (1987). According to Luckett (1978), another wave of proliferating cells grows out from the hypoblast on day 12, produc-ing a new membrane while the old primary yolk sac is pushed away to the abembry-onic pole. This new layer becomes the endodermal lining of the definitive, or secondary yolk sac, and the distal portion of the primary yolk sac is pinched off, to become reduced eventually to a transient collection of vesicles in the abembryonic pole of the chorionic cavity, which gradually degenerate. However, in their recent review, Enders and King (1993) favour an alternative suggestion, namely, that the primary yolk sac breaks up into a number of smaller vesicles, while the endoderm beneath the embryonic disc grows out and extends from the embryo to form the secondary yolk sac. The small secondary yolk sac is initially unilaminar, though remnants of the primary yolk sac may adhere to its wall. By 16 days, the yolk sac consists of three distinct layers: endodermal cells facing towards the yolk sac lumen, splanchnic mesoderm containing blood islands and developing vessels, and an outer layer of extraembryonic mesoderm or mesothelium, which also completely lines the chorionic cavity or exocoelom (Luckett 1978; Enders and King 1993). Over the next few weeks, the secondary yolk sac grows rapidly and by the 37th menstrual day is larger than the amniotic cavity (Jauniaux *et al.* 1991; Jauniaux and Moscoso 1992; Larsen 1993; Enders and King 1993). During the sixth week of gestation, successive foldings of the embryo in combination with the closing up of the embryonic endoderm to form the gut tube, constrict the neck region of the yolk sac, forming the yolk stalk which connects the definitive yolk sac to the ventral part of the embryo, the stalk lumen being continuous with the lumen of the primitive gut tube. The stalk of the yolk sac is progressively reduced to a relatively small duct called the vitelline or omphalomesenteric duct, growth and extension of which causes the yolk sac to be removed away from the body wall (Fig. 11.1). The secondary yolk sac reaches its maximum diameter of between 6 and 7 mm at about 11 weeks' development (Jauniaux *et al.* 1991) but begins to show morphological evidence of a decline in function at around nine weeks of gestation (Jones and Jauniaux 1995). Subsequently, it shrinks in size, usually disappearing by 20 weeks of gestation (Jauniaux and Moscoso 1992).

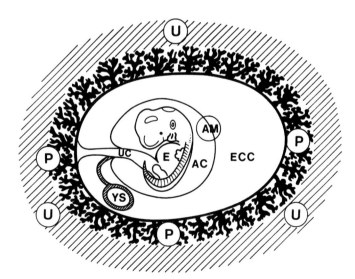

Fig. 11.1 Diagram of a gestational sac at eight weeks of pregnancy, showing the uterine wall (U) and placenta (P), and the embryo (E) with its umbilical cord (UC) and yolk sac (YS). The amniotic membrane (AM), amniotic cavity (AC), and exocoelomic cavity (ECC) are also shown.

MICROSCOPIC ANATOMY

By day 16, the wall of the secondary yolk sac is three-layered, comprising an inner endodermal layer of columnar cells facing the yolk sac cavity, a vascular mesenchyme, and an external mesothelial layer of flattened cells facing the exocoelomic cavity (Jauniaux and Moscoso 1992; Enders and King 1993; Jones and Jauniaux 1995). The thickness of the wall increases with gestational age (Ukeshima *et al.* 1986; Enders and King 1993) due to the development of haematopoietic foci and thickening of the endoderm, although Takashina (1987) stated that the walls stayed approximately the same thickness throughout pregnancy. Large cavities or tubules develop within the endodermal layer (Fig. 11.2), which may drain into the vitelline duct proper; these increase in size and number with age (Ukeshima *et al.* 1986). Some scanning electron microscopy studies have shown orifices of these endodermal tubules, sometimes containing blood cells or droplets of varying sizes, opening out into the cavity of the yolk sac (Ukeshima *et al.* 1986; Takashina 1989, 1993), and Shi *et al.* (1985) described surface pits or indentations at 50 days post-fertilization. Hesseldahl and Larsen (1969) found evidence of tubules communicating with the yolk sac cavity in specimens younger than 52 days, but never in later stages, and they tended to regress after eight weeks. Takashina (1989) suggested that these tubules may have originated from the mesenchyme, a concept disputed by other workers (Enders and King 1993) who found it unsupported by evidence.

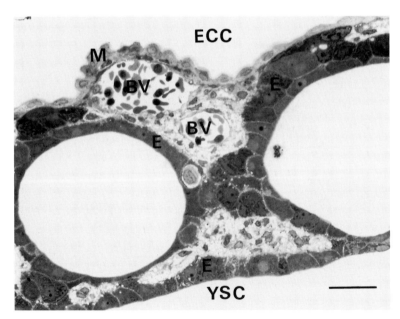

Fig. 11.2   Semi-thin section (0.5 μm) stained with toluidine blue showing a yolk sac at eight weeks' gestation. The mesothelium (M) faces the exocoelomic cavity (ECC) while the endoderm (E) lines the yolk sac cavity (YSC) and contains large ducts. Blood vessels (BV) containing nucleated erythrocytes are present in the mesenchyme. Scale bar represents 100 μm.

ULTRASTRUCTURE OF THE SECONDARY YOLK SAC

Of the various studies describing human yolk sac ultrastructure, the earliest is that of Bourne (1962), who briefly examined the endoderm and mesenchyme of degenerate specimens of about six weeks' gestation. Detailed investigations of specimens between 3 and 11 weeks of pregnancy have been undertaken by Hesseldahl and Larsen (1969), while Fukuda (1973) studied four yolk sacs 4–5 weeks old. Surface morphology of specimens of between five and seven weeks' development has been described by Ukeshima *et al.* (1986), with some transmission electron microscopy, and Shi *et al.* (1985) also used scanning electron microscopy to examine a seven week post-fertilization yolk sac. Haematopoiesis in yolk sacs between 4 and 11 weeks of pregnancy has been described by Takashina (1987, 1989) and Hoyes (1969) gave a detailed description of the yolk sac at 8 and 10 weeks' gestation. A single specimen at eight menstrual weeks was examined by Topilko and Pisarski (1971), and Gonzalez-Crussi and Roth (1976) and Nogales-Fernandez *et al.* (1977) compared the ultrastructure of yolk sac tumours with that of normal yolk sacs of 39 days, and 7 and 12 weeks of pregnancy, respectively. Jones and Jauniaux (1995) have described the ultrastructure of yolk sacs from ectopic pregnancies of 6, 8, and 10 weeks' menstrual age. Many of these and other studies have previously been reviewed by Gonzalez-Crussi (1979), Jauniaux and Moscoso (1992), and Jones and Jauniaux (1995).

In the following sections, the ultrastructure of the yolk sac is described and illustrated with material from nine intact gestational sacs removed from patients with live ectopic pregnancies at 6, 8, and 10 weeks' gestation (menstrual age).

Six weeks' gestation

At this stage, the **endoderm** is irregular in thickness and composed of large cells approximately 10 to 20 μm in diameter (Fig. 11.3), with tight junctions and desmosomes at their apical surfaces (Hesseldahl and Larsen 1969; Fukuda 1973; Gonzales-Crussi and Roth 1976; Ukeshima *et al.* 1986; Takashina 1987, 1993; Jauniaux and Moscoso 1992; Jones and Jauniaux 1995). The endodermal cells are covered by sparse, short microvilli, sometimes club-shaped and uneven in profile, between 0.3 and 2.0 μm in length and 0.1 and 0.4 μm in diameter, with central longitudinal filaments (Hesseldahl and Larsen 1969; Ukeshima *et al.* 1986; Jauniaux and Moscoso 1992) which also form bundles under the apical plasma membrane (Ukeshima *et al.*, 1986) and are probably composed of actin, as in the guinea-pig yolk sac (King 1983). Most subsets of *N*-glycans other than high mannose types, *N*-acetyl lactosamine, sialic acid (especially α2,6-linked residues) and α1,6-*N*-acetyl galactosamine are among those glycans expressed on the microvillous surface (Jones *et al.* 1995). The ciliated cells reported by Takashina (1989, 1993) to be present on the endodermal surface, as seen by scanning electron microscopy, have not been described by other workers using transmission electron microscopy. Lateral and basal plasma membranes tend to form interdigitations with neighbouring cells, and small desmosomes are also present between cells (Hesseldahl and Larsen 1969; Fukuda 1973; Jauniaux and Moscoso 1992; Takashina 1993; Jones and Jauniaux 1995). Nuclei are pale and

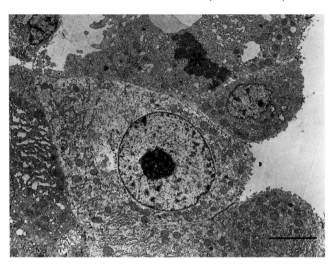

Fig. 11.3 Low power view of the endoderm at six weeks' gestation, showing short surface microvilli, and nuclei with prominent nucleoli. A mitotic figure can also be seen (*). Scale bar represents 5 μm.

round, with one or two prominent and complex nucleoli, and mitotic figures can occasionally be seen (Fig. 11.3). There are many elaborate whorls of rough endoplasmic reticulum in the cytoplasm, some of which have cisternae dilated by electron-lucent contents. Golgi bodies, secretory droplets, and pleomorphic dense bodies, probably lysosomal in nature, are dispersed throughout the cells (Fig. 11.4). Mitochondria are numerous and round to ovoid in shape; according to Hesseldahl and Larsen (1969) they contain few cristae although Jones and Jauniaux (1995) did not find this to be a particularly striking feature. Deposits of glycogen are also present. Intracellular vacuoles lined with small microvilli can occasionally be found inside the endodermal layer (Fig. 11.5). Tenuous fragments of basal lamina are sometimes present between the endodermal and the mesenchymal layers (Bourne 1962; Jones and Jauniaux 1995), as has also been described at 39 days (Gonzalez-Crussi and Roth 1976), at 6–7 weeks (Takashina 1993), and at 7 but not 12 weeks' gestation (Nogales-Fernandez *et al.* 1977). None was found by Fukuda (1973) at 4–5 weeks, by Hoyes (1969) between 8 and 10 weeks, or by Hesseldahl and Larsen (1969) between 3 and 11 weeks. Hesseldahl and Larsen (1969) suggested that this basal lamina may disappear after 4–5 weeks' gestation, and Nogales-Fernandez *et al.* (1977) also maintained that it was a characteristic of the young yolk sac, leading Takashina (1993) to conclude that it is present during a limited period coinciding with the time of maximum yolk sac secretory activity.

At six weeks, the **mesothelium** is thin (Fig. 11.5), with cells joined laterally by tight junctions and desmosomes (Hesseldahl and Larsen 1969; Takashina 1993). The brush border is composed of numerous long, sometimes branched microvilli, 3.0 to 3.5 μm in length (Ukeshima *et al.* 1986), with an internal cytoskeleton and micropinocytotic vesicles often associated with the microvillus base. The surface microvilli are heavily glyco-

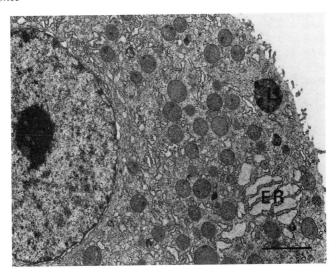

Fig. 11.4 Detail of an endodermal cell at six weeks' gestation, showing numerous mitochondria, dilated cisternae of rough endoplasmic reticulum (ER), and a dense pleomorphic body which may be a lysosome (L). A prominent nucleolus is also evident. Scale bar represents 2 μm.

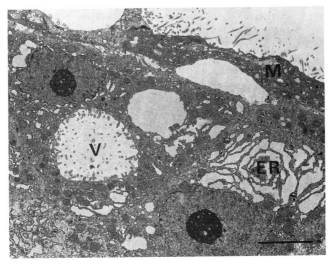

Fig. 11.5 Endodermal cells at six weeks' gestation, with dilated cisternae of rough endoplasmic reticulum (ER); an intracellular vacuole lined with microvilli (V) can be seen, and mesothelial cells (M) bearing long microvilli. There is only a narrow area of mesenchyme between the two cell layers. Scale bar represents 5 μm.

sylated, with an excess of α2,3-linked sialyl residues (Jones *et al.* 1995). Nuclei are often somewhat flattened with dispersed chromatin, and the cytoplasm contains sparse profiles of rough endoplasmic reticulum, free ribosomes, and mitochondria. Hesseldahl and Larsen (1969) described the mitochondria as having bizarre forms, being rather long and sometimes branched. Deposits of glycogen are often found, as well as occasional dense bodies and Golgi saccules. Numerous smooth and coated vesicles are present, especially in the apical cytoplasm, and there are numerous fine cytoplasmic filaments. The basal plasma membrane is often irregular with microvillous processes. A rather thin and discontinuous basal lamina has been described by some workers beneath the mesothelium (Hesseldahl and Larsen 1969; Fukuda 1973; Ukeshima *et al.* 1986; Jones and Jauniaux 1995), though it was not observed by Gonzales-Crussi and Roth (1976), Nogales-Fernandez *et al.* (1977), or Takashina (1987, 1989, 1993).

A layer of **mesenchyme** separates the mesothelium from the endoderm. It is composed of fusiform or stellate cells, free collagen fibrils, and blood vessels lined by endothelial cells which often have very tenuous intercellular connections (Fig. 11.6). The endothelial cells contain a flattened nucleus and a somewhat electron-dense cytoplasm with many strands of rough and smooth endoplasmic reticulum, clusters of free ribosomes, numerous mitochondria, and vacuoles of various sizes (Jones and Jauniaux 1995). No capillary basal lamina is present. At six weeks' gestation, the mesenchymal cells are very scanty. A population of stellate cells, and small round cells with dense nuclei can be seen (Fig. 11.3). Slender cell processes may lie closely apposed to the basal surface of the mesothelium. Often the mesothelium is separated from the endoderm by a thin layer of extracellular matrix only.

Eight weeks' gestation

Between seven and nine weeks' gestation, the cells of the **endoderm** show considerable changes in their architecture. Large cavities develop (Fig. 11.2), and these are lined by

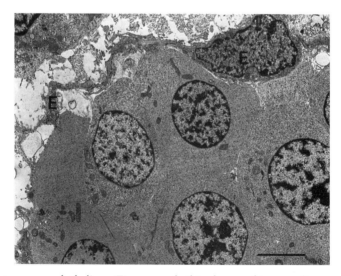

Fig. 11.6   A tenuous endothelium (E) surrounds this cluster of intermediate normoblasts in a yolk sac of six weeks' gestation. Scale bar represents 5 μm.

flattened cells with microvillous surfaces; these cavities may drain ultimately into the vitelline duct proper. Intercellular spaces separating lateral cell membranes show increased complexity in their structure (Fig. 11.7), while intracellular vacuoles are more prominent, features which drew Hoyes (1969) to compare these cells with those of the hepatic parenchyma. Many of the intracellular vacuoles contain cytoplasmic remnants and electron-dense material in the form of concentric rings or aggregates, and some are also lined with microvilli (Fig. 11.8). Cisternae of rough endoplasmic reticulum are now seen as stacks of parallel arrays with masses of glycogen between them (Fig. 11.7), often in close proximity to mitochondria (Takashina 1993). According to Hoyes (1969), five different types of cell may be found in the endoderm at eight weeks, each with varying amounts of glycogen and rough endoplasmic reticulum. Some of these (types 1 to 4) were also found in the mesenchyme and were thought to be red cell precursors, while type 5 was considered to be an early megakaryocyte.

During this period, the **mesothelium** (Fig. 11.9) develops increased amounts of smooth and rough endoplasmic reticulum, Golgi bodies, and mitochondria, and fine skeins of 4 to 6 nm wide filaments may be dispersed through the cytoplasm. Glycogen deposits are sometimes found. Lipid droplets are occasionally seen, as described by Hesseldahl and Larsen (1969). Intercellular contacts between lateral plasma membranes are often very tortuous.

Three types of cell have been described by Hoyes (1969) in the **mesenchyme** at eight weeks' gestation, one of which (type 2) may have been a Hofbauer cell and another (type 3) an early red cell precursor. Enzan (1986) identified macrophages in yolk sacs of 6–7 weeks' gestation, with many heterophagolysosomes and electron-dense bodies

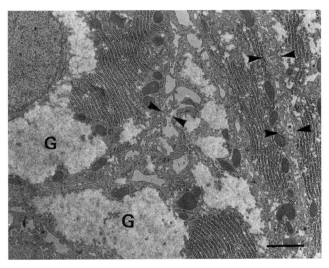

Fig. 11.7 Endodermal cells at eight weeks' gestation, showing stacks of parallel cisternae of rough endoplasmic reticulum with mitochondria in close proximity. Masses of glycogen (G) can be seen, and adjoining plasma membranes form complex microvillous interdigitations (arrowheads). Scale bar represents 2 μm.

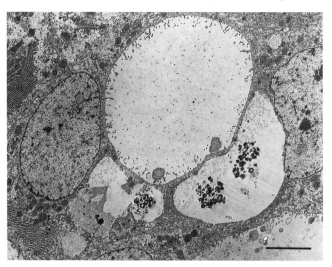

Fig. 11.8 In this eight-week-old yolk sac, a large intracellular vacuole is lined by short microvilli while neighbouring vacuoles have smooth walls and contain electron-dense aggregates. Scale bar represents 5 μm.

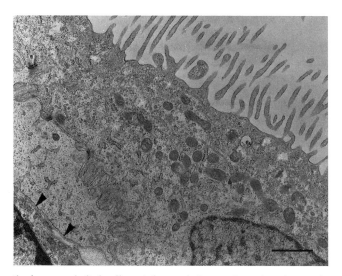

Fig. 11.9 Detail of a mesothelial cell at eight weeks' gestation, showing surface microvilli and numerous organelles. Adjoining plasma membranes follow a convoluted path, and a fine basal lamina may just be discerned (arrowheads). Scale bar represents 1 μm.

in their cytoplasm. He suggested that they arose from mesenchymal cells *in situ* and had a phagocytic function. Takashina (1987, 1993) noted that mesenchymal cells in the vicinity of the endoderm contained organelles similar to those found in the endoderm and suggested that the yolk sac mesenchyme is derived from endoderm. In the mesenchyme, the walls of the blood vessels are thicker and more organized than at six weeks (Fig. 11.10), although Hoyes (1969) reported intercellular spaces to be occasionally present between cells. Extracellular matrix distribution and density does not appear to alter to any significant degree, but Jones and Jauniaux (1995) found the basal lamina to increase slightly in places by nine weeks' gestation, contrary to the findings of some earlier workers (see above). The vitelline duct shows a similar pattern of cellular differentiation around the main collecting ducts and vessels.

Ten weeks' gestation

The secondary yolk sac is now beginning to show evidence of cellular degeneration, with marked changes in the morphology of the cells comprising the **endoderm** (Fig. 11.11) and **mesothelium** (Fig. 11.12) (Hoyes 1969; Topilko and Pisarski 1971; Jauniaux and Moscoso 1992; Jones and Jauniaux 1995). Both layers are considerably thinner and have been progressively replaced by oedematous and fibrotic areas; in the **mesenchyme**, the presence of fibroblasts with dilated cisternae of rough endoplasmic reticulum was seen by Topilko and Pisarski (1971) to be evidence that they were actively engaged in collagenogenesis. Surface microvilli on both endodermal cells and the mesothelium are now much shorter and more widely spaced, and cytoplasmic organelles regress. Endodermal phagolysosomes are more numerous, and many contain large, electron-dense deposits (Fig. 11.11), possibly related to the iron-containing granules seen by Hesseldahl and Larsen (1969) in the regressing yolk sac. Thin-walled blood vessels are present, containing nucleated and mature erythrocytes (Fig. 11.13).

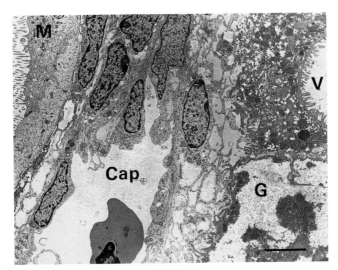

Fig. 11.10 Yolk sac at eight weeks' gestation showing a capillary (Cap) containing a late normoblast; the endothelial cells are well developed at this stage. Part of a mesothelial cell (M) is visible, and endodermal cells with masses of glycogen (G) and an intracellular vacuole (V) can also be seen. Scale bar represents 5 μm.

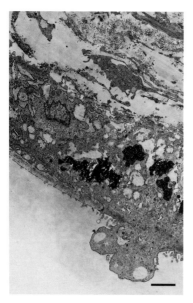

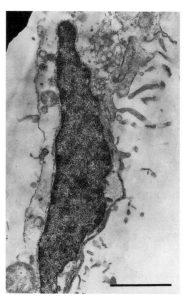

Fig. 11.11 Part of a degenerating endodermal cell at 10 weeks' gestation, containing electron-dense deposits. The surface bears a few, stumpy microvilli and misshapen blebs. Scale bar represents 2 μm.

Fig. 11.12 At 10 weeks' gestation, this mesothelial cell has become detached from the underlying tissue and shows marked signs of degeneration. Scale bar represents 1 μm.

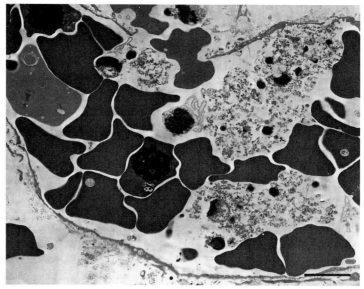

Fig. 11.13 A yolk sac at 10 weeks' gestation with a thin-walled vessel containing erythrocytes, some of which are still nucleated, as well as cell debris. Scale bar represents 5 μm.

FUNCTIONS OF THE SECONDARY YOLK SAC

It is now known that the human secondary yolk sac fulfils many important roles, including protein biosynthesis and secretion, absorption, and haematopoiesis; it is also known to be the source of the primordial germ cells. This is in contrast to earlier ideas, for when, in 1910, Jordan listed possible roles of the yolk sac as including (1) a hepatic function; (2) an absorptive function like the intestine; (3) its presence as a vestigial or rudimentary organ; (4) a primarily haematopoietic function, only the last of these was considered to be of any significance.

It is clear from an examination of the ultrastructure of the yolk sac that, during the first few weeks of embryonic life, the yolk sac acts as a major site of biosynthesis, exchange, and haematopoiesis, as well as being the probable source of the primary germ cells. It supports the developing embryo until its internal organs have matured sufficiently to function independently, and the maternal circulation has been established via the definitive placenta, after which it degenerates. However, there is still much that needs to be elucidated, including the mechanisms relating to the initial formation of the secondary yolk sac as well as the factors which control its growth, differentiation, and subsequent atrophy.

Absorption

Recent studies have once again drawn analogies between the ultrastructure of the mesothelium and that of an absorptive epithelium (Gonzales-Crussi and Roth 1976), pointing out the presence of a well-developed microvillous border, pinocytotic activity, the existence of a potential canalicular system at the bordering cell interfaces, cytoplasmic protrusions, and a tendency to the formation of basal plasmalemmal infoldings. All these are features commonly seen at sites of intense absorptive activity, and Gonzalez-Crussi and Roth speculated the direction of transport to be in a predominantly exocoelomic–vitelline direction, basing their evidence not only on the ultrastructural similarities but on the fact that the exocoelomic fluid rapidly disappears in subsequent development. The mesothelium forms an interface between the coelomic cavity and vitelline capillaries within the mesenchymal layer, which reach the circulation of the embryo via the vitelline duct. Only a tenuous and incomplete basal lamina and scanty extracellular matrix separates these capillaries from the mesothelial layer, facilitating transport between them. Hoyes (1969) also suggested that the coated vesicles in the mesothelium may be related to protein uptake, while King and Wilson (1983) showed that peroxidase was taken up by the cells of the endoderm and mesothelium in the Rhesus monkey yolk sac, with the mesothelium being most active. The comparable ultrastructure of the yolk sac and its vitelline duct suggests that a similar metabolic activity occurs at both levels.

Embryonic nutrition

Hesseldahl and Larsen (1969) discussed evidence of a nutritive role for the yolk sac endoderm, based on morphological similarities between endodermal cells and the cells of the small intestine, and concluded that such a theory was not convincing. However, absorption by either epithelium may provide metabolites important for the function of the epithelial cells or for the cells in the underlying haematopoietic compartment, while transfer of nutrients to the fetus may occur via the yolk sac as an expansion or satellite of the fetal gut. In this context, Nogales *et al.* (1993) noted the possibility of an association between spontaneous abortion and a reduction in the size or complete absence of the yolk sac, and suggested a relation between anomalies in yolk sac development and embryonic development.

Protein biosynthesis and secretion

Many proteins and enzymes involved in energy metabolism and digestion are synthesized by the secondary yolk sac (Shi *et al.* 1985; Buffe *et al.* 1993; Jauniaux *et al.* 1994). Immunohistochemical (Shi *et al.* 1985; Takashina 1993) and *in vitro* studies (Gitlin and Perricelli 1970; Gitlin 1975) have demonstrated the production of plasma proteins such as alpha-fetoprotein (AFP), α1-antitrypsin, albumin, pre-albumin, and transferrin before the embryonic liver has matured sufficiently to produce them, and RNA transcripts of lipoprotein genes AI, AII, B, CII, CIII, and E have been identified in yolk sacs from 6–12 week post-fertilization human embryos (Hopkins *et al.* 1986), as well as in other organs. Enzymes such as acid phosphatase, galactosidase, lactic dehydrogenase, and choline phosphotransferase are also produced in the yolk sac (Buffe *et al.* 1993). Studies of protein biosynthesis by the yolk sac and embryonic liver indicate that they are equally active up to nine weeks' gestation but that most of the biological activities of the yolk sac disappear after this stage. Endodermal cells and liver parenchyma have many ultrastructural features in common, including the presence of glycogen, and microvillus-lined channels between cells, similar to bile canaliculi and which may be important in the secretion of waste products (Hoyes 1969; Gonzales-Crussi and Roth 1976). The presence of features associated with protein biosynthesis as well as an intercellular canalicular system similar to that found in the liver corroborates a secretory function (Jauniaux and Moscoso 1992; Jones and Jauniaux 1995). Hoyes (1969) also proposed a secretory function for the mesothelium, comparing it to the periderm of the skin, suggesting that the uncoated secretory vesicles may contribute to the production of chorionic fluid during early pregnancy. In this context, it appears that both coelomic and amniotic fluid AFP are mainly of yolk sac origin, as shown by analyses of molecular variants of AFP (Jauniaux *et al.* 1993). Such a bidirectional passage of protein is facilitated by the presence of endodermal cell columns in close contact with the mesothelial layer and the absence of a well-formed basal lamina.

Haematopoiesis

One of the major functions of the yolk sac is haematopoiesis, which can be detected between days 16 and 19 of gestation (Luckett 1978; Kelemen *et al.* 1979). Hoyes (1969), Fukuda (1973), and Takashina (1987, 1989, 1993) found early stages in the endoderm and more mature cells in the mesenchyme and vessels, but Hesseldahl and

Larsen (1971) found no evidence of haematopoietic foci in the endoderm in any of their 21 yolk sac specimens. According to Kelemen *et al.* (1979), haematopoiesis is initiated in the mesenchyme below the endoderm, but at six weeks, erythroblasts from the embryo enter the yolk sac and haematopoiesis can then be identified in the endoderm, with which the erythroblasts make intimate contact via gap-like junctions. In the study by Jones and Jauniaux (1995) of yolk sacs between 6 and 10 weeks' gestation, immature blood cells were not recognized outside blood vessels, although intermediate and late normoblasts were present intravascularly. Neither granulocyte nor macrophage precursors were identified at these stages. According to Dommergues *et al.* (1992), both erythroid and granulopoietic progenitors can be found in the yolk sac, but the number of granulopoietic and/or macrophage progenitors is significantly negatively correlated with gestational age, being prominent before day 35 of gestation and rapidly falling off thereafter, which may account for their absence in later specimens. However, Akagi *et al.* (1989) found macrophages intermingled with other haematopoietic cells in yolk sacs ranging from four to seven weeks' gestation, and Enzan (1986) also described macrophages scattered in the mesenchymal tissue and in lumina of blood vessels in specimens of 6–7 weeks' gestation. He suggested that they arose from mesenchymal cells *in situ*, and migrated to blood vessels. Phagocytic endothelial cells were also proposed as intravascular macrophage precursors, after having detached from capillary walls. Janossy *et al.* (1986) used immunocytochemistry to show that antigenic heterogeneity of tissue macrophages was already present in yolk sacs of 4–7 weeks fertilization age, with two populations of cells, one carrying monocyte- and macrophage-associated markers (UCHM1 and RFD7) but no class II (HLA-DR and -DP) antigen, and the other with class II but no UCHM1 or RFD7 markers. The two populations seeded to different microenvironments and underwent additional phenotypic changes. These findings conflict with those of Tavassoli (1991), who claims that the yolk sac is permissive only for erythropoiesis, and not for the development of other cells lines. It has been suggested that blood cells are either discharged from their site of origin into the cavity of the yolk sac via the endodermal tubules and carried to the embryo (Takashina 1987, 1993) or transported via the vasculature. Such a movement is in agreement with the monoclonal model for human embryonic haematopoiesis proposed by Migliaccio *et al.* (1986), based on the migration of stem and early progenitor cells from a generation site (the yolk sac) to a colonization site (the liver).

Germ cell origin

Finally, the yolk sac is though to be the original source of the primordial germ cells (Witschi 1948; Larsen 1993). In 13 somite embryos, they can be seen as a scattered population of ovoid, poorly differentiated cells located in the endoderm near the allantoic invagination, indicating that they may have an endodermal origin, or that they arise from primitive stem cells which also are the source of the endoderm (Witschi 1948). At the 12–14 somite stage, Fujimoto *et al.* (1977, 1989) described cells situated in the endoderm and in the yolk sac stalk, both in the process of separation from the endoderm and in the surrounding mesenchyme, and noted their irregular shape when in the process of migration. Their ultrastructural characteristics include the presence of a large, round cell body often with pseudopods, a large nucleus with prominent reticular nucleoli, a single Golgi body, perinuclear mitochondria with vesicular cristae, rough endoplasmic reticulum, lipid droplets and glycogen, with the cell surface showing alkaline phosphatase activity (Fujimoto *et al.* 1977, 1989; Makabe and Motta 1989). Between four and six weeks, they migrate by amoeboid movement from the yolk sac to the wall of the gut tube and thence via the mesentery to the dorsal body wall, where differentiation of the gonads takes place and the germ cells eventually undergo meiosis (Enders and King 1993; Larsen 1993).

ACKNOWLEDGEMENTS

The author would like to thank Dr E. Jauniaux for his encouragement and assistance in providing the material used in this study, which was supported by a grant from the Fondation Universitaire David et Alice Van Buuren, Free University of Brussels (ULB). The illustrations used in this text, apart from Fig. 11.6, have been reprinted from Jones and Jauniaux (1995) with kind permission of Elsevier Science Ltd, Oxford.

REFERENCES

Akagi, T., Nose, S., Takahashi, K., Yoshino, T., Horie, Y., Motoi, M., *et al.* (1989). Ontogeny of S-100 protein-positive histiocytes and lymphocytes in the human fetal lymphoreticular system. *Acta Medica Okayama*, **43**, 203–10.

Bourne, G. (1962). *The human amnion and chorion.* Lloyd-Luke (Medical Books) Ltd, London.

Buffe, D., Rimbaut, C., and Gaillard, J.A. (1993). Alpha-fetoprotein and other proteins in the human yolk sac. In *The human yolk sac and yolk sac tumors*, (ed. F.F. Nogales), pp. 109–25. Springer, Heidelberg.

Dommergues, M., Aubény, E., Dumez, Y., Durandy, A., and Coulombel, L. (1992). Hematopoiesis in the human yolk sac: quantitation of erythroid and granulopoietic progenitors between 3.5 and 8 weeks of development. *Bone Marrow Transplantation*, **9**, 23–7.

Enders, A.C. and King, B.F. (1993). Development of the human yolk sac. In *The human yolk sac and yolk sac tumors* (ed. F.F. Nogales), pp. 33–47. Springer, Heidelberg.

Enzan, H. (1986). Electron microscopic studies of macrophages in early human yolk sacs. *Acta Pathologica Japonica*, **36**, 49–64.

Fujimoto, T., Miyayama, Y., and Fuyuta, M. (1977). The origin, migration and fine morphology of human primordial germ cells. *Anatomical Record*, **188**, 315–30.

Fujimoto, T., Ukeshima, A., Miyayama, Y., Kuwana, T., Yoshinaga, K., and Nakamura, M. (1989). The primordial germ cells in amniotes: their migration *in vivo* and behaviour *in vitro*. *Progress in Clinical and Biological Research*, **296**, 13–21.

Fukuda, T. (1973). Fetal hemopoiesis 1. Electron microscopic studies on human yolk sac hemopoiesis. *Virchows Archiv. Section B: Cell Pathology*, **14**, 197–213.

Gitlin, D. (1975). Normal biology of alpha-fetoprotein. *Annals of the New York Academy of Sciences USA*, **259**, 7–16.

Gitlin, D. and Perricelli, A. (1970). Synthesis of serum albumin, prealbumin, alphafetoprotein, alpha1-antitrypsin and transferrin by the human yolk sac. *Nature*, **228**, 995–7.

Gonzalez-Crussi, F. (1979). The human yolk sac and yolk sac (endodermal sinus) tumours. A review. *Perspectives in Pediatric Pathology*, 5, 179–215.

Gonzalez-Crussi, F. and Roth, L.M. (1976). The human yolk sac and yolk sac carcinoma: an ultrastructural study. *Human Pathology*, 7, 675–91.

Hesseldahl, H. and Larsen, J.F. (1969). Ultrastructure of human yolk sac: endoderm, mesenchyme, tubules and mesothelium. *American Journal of Anatomy*, 126, 315–36.

Hesseldahl, H. and Larsen, J.F. (1971). Haemopoiesis and blood vessels in human yolk sac. An electron microscopic study. *Acta Anatomica (Basel)*, 78, 274–94.

Hopkins, B., Sharpe, C.R., Baralle, F.E., and Graham, C.F. (1986). Organ distribution of apolipoprotein gene transcripts in 6–12 week postfertilisation human embryos. *Journal of Embryology and Experimental Morphology*, 97, 177–87.

Hoyes, A.D. (1969). The human foetal yolk sac: an ultrastructural study of four specimens. *Zeitschrift für Zellforschung und Mikroskopische Anatomie*, 99, 469–90.

Janossy, G., Bofill, M., Poulter, L.W., Rawlings, E., Burford, G.D., Navarrete, C., *et al.* (1986). Separate ontogeny of two macrophage-like accessory cell populations in the human fetus. *Journal of Immunology*, 136, 4354–61.

Jauniaux, E. and Moscoso, J.G. (1992). Morphology and significance of the human yolk sac. In *The first twelve weeks of gestation* (ed. E. Barnea, J. Hustin, and E. Jauniaux), pp. 192–216. Springer, Heidelberg.

Jauniaux, E., Jurkovic, D., Henriet, Y., Rodesch, F., and Hustin, J. (1991). Development of the secondary human yolk sac: correlation of sonographic and anatomic features. *Human Reproduction*, 6, 1160–6.

Jauniaux, E., Gulbis, B., Jurkovic, D., Schaaps, J.P., Campbell, S., and Meuris, S. (1993). Protein and steroid levels in embryonic cavities in early human pregnancy. *Human Reproduction*, 8, 782–7.

Jauniaux, E., Sherwood, R.A., Jurkovic, D., Boa, F.G., and Campbell, S. (1994). Amino acid concentrations in human embryological fluids. *Human Reproduction*, 9, 1175–9.

Jones, C.J.P. and Jauniaux, E. (1995). Ultrastructure of the materno-embryonic interface in the first trimester of pregnancy. *Micron*, 26, 145–73.

Jones, C.J.P., Jauniaux, E., and Stoddart, R.W. (1995). Glycans of the early human yolk sac. *Histochemical Journal*, 27, 210–21.

Jordan, H.E. (1910). A further study of the human umbilical vesicle. *Anatomical Record*, 4, 341–53.

Kelemen, E., Calvo, W., and Fliedner, T.M. (1979). *Atlas of human hemopoietic development*. Springer, Berlin.

King, B.F. (1983). The organization of actin filaments in the brush border of yolk sac epithelial cells. *Journal of Ultrastructure Research*, 85, 329–37.

King, B.F. and Wilson, J.M. (1983). A fine structural and cytochemical study of the Rhesus monkey yolk sac endoderm and mesothelium. *Anatomical Record*, 205, 143–58.

Larsen, W.J. (1993). *Human embryology*. Churchill Livingstone, New York.

Luckett, W.P. (1978). Origin and differentiation of the yolk sac and extraembryonic mesoderm in presomite human and Rhesus monkey embryos. *American Journal of Anatomy*, 152, 59–98.

Makabe, S. and Motta, P.M. (1989) Migration of human germ cells and their relationship with the developing ovary: ultrastructural aspects. *Progress in Clinical and Biological Research*, 296, 41–54.

Migliaccio, G., Migliaccio, A.R., Petti, S., Mavilio, F., Russo, G., Lazarro, D., *et al.* (1986). Human embryonic hemopoiesis. Kinetics of progenitors and precursors underlying the yolk sac–liver transition. *Journal of Clinical Investigation*, 78, 51–60.

Moore, K.L. (1988). *The developing human: clinically oriented embryology*. Saunders, Philadelphia.

Nogales, F.F., Beltran, E., and Gonzalez, F. (1993). Morphological changes of the secondary human yolk sac in early pregnancy wastage. In *The human yolk sac and yolk sac tumors*, (ed. F.F. Nogales), pp. 174–94. Springer, Heidelberg.

Nogales-Fernandez, F., Silverberg, S.G., Bloustein, P.A., Martinez-Hernandez, A., and Pierce, G.B. (1977). Yolk sac carcinoma (endodermal sinus tumor). Ultrastructure and histogenesis of gonadal and extragonadal tumors in comparison with normal human yolk sac. *Cancer*, 39, 1462–74.

Shi, W.K., Hopkins, B., Thompson, S., Heath, J.K., Luke, B.M., and Graham, C.F. (1985). Synthesis of apolipoproteins, alphafetoprotein, albumin and transferrin by the human fetal yolk sac and other fetal organs. *Journal of Embryology and Experimental Morphology*, 85, 191–206.

Takashina, T. (1987). Haemopoiesis in the human yolk sac. *Journal of Anatomy*, 151, 125–35.

Takashina, T. (1989). Haemopoiesis in the human yolk sac. *American Journal of Anatomy*, 184, 237–44.

Takashina, T. (1993). Histology of the secondary human yolk sac with special reference to hematopoiesis. In *The human yolk sac and yolk sac tumors*, (ed. F.F. Nogales), pp. 48–69. Springer, Heidelberg.

Tavassoli, M. (1991). Embryonic and fetal hemopoiesis: an overview. *Blood Cells*, 1, 269–81.

Topilko, A. and Pisarski, T. (1971). Ultrastructure of the human yolk sac. *Acta Medica Polona*, 12, 127–32.

Ukeshima, A., Hayashi, Y., and Fujimoto, T. (1986). Surface morphology of the human yolk sac: endoderm and mesothelium. *Archivum Histologicum Japonicum*, 49, 483–94.

Vögler, H. (1987). Human blastogenesis. *Bibliotheca Anatomica*, 30, 1–149.

Witschi, E. (1948). Migration of the germ cells of human embryos from the yolk sac to the primitive gonadal folds. *Contributions to Embryology, Carnegie Institute of Washington*, 32, 67–80.

12 | *Mole/chorion genomic imprinting*

Donald P. Marazzo

INTRODUCTION

Description of genomic imprinting and a brief historical review

The phenomenon of genomic imprinting describes, in general, the dichotomous effect of genes which is dependent upon the parent from whom the gene is inherited. If imprinting is operative, the phenotype produced by a certain gene will be different depending on whether it is inherited from the mother or from the father. When referring to a particular gene, the term 'imprinted' is more specific. Genomic imprinting, when applied to a specific gene or gene cluster, means that the particular gene is inactive due to this parent-of-origin effect. The difference between these applications of the term genomic imprinting can be confusing. Remember: the general phenomenon of genomic imprinting implies dichotomous gene expression that is dependent upon the parent of origin; the term genomic imprinting as applied to a specific gene means that the gene is silent due to its parent of origin.

The phenotypic difference exerted by genomic imprinting may be subtle, but most of the differences defined thus far are dramatic. Since the reproductive process requires sexually dimorphic gametes (i.e. sperm and eggs), genomic imprinting can also be described as a gamete-of-origin phenomenon. In fact it is the dichotomous processes of spermatogenesis and oogenesis that re-establish the biological process of genomic imprinting for the next generation. This gamete-determined effect makes genomic imprinting potentially reversible from generation to generation. Therefore if the gene is passed initially by the mother to a male, he will exhibit the maternally influenced phenotype, and the following generation will demonstrate the complementary, paternally inherited phenotype. Due to reversibility the phenotype will revert to the maternally inherited pattern as soon as vertical transmission from a female occurs.

Genomic imprinting is described as an epigenetic phenomenon because the basic genomic structure or DNA sequence is not changed as it is in purely genetic changes. Genomic imprinting violates the basic tenets of Mendelian genetics which state that two copies of a given gene are inherited, one copy from each parent with an equal effect from each copy of each gene. The recognition of phenomena that violate the classic rules of Mendel was the first step in describing the process of genomic imprinting. Accepting that these observations were real and relevant to human reproduction came slowly, in part because of the elegant symmetry of Mendel's laws, which had formed the basis for our understanding of genetic inheritance.

   The recognition that some phenotypes were inherited in relation to the sex of the parent, rather than the classical, parent-irrelevant pattern of Mendelian inheritance, can be traced at least as far back as Spofford's work in *Drosophilia melanogaster* (1961). This work has served as a convenient model for the study of genomic imprinting mechanisms after the initial work demonstrated a clear parent-of-origin effect. The extension of parent-of-origin reproductive phenomena to mammals was pioneered through the identification of late replicating X chromosomes of paternal origin in the somatic tissues of kangaroos by Sharman (1971). Although this preference for inactivation of the paternal X was not present in somatic tissues of placental (eutherian) mammals, it was demonstrated in the extraembryonic membranes of eutherian mammals—initially in mice (Takagi and Sasaki 1975). Preferential paternal X inactivation was subsequently demonstrated in human placentas by Lyon and Rastan using biochemical methods (1984), and later confirmed by Harrison and co-workers (Harrison and Warburton 1986; Harrison 1989). A parentally determined dichotomous phenotype was documented which was associated with the hairpin tail mutation in mice. In this model, the maternally transmitted mutation resulted in fetal death, while the same mutation transmitted by males resulted in hairpin-tailed mice (Johnson 1974*a,b*). Shortly thereafter, evidence for genomic imprinting at the cytogenetic level was demonstrated in a report of asymmetric inheritance patterns of mouse translocations (Searle and Beachey 1978).

Genomic imprinting and other types of non-Mendelian inheritance

At least three other phenomena have been described which may demonstrate different inheritance patterns dependent upon the sex of the parent transmitting the gene. Although these phenomena may superficially mimic genomic imprinting, there are important differences both at the clinical and the molecular levels. These inheritance mechanisms are

(1)   X-linked inheritance;

(2)   mitochondrial inheritance; and

(3)   the sexually dimorphic inheritance patterns of trinucleotide repeat expansions that occur in disorders such as Huntington's disease, fragile X syndrome, and myotonic dystrophy.

   The defining difference between genomic imprinting and these other patterns of inheritance is that with genomic imprinting the identical DNA sequence is passed from generation to generation, but the expression of the DNA is different depending upon the gamete (or parent) that delivers the DNA. The other patterns of inheritance that exhibit sex-of-parent effects lack both the quality of reversibility described for genomic imprinting alone, and differential expression based upon epigenetic phenomena rather than changes in DNA sequences. X-linked inheritance is dependent upon the pairing of X and Y in the male conceptus and the possibility of either hemizygous males or females who exhibit mosaic expression of X-linked genes. Mitochondial inheritance is a result of heterologous mitochondrial DNA inherited solely from the mitochondria within the mother's oocyte. Trinucleotide repeats apparently cause disease when the length of a repetitive portion of the DNA is expanded beyond a critical length. Larger expansions have shown some tendency to worsen the disease expression and the length of the trinucleotide repeat expansion (TRE) tends to increase to a greater or lesser extent, dependent upon the parent who carries a partial expansion or premutation of the trinucleotide repeat.

When investigators were beginning to look for genetic diseases that demonstrated genomic imprinting, some of the first disorders considered as candidates were diseases associated with trinucleotide repeat expansions. Huntington's disease, fragile X syndrome, and myotonic dystrophy were all on the list of suspected diseases associated with genetic imprinting (Clarke 1990). The following characteristics of inheritance in these diseases fuelled this suspicion:

(1)   childhood-onset Huntington's disease is usually inherited from the father;

(2)   congenital myotonic dystrophy is virtually always inherited from the mother; and

(3)   large expansions of the fragile X repeats are never inherited from the father who carries a premutation.

These inheritance patterns are all related to a differential expansion of the trinucleotide repeat in developing sperm versus the expansion in oocytes. While inheritance in TRE is profoundly effected by the distinct processes of spermatogenesis versus oogenesis, it differs from that due to genomic imprinting because the expansion of the triplet repeats are almost never reversible. This property of unidirectional expansion produces the association of triplet repeat expansions with the genetic phenomenon of anticipation, which means that the disease phenotype tends to worsen with each successive generation in terms of severity and age of onset.

TROPHOBLASTIC DISEASE AND GENOMIC IMPRINTING AT THE WHOLE GENOME LEVEL

Contributions of the paternal and maternal genomes in abnormal trophoblastic proliferation

The chromosomal constitution of the complete hydatidiform mole (CHM) was recognized as a product exclusively of the paternal genome in a developing zygote (Kajii and Ohama 1977). Conversely it was recognized that the benign ovarian teratoma was a product exclusively of the maternal genome (Linder *et al.* 1975). These two discoveries taken together represented both a breakthrough in the understanding of human disease and clinical examples of genomic imprinting. Although both processes contain a diploid chromosomal count, the developmental tissues are vastly different, yet complementary: a diploid paternal set leads to disordered placental development and no identifiable embryo, and a diploid maternal complement leads to disordered development of fetal tissues without evidence of placentation. These disparate developmental patterns demonstrate that the paternal genome is somehow programmed toward placental development, while the maternal genome is programmed toward somatic fetal development. The process of genomic imprinting programmes the paternally derived genome toward hyperplastic trophoblastic growth, while the equivalent set of maternally derived chromosomes produces a benign neoplasm, composed of well-differentiated derivatives of the three germ cell layers.

There are several reviews of trophoblastic disease and its pathology (Szulman 1995). I will briefly outline these more comprehensive reviews for the purpose of examining the impact of genomic imprinting on early development. A pathological triad is characteristic of the complete hydatidiform mole:

(1)   generalized and randomly distributed hyperplasia of both the syncytiotrophoblast and cytotrophoblast;

(2)   generalized oedema; and

(3)   the absence of an identifiable embryo.

The usual circumstance for initiation of the complete mole is fertilization of a chromosomally empty egg, followed by duplication of the genome of the haploid sperm (from 23, X to 46, XX), but the complete hydatidiform mole may also result from dual fertilization (with two spermatozoa) of an empty oocyte or rarely from fertilization by a single diploid spermatozoon. The 46,XX karyotype predominates due to the lack of growth potential of any tissue with a 46, YY karyotype. Despite the absence of a developing embryo, the natural history of complete hydatidiform mole is to persist until the second trimester when non-specific bleeding may occur, followed by eventual passage of tissue (Szulman and Surti 1982). Although subclinical embolization and some degree of myometrial invasion are common in CHM, the disease only mimics malignant behaviour. Residual trophoblastic disease (RTD), which is typically non-malignant, occurs in 10–20 per cent of cases, and choriocarcinoma is found in 3–5 per cent of those with RTD (Bagshawe 1992).

The theme that paternal patterns of gene expression favour placental development and maternal patterns of gene expression favour embryonic development is reinforced by reports of variable phenotypes in triploid pregnancies related to their relative paternal and maternal contributions. A triploid pregnancy has three times the haploid number of chromosomes, or 69. Triploidy occurs in approximately 1 per cent of human conceptuses, and 10 per cent of all chromosomally abnormal pregnancies (Fryns and Kleczkowska 1990). A triploid pregnancy with two haploid sets of paternal origin produces a partial hydatidiform mole (PHM), with focal hydatidiform villus changes and focal syncytiotrophoblastic hyperplasia. The placental changes are reminiscent of the complete hydatidiform mole, except that they are milder and focal in distribution (Szulman and Surti 1978; Szulman 1988, 1995). In the partial mole the embryo can be identified but rarely survives beyond eight weeks of gestation. The usual presentation of the partial mole is as a spontaneous or 'missed' abortion. Although the occurrence of diandric triploidy is quite common in first trimester abortions, pathologic examination is frequently required to identify these triploid molar pregnancies because the vesicles may be small and few in number (Szulman and Surti 1982; Szulman *et al.* 1981). When the paternal contribution is doubled, a haploid set from the maternal genome remains in these abnormally fertilized eggs. This doubling of the paternal genome can occur in the same ways as outlined for the paternal diploidy present in CHM, but fertilization with two spermatozoa is considered the most frequent mechanism.

After examining 82 triploid clinical pregnancies of variable gestational age, McFadden and Kalousek (1991) have defined two distinct fetal phenotypes. Type I is an appropriately grown though sometimes microcephalic embryo with a large cystic placenta and type II is growth retarded and relatively macrocephalic with a small noncystic placenta. In the triploid fetus, there is one haploid set from one parent and two haploid or a diploid set from the other parent, referred to as digynic when 46 chromosomes come from the mother and diandric when the paternal contribution predominates. The type I pregnancy correlates with diandry, and type II correlates with digyny, with the digynic conceptus having relatively greater chance of survival. The diandric type rarely survives beyond eight weeks, and the digynic sometimes survives to the third trimester (McFadden *et al.* 1993; Dietzsch *et al.* 1995).

The type I triploidy with diandry differs cytogenetically from the complete hydatidiform mole only in the retention of the normal haploid maternal genomic contribution. The differences between partial hydatidiform mole and the complete hydatidiform mole can therefore be attributable to this maternal contribution. The key differences effected by the maternal genome are simply (1) the presence of an embryo with survival typically limited to the first trimester, and (2) focal syncytiotrophoblastic hyperplasia as compared to the generalized hyperplasia and pronounced oedema of the CHM. The presence of two haploid or a diploid maternal equivalent in a triploid conceptus produces a type II phenotype. The typical parental contribution of the type II triploidy differs from the type I phenotype in two ways: it has one less haploid paternal set and a supernumerary haploid maternal set. This switch of genomic influences from a paternally imprinted diandry to a maternally imprinted digyny has both fetal and placental consequences. Fetal growth retardation may be secondary to a relative decrease in placental function induced through genomic imprinting, or it may be a result of specific imprinting changes that directly affect the growth of somatic tissues. The changes in fetal head size and the changes in placental size and cystic structure are a result of the general phenomenon of imprinting on the two different parentally inherited haploid genome sets. Likewise, since the type II fetus survives longer, despite relative placental insufficiency, we should attribute increased fetal developmental potential to genomic imprinting phenomena. The difference in type I and type II triploidy phenotypes can be attributed to the specific genes whose expression is diminished because they are imprinted, or to the excess expression of non-imprinted genes. Likewise, similar but more extreme differences in expression create the vastly divergent phenotypic differences between CHM and benign cystic teratomas.

Pronuclear transplantation experiments in mice

Although a review of mouse models for genomic imprinting is beyond the scope of this chapter, several features of these mammalian models have predicted the behaviour of imprinting in humans and encouraged researchers and clinicians to define and recognize similar phenomena in humans. Pronuclear transplantation experiments in mice were made possible in the 1980s thanks to the development of relatively non-invasive cell fusion techniques. Researchers produced mouse embryos that had either two maternal or two paternal pronuclei after *in vitro* manipulation of the male and female pronuclei (McGrath and Solter 1984; Surani *et al.* 1984). After replacing the male pronucleus with a female pronucleus (gynogenones) and replacing the female pronucleus with a male pronucleus (androgenones), there was no survival to term. These results were contrasted with pronuclear exchange of the same sex, where there was 5 per cent survival. These simple but elegant experiments demonstrated the necessity of genomes from both parents, transmitted through their respective gametes—eggs (maternal) and sperm (paternal)—for the successful completion of mouse embryogenesis.

Surani and co-workers (Surani *et al.* 1986). Completed similar nuclear transplantation experiments, but examined the developmental potential of the parthenogenones, gynogenones, and androgenones in more detail. These investigators demonstrated advanced fetal development (~25 somites) with growth restriction and poor trophoblast growth in gynogenones, and limited fetal development (~8 somites) with extensive trophoblast growth in androgenones. A review of this mouse work (Surani *et al.* 1990) reveals that androgenones rarely complete pre-implantation development, compared to 85 per cent of gynogenones, some of which advance to 40 somites despite underdeveloped placentae. A broad interpretation of these results reflects the abnormal development in humans of molar pregnancies, and triploidy with a haploid female contribution. In this model, zygotes with an identical karyotype once again vary in phenotype, dependent upon the gamete or parent of origin.

These early investigators speculated that the differential post-gametic function of the androgenones and gynogenones might be essential for embryonic or extraembryonic function or both, and at this time there was uncertainty as to the need for maternal and paternal genome interaction within a single cell, or just the presence of both genomes for specific functions in specific tissues. They suggested that replacement of the inner cell mass or outer cell mass by biparental, gynogenetic, or androgenetic cells should be attempted. An early report of chimeras between normally fertilized mouse embryos and parthenogenetically derived cells was made by Surani *et al.* (1977), which demonstrated survival to term of at least one parthenogenetic and normal chimera, with 10–25 per cent contribution by parthenogenetic cells, and non-survival in mice with greater levels of contribution from digynic cells. Not surprisingly, parthenogenetic cells are eliminated from extraembryonic cells early during development, first from the trophoblast, then from the yolk sac (Clarke *et al.* 1988; Thomson and Solter 1988). These cells continue to proliferate in the fetus until mid-gestation in the mouse, but the selection process is not uniform throughout all tissues (Fundele *et al.* 1989; Nagy *et al.* 1989).

IMPRINTING AT THE CHROMOSOMAL LEVEL

Uniparental disomy: a mouse model of genomic imprinting

An exclusive parental source for a given chromosomal pair is known as uniparental disomy (UPD), a term that was first used by Engel in 1980. The classic work of Searle and Beachey (1978) in mice demonstrated that specific chromosomes or chromosomal segments, when inherited in duplicate solely from one parent, could lead to non-survival, described as non-complementation lethality. This lack of survival when one parent's chromosomal contribution was absent despite the presence of the normal disomic number of copies implies that genomic imprinting is important at the cytogenetic level. This work used complementation studies in mice with chromosomal translocations to show that survival was not possible with maternal duplication and paternal absence of the distal ends of mouse chromosomes 2 and 8. UPD for the other mouse chromosomes studied by Searle and Beachey showed no apparent phenotypic problems. Similar complementation studies in mice have been carried out by Cattanach and Kirk (1985) with particular regard to mouse chromosomes 2 and 11. They observed opposite phenotypes, dependent upon the parental origin of uniparental disomy of mouse chromosome 11. Maternal duplication and paternal absence of chromosome 11 led to developmentally small animals, whereas paternal duplication and maternal absence of chromosome 11 led to larger-than-normal litter mates. By examining fetuses from parents with a different translocation breakpoint they were able to localize this imprinting phenomenon to the proximal portion of chromosome 11. Opposite phenotypes were also observed in neonatal mice with the lethal chromosome 2 UPD. With maternal disomy for the distal portion of chromosome 2 the pups are hyperkinetic with broad flat backs and short square bodies; and with the complementary paternal disomy for distal 2 the pups are hypokinetic with broad flat sides and arched backs. These pioneering studies together demonstrated that different outcomes are produced dependent upon the parental source of genes at the cytogenetic level. Presumably due to the specific genes involved, maternal and paternal patterns of imprinting may cause opposite phenotypes. As will be discussed in the review of uniparental disomy in humans, the gametic source of a pair of chromosomes (or a pair of chromosomal segments) could determine survival, effect pathologic phenotypic change, or may have no discernible effect.

Uniparental disomy and the sequelae of genomic imprinting in humans

UPD can occur in humans through the frequent occurrence of chromosomal aneuploidy in eggs, sperm, and zygotes, when followed by correction to euploidy. Trisomic zygotes can self-correct to the normal disomic pair through loss of one chromosome from the trisomic set (Cassidy *et al.* 1992; Purvis-Smith *et al.* 1992). When this occurs the actual fetal tissues can either remain mosaic, or all trisomic cells may be lost and only disomic cells remain. Since the trisomic cell has two chromosomes from one parent and one from the other parent, there is a one-in-three chance that the disomic cell line that survives has two chromosomes from the same parent, or uniparental disomy. The classification of UPD can be further subdivided, depending on the presence of either two identical chromosomes from one parent (isodisomic) or two different chromosomes from the same parent (heterodisomic). Uniparental disomy may also occur when an aneuploid sperm fertilizes an aneuploid oocyte, if the gametes happen to have a complementary disomy and nulisomy of the same chromosome (Wang *et al.* 1991). In this situation mosaicism would not be anticipated. Both of these phenomena would most probably occur for chromosomes where aneuploidy is most common, such as human chromosomes 13,15,16,21, and 22. In a review of uniparental disomy, Engel (1993) discusses five possible scenarios that can produce uniparental disomy. Beside those already mentioned, he includes monosomy duplication (Spence *et al.* 1988), heterochromosomal substitution (Peterson *et al.* 1992), and heterochromosomal exchange (Cavenee *et al.* 1983 ; Henry *et al.* 1991). In individuals with balanced translocations, the risk for uniparental disomy in offspring would be theoretically increased, due to abnormal chromosomal segregation. A 3:1 segregation could produce UPD from a single non-dysjunction event.

It has been well demonstrated that trisomy and trisomy/disomy mosaicism are common events in human reproduction. Mosaicism has been reported in 15–30 per cent of pre-implantation concepti at the cleavage stage (Plachot *et al.* 1989; Bongso *et al.* 1990). And, while trisomy is common in chromosomally abnormal first trimester abortions mosaicism can be identified in 10 per cent of the trisomic abortuses (Warburton *et al.* 1978). Hogge and colleagues (1986) reported mosaicism confined to the chorionic villi in 1.7 per cent of all viable gestations at the time of chorionic villus sampling. The US collaborative study confirmed a rate of 1–2 per cent for mosaicism from prenatal diagnosis samples (Ledbetter *et al.* 1992).

A report of uniparental disomy for chromosome 7 was the first one of an abnormal phenotype secondary to genomic imprinting at the chromosomal level (Spence *et al.* 1988). Maternal isodisomy was suspected because the proband presented with cystic fibrosis, as the result of an abnormal *CFTR* allele which was presumably inherited from her mother in duplicate. The *CFTR* allele codes for the cystic fibrosis transmembrane conductance regulator protein. The absence of a normally functioning *CFTR* protein results in clinical manifestations of cystic fibrosis. A normal protein inherited from either parent will result in an asymptomatic carrier state. Multiple molecular probes for chromosome 7 established that both chromosomes 7 were identical, and probes for X and other autosomes verified paternity. Although not typical features of cystic fibrosis, short stature (130 cm) with a poor response to growth hormone and asymmetry in leg length were noted. A similar case was reported soon thereafter (Voss *et al.* 1989). In both of these two cases autosomal recessive disease, like cystic fibrosis, is secondary to isodisomic UPD resulting in duplication of a normally recessive mutation. Pathology caused by duplicated expression of a mutant autosomal recessive gene carried by one parent would be restricted to cases of isodisomy; pathology caused by genomic imprinting would occur equally in isodisomic and heterodisomic UPD. Therefore, we must consider both potential sources of pathology in individuals with isodisomic UPD and an unusual phenotype, rather than assume that it is secondary to genomic imprinting. More recently a 30 year old male with short stature (143.7 cm) was homozygous for the COL1A2 gene mutation of type I procollagen, which he inherited from a heterozygous mother (Spotila *et al.* 1992). He was growth retarded at birth, weighing 4.5 lb (2 kg) at term. Although mutations in this gene lead to the highly variable syndrome of osteogenesis imperfecta (OI) with short stature and bone deformities, his two brothers who were heterozygous for the mutation were tall (> 6 feet or 1.8 m). Also, unlike short stature in OI his limbs were symmetrical.

These three case reports provide compelling evidence for imprinted genes on (the long arm of) chromosome 7 which lead to congenital growth retardation and short stature. In all three cases a mutated gene on chromosome 7 was the clue to uniparental isodisomy, but the syndrome of symmetrical growth retardation seems to be the result of imprinting of the maternal allele and the absence of paternal alleles on chromosome 7. A subsequent report suggested that a genetic short stature syndrome with right–left facial and body asymmetry, known as Silver–Russell syndrome, may sometimes be caused by imprinted genes on chromosome 7 when there is absence of paternal alleles (Kotzot *et al.* 1995). Four of 35 individuals with either Silver–Russell syndrome (3/25) or primordial growth retardation (1/10) had maternal UPD 7, three isodosomic and one heterodisomic. These authors recommend screening for maternal UPD 7 in all growth retarded fetuses and all offspring with Silver–Russell syndrome. Indeed the incidence of UPD may be more common than generally recognized considering the high rate of human aneuploidy (Warburton *et al.* 1978). The previous cases described above have been identified because of homozygous mutations that have been inherited from one heterozygous parent. Additionally, imprinting as a result of UPD should be sought whenever autosomal recessive disorders are identified with unusual features.

The complementary syndromes of Prader–Willi (PWS) and Angelman (AS) are a result of genomic imprinting on the long arm of chromosome 15 (locus 15q11-13). PWS is marked by hypotonia, lethargy, obesity, mental retardation, and overeating; Angelman syndrome by hyperactivity, behavioural problems, seizures, and unusual laughter. At 15q11-13, absence of paternal alleles due either to deletion of paternal alleles or maternal UPD both result in Prader–Willi syndrome; absence of maternal alleles due to either deletion of maternal alleles or paternal UPD both result in Angelman syndrome. The maternally imprinted gene, *SNRPN*, is the leading candidate for the PWS gene. *SNRPN* is the small nuclear ribonucleotide polypeptide N. While the function of the different SNRP proteins (5) are poorly understood, their physical association with mRNA and tissue-specific expression patterns suggest involvement in tissue-specific mRNA splicing. Mutations of this gene could affect mRNA splicing patterns in the brain with pleiotropic effects on the development of the nervous system. One of the initial cases of PWS due to maternal UPD was recognized because of a maternally inherited 13/15 balanced translocation (Nicholls *et al.* 1989). As noted above, 3:1 segregation of balanced translocations can increase the risk for UPD and abnormal phenotype related to imprinting.

Imprinting on human chromosome 14 has been recognized through ascertainment of both paternal UDP (Wang *et al.* 1991) and maternal UDP (Temple *et al.* 1991; Antonarakis *et al.* 1993) after inheritance of a balanced Robertsonian translocation. The syndrome of maternal UDP 14 is not well defined but includes short stature, learning disability, and mild hydrocephalus. Paternal UDP 14 has shown multiple congenital anomalies but is even less well defined. Despite an increased risk for uniparental disomy in carriers of balanced Robertsonian translocations, neither the precise phenotype nor the frequency of occurrence can be provided (Antonarakis *et al.* 1993).

Intrauterine fetal development and confined placental mosaicism: its relationship to genomic imprinting

The phenomenon and effect of CPM was first described in term placentas with chromosomally normal fetuses by Kalousek and Dill (1983). Confined placental mosaicism represents a dichotomy between the chromosomal constitution of the placental tissues and the fetus (or embryo), in which a true mosaicism affects the placenta only. Excellent reviews exist on the association of confined placental mosaicism (CPM) with abnormal pregnancy outcome (Kalousek 1994). In this section our focus will be on the relationship of genomic imprinting to CPM. Possible inferences regarding genomic imprinting and UPD will be made, as they relate to CPM and its effect on intrauterine development. The major complications that have been associated with CPM are fetal growth retardation and fetal death. The determinant factors that have been evaluated with regard to outcome are

(1)   the specific cell lineages involved in the mosaicism;

(2)   the specific chromosomes involved in the mosaicism; and

(3)   the 'ill-defined' placental–embryo interaction (Kalousek 1994).

The three types of placental involvement in confined placental mosaicism are type I CPM with trisomic cytotrophoblast and disomic chorionic stroma; type II CPM with disomic cytotrophoblast and trisomic chorionic stroma; and type III CPM with trisomic cytotrophoblast and chorionic stroma. General trends have been suggested between the various cell types involved in CPM, the specific chromosomes involved, and outcome. For instance, survival of fetuses trisomic for chromosomes 13 and 18 almost always occur in association with disomic cytotrophoblast and trisomic chorionic stroma, amnion, and fetal tissues (Kalousek *et al.* 1989; Lilford *et al.* 1991; Wirtz *et al.* 1991). However, both survival and normality of growth and development are difficult to predict in specific cases of CPM (Kalousek 1994). An important limitation in available data is that the presence or absence of uniparental disomy in the disomic cell lines is usually unknown. The abnormal outcomes associated with CPM may be due to the phenomenon of genomic imprinting when UPD occurs, or they may be due to the persistence of trisomic cell lines. The relative contributions of genomic imprinting and trisomic mosaicism to abnormal outcomes in CPM vary depending upon the chromosomes involved and the degree of mosaicism. Statistically, UPD is a factor in one of three pregnancies with CPM. Molecular polymorphisms can define the parental source of the disomic cells so that researchers can know when paternal or maternal disomy is a factor in normal and abnormal phenotypes.

Chromosome 16 is the most commonly reported chromosome involved in trisomic abortions and in CPM (Kalousek 1994; Wolstenholme 1994). A theoretical audit of outcome based upon trisomy 16 zygotes has been made from the relatively vast amount of available information on this chromosome (Wolstenholme 1994). The number of cases in which the parental source of chromosomes in the disomic cell lines was determined is small, even for chromosome 16. Table 12.1 compares fetal weights in all fetuses between 35 and 37 weeks, with and without UPD. The sample was limited to these three weeks because no surviving fetuses with maternal UPD 16 were

Table 12.1 CPM in trisomy 16—outcome at 35–37 weeks based on presence or absence of maternal UDP

Maternal UPD		No Maternal UPD	
Weeks gestation	Fetal weight (g)	Weeks gestation	Fetal weight (g)
35	1800	35	1578
35	1600	36	1631
37	1875	36	2660
		36	2280
		37	2440
Mean 35.7	Mean 1758.3	Mean 36	Mean 2117.8

Data from Wolstenholme 1994.

described beyond 37 weeks. Also, no adverse pregnancy outcomes without UPD were identified prior to 35 weeks. All cases of CPM 16 with UPD identified prior to 35 weeks resulted in severe growth retardation with or without fetal death. The results presented in Table 12.1 were therefore the best outcomes reported for CPM pregnancies that were complicated by UPD 16. Nevertheless, the average fetal weight is still lower with UPD 16 than for those pregnancies without UPD 16. This compilation of reported results for CPM 16 suggests that the presence of maternal UPD indicates a significantly worse prognosis. The ascertainment and the methods of determining UPD are not uniform, so that further studies of UPD/CPM 16 are needed to verify this impression. Furthermore, these data only pertain to one chromosome, albeit the most common one associated with aneuploidy and CPM. Kalousek and others have documented the frequent association between CPM of specific chromosomes and intrauterine growth retardation or fetal death (Kalousek 1994; Kalousek and Barrett 1994; Gosden *et al.* 1995). Untangling the effect of genomic imprinting in this phenomenon will require an ongoing effort to determine the parental source of the disomies in complicated and uncomplicated pregnancies.

Summary: effects of UPD in human reproduction

Clearly genomic imprinting has an impact on pregnancy outcomes as a result of uniparental disomy for specific chromosomes. Growth retardation has been reported consistently in association with maternal UPD 7 and 16. Paternal UPD appears to be less deleterious to fetal growth specifically with regard to chromosome 7 (Hoglund *et al.* 1994), and perhaps in other circumstances as well. Significant fetal dysmorphology and reduced survival are associated with the finding of maternal UPD 2 or 14. Paternal UPD 14 produces an ill-defined syndrome with multiple congenital anomalies. Prader–Willi syndrome would be anticipated for maternal UPD 15, or Angelman syndrome for paternal UPD 15. When CPM for chromosomes 2,7,14,15, or 16 is identified by CVS, maternal UPD for those chromosomes indicates a high risk for an abnormal outcome. Maternal UPD for chromosomes 13 and 22 apparently has no deleterious effect as demonstrated in single case reports of an inherited isochromo-some (Schinzel *et al.* 1994; Stallard *et al.* 1995).

Couples who carry a balanced translocation, in particular maternal Robertsonian translocations involving chromosome 14 or 15, have an increased risk for adverse outcomes secondary to UPD. Extensive mouse studies have demonstrated the effect of imprinting on development (Surani *et al.* 1990), and homologous chromosomal regions between mouse and man have been identified (Searle *et al.* 1994). By using this information in evaluating the potential for adverse outcomes in humans we should become better at identifying high risk situations. By continuing to look for clues to uniparental disomy and documenting it when suspected, we can begin to gauge its importance and develop programmes to anticipate adverse effects.

IMPRINTING OF SPECIFIC GENES IN EARLY DEVELOPMENT

DNA methylation and imprinting during embryonic development

The precise molecular mechanism by which genes are imprinted is unknown, but dif-ferential patterns of DNA methylation apparently play a role. DNA methylation occurs at cytosine in CpG dinucleotide sequences and has been known to affect gene expression even prior to the discovery of genomic imprinting. The DNA methylation status affects transcriptional activity of a gene at promoter regions in a differentiation and tissue specific manner (Cedar 1988).

At least four criteria must be fulfilled by the imprinting mechanism:

(1) the imprint must be physically linked to the pronucleus;

(2) the imprint must persist through somatic cell replication;

(3) the mechanism must be capable of affecting gene expression; and

(4) the mechanism must be capable of switching identity from one sex to the other in successive generations (Sapienza *et al.* 1987).

Surani and co-workers (Swani *et al.* 1986*a,b*) have linked differential DNA methyla-tion with the first three criteria. The methylation patterns of transgenes in mice satisfy the fourth criterion as they have been shown to vary depending upon the gamete of origin, and to be reversible between successive generations (Reik *et al.* 1987; Sapienza *et al.* 1987). In both of these studies transgenes were microinjected into new embryonic cell lines and the relative methylation pattern studied through successive generations. Methylation-sensitive restriction endonucleases cleaved the DNA in question, so that banding patterns were dependent upon the methylation status at the cleavage sites. Despite the use of different methylated transgenes in the two experiments the CpG sites showed a greater degree of methylation when inherited from females than when inher-ited from males. Subsequent studies indicate that methylation status is not always greater in the male-inherited gene though this is the typical status.

Chaillet and co-workers (1991) followed the methylation patterns of transgenes in mice through gametogenesis and embryogenesis. Maternally and paternally inherited methylation patterns are entirely erased in primordial germ cells. The methylation pattern of the maternal allele is fully matured during oogenesis, but the methylation pattern of the paternal allele develops partially during spermatogenesis and undergoes further maturation during embryogenesis. In agreement with previous studies, the transgene determined its own methylation pattern, which was independent of its insertional site in the genome, and methylation did not spread into the surrounding site of DNA insertion.

DNA methyltransferase (DNMT) is responsible for maintenance of the methylation status of CpG dinucleotides in cells throughout the cell cycle. Homozygous mouse mutants deficient for DNA methyltransferase have been studied to determine the association between methylation patterns and gene expression in murine genes known to be imprinted (Li *et al.* 1993). Expression of the imprinted genes *H19*, *Igf2*, and *Igf2r*, as well as their methylation patterns were studied using the DNMT homozygous mutation mouse model. *H19* and *Igf2* are closely linked and reciprocally imprinted. Demethylation of the normally silent paternal *H19* allele correlated with increased activity of the *H19* gene to the same level as the normally active maternal allele. Demethylation of the normally active paternal allele repressed its expression. *Igf2r* is on a different chromosome than *H19* and *Igf2*, and is normally imprinted or inactive on the paternal allele. This imprinted locus required a functionally less active DNMT mutation before demethylation-induced changes in expression could be verified. Like the *H19* allele, which is also relatively inactive from the paternal homologue, demethylation eventually led to greater expression from the paternal allele.

The *IGF2* and *H19* system in placenta and early development

The *IGF2* and *H19* gene system comprises a reciprocally expressed pair of imprinted genes that are expressed early in embryological development and in the differentiating placenta. The usual pattern of imprinting in this pair of genes is crucial to the normal growth and development of the placenta and early embryo. Indeed these two genes, along with other genes that are functionally interrelated, provide a useful paradigm for the role of genomic imprinting in placental development and early human embryogenesis. *IGF2* and *H19* are imprinted genes that are physically linked on human chromosome 11q15.5, with homologous imprinted genes on mouse chromosome 7 (*Igf2* and *H19*).

IGF2 is a protein growth factor structurally related to IGF1 and proinsulin (Ohlsson *et al.* 1989). IGF2 is primarily expressed amongst proliferative cytotrophoblast columns that protrude from chorionic villi in the first trimester. IGF2 transcripts are found at much reduced levels of expression in villus cytotrophoblast and mesenchymal stroma. Although IGF2 expression is also high in term placentae, there is a lack of proliferative transformation in these differentiated structures. Insulin-like growth factor type 2 is the first mammalian gene noted to exhibit imprinting behaviour (DeChiara *et al.* 1991). Mice with a targeted disruption of the homologous gene, *igf2*, were followed through several generations. When the mutated gene was transmitted through the male line the offspring were small and indistinguishable from homozygous mice which have inherited two copies of the mutated growth factor gene. In contrast, when one copy of the mutated gene was inherited from a female, the offspring reached normal size, demonstrating that only the paternally inherited gene is expressed and the maternal gene is imprinted. A normal gene from the father is necessary and sufficient for normal growth because it is normally the only allele expressed during growth of the embryo. The same pattern of parental imprinting and expression was documented in humans, using a structural polymorphism of human IGF2 mRNA (Giannoukakis *et al.* 1993). Type 2 IGF receptor, and type 1 IGF receptor are also known as IGF2 receptor (IGf2R) and IGF1 receptor (IGF1R) respectively. These names can be deceptive, however, because IGF2 receptor is not the primary functional receptor for IGF2, and IGF1 receptor is not exclusively the receptor for IGF1. Rather, the overall interaction between insulin-like growth factors, their receptors, and their binding proteins is complex, with no imprinting of IGF1 nor of the type 1 IGF receptor. IGF2 receptor is maternally imprinted. The most likely function of this type 2 IGF receptor is to act as a sponge for active IGF2, which inhibits the effect of this growth-promoting hormone by binding to it (Haig and Graham 1991). This hypothesis finds support in the description of the phenotype of mice with a non-functional mutation of the *Igf2r* gene (Lau *et al.* 1994). This report also confirms paternal imprinting of the IGF2 receptor gene. When the mutated IGf2 receptor gene is inherited from a female there is a lack of IGF2R expression, the mice are 25–30 per cent larger than normal, and they have elevated levels of IGF2 and IGF-binding proteins. They also die from major cardiac abnormalities. When the mutated gene is inherited from a male, the phenotype is normal, because the paternally inherited allele is silent.

H19 is not translated into a protein and probably functions in its RNA form (Brannan *et al.* 1990). The *H19* gene was initially identified as a structurally unusual gene whose mRNA is regulated by the same *trans*-acting loci as alpha-fetoprotein (Pachnis *et al.* 1988). Tissue culture of mesodermal cell lines demonstrated activation very early during embryonic muscle differentiation. Activation of the murine equivalent of *H19* was documented throughout development, from embryonic stem (ES) cells to embryoid bodies (EB) (Poirier *et al.* 1991). ES cells that are cultured *in vitro* develop into EBs by a process that partially mimics the formation of the embryo. Poirier and co-workers found that the *H19* gene is activated in the outer layers of the embryoid body *in vitro* and at the time of implantation in the extraembryonic cell lineages, but is not activated in the embryo proper *in vivo*.

The timing of expression and the cell lineages where expression initially occurs suggest that *H19* may participate in the implantation process (Poirier *et al.* 1991). *H19* transcripts are not identifiable from the time of fertilization and for three days of cleavage. Detectable levels are first identified in the trophectoderm of the expanded blastocyst. After implantation the expression of *H19* becomes more diffuse and abundant, but is not expressed in the primitive ectoderm, which is destined to develop into the embryo proper. At this stage the expression of *H19* in nutritive support cells of the newly formed embryo coincides with terminal differentiation of these cells, while the embryonic streak remains pluripotent. By mid-gestation the expression of this gene is widespread, except for limited expression in the central nervous system. First identified in developing muscle and fetal liver, *H19* expression is abundant in other developing tissues. After birth, the gene is rapidly downregulated and found in few tissues of the adult. As such, *H19* can be classified as an embryonic gene.

Imprinting of the paternal *H19* gene in human placenta has been shown to increase from seven to ten weeks of gestation, such that biallelic expression of *H19* essentially ceased after nine weeks of gestation (Jinno *et al.* 1995). The only exception, where the paternal allele continued to be expressed after ten weeks gestation, was in a 15-week placenta from a spontaneously aborted pregnancy obtained from a recurrent spontaneous aborter. In this study *IGF2* was always monoallelically expressed in the placenta from the paternal homologue. This finding agrees with previous work (Ohlsson *et al.* 1993) which demonstrated paternal-only expression of *IGF2* in embryonic and extraembryonic tissues. A study of *H19* expression in cultured human cytotrophoblast demonstrated a correlation with the stage of cell differentiation (Rachmilewitz *et al.* 1992). The authors suggested that *H19* plays a role in cytotrophoblast differentiation. Thus, in the normal development of the placenta and embryo, the reciprocally imprinted *IGF2* and *H19* genes on chromosomal region 11p15.5 appear to participate in the complementary processes of proliferation and differentiation, respectively. The pattern of imprinting agrees neatly with the theory that paternal genes promote growth and maternal genes limit growth. In an evolutionary model of competition the father has a genetic stake in his progeny outgrowing competitors, and the mother has a stake in limiting the growth of any single offspring in order to provide for all of her children. This model of competition is often evoked to explain the central evolutionary role of genomic imprinting. The expression of *H19* and *IGF2* in human tissues is summarized in Table 12.2.

Beckwith–Wiedemann as a relevant model of genomic imprinting

Beckwith–Wiedemann syndrome (BWS) is a syndrome of multiple organ overgrowth, most frequently involving the tongue and abdominal viscera. Infants with BWS are macrosomic, and frequently have hemihypertrophy secondary to asymmetric growth. Other commonly recognized features include anterior abdominal wall defects and neonatal hypoglycaemia in the more severe cases. Paediatric neoplasms occur in 7.5 per cent and include Wilms' tumour, adrenocortical carcinoma, and hepatoblastoma (Sotelo-Avila *et al.* 1980). Familial Beckwith–Wiedemann syndrome occurs in 15 per cent of the cases. In these families and in individuals with chromosomal abnormalities the disorder has been linked to chromosome 11p15.

IGF2 has been proposed as a candidate gene in BWS because

(1)   imprinting phenomena appear to play a role in the pathology of BWS; and

(2)   11p15 has been identified as the region responsible for BWS; and

(3)   excess expression of *IGF2* promotes excess growth (Little *et al.* 1991).

Ramesar and co-workers (1993) reported a family in which BWS was expressed only when the same region of 11p15 was maternally derived, and argued that this family provided evidence that a paternally imprinted growth suppressor was involved. They suggested that a maternally inherited and non-functional *H19* was the gene that caused BWS in this family. An alternative interpretation, however, is that excess expression of *IGF2* due to failure of imprinting at the maternal *IGF2* gene was

Table 12.2 Expression of *H19* and *IGF2* in human tissues

Tissue	*H19* expression	*IGF2* expression
First trimester placenta	Monoallelic maternal (1) imprinting of the paternal H19 gene increases from seven to ten weeks of gestation (2) biallelic expression essentially ceases after nine weeks (Jinno *et al.* 1995) (3) correlated with stage of cytotrophoblast differentiation (Rachmilewitz *et al.* 1992)	Monoallelic paternal (1) highest expression in proliferative cytotrophoblast (2) reduced levels of expression in villous cytotrophoblast and mesenchymal stroma (Giannoukakis *et al.* 1993)
Full term placenta	Monoallelic maternal, predominantly (Jinno *et al.* 1995)	Monoallelic paternal expression high (Giannoukakis *et al.* 1993; Ohlsson *et al.* 1993)
Complete hydatidiform mole	Significant *H19* expression, despite androgenic source of genes (Ariel *et al.* 1994)	High levels of expression of both *IGF2* and *H19* were documented in two of four CHMs that progressed to choriocarcinoma (Walsh *et al.* 1995)
Partial hydatidiform mole	Similar pattern to normal placenta (Ariel *et al.* 1994)	Similar pattern to normal placenta (Ariel *et al.* 1994)
Choriocarcinoma	Prominent expression of *H19* in choriocarcinoma and placental site trophoblastic tumour (Ariel *et al.* 1994)	High levels of expression of both *IGF2* and *H19* were documented in two of four CHMs that progressed to choriocarcinoma (Walsh *et al.* 1995)
Embryonal and adult somatic tissue	(1) Abundant in developing tissues (2) The gene is rapidly downregulated after birth (3) Found in few tissues of the adult (Jinno *et al.* 1995)	Monoallelic paternal (Giannoukakis *et al.* 1993; Ohlsson *et al.* 1993)
Wilms' tumour/ BWS	Diminished expression (Taniguchi *et al.* 1995)	Biallelic expression (Taniguchi *et al.* 1995)
Testicular tumour	Biallelic expression (van Gurp *et al.* 1994)	Biallelic expression (van Gurp *et al.* 1994)

responsible. Theoretically, a paternal pattern of methylation in the maternally derived allele would lead to both decreased *H19* expression and increased *IGF2* expression. Slatter and associates (1994) presented further evidence for an excess expression of *IGF2* from the non-imprinted paternally derived genes. These researchers identified mosaic UPD for 11p15 in nine of 32 (28 per cent) informative individuals with sporadic BWS, using linkage. These findings would suggest that a paternal pattern of expression for *IGF2* and *H19* from the maternally inherited allele could produce BWS. This 'reversal' of maternal imprinting patterns should correlate with increased methylation. Conflicting data have been reported. Reik and colleagues (1994) could not demonstrate an abnormal methylation pattern in a group of 42 BWS patients. Taniguchi and co-workers (1995), in contradiction, demonstrated abnormal methylation patterns restricted to the *IGF2/H19* region of 11p15. In this study biallelic expression of *IGF2* and diminished expression of *H19* were both demonstrated in Wilms' tumour tissue. This loss of normal imprinting patterns is known as relaxation of imprinting, and is associated with development of neoplasia and malignant potential in Wilms' tumour.

Relaxation of imprinting has been documented in trophoblastic disease, specifically with regard to *H19* expression (Ariel *et al.* 1994). In normal placenta, *H19* expression in the trophoblast and stroma is prominent, with greatest abundance in the intermediate trophoblast, decreasing in the cytotrophoblast down through the syncytiotrophoblast. Not surprisingly, partial hydatidiform mole shows a similar pattern to normal placenta. Since complete hydatidiform mole is strictly androgenetic, no *H19* expression would be anticipated from paternally imprinted genes. CHM, however, did show significant H19 expression. Prominent expression of *H19* found in choriocarcinoma (CC) and placental site trophoblastic tumour (PSTT) suggests that relaxation of imprinting may also be related to malignant potential in trophoblastic disease. In another recent study, high levels of expression of both *IGF2* and *H19* were documented in two of four CHMs that progressed to choriocarcinoma (Walsh *et al.* 1995). Both of these studies documented relaxation of imprinting for the *IGF2/H19* locus in the progression to malignancy from CHM to CC. Relaxation of imprinting, with regard to the *H19/IGF2* locus, is a common feature of malignant transformation in both trophoblastic disease and Wilms' tumour. Appropriate expression of this locus may also prevent testicular tumours and breast cancer, as evidenced by reports of abnormal expression in both conditions. The precise function of *H19*, and its interaction with *IGF2*, remains incompletely described.

FUTURE RESEARCH: THE ROLE OF IMPRINTING IN EARLY HUMAN DEVELOPMENT

Mouse models have been useful in predicting the general behaviour and mechanisms of imprinting in humans. The development of mouse zygotes in pronuclear transplantation experiments correlates with the fate of human zygotes following abnormalities of fertilization as in complete and partial hydatidiform moles. Mouse experiments in translocation carriers have anticipated some of the effects of uniparental disomy in humans. Specific homologous genes appear to be imprinted in both man and mouse, and participate in early development through parentally defined regulation of expression. Mouse models will continue to be useful in examining pathophysiologic changes due to abnormalities in imprinting.

Genomic imprinting plays a central role in placental–fetal development, as first recognized by the parental genomic source for complete and partial hydatidiform moles. *H19* and *IGF2*, imprinted genes at the 11p15 locus, appear to be crucial in the regulation of implantation and embryogenesis. While the pattern of expression for this conversely imprinted gene pair has been described in some clinical situations and during development in mice and humans, the precise genomic regulation is unknown. How these genes affect downstream effectors is also unknown. These genes are finely regulated in trophoblast and decidua, along with other growth factors and their receptors. Additional murine genes near this locus have been identified, which are also imprinted and play roles in trophoblast development (*Mash2*, Guillemot *et al.* 1995), and possibly tumour suppressors (*p57KIP2*, Hatada and Mukai 1995). The fetal overgrowth syndrome BWS is related to disturbances in expression of these genes, and relaxation of imprinting within this locus apparently contributes to neoplasia in the development of Wilms' tumour, other somatic malignancies, and possibly choriocarcinoma. Continued basic research in the regulation of this important embryonic gene pair will be crucial to our understanding of embryogenesis and neoplastic processes, as well as continued comparison with other imprinted homologous mouse genes. Careful attention to human syndromes in which imprinting abnormalities of these and similar related genes will give further insight into the role of imprinting in human reproduction, and mouse models will be developed to mimic the pathophysiology in clinical situations in man.

Polymorphisms in expressed genes can be used to determine allelic expression, and methylation-sensitive restriction endonucleases can be used to determine the methylation status of genes where the relevance of imprinting is suspected. Clinical problems that may be related to imprinted genes include developmental problems, cancer, and implantation abnormalities associated with recurrent pregnancy loss or infertility. Individuals with these problems should be screened for abnormal expression of *H19*, *IGF2*, and similar genes. Likewise, specific cancers and cancer-predisposing syndromes should be evaluated for abnormalities in imprinting and control of gene expression in imprinted loci. For example, a recent study demonstrated biallelic expression of *IGF2* and *H19* in most testicular germ cell tumours (van Gurp *et al.* 1994). Other growth and development genes should be evaluated for the importance of imprinting phenomena. The Wilms' tumour gene 1 (*WT1*) is one possible candidate gene for cancer-related imprinting. Syndromes with developmental abnormalities and early-onset tumours, such as Denys–Drash syndrome, should be examined for abnormalities in imprinting phenomena.

Uniparental disomy is a common human phenomenon due to a high propensity for aneuploid gametes. UPD and its heterodisomic or isodisomic source should be determined in pathologic situations whenever it is suspected to help in the identification of imprinted genes. Linkage studies, using restriction fragment length polymorphisms or the more powerful tool of microsatellites, will allow researchers to identify sites of clinically significant genomic imprinting. UPD should be suspected whenever an abnormal outcome occurs related to confined placental mosaicism. Isodisomic UPD should also be suspected whenever an autosomal recessive disorder is associated with atypical features. Suspicion is especially high when only one parent can be identified as a heterozygous carrier for the autosomal recessive disease. Since CPM is so commonly identified by chorionic villus sampling, a collaborative registry should be developed to track outcomes following CPM and the presence or absence of UPD.

Typically in the evolution of our understanding of genetic disease the most obviously abnormal adverse outcomes are identified first. For that reason we should sharpen our view and now begin to search more closely for subtle effects of genomic imprinting. In human reproduction, on the other hand, the most extreme outcome is early pregnancy loss or even developmental failure prior to implantation. These severe outcomes tend to attract less attention, however, because there is so little development. Now is the time to search for problems associated with abnormal imprinting in those couples who suffer recurrent miscarriages or who are infertile. More complete evaluations for the role of imprinting (as well as the opportunity to affect the imprinting process) will eventually require investigation of human embryos. The imperative for ethical and well-reasoned embryo research is becoming greater as we address basic areas of human reproduction, such as genomic imprinting.

REFERENCES

Antonarakis, S.E., Blouin, J.L., Maher, J., Avramopolous, D., Thomas G., and Talbot Jr, G.G. (1993). Maternal uniparental disomy for chromosome 14, due to loss of a chromosome 14 from somatic cells with t(13;14) trisomy. *American Journal of Human Genetics*, 52, 1145–52.
Ariel, I., Lustig, O., Oyer, C.E., Elkin, M., Gonik, B., Rachmilewitz, J., *et al.* (1994). Relaxation of imprinting in trophoblastic disease. *Gynecologic Oncology*, 53, 212–19.
Bagshawe, K.D. (1992). Choriocarcinoma: a model for tumor markers. *Reviews in Oncology*, 5, 99–106.
Bongso, A., Ng, C.S., Lim, J., Fong, C.Y., and Ratnam, S. (1990). Preimplantation genetics: chromsomes of fragmented human embryos. *Fertility and Sterility*, 56, 66–70.
Brannan, C.I., Dees, E.C., Ingram, R.S., and Tilghman, S.M. (1990). The product of the *H19* gene may function as an RNA. *Molecular and Cellular Biology*, 10, 28–36.
Cassidy, S.B., Li-Wen, L., Erickson, R.P., Magnusson, L., Thomas, E., Gendron, R., and Hermann, R. (1992). Trisomy 15 with loss of the paternal 15 as a cause of Prader–Willi syndrome due to maternal disomy. *American Journal of Human Genetics*, 51, 701–8.
Cattanach, B.M. and Kirk, M. (1985). Differential activity of maternally and paternally derived chromosome regions in mice. *Nature*, 315, 496–8.
Cavenee, W.K., Dryja, T.P., Phillips, R.A., Benedict, W.F., Godbout, R., Gallie, B.L., *et al.* (1983). Expression of recessive alleles by chromosomal mechanism in retinoblastoma. *Nature*, 305, 779–84.
Cedar, H. (1988). DNA methylation and gene activity. *Cell*, 53, 3–4.
Chaillet, J.R., Vogt, T.F., Beier, D.R., and Leder, P. (1991). Parental-specific methylation of an imprinted transgene is established during gametogenesis and progressively changes during embryogenesis. *Cell*, 66, 77–83.
Clarke, A. (1990). Genetic imprinting in clinical genetics. *Development (Suppl.)*, 89, 131–9.

Clarke, H.J., Varmuza, S., Prideaux, V.R., and Rossant, J. (1988). The developmental potential of parthenogenetically-derived cells in chimeric mouse embryos: implications for action of imprinted genes. *Development*, **104**, 175–82.

DeChiara, T.M., Robertson, E.J., and Afstratiadis, A. (1991). Parental imprinting of the mouse insulin-like growth factor II gene. *Cell*, **64**, 849–59.

Dietzsch, E., Ramsay M., Christianson, A.L., Henderson, B.D., and de Ravel, T.J.L. (1995). Maternal origin of extra haploid set of chromosomes in the third trimester triploid fetuses. *American Journal of Medical Genetics*, **58**, 360–4.

Engel, E. (1980). A new genetic concept: uniparental disomy and its ptoential effect, isodisomy. *American Journal of Medical Genetics*, **6**, 137–43.

Engel, E. (1993). Uniparental disomy revisited: the first twelve years. *American Journal of Medical Genetics*, **46**, 670–4.

Fryns, J.P. and Kleczkowska, A. (1990). Chromosome triploidy. In *Birth defects encyclopedia*, (ed. M.L. Buyse), pp. 398–9. Blackwell, Dover.

Fundele, R.H., Norris, M.L., Barton, S.C., Reich, W., and Surani, M.A. (1989). Systematic elimination of parthenogenetic cells in mouse chimeras. *Development*, **106**, 20–35.

Giannoukakis, N., Deal, C., Paguette, J., Goodyer, C.G., and Polychronakos, C. (1993). Parental genomic imprinting of the human *IGF2* gene. *Nature Genetics*, **4**, 98–101.

Gosden, C.M., Harrison, K., and Kalousek, D.K. (1995). Chromosomal mosaicism. In *Diseases of the fetus and newborn: pathology, genetics, imaging and management*, Vol. 1, (2nd edn), (ed. G.B. Reed, A.E. Claireaux, and F. Cockburn), pp. 1099–114. Chapman and Hall, London.

Guillemot, F., Caspary, T., Tilghman, S.M., Copeland, N.G., Gilbert, D.J., Jenkins, N.A., *et al.* (1995). Genomic imprinting of *Mash2*, a mouse gene required for trophoblast development. *Nature Genetics*, **9**, 235–42.

Haig, D. and Graham, C. (1991). Genomic imprinting and the strange case of the insulin-like growth factor II receptor. *Cell*, **64**, 1045–6.

Harrison, K.B. (1989). X-chromosome inactivation in the human cytotrophoblast. *Cytogenetics and Cell Genetics*, **52**, 37–41.

Harrison, K.B. and Warburton, D. (1986). Preferential X-chromosome activity in human female placental tissues. *Cytogenetics and Cell Genetics*, **41**, 163–8.

Hatada, I. and Mukai, T. (1995). Genomic imprinting of p57KIP2, a cyclin-dependent kinase inhibitor, in mouse. *Nature Genetics*, **11**, 204–6.

Henry, I., Bonaite-Pellie, C., Chenhensse, V., Beldjord, P., Schwartz, C., Utermann, G., and Junien, C. (1991). Uniparental paternal disomy in a genetic, cancer predisposing syndrome. *Nature*, **351**, 665–7.

Hogge, W.A., Schonberg, S.A., and Golbus, M.A. (1986). Chorionic villus sampling: experience of the first 1000 cases. *American Journal of Obstetrics and Gynecology*, **154**, 1249–52.

Hoglund, P., Holmberg, C., de la Chappelle, A., and Kere, J. (1994). Paternal isodisomy for chromosome 7 is compatible with normal growth and development in a patient with congenital chloride diarrhea. *American Journal of Human Genetics*, **55**, 747–52.

Jinno, Y., Ikeda, Y., Yun, K., Maw, M., Masuzaki, H., Fukuda, H., *et al.* (1995). Establishment of functional imprinting of the *H19* gene in human developing placentae. *Nature Genetics*, **10**, 318–24.

Johnson, D.R. (1974*a*). Hairpin-tail: a case of post-reductional gene action in the egg? *Genetics*, **76**, 795–805.

Johnson, D.R. (1974*b*). Further observations on the hairpin-tail (T^{hp}) mutation in the mouse. *Genetic Research*, **24**, 207–13.

Kajii, T. and Ohama, K. (1977). Androgenetic origin of hydatidiform mole. *Nature*, **268**, 633–4.

Kalousek, D.K. (1994). Current topic: confined placental mosaicism and intrauterine fetal development. *Placenta*, **15**, 219–30.

Kalousek, D.K. and Barrett, I.J. (1994). Confined placental mosaicism and stillbirth. *Pediatric Pathology*, **14**, 151–9.

Kalousek, D.K. and Dill, F.J. (1983). Chromosomal mosaicism confined to the placenta in human conceptions. *Science*, **221**, 665–7.

Kalousek, D.K., Barret, I.J., and McGillivray, B.C. (1989). Placental mosaicism and intra-uterine survival of trisomies 13 and 18. *American Journal of Human Genetics*, **44**, 338–43.

Kotzot, D., Schmitt, S., Bernasconi, F., Robinson, W.P., Lurie, I.W., Ilyina, H., *et al.*, (1995). Uniparental disomy 7 in Silver–Russell syndrome and primordial growth retardation. *Human Molecular Genetics*, **4**, 583–7.

Lau, M.M.H., Stewart, C.E.H., Liu, Z., Bhatt, H., Rotwein, P., and Stewart, C.L. (1994). Loss of the imprinted IGF2/cation-independent 6-phosphate receptor results in fetal overgrowth. *Genes and Development*, **8**, 2953–63.

Ledbetter, D., Zachery, J.M., Simpson, J.L., Golbus, M.S., Pergament, E., Jackson, L. (1992). Cytogenetic results from the US collaborative study on CVS. *Prenatal Diagnosis*, **12**, 317–54.

Li, E., Beard, C., and Jaenish, R. (1993). Role for DNA methylation in genomic imprinting. *Nature*, **366**, 362–5.

Lilford, R.J., Caine, A., Linton, G., and Mason, G. (1991). Short-term culture and false-negative results for Down's syndrome on chorionic villus sampling. *Lancet*, **337**, 861.

Linder, D., McCaw, B.K., and Hecht, F. (1975). Parthenogenetic origin of benign ovarian teratomas. *New England Journal of Medicine*, **292**, 63–6.

Little, M., Van Heynigen, V., and Hastie, N. (1991). Dads, disomy and disease. *Nature*, **351**, 609–10.

Lyon, M.F. and Rastan, S. (1984). Parental source of chromosome imprinting and its relevance of X-chromosome inactivation. *Differentiation*, **26**, 63–7.

McFadden, D.E. and Kalousek, D.K. (1991). Two different phenotypes of fetuses with chromo-somal triploidy: correlation with parental origin of the extra haploid set. *American Journal of Medical Genetics*, **38**, 535–8.

McFadden, D.E., Kwong, L.C., Yam, I.Y.L., and Langois, S. (1993). Parental origin of triploidy in human fetuses: evidence for genomic imprinting. *Human Genetics*, **92**, 465–9.

McGrath, J. and Solter, D. (1984). Completion of mouse embryogenesis requires both the maternal and paternal genomes. *Cell*, **37**, 179–83.

Nagy, A., Sass, M., and Markkula, M. (1989). Systematic nonuniform distribution of parthenogenetic cells in adult mouse chimeras. *Development*, **106**, 321–4.

Nicholls, R.D., Knoll, J.H.M., Butler, M.G., Karam, S., and Lalande, M. (1989). Genetic imprinting suggested by maternal heterodisomy in non-deletion Prader–Willi syndrome. *Nature*, **342**, 281–5.

Ohlsson, R., Hohlmgren, L., Glaser, A., Szpecht, A., and Pfeifer-Ohlsson, S. (1989). Insulin-like growth factor 2 and short-range stimulatory loops in control of human placental growth. *EMBO Journal*, **8**, 1993–9.

Ohlsson, R., Nystrom, A., Pfeifer-Ohlsson, S., Tohonen, V., Hedborg, F., Schofield, P., *et al.* (1993). IGF2 is parentally imprinted during human embryogenesis and in the Beckwith–Wiedemann syndrome. *Nature Genetics*, **4**, 94–7.

Pachnis, V., Brannan, C.I., and Tilghman, S.M. (1988). The structure and expression of a novel gene activated in early mouse embryogenesis. *EMBO Journal*, **7**, 673–81.

Peterson, M.B., Bartsch, O., Adelsberger, P.A., Mikkelsen, M., Schwinger, E., and Antonarakis, E. (1992). Uniparental disomy due to duplication of chromosome 21 occuring in somatic cells monosomic for chromosome 21. *Genomics*, **13**, 269–74.

Plachot, M., Mandelbaum, J., Junca, J.M., deGrouchy, J., Salat-Baraoux, J. and Cohen, J. (1989). Cytogenetic analysis and developmental potential of normal and abnormal embryos of the IVF. *Human Reproduction (Suppl. ment)*, **4**, 99–103.

Poirier, F., Chan C.-T.J., Timmons, P.M., Robertson, E.J., Evans P.J., and Rigby, P.W.J. (1991). The murine *H19* gene is activated during embryonic stem cell differentiation *in vitro* and at the time of implantation in the developing embryo. *Development*, **113**, 1105–14.

Purvis-Smith, S.G., Saville, T., Manass, S., Yip, M.-Y., Lam-Po-Tang, P.R.L., Duffy, B., *et al.* (1992). Uniparental disomy 15 resulting from 'correction' of an intitial trisomy 15. *American Journal of Human Genetics*, **50**, 1348–50.

Rachmilewitz, J., Gileadi, O., Eldar-Geva, T., Schneider, T., deGroot, N., and Hochberg, A. (1992). Transcription of the *H19* gene in differentiating cytotrophoblast from human placenta. *Molecular Reproduction and Development*, **32**, 196–202.

Ramesar, R. Babaya, M., and Viljoen, D. (1993). Molecular investigation of familial Beckwith–Wiedemann syndrome: a model for paternal imprinting. *European Journal of Human Genetics*, **1**, 109–13.

Reik, W., Collick, A., Norris, M.L., Barton, S.C., and Surani, M.L. (1987). Genomic imprinting determines methylation of parental alleles in transgenic mice. *Nature*, **328**, 248–50.

Reik, W., Brown, K.W., Slatter, R.E., Sartori, P., Elliot, M., and Maher, E.R. (1994). Allelic methylation of *H19* and *IGF2* in the Beckwith–Wiedemann syndrome. *Human Molecular Genetics*, **3**, 1297–301.

Sapienza, C., Peterson, A.C., Rossant, J., and Balling, R. (1987). Degree of methylation of transgenes is dependent of gamete of origin. *Nature*, **328**, 251–4.

Schinzel, A.A., Basaran, S., Bernasconi, F., Karaman, B., Yuksel-Apak, M., and Robinson, W.P. (1994). Maternal uniparental disomy 22 has no impact on the phenotype. *American Journal of Human Genetics*, **54**, 21–4.

Searle, A.G. and Beachey, C.V. (1978). Complementation studies with mouse translocations. *Cytogenetics and Cell Genetics*, **20**, 282–303.

Searle, A.G., Edwards, J.H., and Hall, J.G. (1994). Mouse homologues of human hereditary disease. *Journal of Medical Genetics*, **31**, 1–19.

Sharman, G.B. (1971). Late DNA replication in paternally derived X-chromosome of female kangaroos. *Nature*, **230**, 231–2.

Slatter, R.E, Elliott, M., Welham, K., Carrera, M., Schofield, P.N., Barton, D.E., *et al.* (1994). Mosaic uniparental disomy in Beckwith–Wiedemann syndrome. *Journal of Medical Genetics*, **31**, 749–53.

Sotelo-Avila, C., Gonzalez-Crussi, F., and Fowler, J. (1980). Wilms' tumor in a patient with an incomplete form of Beckwith–Wiedemann syndrome. *Pediatrics*, **66**, 121–3.

Spence, J.E., Perciaccante, R.G., Grieg, G.M., Willard, H.F., Ledbetter, D.H., Hejtmancik, J.F., *et al.* (1988). Uniparental disomy as a mechanism for human disease. *American Journal of Human Genetics*, **42**, 217–26.

Spofford, J.B. (1961). Parental control of position–effect variegation. II Effect of sex of parent contributing white-mottled rearrangement in *Drosophilia melanogaster*. *Genetics*, **46**, 1151–67.

Spotila, L.D., Sereda, L., and Prockop, D.J. (1992). Partial isodisomy for chromosome 7 and short stature in an individual with a mutation at the *COL1A2* locus. *American Journal of Human Genetics*, **51**, 1396–405.

Stallard, R., Krueger, S., James, R.S., and Schwartz, S. (1995). Uniparental isodisomy 13 in a normal female due to transmission of a maternal t(13q;13q). *American Journal of Medical Genetics*, **57**, 14–18.

Surani, M.A.H., Barton, S.C., and Kaufmann, M.H. (1977). Development to term of chimeras between diploid parthenogenetic and fertilized embryos. *Nature*, **270**, 601–3.

Surani, M.A.H., Barton, S.C., and Norris, L. (1984). Development of reconstituted mouse eggs suggests imprinting of the genome during gametogenesis. *Nature*, **308**, 548–50.

Surani, M.A., Barton, S.C., and Norris, M.L. (1986). Nuclear transplantation in the mouse: hereditable differences between parental genomes after activation of the embryonic genome. *Cell*, **45**, 127–36.

Surani, M.A.H., Barton, S.C., and Norris, L. (1986*b*). Nuclear transplantation in the mouse: heritable differences between parental genomes after embryonic activation of the embryonic genome. *Cell*, **45**, 127–36.

Surani, M.A.H., Kothary R., Allen, N.D., Singh, P.B., Fundele, R., Ferguson-Smith, A.C., and Barton, S.C. (1990). Genome imprinting and development in the mouse. *Development (Suppl.)*, **89**, 89–98.

Szulman, A.E. (1988). Trophoblastic disease: clinical pathology of hydatidiform mole. *Obstetrical and Gynecological Clinics of North America*, **15**, 443–56.

Szulman, A.E. (1995). Trophoblastic disease: pathology of complete and partial moles. In *Diseases of the fetus and newborn: pathology, genetics, imaging and management*, Vol. 1, (2nd edn), (ed. G.B. Reed, A.E. Claireaux, and F. Cockburn), pp. 187–99. Chapman and Hall, London.

Szulman, A.E. and Surti, U. (1978). The syndromes of hydatidiform moles. I. Cytogenetic and morphologic correlations. *American Journal of Obstetrics and Gynecology*, **132**, 665–71.

Szulman, A.E. and Surti, U. (1982). The clinicopathologic profile of the partial hydatidiform mole. *Obstetrics and Gynecology*, **59**, 597–602.

Szulman, A.E., Philippe, E., Boue, J.G., and Boue, A. (1981). Human triploidy: association with partial hydatidiform moles and non-molar conceptuses. *Human Pathology*, **12**, 1016–21.

Takagi, N. and Sasaki, M. (1975). Preferential inactivation of the paternally derived X chromosomein the extraembryonic membrane of the mouse. *Nature*, **256**, 640–1.

Taniguchi, T., Sullivan, M.J., Ogawa, O., and Reeve, A.E. (1995). Epigenetic changes encompassing the *IGF2/H19* locus associated with relaxation and silencing of *H19* in Wilms tumor. *Proceedings of the National Academy of Science, USA*, **92**, 2159–63.

Temple I.K., Cockwell, A., Hassold, T., Pettay, D., and Jacobs, P. (1991). Maternal uniparental disomy for chromosome 14. *Journal of Medical Genetics*, **28**, 511–14.

Thomson, J.A. and Solter, D. (1988). The developmental fate of androgenetic, partenogenetic, and gynogenetic cells in chimeric gastrulating mouse embryos. *Genes and Development*, **2**, 1344–51.

Van Gurp, R.J., Oosterhuis, J.W., Kalschever, V., Mariman, E.C., and Looijenga, L.H. (1994). Biallelic expression of the H19 and IGF2 genes in human testicular germ cell tumors. *Journal of the National Cancer Institute*, **86**, 1070–5.

Voss, R., Ben-Simon, E., Avita, A., Godfrey, S., Zlotogora, J., Dagan, J., *et al.* (1989). Isodisomy of chromosme 7 in a patient with cystic fibrosis: could uniparental disomy be common in humans? *American Journal of Human Genetics*, **45**, 373–80.

Walsh, C., Miller, S.J., Flam, F., Fisher, R.A., and Ohlsson, R. (1995). Paternally derived *H19* is differentially expressed in malignant and nonmalignant trophoblast. *Cancer Research*, **55**, 1111–16.

Wang, J.C., Passage, M.B., Yen P.H., Shapiro, L.J., and Mohandas, T.K. (1991). Uniparental heterodisomy for chromosome 14 in a phenotypically abnormal familial balanced 13/14 Robertsonian translocation carrier. *American Journal of Human Genetics*, **48**, 1069–74.

Warburton, D., Yu, C.-Y., Kline, J., and Stein, Z. (1978). Mosaic autosomal trisomy in cultures from spontaneous abortions. *American Journal of Human Genetics*, **30**, 609–17.

Wirtz, A., Gloning, K.P.H., and Murken, J. (1991). Trisomy 18 in chorionic villus sampling: problems and consequences. *Prenatal Diagnosis*, **11**, 563–7.

Wolstenholme, J. (1994). An audit of trisomy 16 in man. *Prenatal Diagnosis*, **15**, 109–21.

III | *Development of the embryo and early fetus*

Embryonal physiology

Eric Jauniaux and Beatrice Gulbis

INTRODUCTION

Embryonal physiology is treated only incidentally in embryology textbooks and has been overshadowed by the extraordinary profusion of anatomical descriptions of embryos and early fetuses. The developmental physiology of most embryonic organs remains largely unknown because of the limited access to these organs *in vivo* and *in vitro* for experimentation. The most prominent organs of the embryonic period of human pregnancy are the heart, the liver, the brain, the secondary yolk sac, and the placenta. The other organs and, in particular, endocrinological organs such as the thyroid gland or the pancreas are known to be only functional after 12 weeks of gestation. Up to mid-pregnancy the placenta and its membranes are larger than the fetus and, therefore, more accessible for research—it is thus not surprising that most of our knowledge on the physiology of the embryo and early fetus is essentially that of its adnexae which provide the habitat in which the embryo and its functions develop. For a more comprehensive view of the anatomy and potential roles of the human yolk sac, the reader is referred to Chapter 11. Rather than restricting the discussion to isolated findings on individual fetal organs which have been described elsewhere (Moscoso 1992), we present here the current knowledge on the developmental physiology of the materno-embryonic interface and the embryonic fluid compartments.

THE MATERNO-EMBRYONIC INTERFACE

Human placentation is theoretically haemochorial and mainly characterized by diffuse infiltration of the uterine endometrium and superficial myometrium by extra-villous trophoblastic cells (see Chapters 8 and 9). Up to 10 weeks of gestation, the chorionic sac surface is entirely covered by villous tissue (Fig. 13.1). From 8–9 weeks, the villi associated with the decidua capsularis degenerate forming an avascular shell known as the chorion laeve, or smooth chorion, whereas the villi associated with the decidua basalis proliferate forming the chorion frondosum or definitive placenta (Jauniaux *et al.* 1992*a*). At the time of gestation, the decidua capsularis and decidua parietalis fuse, obliterating completely the uterine cavity and inducing irreversible changes in gestational sac morphology and in its spacial relationship with the uterine environment (Jones and Jauniaux 1995).

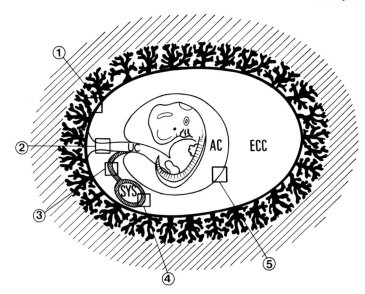

Fig. 13.1 Diagram of the first trimester gestational sac showing the possible route of transfer between fetal compartments. 1 = Chorionic plate; 2 = Umbilical cord (UC); 3 = Vitelline duct; 4 = Secondary yolk sac (SYS) wall; 5 = Amniotic membrane separating the amniotic cavity (AC) from the exo-coelomic cavity (ECC).

Development of materno-placental circulation

The new concept

Classically, immediately after implantation, a number of endometrial vessels are opened by the phagocytic activity of the extravillous trophoblastic cells and the maternal circulation starts in the intervillous space (Ramsey and Donner 1980). This theory has been challenged by the data presented by Hustin and Schaaps which show that during the first trimester of pregnancy, the intervillous space of the definitive placenta is separated from the uterine circulation by trophoblastic plugs obliterating the tip of the utero-placental arteries (Hustin and Schaaps 1987; Hustin *et al.* 1988). At the end of the first trimester, these plugs are progressively dislocated allowing maternal blood to flow freely and continuously in the intervillous space. This hypothesis is first based on *in vivo* findings which include the visualization of the intervillous space by hysteroscopy showing only a clear fluid (and transvaginal ultrasound imaging showing no or fewer moving echoes) inside the placenta during the first trimester. This concept was prompted by the fact that the investigators were surprised to find few chorion villous samples tinted by maternal blood before 12 weeks of gestation compared with later in pregnancy (Hustin and Schaaps 1987). In addition to these experiments, they were able to perfuse with barium sulphate hysterectomy specimens containing pregnancies at 8, 9, and 13 weeks of gestation. X-ray examination of the uteri and spacial reconstruction of the corresponding utero-placental vascular network (Fig. 13.2) shows clearly the presence of a continuous trophoblastic shell at

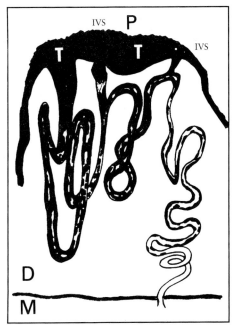

Fig. 13.2 Reconstruction of the course of a spiral artery through the placental bed based on seriel sections of a hysterectomy specimen containing a 9-week pregnancy. Average length irrespective of numerous coils varies between 0.5 and 0.7 mm. The trophoblast (T) forms a continuous shell between the spiral arteries and the intervillous space (IVS). The trophoblast also forms plugs which occlude the lumen of the spiral arteries. P = Placenta; D = Decidua; M = Myometrium (Modified from Hustin *et al.* 1988.)

the level of the uterine–intervillous interface and no direct entry of the medium into the intervillous space at eight and nine weeks (Hustin and Schaaps 1987).

Boyd and Hamilton (1970) and Ramsey and Donner (1980) had previously observed that spiral arteries contain plugs of trophoblastic cells that became loosely arranged as pregnancy developed. The findings of Boyd and Hamilton (1970), using India ink to perfuse their specimens, also suggested that the first trimester utero-placental interface, with its intravascular trophoblastic plugs, acts like a labyrinthine organ which filters maternal blood, leaving a slow but continuous seepage of plasma into the intervillous space. In the remarkable book by Ramsey and Donner (1980) which summarizes their findings of more than 20 years of studying the placental vasculature and circulation in Rhesus monkeys and humans, one can read some surprising statements regarding the utero-placental circulation. In particular, discussing the action of the trophoblast, they ask themselves at what stage full, effective utero-placental circulation is established in the human. Since they found that in human pregnancy, the intra-arterial trophoblast is present until about the 12th week and thereafter disappears, they assume that free circulation is not achieved until after that time. The concept of plugs of cytotrophoblast occluding the lumina of utero-placental arteries during the first trimester is still misunderstood by recent authors (Merce *et al.* 1996; Valentin *et al.* 1996). This is not surprising when one considers the rather poor methodology used by these authors to compare *in vivo* with *in vitro* findings (Valentine *et al.* 1996).

In vivo studies

Before the study by Hustin and Schaaps there had been a few other attempts to invest-igate the utero-placental circulation *in utero*, most of them only reported in proceedings of conferences. In 1967 Burchell injected contrast medium directly into the femoral artery of pregnant women to study the maternal arterial blood supply to the human pla-centa at various gestational ages. He recruited patients with pregnancies complicated by heavy vaginal bleeding or fetal death or patients requesting termination. In a few cases studied before 10 weeks of gestation and which were not complicated by bleeding, he noted that diffusion in the intervillous space occurs only at a few entry sites and for a very short time. No pregnancy between 12 and 20 weeks was studied.

The ability of Doppler ultrasound to detect flow velocity waveforms within the dif-ferent branches of the uterine and feto-placental circulations has enabled *in vivo* studies of large numbers of early pregnancies (Jauniaux *et al.* 1991*a*). Our initial studies were performed using the first available colour Doppler imaging equipment. At that time, a non-pulsatile flow corresponding to maternal intervillous blood flow could only be identified by colour mapping in the placenta of second trimester normal pregnancies (Jauniaux *et al.* 1991*a,b*, 1992*b*). Our findings were rapidly confirmed by independent authors, using similar equipment (Jaffe and Woods 1993; Coppens *et al.* 1996). However, the resolution and characteristics of our early ultrasound equipment may have been a limiting factor for the detection of slow flows. More recently, using new equipment with more sensitive ultrasound probes, we observed inside some areas of placenta between 10 and 12 weeks, intervillous blood flow patterns suggesting that a limited (slow and discontinuous) intervillous circulation may be present from around 10 weeks of gestation (Jauniaux 1996*a*). A recent longitudinal study of uterine blood flow has demonstrated that uterine artery blood flow volume and velo-city increase gradually until 10 weeks and rapidly thereafter (Dickey and Hower 1995). Overall, these finding indicate that in normal pregnancies the development of the intervillous circulation is a progressive phenomenon which is only fully estab-lished at the end of the first trimester (Jaffe *et al.* 1997). Very slow flows will prob-ably never be detected by Doppler ultrasound. By contrast, false positive intervillous signals can be generated by the placental area transforming into the chorion laeve. There is little doubt that the dislocation of two-thirds of the original placental ring may be a common source of intervillous flow signals. At the same time maternal vessels become closer to the gestational sac periphery and the signal obtained from uterine venous vessels may be misinterpreted as belonging to the intervillous circula-tion (Merce *et al.* 1996; Valentin *et al.* 1996). Individual anatomical variations such as the area inside the placenta containing less villous tissue or a thinner trophoblastic layer may result in focal premature entry of maternal blood into the intervillous space. This may explain some of the benign 'maternal lakes' commonly found during the second trimester (Jauniaux and Campbell 1990).

The impact of this new concept on early pregnancy physiology

The new concept challenges not only the classic anatomical doctrine but also questions our understanding of early pregnancy physiology. The first-trimester trophoblastic shell at the materno-embryonic interface may first serve to protect the early gestational sac from the forces of maternal arterial blood flow until the definitive placenta is formed and well implanted. Rodesch *et al.* (1992) measured placental and endometrial p_{O_2} levels and found that a significant increase in placental p_{O_2} occurred at 12–13 weeks' gestation. This was thought to be related to the full establishment of the intervillous circulation and can explain some of the metabolic and endocrinologic changes observed during this important transition period (Jauniaux *et al.* 1994a; Meuris *et al.* 1995). These findings and the fact that most of the mechanisms of defence against the deleterious effect of oxygen, such as superoxide dismutase enzymes, are absent or in small amounts in embryonic tissues (Umaoka *et al.* 1992) and in particular in trophoblastic tissue (Watson *et al.* 1997) suggest that the embryo develops in an environment lower in oxygen than the fetus. The results of a recent study by Genbacev *et al.* (1996) support this proposal and show that during early pregnancy, allocation of the trophoblast lineage, differentiation and invasion can occur in a relatively hypoxic environment.

Development of embryo–placental circulation

During the fourth gestational week, the primitive villi become branched and the mesenchymal cells within the villous mesoblastic core differentiate into blood capillaries, forming the primitive villous capillary network (Jauniaux *et al.* 1992a). Around 28 days post-ovulation (six completed menstrual weeks), the villous vasculature is connected with the primitive heart and the vascular plexus of the yolk sac via the vessels of connecting stalk (Boyd and Hamilton 1970). At this stage, the blood circulation is probably limited to the embryo and its secondary yolk sac. The number of fetal capillaries per villous profile and the proportion of the villi (volume fraction) occupied by the fetal capillaries increases progressively from the second month of pregnancy (Jauniaux *et al.* 1991c) thus increasing rapidly the mean radius of the villous vascular system. Cardiac organogenesis ends by the formation of the membranous portion of interventricular septum which is complete by 11 weeks of gestation (Moscoso 1992). Changes in fetal cardiac output seem to be directly related to fetal heart rate changes (Blackburn and Loper 1992). Due to the lack of autonomic control of the feto-placental circulation, locally produced factors play an important role in the maintenance of the low resistance of this vascular bed during the second half of pregnancy (Kingdom *et al.* 1994). Maternal factors such as thyroxine (T$_4$) or relaxin which can cross the first trimester placenta could have an influence on the regulation of embryonic heart rate and circulation (Johnson *et al.* 1994a,b).

Embryonic vascular haemodynamics can be investigated *in utero* as soon as the primitive heart starts to beat (see Chapter 19). The resistance to flow in the umbilical arteries is high during the first trimester and shows little variation until 11–12 weeks when end-diastolic flow (EDF) velocities start to appear. Between 12 and 14 weeks, the EDF develops rapidly but remains incomplete and/or inconsistently present. From

14 weeks onward, diastolic frequencies throughout the entire cardiac cycle are recorded in the umbilical artery of all normally developing fetuses (Jauniaux *et al.* 1991*a,b*; Coppens *et al.* 1996). After that period, the trend in the umbilical artery resistance to flow shows a gradual decrease until the end of the third trimester. End-diastolic velocities are present at the level of intracerebral arteries two weeks earlier than in the umbilical artery (Huisman *et al.* 1992). There is no correlation between umbilical artery Doppler indices and fetal heart rate in early pregnancy or fetal blood haematocrit and umbilical cord length later in pregnancy (Wright and Ridgway 1990; Huisman *et al.* 1992). The progressive increase in the number of villous vessels and their surface area must have a key role in the gradual fall in blood flow impedance in the umbilical circulation. We have hypothesized that the rapid increase in diastolic velocities in the umbilical arteries at the end of the first trimester is also related to the establishment of the intervillous circulation (Jauniaux *et al.* 1991*b*; 1992*b*). A change in the pressure gradient due to the expansion of the intervillous space and/or a modification of the local concentration of vasodilators could also influence relaxation of the small placental arteries.

EARLY PLACENTAL TRANSPORT PHYSIOLOGY

Materno-fetal exchanges occur between maternal plasma in the intervillous space and fetal plasma in the villous capillaries (Fig. 13.3). Placental transfers have been mainly studied in experimental animals such as guinea-pigs and monkeys because they have haemochorial placentas similar to those of humans (Burton 1992). In lower vertebrates, the yolk sac serves as the principal membrane for placental exchanges. In particular, rodents have a subsidiary yolk sac placenta which completely envelops the fetus throughout gestation and serves as the principal site for acquisition of protein by the fetus. Due to the complexity of the experimental situation in the intact animal and the considerable embryological differences between human and some animal species, the precise mechanism of transfer of many substances across the human placenta has not been elucidated. Transfer of protein across the human placenta has been studied *in vivo* by the injection of radiolabelled albumin or immunoglobin in the maternal circulation before delivery (Dancis *et al.* 1961; Gitlin *et al.* 1964). This type of investigation was subsequently abandoned because of the damage that radioactive substances can cause to the developing fetal organs. Materno-fetal transfer in humans has been more satisfactorily investigated *in vitro* by using isolated, dually perfused placentae (Sibley and Boyd 1992).

The recent possibility of obtaining pure fetal blood *in utero* by percutaneous blood sampling has allowed a better understanding of the materno-fetal metabolic exchanges in the second and third trimesters of pregnancy (Cetin *et al.* 1990). Due to technical limitations, similar studies are not feasible during the first trimester. However, the selective sampling of fluid from the exocoelomic cavity which separates the placental chorionic plate from the amniotic cavity between 5 and 12 weeks of gestation offers a novel approach to the study of transfer across the early human placenta (Jauniaux *et al.* 1991*d*). When the biochemistry of coelomic and amniotic fluids

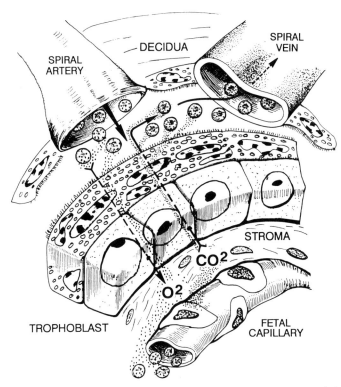

Fig. 13.3 Diagram showing the utero-placental and villous circulations and the trophoblastic barrier.

is compared it is found that they differ in relative composition. In particular, their protein pattern varies widely (Table 13.1) suggesting that they have a different origin. Overall these studies indicate that coelomic fluid contains numerous specific trophoblastic proteins and that the exocoelomic cavity is to be considered as the physiologic liquid extension of the placental villous mesenchyme (Gulbis *et al.* 1992; Jauniaux *et al.* 1994*a*, 1996*b*).

Proteins

The trophoblastic villous membrane of the definitive human placenta has been identified as a highly selective route for plasma protein transport from mother to fetus (Sibley and Boyd 1992). Furthermore, the trophoblast produces a variety of specific proteins such as human chorionic gonadotrophin (hCG), human placental lactogen (hPL), or pregnancy-associated protein A which are excreted in both the maternal and embryonic compartments (Jauniaux *et al.* 1993; Iles *et al.* 1994). The endodermal layer of the secondary yolk sac has also all the features of an absorptive and secretory tissue (Jones and Jauniaux 1995) and is known to synthesize several serum proteins in

Table 13.1 Comparison of total and individual protein mean concentration in embryonic fluids between 7 and 11 weeks of gestation

Protein	Coelomic fluid	Amniotic fluid
Total protein (g/l)	3.5	0.07
AFP (g/l)	19.63	24.29
Albumin (g/l)	1.7	ND
Pre-albumin (g/l)	0.04	ND
Transferrin (g/l)	0.22	ND
IgG (mg/dl)	32	ND
Creatinine (μmol/l)	43.6	27.7
Erythropoietin (mU/ml)*	15.5	5
IL-6 (pg/ml)	72.5	13.6
hCG (mIU/ml)	165 607	1752
hCG/α (mIU/ml)	12 534	241
hCG/βb (mIU/ml)	1395	24
Oestradiol (pg/ml)	8372	1993
Oestriol (pmol/ml)[+]	2.6	< 1.2
hPL (ng/ml)[+]	80	30
PP14 (μg/l)[+]	4416	77
Prolactin (U/ml)[+]	371	40

ND = not detectable. * from Campbell *et al.* 1992; [+] from Iles *et al.* 1994.

common with the fetal liver such alpha-fetoprotein (AFP), α1 antitrypsin, albumin, pre-albumin, and transferrin (Gitlin and Perricelli 1970; Shi *et al.* 1985). With rare exceptions, the synthesis of most of these proteins is confined to embryonic compartments and the contribution of the yolk sac to the protein pool of the mother is limited.

Albumin, Pre-albumin, and AFP

These large proteins are essential proteins initially produced inside the gestational sac by the secondary yolk sac until the embryonic liver has matured sufficiently to carry out this function (Table 13.2). Between 6 and 12 weeks of gestation, the mean level of total protein is 18 times lower in the coelomic fluid than in maternal serum (Table 13.3) and 54 times higher in the coelomic cavity than in the amniotic cavity (Table 13.1). The physiologic decrease in total maternal serum protein which occurs mainly in the first three months of gestation ranges from 10 to 14 per cent of non-pregnant values (Blackburn and Loper 1992) and is not related to similar changes in the embryonic fluids. During the first trimester, albumin concentration in maternal serum demonstrates a relative decrease due to increased maternal blood volume and haemodilution, while globulin and fibrinogen concentrations demonstrate both absolute and relative increases. During the same period, the levels of total protein and pre-albumin increase in coelomic fluid, whereas the levels of albumin do not varie significantly (Table 13.3). There is no difference in fetal size, yolk sac volume, and the

Table 13.2 Tissue sources of embryonic and fetal proteins

Protein	Molecular weight (Daltons)	Tissue source
AFP	69 000	SYS/fetal liver/gut
Albumin	66 000	SYS/fetal liver/maternal?
Pre-albumin	54 000	SYS/fetal liver/maternal?
Creatinine	116	Maternal/fetal (> 11 weeks)
Transferrin	77 000	SYS/fetal liver/maternal
IgG	160 000	Maternal/fetal blood (> 12 weeks)
Thyroxine (T_4)	777	Maternal/fetal thyroid (> 12 weeks)
IL-6	20 000	Decidua > placenta
hCG	36 000	Placenta

SYS = Secondary yolk sac

Table 13.3 Comparison of total and individual protein mean concentration in coelomic fluid, fetal blood, and first trimester maternal serum

Protein	Maternal serum ($n = 35$)	Coelomic fluid			Fetal serum 13–14 wks ($n = 5$)[*]
		6–7 wks ($n = 18$)	8–9 wks ($n = 24$)	10–12 wks ($n = 15$)	
Total (g/L)	70	3.3	3.7	4.2	35.1
AFP (g/L)	0.002	22.2	20.6	18.0	4.1
Albumin (g/L)	45	1.6	2.1	2.1	16.6
Pre-albumin (g/L)	1.3	0.03	0.04	0.05	0.18
Transferrin (g/L)	2:5	0.16	0.19	0.28	1.02
IgG (mg/dL)	907	18.2	34.8	47.3	N/A
IgA (mg/dL)	122	0.72	1.09	1.54	N/A
Creatinine (μmol/L)	49.2	44.3	45.0	42.7	N/A
hCG (mIU/mL)	98 456	149 734	115 199	108 981	N/A

N/A = not available. [*] From Fryer et al., 1993.

level of protein in the coelomic fluid between mothers with low serum pre-albumin levels and mothers with high serum pre-albumin levels (Jauniaux et al. 1994b). These results suggest that the total protein concentration in the coelomic fluid is not influenced by changes in maternal serum protein levels during the first trimester. The increase of most proteins' concentration observed in the exocoelomic cavity during the first trimester can be explained by the slow turnover of the coelomic fluid and/or the increased production of these proteins by fetal organs.

During the first trimester of pregnancy, AFP is produced by the secondary yolk sac up to 10 weeks of gestation and by the embryonic liver from six weeks until delivery (Gitlin and Perricelli 1970). AFP has a high molecular weight (Table 13.2) and the mean AFP concentration is about 10 000 higher in embryonic fluid than in maternal serum (Jauniaux *et al.* 1993). The presence on the external surface of the secondary yolk sac of mesothelial cells showing a well developed microvillous border, numerous pinocytic vesicles within their cytoplasm, and a canalicular system at the cell interface implies that these cells have a very active absorptive function (Jones and Jauniaux 1995). Analysis of concanavalin A affinity molecular variants of AFP have demonstrated that both coelomic and amniotic fluid AFP molecules are mainly of yolk sac origin whereas maternal serum AFP molecules are mainly of fetal liver origin (Fig. 13.4). These results show that the human secondary yolk sac has also an excretory function and secretes AFP into the embryonic and extraembryonic compartments. In contrast, AFP molecules of fetal liver origin are probably transferred from the embryonic circulation to the maternal circulation, mainly across the placental villous membrane.

hCG, oestradiol, and progesterone

Higher hCG, oestrodiol, and progesterone levels in the exocoelomic fluid compared to maternal serum can be explained by the close anatomical relationship existing between the exocoelomic cavity and the trophoblast, as these structures are only separated by the loose mesenchymal tissue of the chorionic placental plate (Jauniaux *et al.* 1995*a*; Jones and Jauniaux 1995). Similar features have been observed for placental protein 14 and human placental lactogen (Wathen *et al.* 1992), which are produced by the placenta only. So far the only exception is PAPP-A which is found in a higher concentration in the maternal serum than in coelomic fluid (Iles *et al.* 1994).

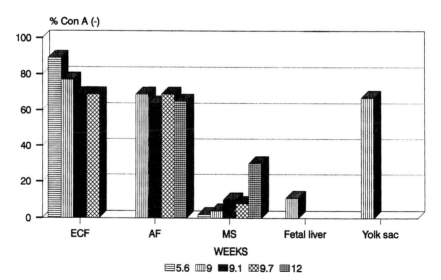

Fig. 13.4 Percentage of concanavalin A non-reactive AFP (% Con A (–)) found in samples of coelomic fluid (ECF), amniotic fluid (AF), maternal serum (MS), fetal liver, and yolk sac collected during the first trimester. (From Jauniaux *et al.* 1993.)

Free hCGα and free hCGβ levels are respectively 185 and 33 times higher in the coelomic fluid of normal pregnancy than in the corresponding maternal serum samples. This finding supports the hypothesis that, in the first trimester, there is an excess of α over β subunit secretion by the villous trophoblast (Nagy *et al.* 1994) and suggests that the hCG clearance rate is slower in the coelomic cavity than in maternal circulation. It is likely that maternal serum hCG levels are influenced by both villous and extravillous trophoblastic synthesis, whereas the coelomic cavity, being completely surrounded by villous tissue, causes coelomic hCG levels to be influenced only by villous trophoblastic secretion.

In contrast to maternal serum, coelomic levels of intact hCG and free hCGα decrease progressively between 8 and 12 weeks of gestation and free hCGβ levels do not vary (Jauniaux *et al.* 1995a). Oestradiol and progesterone concentrations also decrease in coelomic fluid between the second and third months of gestation whereas these levels vary in an opposite manner in maternal serum. These changes in coelomic hormonal concentration are probably secondary to a decrease in the exchange surface as two-thirds of the primitive placental ring start to degenerate during the third month of gestation (Jauniaux *et al.* 1993). The decrease in intact hCG and free hCG coelomic levels with advancing gestation may also be secondary to a simultaneous decline in the number of differentiating cytotrophoblastic cells and/or to the disappearance of two-thirds of the original placental tissue occurring during the same period.

Thyroxine (T_4) and immunoglobulins (Ig)

Thyroid hormones are theoretically not synthesized by embryonic tissue during the first trimester of pregnancy (Table 13.2). These proteins are found in low concentration in the exocoelomic cavity and this must be the result of materno-embryonic transfer.

Although synthesis of thyroid hormones by the fetal thyroid may begin between the 10th and 12th weeks of gestation, their secretion *in vivo* is believed to start after the development of the median eminence portal system which occurs at mid-gestation (18–22 weeks), when there is a generalized maturation of anterior pituitary secretory cells (Contempre *et al.* 1993). Therefore, there is little doubt that the fetal thyroid is not yet functioning during the first trimester and that the iodothyronines found in the embryonic cavities are of maternal origin. Notable concentrations of thyroxine (or tetraiodothyronine, T_4) and reverse T_3 (triiodothyronine) have been found in coelomic fluid samples suggesting that maternal thyroid hormones are potentially available to the embryo as early as five weeks of gestation (Contempre *et al.* 1993). T_4 molecules found in the exocoelomic cavity could be bound to pre-albumin or transthyretin (TTR) also present in representative amounts in the coelomic fluid (Table 13.1). T_4 transfer to the embryo could be facilitated by TTR secreted by the yolk sac epithelium preferentially towards the embryo (Jauniaux *et al.* 1994a). TTR is also synthesized very early by the choroid plexus (Jacobsson 1989) suggesting that the thyroid hormones detected in the exocoelomic cavity may also reach the embryonic brain.

IgG molecules are selectively transferred across the villous tissue thus contributing to fetal passive immunity in the second half of pregnancy. *In vitro* experiments have shown that the transport of intact proteins through the trophoblastic layer involves pinocytosis and endocytosis and probably exocytosis to allow expulsion of the protein into the fetal circulation (Sibley and Boyd 1992). The only proteins transported in notable quantities are immunoglobins of the IgG class and retinol-binding proteins. However, *in vitro* studies have also indicated that IgA can cross the placental barrier in small quantities (Gitlin and Biasucci 1969). Trace levels of IgG and IgM have been found in cultures of human fetal liver and spleen only from the end of the third trimester (Gitlin and Biasucci 1969). IgA synthesis has not been demonstrated *in vitro* until after 30 weeks of gestation and only very low levels of IgG and IgM have been detected in the plasma of 12–14 week fetuses (Gitlin 1984). IgG and IgM levels rise during the second half of pregnancy to be equivalent to maternal levels by 26 weeks for IgG and after birth for IgM (Gitlin and Biasucci 1969; Gitlin 1984). Levels of IgG, including specific IgG against *Toxoplasma gondii*, cytomegalovirus, and rubella virus and levels of IgA are measurable in coelomic fluid samples collected between 6 and 12 weeks of gestation whereas IgM is not (Jauniaux *et al.* 1995b). This suggests that the placental transfer of IgG and IgA starts very early in pregnancy, probably when the first placental villi are formed. IgG and IgA molecules in coelomic fluid could play a role in the initial antigenic challenge of blood cell precursors to early congenital infection and in limiting the potentially devastating effects of congenital infections.

Iron storage proteins

In primates, including humans, the greatest source of iron transferable to the fetus is maternal transferrin and the amount of iron needed by the fetal tissues is an obligatory requirement that is met regardless of maternal iron stores. Iron is known to pass rapidly through the placental barrier, against a concentration gradient from mother to fetus, but the mechanisms by which iron is transferred accross the human trophoblast are a little uncertain (Sibley and Boyd 1992). If transferrin molecules may traverse the placenta in very small amounts and very slowly, *in vitro* experiments have demonstrated that most maternal iron is released into the intervillous space and rapidly taken up by transferrin receptors located on the surface of the syncytiotrophoblast. Cellular iron is probably transported in an uncharacterized low molecular weight form to iron storage granules in the syncytiotrophoblast or to ferritin (Sibley and Boyd 1992) and is released into the fetal circulation to be bound to transferrin. The rate of iron transfer across the placenta increases with fetal growth and has been related to the development of its haematopoiesis (Bentley 1985). Investigations of fetal cord blood obtained *in utero* and at delivery have shown that in the second half of human pregnancies, iron and transferrin are in lower concentration and ferritin is in higher concentration in fetal blood than in maternal blood (Carpani *et al.* 1992; Fryer *et al.* 1993). In the first trimester the distribution of iron and iron-binding proteins between the maternal and exocoelomic compartments is comparable (Gulbis *et al.* 1994) suggesting that the iron transfer mechanisms are functional soon after implantation. Very high levels of ferritin in the coelomic fluid demonstrate that the exocoelomic cavity is an important iron reservoir in early pregnancy for yolk sac haematopoiesis and the numerous enzymatic activities of the developing embryo.

Amino acids (AA)

In vitro studies have shown that the transplacental transport of most AA in the materno-fetal direction occurs mainly via an active mechanism of the pump/leak type (Sibley and Boyd 1992). The active step is located at the level of the microvillous membrane of the syncytiotrophoblast and generates a higher concentration of AA in the placental tissue than in either maternal or fetal plasma. Energy is required to transport AA in the trophoblast followed by a passive leak down the concentration gradient to fetal plasma (Sibley and Boyd 1992), resulting in higher concentrations of most AA in fetal than in maternal plasma. In early pregnancy the total molar AA concentration is also higher in the coelomic fluid than in maternal serum (Jauniaux *et al.* 1994*c*). The levels of 12 out of 18 individual AA measured are more than twice as high in the coelomic fluid than in maternal serum and only two are present with similar levels in both compartments (Fig. 13.5). The total molar amino acid concentration in both maternal venous blood and coelomic fluid decreases between 7 and 12 weeks gestation (Jauniaux *et al.* 1994*c*). The analysis of the variation of individual amino acid concentrations during that period has demonstrated that only methionine decreases with advancing gestation in maternal blood whereas the concentration of 8 out of 18 amino acids measured decrease in the coelomic fluid. This decrease may reflect changes in the exchange surface between the placenta and the exocoelomic cavity when two-thirds of the placental mass degenerate to form the chorion laeve at

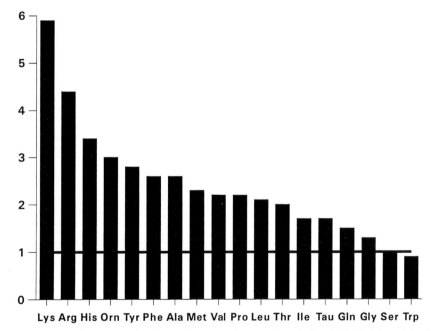

Fig. 13.5 Ratios of mean coelomic and maternal serum levels for 18 individual AA. (From Jauniaux *et al.* 1994*b*).

the end of the first trimester (Jauniaux *et al.* 1992*a*) and/or the increased use of these AA by the fetal tissues with advancing gestation.

Acid–base balance and oxygen levels

As a consequence of respiratory alkalosis of pregnancy, maternal renal excretion of bicarbonate secondarily increases and the overall maternal blood pH remains relatively unchanged (Blackburn and Loper 1992). Except for the total protein and lactate levels, there is no significant variation in the biochemical composition of the coelomic fluid between 7 and 11 weeks of gestation and no correlation for the different variables between coelomic fluid and maternal serum, suggesting that the coelomic fluid's acid–base regulation is not directly influenced by maternal physiological changes. During that period, the coelomic fluid has a lower pH, base excess, and bicarbonate level than maternal venous blood and has higher levels of p_{CO_2}, lactate, and phosphate and lower levels of protein than the maternal serum. These findings are consistent with a metabolic anaerobic acidosis status which is mainly due to the accumulation of acid biological products of the placental metabolism in the exocoelomic cavity (Jauniaux *et al.* 1994*a*).

Transport across the placenta is known to increase during the course of gestation due to a decrease in thickness of the villous barrier and a simultaneous increase of maternal and fetal placental blood flow (Blackburn and Loper 1992). According to Hustin's hypothesis, the villi of the first trimester placenta are only bathed by a clear fluid probably made of filtered maternal plasma and uterine gland secretions and not by a true and continous maternal blood circulation (Hustin 1995). Furthermore, if the villous barrier thickness and trophoblastic layer thickness of branching villi demonstrate an important decrease during the first half of pregnancy, these anatomical changes take place mainly after 10 weeks (Jauniaux *et al.* 1991*c*). These findings suggest that materno-embryonic gaseous exchanges are regulated differently from those of the fetal period. Using polarographic electrodes, inserted *in vivo* in different parts of the gestational sac, we found that between 8 and 10 weeks of gestation, placental p_{O_2} levels are notably lower than those of the endometrium (Rodesch *et al.* 1992). Placental p_{O_2} levels only become similar to those of the endometrial p_{O_2} after 12 weeks (Fig. 13.6). These results and the fact that neither the copper/zinc nor manganese forms of superoxide dismutase are present in detectable quantities within the syncytiotrphoblast of 8 and 9 week placental tissues and only in certain areas of 10–12 week tissue (Watson *et al.* 1996) support the proposal that the first trimester of gestation occurs under a low oxygen tension.

FORMATION OF THE AMNIOTIC FLUID

The amniotic cavity develops during the third week of pregnancy from the inner cell mass of the implanted blastocyst and grows inside the exocoelomic cavity, fusing with the placental chorionic plate at the end of the first trimester (Jones and Jauniaux 1995). Until recently, the amniotic fluid was the only relatively accessible fetal milieu

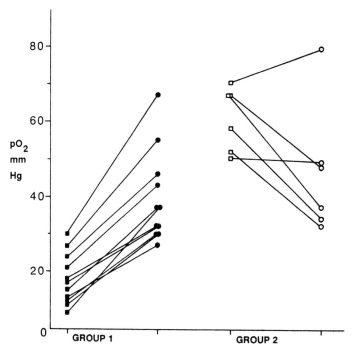

Fig. 13.6 Individual pO_2 values within the placenta (solid and open squares) and at the level of the decidua (solid and open circles) at 8–10 weeks (group 1) and at 12–13 weeks (group 2). (Modified from Rodesch *et al*. 1992.)

in early pregnancy. Amniotic fluid analyses have been performed from the third month of gestation onwards and have demonstrated important variations in gas tension, acid–base status, and biochemical composition with gestational age and differences compared with maternal blood (Lind 1978). The biochemistry of the amniotic fluid has been occasionally investigated in the first trimester (Sinha and Carlton 1970) but the changes occurring with advancing gestation were never evaluated at the time of the shift from the embryonic to the fetal period. Due to technical difficulties in recognizing accurately the different anatomical structures of the early gestational sac *in utero*, it is likely that some of the rare samples obtained in these studies before 12 weeks of gestation were a mixture of coelomic and amniotic fluids.

Early amniotic fluid composition

During the second and third trimesters, the pool of amniotic fluid is subject to a constant turnover, being added to by fetal lung fluid and urine and being removed by fetal swallowing (MacCarthy and Saunders 1978). When the definitive placenta has formed, movements of water and electrolyte also take place across the free placental membranes. During the first trimester, the amniotic membrane floats freely between the embryonic cavities. Despite its apparent simplicity (Jones and Jauniaux

1995), direct transfer from the exocoelomic to the amniotic cavity via the amniotic membrane is limited and the amniotic fluid contains very low levels of proteins (Gulbis *et al.* 1992; Jauniaux *et al.* 1993). The total amniotic fluid protein concentration is respectively 50 and 900 times lower than in coelomic fluid and maternal serum (Tables 13.1 and 13.3). Almost all individual proteins, except AFP, are in very low concentration in the amniotic fluid. The vitelline duct has the same cellular constitution as the secondary yolk sac (Jones and Jauniaux 1995) and AFP and other yolk sac proteins found in the early amniotic fluid could be excreted at the level where the duct fuses with the primitive umbilical cord. Yolk sac AFP could also be shifted in the amniotic fluid via the vitelline duct and the embryonic gut when the anal membranes break down around 10 weeks post-menstruation (Boyd and Hamilton 1970).

The amniotic fluid collected before 11 weeks of gestation has a higher pH and base excess, higher levels of lactate and bicarbonate, and lower levels of total protein, phosphate, chloride, sodium, and potassium than the coelomic fluid collected during the same period of gestation (Jauniaux *et al.* 1994c). Of these biological parameters, only the pH and the bicarbonate levels varied between 7 and 11 weeks of gestation. The metabolic alkalosis of the amniotic fluid observed in the first trimester probably arises from the accumulation of bicarbonate and the increased consumption of organic anions such as lactate by the embryonic tissue. The embryonic skin, which becomes keratinized only during the second trimester, is probably the major source of amniotic fluid in early pregnancy (MacCarthy and Saunders 1978). These results indicate that in contrast to the coelomic fluid composition which is mainly influenced by placental and yolk sac by-products, the first trimester amniotic fluid composition is mainly influenced by fetal bioproducts which may diffuse through the fetal skin or through the oropharyngeal and cloacal membranes (Jauniaux *et al.* 1994c; Gulbis *et al.* 1996). The latter two rupture around the end of the 5th and 7th weeks of gestation, respectively, allowing free circulation between fetal digestive and respiratory tracts and the amniotic cavity (O'Rahilly and Muller 1992).

Switch of the mesonephros to the metanephros

It is clear that fetal urine is a major source of amniotic fluid in the latter half of pregnancy. The amniotic fluid's electrolyte composition, protein patterns, and acid–base balance change rapidly at the end of the first trimester (Gulbis *et al.* 1992, 1996; Jauniaux *et al.* 1993, 1994c). Various mechanisms must also be considered to explain these changes and, in particular, the metabolic activity of the definitive kidneys, the lungs, and the digestive tract. The development of nephrons starts around the beginning of the third month of gestation and theoretically, the metanephros or definitive kidney produces urine from 10 weeks onwards (O'Rahilly and Muller 1992). Around 11 weeks, we have observed an abrupt increase in β2-microglobulin and τ-glutamyl transferase (τGT) amniotic fluid concentrations (Fig. 13.7) and we suggest that it reflects the maturation of the fetal renal glomerular function (Gulbis *et al.* 1996). In particular, the β2-microglobulin level found in the amniotic cavity during the second trimester is linked with the establishment of glomerular filtration in the definitive fetal

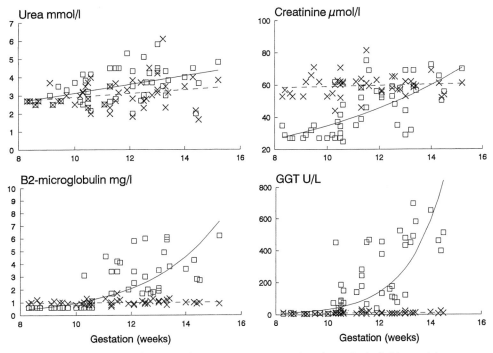

Fig. 13.7 Comparison of maternal serum (open squares) and amniotic fluid asterisks concentrations of urea, creatinine, τGT and β2-microglobulin between 9 and 16 weeks of gestation. (Modified from Gulbis *et al.* 1996.)

kidneys at a time when tubular function is still immature. The amniotic fluid β2-microglobulin level decreases during the third trimester as a consequence of the increasing reabsorption capacity of the proximal tubular cells. τGT is the only molecule that we have found in higher concentration in the amniotic fluid compared to both coelomic fluid and maternal serum. The very low activity of this enzyme in the coelomic fluid suggests that the placental villi are not a main source for this enzyme. τGT activity in the early amniotic fluid is not a specific marker of kidney maturation as it can also be influenced by enzymes released from the cellular debris by other organs such as fetal digestive and respiratory tracts and by the amniotic membrane.

The changes observed in the amniotic fluid composition at the end of the first trimester are also characterized by a decrease of pH, base excess, and bicarbonate level and an increase in p_{CO_2} and chloride levels (Table 13.4). It is of interest that except for the total protein level, which remained lower, the mean value of the other amniotic biological parameters obtained after 11 weeks of gestation became similar to those found in the coelomic fluid before 11 weeks (Tables 13.1 and 13.4). These changes continue during the second and third trimesters (Sinha and Carlton 1970) and probably reflect the increasing contribution of the different fetal organs to the amniotic fluid composition.

Table 13.4 Comparison of the mean value (± SD) of the different biochemical variables obtained in amniotic fluid between 7–10 weeks and 11–13 weeks of gestation (from Jauniaux *et al.* 1994*a*)

Variables	7–10 weeks ($n = 23$)	11–14 weeks ($n = 24$)	Rank test p value
pH	7.45 ± 0.06	7.23 ± 0.09	< 0.0001
pCO$_2$ (mmHg)	50 ± 7	55 ± 10	< 0.05
Base excess (mmol/l)	12.4 ± 3.8	−5.1 ± 6.2	< 0.0001
Glucose (mmol/l)	2.7 ± 0.6	2.8 ± 0.5	NS
Lactate (mmol/l)	1.0 ± 0.2	0.9 ± 0.4	NS
Bicarbonate (mmol/l)	39 ± 5.6	21.1 ± 5.6	< 0.0001
Protein (g/l)	0.05 ± 0.04	0.36 ± 0.4	< 0.0001
Chloride (mmol/l)	90 ± 9.3	102 ± 8.2	< 0.0001
Potassium (mmol/l)	3.6 ± 0.5	3.6 ± 0.6	NS
Sodium (mmol/l)	129 ± 14	131 ± 8	NS

p = statistical significance; NS = non-significant.

REFERENCES

Bentley, D.P. (1985). Iron metabolism and anaemia in pregnancy. *Clinical Haematology*, **14**, 613–19.

Blackburn, S.T. and Loper, D.L. (1992). *Maternal, fetal and neonatal physiology: a clinical perspective*. Saunders, Philadelphia.

Boyd, J.D. and Hamilton, W.J. (1970). *The human placenta*. Heffer, Cambridge.

Burchell, R.C. (1967). Arterial blood flow into the human intervillous space. *American Journal of Obstetrics and Gynecology*, **98**, 303–11.

Burton, G.J. (1992). Human and animal models: limitations and comparisons. In *The first twelve weeks of gestation*, (ed. E. Barnea, J. Hustin, and E. Jauniaux), pp. 469–85. Springer, Heidelberg.

Campbell, J., Wathen, N., Lewis, M., Fingerova, H., and Chard, T. (1992). Erythropoietin levels in amniotic fluid and extraembryonic coelomic fluid in the first trimester of pregnancy. *British Journal of Obstetrics and Gynaecology*, **9**, 974–6.

Carpani, G., Marini, F., Ghisoni, L., Buscaglia, M., Sinigaglia, E., and Moroni, G. (1992). Red cell and plasma ferritin in a group of normal fetuses at different ages of gestation. *European Journal of Haematology*, **49**, 260–2.

Cetin, I., Corbetta, C., Serini, L., Marconi, A., Bozzetti, P., Pardi, G., and Battaglia F.C. (1990). Umbilical amnio acid concentrations in normal and growth retardated fetuses sampled *in utero* by cordocentesis. *American Journal of Obstetrics and Gynecology*, **162**, 253–61.

Contempre, B., Jauniaux, E., Calvo, R., Jurkovic, D., Campbell, S., and Morreale de Escobar, G. (1993). Detection of thyroid hormones in human embryonic cavities during the first trimester of pregnancy. *Journal of Clinical Endocrinology and Metabolism*, **77**, 1719–22.

Coppens, M., Loquet, P., Kollen, M., De Neubourg, F., and Buytaert, P. (1996). Longitudinal evaluation of uteroplacental and umbilical blood flow changes in normal early pregnancy. *Ultrasound in Obstetrics and Gynecology*, **7**, 114–21.

Dancis, J., Lind, J., Oratz, M., Smolens, J., and Vara, P. (1961). Placental transfer of proteins in human gestation. *American Journal of Obstetrics and Gynecology*, **82**, 167–71.

Dickey, R.P. and Hower, J.F. (1995). Ultrasonographic features of uterine blood flow during the first 16 weeks of pregnancy. *Human Reproduction*, **10**, 2448–52.

Fryer, A.A., Jones, P., Strange, R., Hume, R., and Bell, J.E. (1993). Plasma protein levels in normal human fetuses: 13 to 41 weeks' gestation. *British Journal of Obstetrics and Gynaecology*, **100**, 850–5.

Genbacev, O., Joslin, R., Damsky, C.H., Polliotti, B.M., and Fisher, S.J. (1996). Hypoxia alters early gestation human cytotrophoblast differenciation/invasion *in vitro* and models the placental defects that occur in preeclampsia. *Journal of Clinical Investigation*, **97**, 540–50.

Gitilin, D. (1984). Protein transport across the placenta and protein turnover between amniotic fluid, maternal and fetal circulation. In *The placenta*, (ed. K.S. Moghissi and E.S.E. Hafez), pp. 151–72. Charles C. Thomas, Springfield.

Gitlin, D. and Biasucci, A. (1969). Development of IgG, IgA, IgM, β1C/β1a, C'1 esterase inhibitor, ceruloplasmin, haptoglobin, fibrinogen, plasminogen, α1-antitrypsin, orosomucoid, β-lipoprotein, α2-macroglobulin and prealbumin in the human conceptus. *Journal of Clinical Investigation*, **48**, 1433–46.

Gitlin, D. and Perricelli, A. (1970). Synthesis of serum albumin, prealbumin, alphafetoprotein, alphal-antitrypsin and transferrin by the human yolk sac. *Nature*, **228**, 995–7.

Gitlin, D., Kumate, J., Urrusti, J., and Morales, C. (1964). The selectivity of the human placenta in the transfer of plasma proteins from mother to fetus. *Journal of Clinical Investigation*, **10**, 1938–51.

Gulbis, B., Jauniaux, E., Jurkovic, D., Thiry, P., Campbell, S., and Ooms, H.A. (1992). Determination of protein pattern in embryonic cavities of early human pregnancies: a model to understand materno-embryonic exchanges. *Human Reproduction*, **7**, 886–9.

Gulbis, B., Jauniaux, E., Decuyper, J., Thiry, P., Jurkovic, D., and Campbell, S. (1994). Distribution of iron and iron-binding proteins in first trimester human pregnancies. *Obstetrics and Gynecology*, **84**, 289–93.

Gulbis, B., Jauniaux, E., Gervy, C., Jurkovic, D., Campbell, S., and Ooms, H.A. (1996). Biochemical investigation of kidney functional maturation in early human pregnancy. *Pediatric Research*, **39**, 1–5.

Huisman, T.W.A., Stewart, P.A., and Wladimiroff, J.W. (1992). Doppler assessment of normal early fetal circulation. *Ultrasound in Obstetrics and Gynecology*, **2**, 300–5.

Hustin, J. and Schaaps, J.P. (1987). Echographic and anatomic studies of the maternotrophoblastic border during the first trimester of pregnancy. *American Journal of Obstetrics and Gynecology*, **157**, 162–8.

Hustin, J., Schaaps, J.P., and Lambotte, R. (1988). Anatomical studies of the utero-placental vascularization in the first trimester of pregnancy. *Trophoblast Research*, **3**, 49–60.

Hustin, J. (1995). Vascular physiology and pathophysiology of early pregnancy. In *Transvaginal colour Doppler*, (ed. T. Bourne, E. Jauniaux, and D. Jurkovic), pp. 47–56. Springer, Heidelberg.

Iles, R.K., Wathen, N.C., Sharma, K.B., Campbell, J., Gruzinskas, J.G., and Chard, T. (1994). Pregnancy-associated plasma protein A levels in maternal serum, extraembryonic coelomic and amniotic fluids in the first trimester. *Placenta*, **15**, 693–9.

Jacobsson, B. (1989). Localisation of transthyretin-mRNA and immunoreactive transthyretin in the human fetus. *Virchows Archivs A. Pathologie, Anatomie*, **415**, 259–63.

Jaffe, R. and Woods, J.R. (1993). Color Doppler imaging and *in vivo* assessment of the anatomy and physiology of the early uteroplacental circulation. *Fertility and Sterility*, **60**, 293–7.

Jaffe, R., Jauniaux, E. and Hustin, J. (1997). Maternal circulation in the first trimester human placenta: Myth or reality. *American Journal of Obstetrics and Gynecology*, **176**, 695–705.

Jauniaux, E. and Campbell, S. (1990). Sonographic assessment of placental abnormalities. *American Journal of Obstetrics and Gynecology*, **163**, 1650–8.

Jauniaux, E., Jurkovic, D., Campbell, S., Kurjak, A., and Hustin, J. (1991*a*). Investigation of placental circulations by color Doppler ultrasound. *American Journal of Obstetrics and Gynecology*, **164**, 486–8.

Jauniaux, E., Jurkovic, D., and Campbell, S. (1991*b*). *In vivo* investigations of anatomy and physiology of early human placental circulations. *Ultrasound in Obstetrics and Gynecology*, **1**, 435–45.

Jauniaux, E., Burton, G.J., Moscoso, G.J., and Hustin, J. (1991*c*). Development of the early human placenta: a morphometric study. *Placenta*, **12**, 269–76.

Jauniaux, E., Jurkovic, D., Gulbis, B., Gervy, C., Ooms, H.A., and Campbell, S. (1991*d*). Biochemical composition of coelomic fluid in early human pregnancy. *Obstetrics and Gynecology*, **78**, 1124–8.

Jauniaux, E., Burton, G.J., and Jones, C.P.J. (1992*a*). Early human placental morphology. In *The first twelve weeks of gestation*, (ed. E. Barnea, J. Hustin, and E Jauniaux), pp. 45–64. Springer, Heidelberg.

Jauniaux, E., Jurkovic, D., Campbell, S., and Hustin, J. (1992*b*). Doppler ultrasound features of the developing placental circulations: correlation with anatomic findings. *American Journal of Obstetrics and Gynecology*, **166**, 585–7.

Jauniaux, E., Gulbis, B., Jurkovic, D., Schaaps, J.P., Campbell, S., and Meuris, S. (1993). Protein and steroid levels in embryonic cavities of early human pregnancy. *Human Reproduction*, **8**, 782–7.

Jauniaux, E., Jurkovic, D., Gulbis, B., Collin, W.P., Zaidi, J., and Campbell, S. (1994*a*). Investigation of the acid–base balance of coelomic and amniotic fluids in early human pregnancy. *American Journal of Obstetrics and Gynecology*, **170**, 1359–65.

Jauniaux, E., Gulbis, B., Jurkovic, D., Campbell, S., Collins, W.P., and Ooms, H.A. (1994*b*). Relationship between protein levels in embryological fluids and maternal serum and yolk sac size during early human pregnancy. *Human Reproduction*, **9**, 161–6.

Jauniaux, E., Sherwood, R., Jurkovic, D., Boa, A., and Campbell, S. (1994*c*). Amino acids concentration in human embryological fluids. *Human Reproduction*, **9**, 1175–9.

Jauniaux, E., Gulbis, B., Nagy, A.M., Jurkovic, D., Campbell, S., and Meuris, S. (1995*a*). Coelomic fluid chorionic gonadotropin and protein levels in normal and complicated first trimester human pregnancies. *Human Reproduction*, **10**, 214–20.

Jauniaux, E., Jurkovic, D., Gulbis, B., Liesnard, C., Lees, C., and Campbell, S. (1995*b*). Materno-fetal immunoglobulin transfer and passive immunity during the first trimester of human pregnancy. *Human Reproduction*, **10**, 3297–300.

Jauniaux, E. (1996*a*). Intervillous circulation in the first trimester: the phantom of the color Doppler obstetrics opera. *Ultrasound in Obstetrics and Gynecology*, **8**, 763–6.

Jauniaux, E., Gulbis, B., Schandene, L., Colette, J., and Hustin, J. (1996*b*). Distribution of interleukin-6 in maternal and embryonic tissues during the first trimester. *Molecular Human Reproduction*, **2**, 239–43.

Johnson, M.R., Jauniaux, E., Ramsay, B., Jurkovic, D., and Meuris, S. (1994*a*). The relationship between fetal heart rate, maternal endocrinology and the development of placental circulations. *British Journal of Obstetrics and Gynaecology*, **101**, 1003–4.

Johnson, M.R., Jauniaux, E., Jurkovic, D., Campbell, S., and Nicolaides, K.H. (1994*b*). Relaxin levels in embryonic fluids during the first trimester. *Human Reproduction*, **9**, 1561–2.

Jones, C.P.J. and Jauniaux, E. (1995). Ultrastucture of the maternoembryonic interface in the first trimester of pregnancy. *Micron*, **2**, 145–73.

Kingdom, J.C.P., Macara, L.M., and Whittle, M.J. (1994). Fetoplacental circulation in health and disease. *Archives of Disease in Childhood*, **70**, F161–5.

Lind, T. (1978). The biochemistry of amniotic fluid. In *Amniotic fluid: research and clinical application*, 2nd edn, (ed. D.V.I. Fairweather and T.K.A.B. Eskes), pp. 59–80. Excerpta Medica, Amsterdam.

MacCarthy, T. and Saunders, P. (1978). The origin and circulation of the amniotic fluid. In *Amniotic fluid: research and clinical application*, 2nd edn, (ed. D.V.I. Fairweather and T.K.A.B. Eskes), pp. 1–18. Excerpta Medica, Amsterdam.

Merce, L.T., Barco, M.J., and Bau, S. (1996). Colour Doppler sonographic assessment of placental circulation in the first trimester of normal pregnancy. *Journal of Ultrasound Medicine*, **15**, 135–42.

Meuris, S., Nagy, A.M., Delogne-Desnoeck, Jurkovic, D., and Jauniaux, E. (1995). Relationship between the establishment of intervillous blood flow and the human chorionic gonadotrophin early pregnancy peak. *Human Reproduction*, **10**, 947–50.

Moscoso, J.G. (1992). Functional aspects of embryology. In *The first twelve weeks of gestation*, (ed. E. Barnea, J. Hustin, and E. Jauniaux), pp. 167–91. Springer, Heidelberg.

Nagy, A.M., Jauniaux, E., Jurkovic, D., and Meuris, S. (1994). Placental overproduction of human chorionic gonadotropin α-subunit in early pregnancy as evidenced in exocoelomic fluid. *Journal of Endocrinology*, **142**, 511–16.

O'Rahilly, R. and Muller, F. (1992). Human embryology and teratology. Wiley–Liss, New York.

Ramsey, E.M. and Donner, N.W. (1980). *Placental vasculature and circulation*. Georg Thieme, Stuttgart.

Rodesch, F., Simon, P., Donner, C., and Jauniaux, E. (1992). Oxygen measurements in the maternotrophoblastic border during early pregnancy. *Obstetrics and Gynecology*, **80**, 283–5.

Shi, W.K., Hopkins, B., Thompson, S., Heath, J.K., Luke, B.M., and Graham, C.F. (1985). Synthesis of apolipoproteins, alphfoetoprotein, albumin and transferrin by the human foetal yolk sac and other foetal organs. *Journal of Embryology and Experimental Morphology*, **85**, 191–206.

Sibley, C.P. and Boyd, R.D.H. (1992). Mechanisms of transfer across the human placenta. In *Fetal and neonatal physiology*, Vol. 1, (ed. R.A. Polin and W.W. Fox), pp. 62–74. Saunders, Philadelphia.

Sinha, R. and Carlton, M. (1970). The volume and composition of amniotic fluid in early pregnancy. *Journal of Obstetrics and Gynaecology of the British Commonwealth*, **77**, 211–14.

Umaoka, Y., Noda, Y., Narimoto, K., and Mori, T. (1992). Effects of oxygen toxicity on early development of mouse embryo. *Molecular Reproduction and Development*, **31**, 28–33.

Valentin, L., Sladkevicius, P., Laurini, R., Soderberg, H., and Marsal, K. (1996). Uteroplacental and luteal circulation in normal first-trimester pregnancies: Doppler ultrasonographic and morphologic study. *American Journal of Obstetrics and Gynecology*, **174**, 768–75.

Wathen, N.C., Cass, P.L., Campbell, J., Kitau, M.J., and Chard, T. (1992). Levels of placental protein 14, human placental lactogen and unconjugated oestriol in extraembryonic coelomic fluid. (Letter.) *Placenta*, **13**, 195–7.

Watson, A.L., Palmer, M.E., Jauniaux, E., and Burton, G.J. (1997). Variation in expression of copper/zinc superoxide dismutase in villous trophoblast of the human placenta with gestational age. *Placenta*, (in press).

Wright, J.W. and Ridgway, L.E. (1990). Sources of variability in umbilical artery systolic/diastolic ratios: implication of the Poiseuille equation. *American Journal of Obstetrics and Gynecology*, **163**, 1788–91.

14 | *Maternal endocrine changes in early pregnancy*

J.G. Grudzinskas, I. Apaolaza, and T. Chard

INTRODUCTION

The endocrine and metabolic events that follow fertilization can be observed in the mother once implantation commences, the major endocrine event being the extraordinary rapid rise in the production of human chorionic gonadotrophin (hCG). The hypothalamic pituitary axis has a varied response, for example, gonadotrophin production appears to decrease whilst prolactin synthesis is increased. Thereafter, there is an increase in several hormones and proteins (Table 14.1). The hormonal assessment of early pregnancy and common disorders such as miscarriage and ectopic pregnancy have been extensively reviewed elsewhere (Grudzinskas 1995). Here we review endocrine and metabolic changes in early pregnancy which may be relevant in implantation, embryonic development, and the identification of women at increased risk of trisomy 21 and other aneuploidies.

Table 14.1 Principal fetal, trophoblast, and maternal proteins and hormones in early pregnancy

Trophoblast	Human chorionic gonadotrophin (hCG)
	Human placental lactogen (hPL)
	Schwangerschaftsprotein 1 (SP1)
	Pregnancy-associated plasma protein A (PAPP-A)
	Oestriol
	Progesterone
Fetal	Alpha-fetoprotein (AFP)
	Fetal antigen 1 (FA1)
	Fetal antigen 2 (FA2)
Decidual/endometrial	Insulin-like growth factor binding protein 1 (IGF-BP; IGF-BP1) or placental protein 12 (PP12)
	Glycodelin or progesterone-dependent endometrial protein (PEP) or placental protein 14 (PP14)

TROPHOBLAST PROTEINS AND HORMONES

Human chorionic gonadotrophin (hCG)

Human chorionic gonadotrophin is a glycoprotein with close structural similarities to pituitary luteinizing hormone (LH), follicle-stimulating hormone (FSH), and thyroid-stimulating hormone (TSH). It consists of two protein chains, the α and β subunits. The chains are joined by non-covalent bonds. Both subunits have side chains of carbohydrate residues, principally sialic acid, which constitute some 12 per cent of the molecule on a weight basis. The α subunit has 92 amino acid residues and is virtually identical with the α subunits of LH, FSH, and TSH. The β subunit has 145 amino acid residues. Thirty of these, at the carboxy terminus of the molecule, are unique to hCG. The remaining 115 residues are very similar to the 115 residues of the β subunit of LH; 80 per cent of the sequence is identical. The molecular weights of the α subunit, the β subunit, and the whole molecule are 14 930, 23 470, and 38 400 respectively (Bahl *et al.* 1972; Morgan *et al.* 1975; Fiddes and Goodman 1981).

Within the trophoblast the synthesis of the α and β subunits of hCG is independent, the α subunit being encoded by a single gene on chromosome 6 (6q 12–21) (Fiddes and Goodman 1981) and the β subunit by a family of six genes on the long arm of chromosome 19 (Graham *et al.* 1987). The two subunits combine in the cell prior to release as intact hCG, and for this reason only small quantities of the free subunits appear in the circulation. The production of β subunit appears to be the rate-limiting factor; the trophoblast can synthesize much greater quantities of α subunit than β subunit, but combination of the two is essential for release from the cell. The β subunit production peaks at 8–10 weeks, declining thereafter, but α subunit levels increase until term (Hoshina *et al.* 1984).

The main proposed function for hCG is maintenance of the corpus luteum in early pregnancy. The mechanisms that control hCG synthesis are still largely unknown. It is suggested that in early pregnancy some factor stimulates trophoblastic hCG synthesis. Later in pregnancy this factor either declines or is replaced by another which actively reduces hCG production. No hypothesis as to what such factors must be has been put forward. There is some evidence that cyclic adenosine monophosphate (cAMP) or luteinizing hormone releasing factor will stimulate hCG production in placental explants, but it is difficult to relate this to control *in vivo*.

The measurement of hCG has an established place in the diagnosis of pregnancy, screening for ectopic pregnancy, Down syndrome and other aneuploidies, and monitoring trophoblastic disease.

Human placental lactogen (hPL)

Placental lactogen (hPL) is a protein with close similarities to pituitary prolactin and growth hormone (96 per cent homology). It consists of a single chain of 191 amino acids without carbohydrate residues. There are two intrachain disulphide (–S–S–) links. The molecular weight is 21 600 (Chard 1982).

In common with many other proteins, hPL is initially synthesized in the form of a somewhat larger molecule, having an additional 20 amino acids at the NH_2 terminus. This extra 'signal' sequence is removed as part of the process of secretion. hPL is encoded by a gene cluster on chromosome 17 (George *et al.* 1981).

hPL is produced by syncytiotrophoblast, and fits very well to the model of control by mass of trophoblast, i.e. the concentrations in maternal blood increase slowly and appear to parallel the size of the placental mass. Maximum levels are reached at 32 weeks. Most investigators agree that hPL levels are related to placental mass, and secondarily to fetal weight. Serum hPL levels are no longer used in the assessment of fetal well-being, as other biophysical methods of fetal assessment are far superior (Chard 1982).

Schwangerschaftsprotein 1 (SP1)

This protein has a molecular weight of 90 000 and the electrophoretic mobility of a β1-globulin. A large part (30 per cent) of the molecule consists of carbohydrate containing sialic acid. Its biological activity is unknown, although it forms part of a large family of proteins of which carcinoembryonic antigen (CEA) is the most familiar (Grudzinskas *et al.* 1982). SP1 is coded by a gene on chromosome 19 (19q13.1) (Barnett *et al.* 1989; Niemann *et al.* 1989). SP1 levels are significantly lower in ectopic and failing pregnancies than gestational age-matched normal pregnancies and threatened abortions of good outcome (Seppala *et al.* 1980; Mantzavinos *et al.* 1991; Johnson *et al.* 1993). SP1 measurements in the first and second trimester of pregnancy are currently being evaluated as a secondary screening test for Down syndrome (Macintosh *et al.* 1993).

Pregnancy-associated plasma protein A (PAPP-A)

PAPP-A is a pregnancy-specific glycoprotein produced by trophoblast. It is detectable in maternal serum from 28 days after conception and increases throughout gestation with a doubling time of 4–5 days in the first trimester (Figure 2). PAPP-A is a glycoprotein with α_2 electrophoretic mobility and a molecular weight of 750 000–820 000. Various functions have been proposed, notably as an inhibitor of enzymes such as granulocyte elastase. No specific control mechanisms are known (Stabile *et al.* 1988). The gene for PAPP-A is located on the distal part of the long arm of chromosome 9 (9q33.1) (Silahtaroglu *et al.* 1993). Depressed serum PAPP-A levels are seen in association with early pregnancy failure (spontaneous miscarriage and ectopic pregnancy) Grudzinskas *et al.* 1985 and in association with fetal aneuploidy (El-Farra and Grudzinskas 1995). A number of retrospective studies has defined a relationship between low levels of PAPP-A in the first trimester and Down syndrome and other trisomies (Spencer *et al.* 1992; Wald *et al.* 1992; Brambati *et al.* 1993a,b, 1994). This difference is greatest at the earliest gestations, and decreases rapidly towards the second trimester. Serum PAPP-A levels in affected pregnancies at 6–11 weeks are substantially lower (0.27 multiples of the normal median, MOM) than those seen in normal pregnancies (Brambati *et al.* 1993a). By the second trimester the difference is no longer evident (Aitken *et al.* 1993). It has been suggested that using first trimester measurements of maternal serum PAPP-A and maternal age to define the 5 per cent of women at highest risk of Down syndrome, and offering karyotyping to this 5 per cent, it may be possible to detect 71 per cent of cases of Down syndrome.

Oestriol

The principal oestrogen in human pregnancy is oestriol, which has hydroxyl groups at C3, C16, and C17. The first step of synthesis involves the removal of six carbon atoms from the side chain of cholesterol leaving the 21-carbon steroid pregnenolone. In the fetal adrenal gland pregnenolone is converted into the C_{19} steroid dehydroepiandrosterone (DHEA) which passes to the fetal liver where it is hydroxylated to 16-OH-DHEA. In turn, this passes to the placenta where an aromatase confers the characteristic oestrogen A-ring to produce oestriol. In the fetal circulation the bulk of these steroids exist as sulphate conjugates. The placenta has a high content of a sulphatase enzyme which is essential for the conversion of 16-OH-DHEA-SO$_4$ in the trophoblast prior to aromatization (Siiteri and MacDonald 1966; France and Liggins 1969; Shearman 1979). In cases of sulphatase deficiency little or no oestriol is secreted into the mother. In maternal blood, half or more of oestriol circulates in the form of 16-glucosiduronate conjugates, and this is also the principal form in urine. Around one-half of oestrogens are directed through the enterohepatic circulation. In the bile the main form is oestriol-3-sulphate-16-glucosiduronate.

There is no information on the function of oestriol in pregnancy; an almost complete deficiency, in the absence of placental sulphatase, seems to have no effect on maternal or fetal well-being. Similarly, there is little information on control mechanisms, other than the general mechanisms already proposed. Certain specific factors affect oestriol synthesis. It is deficient in the absence of placental sulphatase, in adrenal hypoplasia, in anencephaly, and following administration of corticosteroids. The last three situations all have in common a reduction in the synthesis of the main precursor, DHEA. Depressed serum levels are also seen in association with trisomy 21 (Canick *et al.* 1988). The measurement of oestriol in maternal blood was introduced to assess fetal well-being in the third trimester. Currently, serum oestriol measurements in the second trimester are used in conjunction with hCG and AFP to identify women at increased risk of having a Down syndrome baby (Spencer 1994).

Progesterone

This trophoblast steroid does not depend upon fetal precursors. After six weeks of pregnancy the placental secretion of progesterone takes over from that of the corpus luteum. The major excretion product in urine is pregnanediol. Progesterone is believed to play a major role in the maintenance of early pregnancy, especially in the transformation of the endometrium to the decidua. Progesterone concentrations are depressed in women with spontaneous miscarriages and ectopic pregnancy and this, in conjunction with hCG levels, may be useful in the diagnosis of this condition (Stabile and Grudzinskas 1994).

FETAL PROTEINS

Alpha-fetoprotein (AFP)

AFP is a protein synthesized by the fetal liver and yolk sac, which is believed to serve an oncotic function in the fetus similar to that of albumin in the adult. AFP is a glycoprotein in which more than 39 per cent of the amino acid sequence resembles albumin. The gene for AFP is coded on the long arm of chromosome 4 (4q11.22) (Harper and Dugaiczyk 1983). Serum AFP levels in ectopic pregnancy tend to be higher than in intrauterine pregnancies (Grosskinsky *et al.* 1993). Serum AFP levels are measured in screening for open neural tube defects (elevated levels) and Down syndrome (depressed levels). Maternal serum levels of AFP (MS-AFP) in the second trimester tend to be lower in pregnancies affected by Down syndrome, the median level in an affected pregnancy is 0.75 multiples of the normal median (MOM) of normal pregnancies. In the first trimester, the situation is very similar: a number of studies report MS-AFP in Down syndrome as 0.7 to 0.8 MOM of normal pregnancies (Brambati *et al.* 1986; Crandall *et al.* 1993). Current research is addressing whether determination of MS-AFP in first trimester serum will be as useful as it is in the second trimester.

Fetal antigen 1 (FA1)

Fetal antigen 1, like its partner FA2, was first identified in second trimester amniotic fluid and the fetal origin was suggested by its distribution in fetal and maternal compartments and tissues (Fay *et al.* 1988; Tornehave *et al.* 1989). High concentrations of FA1 were found in second trimester amniotic fluid and in fetal serum, whereas the concentration in normal human serum was found to be approximately 20 ng/ml, which is 1000 times less than in second trimester fetal serum (Fay *et al.* 1988). Studies on fetal tissues (week 7) have demonstrated FA1 immunoreactivity in the hepatocytes of the fetal liver (Tornehave *et al.* 1989). Subsequently, the presence of FA1 was observed within the cytoplasm of nearly all glandular cells of the first trimester anlage of the fetal pancreas (Tornehave *et al.* 1993), the relative number of FA1-positive glandular cells decreasing as the development of the fetal pancreas progresses. Postnatally, the expression of FA1 is restricted to the insulin-producing β cells of the islets of Langerhans (Tornehave *et al.* 1993; Jensen *et al.* 1993). It is suggested that FA1 is synthesized as a membrane-anchored protein and released into the circulation after enzyme cleavage, and that circulating FA1 represents the post-translationally modified gene product of the human *dlk* gene which, in turn, is identical to human adrenal-specific mRNA of the *pG2* gene (Jensen *et al.* 1994). FA1 has the potential to be an index of organ specific or general embryonic or fetal development.

Fetal antigen 2 (FA2)

FA2 was first identified in amniotic fluid (Fay *et al.* 1988; Tornehave *et al.* 1989) and has been shown to be identical to the aminopropeptide of the α1 chain of collagen type I (Teisner *et al.* 1992). Biochemical characterization has revealed several molecular forms of the protein which differ in both size (Fay *et al.* 1988; Rasmussen *et al.* 1992*a*) and charge (Price *et al.* 1995*a*). An enzyme-linked immunosurbent assay (ELISA) has been developed and used to demonstrate the presence of FA2 in normal serum (Rasmussen *et al.* 1992*b*). A radioimmunoassay has also been described (Price *et al.* 1995*b*) and a standard prepared (Price *et al.* 1994). In amniotic fluid there are two major high molecular mass FA2 types and several low molecular mass forms (Price *et al.* 1995*a*). Levels rise steeply from 10 to 14 weeks, peak at 17 weeks, and then fall slightly by 23 weeks. FA2 holds the promise of being a marker of fetal mesodermal activity, tumour activity, or tissue regeneration. A comparison of amniotic fluid FA2 levels between 10 and 23 weeks gestation in normal pregnancies and pregnancies affected by trisomy, showed significantly higher FA2 levels in trisomy 21 and significantly lower levels in trisomy 18 (Figure 3) (Price *et al.* 1995*b*).

DECIDUAL–ENDOMETRIAL PROTEINS

Insulin-like growth factor binding protein 1 (IGF-BP1) (also known as PP12, placental protein 12)

The identification of IGF-BP1 as a major secretory product of decidualized endometrium suggests that studies of the IGFs and their binding proteins may contribute to implantation. IGF-BP1 is a 25 kDa growth-hormone independent, acid-stable protein found in fetal and adult serum and also in amniotic, follicular, and cerebrospinal fluid. IGF-BP3 is the main serum IGF-BP with a molecular weight of 29 kDa and is growth-hormone dependent. In the peripheral circulation, IGF-BP3 forms a 150 kDa complex and in pregnancy both IGF-BP3 and IGF-BP2 are present in the peripheral circulation but in reduced concentrations. However, IGF-BP1 increases steadily throughout pregnancy (Seppala *et al.* 1992). Maternal serum IGF-BP1 levels greater than those in non-pregnant women are observed from week 7 onward. The maximum levels are reached at 22–23 weeks. There is a correlation between endometrial IGF-BP1 and progesterone levels (Rutanen *et al.* 1982, 1984)

The primary stucture of IGF-BP1 has been determined and the single gene encoding IGF-BP1 located on the short arm of chromosome 7 (7p12.13) (Jalkunen *et al.* 1989). The gene encodes a single 1.6 kb mRNA species expressed in gestational endometrium from the first and third trimesters of pregnancy, secretory endometrium, liver and hepatoma cell lines, but not in proliferative endometrium or trophoblastic tissue obtained at term (Julkunen *et al.* 1988). Using *in situ* hybridization, the mRNA for IGF-BP1 has been identified in a population of stromal cells in late secretory phase endometrium and decidua (Julkunen *et al.* 1990). The production by the decidualized endometrium of a peptide that controls the bioavailability of growth factors suggests that the human endometrium may exert local control on the development and growth of the placenta and influences fetal metabolism, since it is present in the amniotic cavity (Rutanen *et al.* 1982; Giudice *et al.* 1990). Hustin and colleagues (1994) have recently reported the apparent selective expression of IGF-BP1 at the implantation site in humans in the earliest days of pregnancy.

Glycodelin (also known as placental protein 14 (PP14) and progesterone-dependent endometrial protein)

Biochemical and immunohistochemical observations (Wahlstrom *et al.* 1985) have shown that glycodelin is the most abundant protein derived from glandular epithelium of late secretory endometrium. The protein is actively secreted into the uterine cavity (Bell and Dore-Green 1987). Glycodelin is a glycoprotein which expresses polymorphism with a molecular weight of 42–43 kDa, containing 17.5 per cent carbohydrate (Bohn *et al.* 1982), the gene being located on chromosome 9 (Van Cong *et al.* 1991).

Circulating levels increase 20-fold from the late secretory phase to the early first trimester whereas tissue levels increase only two fold, suggesting that much of the rise is due to the increase in the mass of the decidua (Bell 1988). Significant amounts of Glycodelin have not been detected in any tissue in the adult or fetus, except the reproductive organs (Tornehave *et al.* 1989; Waites *et al.* 1990; Karamarainen *et al.* 1996).

Serum glycodelin levels are high in the late luteal and menstrual phase of the normal menstrual cycle. A number of observations suggest that progesterone might be an important control factor (Fay *et al.* 1990). Circulating levels of glycodelin start to rise one week after ovulation. In a conceptual cycle, the rise continues with a doubling time of 2.5 days; the levels peak within four weeks (Joshi 1987). The levels remain high for up to 8–10 weeks after which there is a fall, a pattern similar to hCG (Joshi *et al.* 1982; Bell *et al.* 1985; Julkunen *et al.* 1985; Than *et al.* 1987). A similar pattern is observed by quantitative immunohistochemistry of the endometrium (Bolton *et al.* 1988). The correlation suggests that fetal PP14 originates from the mother, although it is surprising that a protein of this size would cross the placenta. At term, glycodelin levels in the fetus correlate with but are 10-fold less than those in the mother (Bell *et al.* 1985). The glycodelin concentration in amniotic fluid is 100 to 1000-fold higher than that in maternal blood. The highest levels in amniotic fluid are found at 8 to 10 weeks. Serum glycodelin levels are lower in ectopic than in non-complicated intrauterine pregnancies, and when used in combination with hCG concentration, may distinguish between normal and abnormal implantation (Nylund *et al.* 1992; Ruge *et al.* 1992).

CONCLUDING REMARKS

The measurement of hormones and proteins in maternal and fetal blood, amniotic and coelomic fluids provides useful information about the intrauterine environment and embryonic and fetal development in addition to that obtained by high resolution ultrasonography. This is certainly the case in relation to subsequent miscarriage of a live fetus and the detection of women at increased risk of trisomy 21 and other aneuploidies. The further study of metabolic and endocrine events in early pregnancy will continue to improve our ability to manage early pregnancy problems.

REFERENCES

Aitken, D.A., McCaw, G., and Crossley, J.A. (1993). First trimester biochemical screening for fetal chromosome abnormalities and neural tube defects. *Prenatal Diagnosis*, **13**, 68–9.

Bahl, O.P., Carlson, R.B., Bellisario, R., and Swaminathan, N. (1972). Human chorionic gonadotrophin amino acid sequence of the alpha and beta subunits. *Biochemical and Biophysical Research Communications*, **48**, 416–22.

Barnett, T.R., Pickle, W., Rae, P.M., Hart, J., Kamarck, M., and Elting, J. (1989). Human pregnancy-specific beta-1-glycoproteins are coded within chromosome 19. *American Journal of Human Genetics*, **44**, 890–3.

Bell, S.C., Hales, M.W., Patel, S.R., Kirwan, P.H., and Drife, J.O. (1985). Protein synthesis and secretion by the human endometrium and decidua during early pregnancy. *British Journal of Obstetrics and Gynaecology*, **92**, 793.

Bell, S.C. (1988). Secretory/endometrial decidual proteins and their function in early pregnancy. *Journal of Reproduction and Fertility*, (Suppl.), **36**, 109.

Bell, S.C. and Dore-Green, F. (1987). Detection and characterization of human secretory pregnancy-associated and endometrial alpha-2-globulin (α2-PEG) in uterine luminal fluid. *Journal of Reproduction and Fertility*, **11**, 13.

Bohn, H., Kraus, N. and Winkler, W. (1982). New soluble placental tissue problems: Their solution, characterization, localisation, and quantification. *Placenta*, **4** (Suppl.), 67–81.

Bolton, A.E., Pockley, A.G., Mowles, R., Stoker, R.J., Westwood, O., and Chapman, M.G. (1988). Biological activity of placental protein 14. In *Implantation: biological and clinical aspects*, (ed.) M. Chapman, J.G., Grudzinskas, and T. Chard), pp. 135–44. Springer, London.

Brambati, B., Simoni, G., Bonacchi, I., and Piceni, I. (1986). Fetal chromosomal aneuploidies and maternal serum alphafetoprotein levels in the first trimester. *Lancet*, ii, 165–6.

Brambati, B., Macintosh, M.C.M., Teisner, B., Shrimanker, K., Lanzani, A., Maguiness, S., *et al.* (1993*a*). Low maternal serum levels of pregnancy associated plasma protein A in the first trimester in association with abnormal karyotype. *British Journal of Obstetrics and Gynaecology*, **100**, 324–6.

Brambati, B., Tului, L., Bonnachi, I., Shrimanker, K., Suzuki, Y., and Grudzinskas, J.G. (1993*b*). Serum PAPP-A and free beta hCG are first trimester screening markers for Down syndrome. (Abstract.) *Human Reproduction*, **8**, (Suppl. 1), 183.

Brambati, B., Tului, L., Bonnachi, I., Suzuki, Y., Shrimanker, K., and Grudzinskas, J.G. (1994). Biochemical screening for Down syndrome in the first trimester. In *Screening for Down syndrome*, (ed.) J.G., Grudzinskas, T., Chard, M. Chapman, and H. Cuckle, pp. 289–94. Cambridge University Press.

Canick, J.A., Knight, G.J., Palomaki G.E., Haddon, J.E., Cuckle, H., and Wald, N.J. (1988). Low second trimester maternal serum unconjugated oestriol in pregnancies with Down's syndrome. *British Journal of Obstetrics and Gynaecology*, **95**, 330–3.

Chard, T. (1982). Placental lactogen: biology and clinical applications. In *Pregnancy proteins: biology, chemistry and clinical applications*, (ed.) J.G. Grudzinskas, B. Turner, and M. Seppala), pp. 101–18. Academic Press, Sydney.

Crandall, B.F., Hansen, F.W., Hansen, F.W., Keener, M.S., Matsumo, B.S., and Miller, W. (1993). Maternal serum screening for alpha-fetoprotein, unconjugated oestriol and human chorionic gonadotrophin between 11 and 15 weeks of pregnancy to detect fetal chromosome abnormalities. *American Journal of Obstetics and Gynecology*, **168**, 1864–9.

El-Farra, K. and Grudzinskas, J.G. (1995). Will PAPP-A be a biochemical marker for screening of Down's syndrome in the first trimester? *Early Pregnancy Biology and Medicine*, **1**, 4–12.

Fay, T., Jacobs, I., Teisner, B., Poulsen, O., Chapman, M., Stabile, I., *et al.* (1988). Two fetal antigens (FA1 and FA2) and endometrial proteins (PP12 and PP14) isolated from amniotic fluid. Preliminary observations in fetal and maternal issues. *European Journal of Gynaecological Biology*, **29**, 73–5.

Fay, T.N., Jacobs, I.J., Teisner, B., Westergaard, J.G., and Grudzinskas (1990). A biochemical test for the direct assessment of endometrial function: measurement of the major secretory endometrial protein PP14 in serum during menstruation in relation to ovulation and luteal function. *Human Reproduction*, **5**, 382.

Fiddes, J.C. and Goodman, H.M. (1981). The gene encoding the common alpha-subunit in the four human glycoprotein hormones. *Journal of Molecular and Applied Genetics*, **1**, 3–18.

France, J.T. and Liggins, G.C. (1969). Placental sulphatase deficiency. *Journal of Clinical Endocrinology and Metabolism*, **29**, 138–41.

George, D.L., Phillips, J.A., Francke, U., and Seeburg, P.H. (1981). The genes of growth hormone and chorionic somatomammotrophin are on the long arm of human chromosome 17 in region q21 to qter. *Human Genetics*, **57**, 138–41.

Giudice, L.C., Farrell, E.M., Pham, H., Lamson, G., and Rosenfeld, R.G. (1990). Insulin-like growth factor binding proteins in the maternal serum throughout gestation and in the puerperium: effects of a pregnancy-associated serum protease activity. *Journal of Clinical Endocrinology and Metabolism*, **71**, 806–16.

Graham, M.Y., Otani, T., Boime, I., Olsen, M.V., Carle, G.F., and Chaplin, D.D. (1987). Cosmid mapping of the human chorionic gonadotrophin beta subunit genes by field-inversion gel electrophoresis. *Nucleic Acids Research*, **15**, 443–7.

Grosskinsky, C.M., Hage, M.L., Tyrey, L., Christakos, A.C., and Hughes, C.L. (1993). hCG, progesterone, alpha-fetoprotein, and estradiol in the identification of ectopic pregnancy. *Obstetrics and Gynecology*, **81**, 705–9.

Grudzinskas, J.G. (1995). Endocrinological and metabolic assessment of early pregnancy. In *Turnbull's obstetrics*, (ed.) G. Chamberlain), p. 185–94. Churchill Livingstone, Edinburgh.

Grudzinskas, J.G., Teisner, B., and Seppala, M. (eds) (1982). Pregnancy specific beta glycoprotein. In *Pregnancy proteins; biology, chemistry and clinical applications*. pp. 179–262. Academic Press, Sydney.

Grudzinskas, J.G., Westergaard, J.G., and Teisner, B. (1985). Pregnancy-associated plasma protein A in normal and abnormal pregnancies. *Proteins of the placenta. Biochemistry, biology and clinical application*, (ed.), p. 184. P. Bischof and A. Klopper Karger, Basel. Basel.

Harper, M.E., and Dugaiczyk, A. (1983). Linkage of evolutionary related serum albumin and AFP genes within q11–22 of chromosome 4. *American Journal of Human Genetics*, **35**, 565–72.

Hoshina, M., Hussa, R., Paltillo, R., Camel, M.H., and Boime, I. (1984). The role of trophoblast differentiation in the control of the hCG and hPL genes. *Advances in Experimental Medicine and Biology*, **176**, 299–311.

Hustin, J., Philippe, E., Teisner, B., and Grudzinskas, J.G. (1994). Immunohistochemical localization of two endometrial proteins in the early days of human pregnancy. *Placenta*, **7**, 701–8.

Jalkunen, M., Suikkari, A.M., Koistinen, R., Butzow, W., Ritzos, O., Seppala, M., and Ranta T. (1989). Regulation of insulin-like growth factor-binding protein 1: production by human granulosa luteal cells. *Journal of Clinical Endocrinology and Metabolism*, **69**, 1174–9.

Jensen, C.H., Teisner, B., Hojrup, P., Rasmussen, H.B., Madsa, O.D., Nielsen, B., and Skojodt, K. (1993). Studies on the isolation, structural analysis and tissue localisation of fetal antigen 1 and its relation to human adrenal-specific cDNA, pG2. *Human Reproduction*, **8**, 635–41.

Jensen, C.H., Krogh, T.N., Hojrup, P., Clausen, P.P., Skjodt, K., Larsson, L-I., *et al.* (1994). Protein structure of fetal antigen 1 (FA1), a novel circulating human epidermal growth factor-like protein expressed in neuroendocrine tumours and its relation to the gene products of dlk and pG2. *European Journal of Biochemistry*, **225**, 83–92.

Johnson, M.R., Riddle, A.F., Irvine, R., Sharma, V., Collins W.P., Nicolaides, K.H., and Grudzinskas J.G. (1993). Corpus luteum failure in ectopic pregnancy. *Human Reproduction*, **8**, 1491–5.

Joshi, S.G. (1987). Progestogen-dependent human endometrial protein: a marker for monitoring human endometrial function. *Advances in Experimental Medicine and Biology*, **230**, 167.

Joshi, S.G., Bank, J.G., Henriques, E.S., Makarachi, A., and Matties, G. (1982). Serum levels of progestogen-associated endometrial protein during the menstrual cycle and pregnancy. *Journal of Clinical Endocrinology and Metabolism*, **55**, 642.

Julkunen, M., Rutanen, E.M., Koskimies A., Ranta, T., Bohn, H., and Seppala, M. (1985). Distribution of placental protein 14 in tissues and body fluids during pregnancy. *British Journal of Obstetrics and Gynaecology*, **92**, 1145.

Julkunen, M., Koistinen, R., Aalto-Setala K., Seppala, M., Janne, O.A., and Kontula, K. (1988). Primary structure of human insulin-like growth factor-binding protein/placental protein 12 and tissue-specific expression of its mRNA. *FEBS Letters*, **236**, 295–302.

Julkunen, M., Koistinen, R., Suikkari, A-M., Seppala, M., and Janne, O.A. (1990). Identification by hybridization histochemistry of human endometrial cells expressing mRNAs encoding a uterine betalactoglobulin homologue and insulin-like growth factor-binding protein-1. *Molecular Endocrinology*, **4**, 700–7.

Karmarainen, M., Leivo, I., Koistinen, R., Julkunen, M., Karronen, U., Rutanen, E-M., and Seppala, M. (1996). Normal human ovary and ovarian tumours express glycodelin, a glycoprotein with immunosuppressive and contraceptive properties. *American Journal of Pathology*, **148**, 1435–43.

Macintosh, M.C.M., Brambati, B., Chard, T., and Grudzinskas, J.G. (1993). First trimester maternal serum Schwangerschafts protein 1 (SP1), in pregnancies associated with chromosomal abnormalities. *Prenatal Diagnosis*, **13**, 567–8.

Mantzavinos, T., Phocas, I., Chrelias, H, Sarandakou, A., and Zourlas, P.A. (1991). Serum levels of steroids and placental proteins in ectopic pregnancy. *European Journal of Obstetrics Gynecology and Reproductive Biology*, **39**, 117–22.

Morgan, F.J., Birkan, S. and Canfield, R.E. (1975). The amino acid sequence of human chorionic gonadotrophin. The alpha and beta subunit. *Journal of Biological Chemistry*, **250**, 5247–58.

Niemann, S.C., Schonk, D., van Dijk, P., Wieinga, B., Graeschizk, K.H., Bartels, I. (1989). Regional localization of the gene encoding pregnancy specific beta 1 glycoprotein (PSBG-1) to human chromosome 19q 13.1. *Cytogenetics and Cellular Genetics*, **52**, 95–7.

Nylund, L., Gustafson, O., Lindblom, B., Pousette, A., Seppala, M., Riittinen, L., and Akerlof, E. (1992). Placental protein 14 in human *in-vitro* fertilization early pregnancies. *Human Reproduction*, **7**, 128–30.

Price, K.M., Silman, R., and Grudzinskas, J.G. (1994). Isolation of fetal antigen 2 assay standard. *Clinical et Chimica Acta*, **226**, 83–8.

Price, K.M., Silman, R., Armstrong, P., Teisner, B., and Grudzinskas, J.G. (1995*a*). The typing of fetal antigen 2 in human amniotic fluid. *Clinical et Chimica Acta*, **236**, 181–94.

Price, K., Silman, R., Armstrong, P., and Grudzinskas (1995*b*). Abnormal amniotic fetal antigen 2 levels in trisomy 18 and 21. *Human Reproduction*, **10**, 2438–40.

Rasmussen, H.B., Teisner, B., Andersen, J.A., Yde-Andersen, E., and Leigh, I. (1992*a*). Fetal antigen 2 (FA2) in relation to wound healing and fibroblast proliferation. *British Journal of Dermatology*, **126**, 148–53.

Rasmussen, H.B., Teisner, B., Bangsgaard-Petersen, F., Yde-Andersen, E., and Kassem M. (1992*b*). Quantification of fetal antigen 2 (FA2) in supernatants of cultured osteoblasts, normal human serum, and serum from patients with chronic renal failure. *Nephrology Dialysis and Transplantation*, **7**, 902–7.

Ruge, S., Sorensen, S., Vejtorp, M., and Vejerslev, L.O. (1992). The secretory endometrial protein, placental protein 14, in women with ectopic pregnancy. *Fertility and Sterility*, **57**, 102–6.

Rutanen, E-M., Bohn, H., and Seppala, M. (1982). Radioimmunoassay of placental protein 12: levels in amniotic fluid, cord blood and serum of healthy adults, pregnant women and patients with trophoblastic disease. *American Journal of Obstetrics and Gynecology*, **144**, 460–3.

Rutanen, E-M., Koistinen, R., Wahlstrom, T., Sjoberg, J., Stenman, UH., and Seppala M. (1984). Placental protein 12 (PP12) in the human endometrium: tissue concentration in relation to histology and serum levels of PP12, progesterone and oestradiol. *British Journal of Obstetrics and Gynaecology*, **91**, 377–81.

Seppala, M, Venesmma, P., and Rutanen, E-M. (1980). Pregnancy-specific beta-1 glycoprotein in ectopic pregnancy. *American Journal of Obstetrics and Gynaecology*, **136**, 189–93.

Seppala, M., Julkunen, M., Riittinen, L., and Koistinen, R. (1992). Endometrial proteins: a reappraisal. *Human Reproduction*, **7**, 31–40.

Shearman, R.P. (1979). Endocrinology of the feto-maternal unit. In *Human reproductive physiology*, (ed. R.P. Sherman), pp. 97–126. Blackwell, Oxford.

Siiteri, P.K. and MacDonald, P.C. (1966). Placental oestrogen biosynthesis during human pregnancy. *Journal of Clinical Endocrinology and Metabolism*, **26**, 751–62.

Silahtaroglu, A.N., Tumer, Z., Kristensen, T., Sottrup-Jensen, L., and Tommerup, N. (1993). Assignment of the human gene for pregnancy-associated plasma protein A (PAPP-A) to 9q33.1 by fluorescence in situ hybridization to mitotic and meiotic chromosomes. *Cytogenetics and Cellular Genetics*, **61**, 214–16.

Spencer, K. (1994). Is the measurement of unconjugated oestriol of value in screening for Down's syndrome? In *Screening for Down's syndrome*, (ed.) J.G. Grudzinskas, *et al.*), pp. 141–61. Cambridge University Press.

Spencer, K., Macri, J.N., Aitken, D., and Connor, J.M. (1992). Free beta hCG as a first trimester marker for fetal trisomy. *Lancet*, **339**, 1480.

Stabile, I. and Grudzinskas, J.G. (1994). Ectopic pregnancy: what's new? In *Progress in obstetrics and gynaecology*, (ed. J.W. Studd), vol. 11, pp. 291–309. Churchill Livingstone, London.

Stabile, I., Grudzinskas, J.G., and Chard, T. (1988). Clinical applications of pregnancy protein estimations with particular reference to PAPP-A. *Obstetric and Gynaecological Surveys*, **49**, 73–89.

Teisner, B., Rasmussen, H.B., Hojrup, P., Yde-Andersen, E., and Skjodt, K. (1992). Fetal antigen 2: an amniotic protein identified as the aminopropeptide of the α1 chain of human procollagen type I. *Acta Pathologica Microbiologica Immunologica Scandinavica*, **100**, 1106–14.

Than, G.N., Tatra, G., Bohn, H., and Csaba, F. (1987). Placental protein 14 serum levels following conception. *Medical Sciences Research*, **15**, 1243.

Tornehave, D., Fay, R.N., Teisner, B., Chemnitz, J., Westergaard, J.G., and Grudzinskas, K.G. (1989). Two fetal antigens (FA-1 and FA-2) and endometrial proteins (PP12 and PP14) isolated from amniotic fluid: localisation in the fetus and adult female genital tract. *European Journal of Obstetrics, Gynecology and Reproductive Biology*, **30**, 221–32.

Tornehave, D., Jensen, P., Teisner, B., Rasmussen, H.B., Chemnitz, J., and Moscoso, G. (1993). Fetal antigen 1 (FA-1) in the human pancreas. Cell type expression, topological and quantitative variations during development. *Anatomical Embryology*, **187**, 335–46.

Van, Cong N., Vaisse, C., Gross, M.S., Slim, R., Milgrom, E., and Bernheim, A. (1991). The human placental protein 14 gene is localised to chromosome 9q34. *Human Genetics*, **86**, 515–18.

Wahlstrom, T., Koskimies, A.I., Tenhunen, A., *et al.* (1985). Pregnancy proteins in the endometrium after follicle aspiration for *in vitro* fertilisation. *Annals of the New York Academy of Science*, **442**, 402.

Waites, G.T., James, R.F., and Bell SC (1988*a*). Immunohistological localisation of human endometrial secretory protein pregnancy-associated endometrial alpha₁ globulin, an insulin-like growth factor binding protein, during the menstrual cycle. *Journal of Clinical Endocrinology and Metabolism*, **67**, 1100–4.

Waites, G.T., Wood, O.L., Walker, R.A., *et al.* (1988*b*). Immunohistological localization of human endometrial secretory protein, pregnancy-associated endometrial alpha-2-globulin (α2-PEG) during the menstrual cycle. *Journal of Reproduction and Fertility*, **82**, 665.

Waites, G.T., Bell, S.C., Walker, R.A., and Wood, P.L. (1990). Immunohistological distribution of the secretory endometrial protein, 'pregnancy-associated endometrial α2-globulin', a glycosylated β-lactoglobulin homologue, in the human fetus and adult employing monoclonal antibodies. *Human Reproduction*, 5, 105.

Wald, N.J., Stone, R., Cuckle, HS., Grudzinskas J.G., Barkai G., Brambati B., (1992). First trimester concentrations of pregnancy associated plasma protein A and placental protein 14 in Down's syndrome. *British Medical Journal*, 305, 28.

Wood, P.L., Waites, G.T., MacVicas, J., Davidson, A.C., Walker, R.A., and Bell, S.C. (1988). Immunohistochemical localisation of pregnancy associated endometrial α_2 globulin (α_2 PEG) in endometrial adenocarnoma and effect of MPA. *British Journal of Obstetrics and Gynaecology*, 95, 1292–8.

15 | *The embryo/trophoblastic paradox*

Eytan R. Barnea and Jean-David Barnea

INTRODUCTION

Conception in mammals is a unique and singular event. It requires the merging of genetic material from two distinctly different individuals leading to the formation of a sturdy union between their gametes in such a manner that the conceptus' resemblance to the individual entities from which it originated is lost forever. Following a few replication cycles, the blastocyst separates into embryoblast and extraembryonic structures, including the trophoblast which completely surrounds the embryonal cells. The rate-limiting step in reproduction is implantation, in which the partial xenograft implants into the host, through immunomodulation and embryo-derived recognition signals (see Chapter 4) coupled with endometrial receptivity (Strowitzki *et al.* 1994; see Chapter 7). During implantation, the trophoblast plays a leading role in attaching the conceptus to the uterine decidua, and subsequently invades the decidua to link with the maternal circulation. Meanwhile, embryoblast proliferation continues rather slowly in comparison to the trophoblast. Our knowledge on this period in humans is very limited and the mechanisms responsible for this preferential growth are not known; it is, however, critical for understanding embryogenesis.

Current evidence indicates that trophoblast development is largely controlled by the paternal genome, while that of the embryo is controlled mainly by maternal influences (see Chapter 12). The questions that arise are: why there is such a differential expression and what are the associated long-term consequences of such a complex interaction? Is the role of the paternal genome-derived trophoblast (representing aggressivity, required for implantation) to shield and protect the vulnerable embryo from a potentially adverse maternal environment, in addition to having a trophic role? If this is the case, why does nature go to such lengths to fuse the two genomes in the first place? Evidently, mixing the genes enormously increases phenotypic diversity, thereby leading to the development of much better adapting individuals, postnatally.

Once a critical mass of cells, a critical level of trophoblastic penetration of the endometrium, highly specific signals, and the maternal recognition of pregnancy are reached, then and only then, will the embryoblast start to proliferate rapidly. At this stage, the speed of proliferation is incredible and the coordination is phenomenal since embryonal development is completed in approximately four weeks.

Embryogenesis is characterized by the highly coordinated processes of cell proliferation and differentiation that rapidly result in complete embryo formation. This is intimately combined with a modulation of cell migration and an inhibition of excessive cell growth, which require the activation of a large number of genes following a specific sequence. Earlier studies on the theory of complexity and self-organization have greatly helped to shed light on this incredibly intricate process (Kauffman 1992). For example, the brain can not develop before the heart initiates circulation, which in turn is required to provide oxygenated blood to the encephalus.

Successful completion of embryogenesis is the result of an interplay between genetic and epigenetic phenomena, allowing for a great phenotypic diversity, making each individual unique despite being derived from very similar blueprints. Overall, the fully formed embryo is the culmination of a complex series of 'on' and 'off' expressions of gene products in a highly precise, sequential manner, from which even slight deviations may lead to embryonal dysfunction or demise. Numerous interacting transcription factors, homeobox genes, the c-*erb*A/thyroid hormone/retinoic acid receptor family proteins, and the c-*Fos*/c-*Jun* genes appear to be important in this process (Karin 1990; Kessel and Gruss 1990). Present information on the expression of embryonal period-specific suppressor genes and their products is very limited.

The trophoblast is not a static organ and has several important functions (see Chapter 10), it implants and invades the decidua reaching the maternal circulation. Subsequently, it anchors the conceptus to the uterus and serves as a metabolic and immunological shield, allowing passage of nutrients almost exclusively through a process of diffusion (Hustin 1992). When the trophoblast becomes metabolically competent, shortly before embryogenesis begins, it acquires paracrine hormonal control of human chorionic gonadotropin (hCG) and perhaps of other hormones (see Chapter 10).

The cytotrophoblast (CT) is a mononuclear cell which has both proliferative and invasive potential, and can differentiate into villous syncytiotrophoblast (ST) (hormone-dependent) which anchors the trophoblast, or invades the placental bed-lining maternal blood vessels (invading trophoblast) and can even migrate to the lung (see Chapter 8). Each of these types has specific cellular markers whose expression appears to be dependent on the local environment (Kliman and Feinberg 1992). The villous CT, which for strategic reasons is covered by the ST, is a terminal cell aggregate which lacks proliferative potential. With advancing embryogenesis, the apparent aggressivity of the trophoblast decreases, the levels of its major functional marker, hCG, plateau, and the rate of CT differentiation into ST accelerates.

Examination of the conceptus shows that the embryo, starting from a few-cell stage, proliferates while differentiating, creating great cell and organ diversity which are linked in a highly coordinated manner. In contrast, the trophoblast, from monocellular elements through brief intermediate stages, loses its proliferative potential and becomes ST.

Our central hypothesis is that the embryo has important control mechanisms which provide a careful balance between proliferative and differentiative processes, thus allowing embryonal development. On the other hand, although the trophoblast has a certain autonomy over its proliferation and differentiation, it is also maintained in check and is prevented from becoming overly aggressive and developing neoplastic features; such an occurrence would be clearly detrimental for the maternal host and the embryo itself. If this control system fails, instead of the trophoblast acting as a shield and support it interferes and impairs embryo development, leading to its inevitable demise.

In this chapter, we will discuss the biological rationale for embryo and trophoblast development, analogies and differences between the trophoblast and cancer, embryo/trophoblast dependence in mammals, and our very recent data supporting the role of the embryo in trophoblast hormone modulation and control of embryo and malignant cell proliferation.

THE PROPERTIES OF TROPHOBLAST CELLS

In early pregnancy, the trophoblast may become aggressive, defying its own purpose of existence, namely to support the embryo (Loke 1983). In the case of a mole or choriocarcinoma, the trophoblast, caused by over-expression of the male genome (Szulman 1992; Goshen *et al.* 1994; see Chapter 12), utilizes resources for its own benefit thereby damaging both the embryo (rarely present) and the host. The properties of trophoblastic neoplasia are beyond the scope of this chapter and will not be further discussed (see Maruo and Mochizuki 1994).

It is evident that in order to allow the conceptus to implant and develop, the trophoblast must have certain neoplastic-like features (p. 00). It is not yet clear whether the controlled invasivity by the trophoblast during normal pregnancy is a battle won or a cooperation between the host and the partial allograft, although in our view the latter is more likely. The balance is, however, precarious since if invasion is too shallow or too deep, or if angiogenesis is poor, severe pregnancy complications may ensue. Evidently, in normal pregnancies the host is not damaged and the fetus is sustained until delivery.

In normal pregnancy, the following sequence of events takes place: implantation involves the attachment of the conceptus, proliferation of the trophoblast, invasion of the endometrium, and degradation of the basement membrane and extracellular matrix. Subsequently, the cells migrate into the decidua reaching uterine blood vessels, occupy their lumen, develop functional blood vessels, and even metastasize to the lung (Boyd and Hamilton 1970). It is of note that the presence of microvilli in the lung do not cause an inflammatory response or local inflammation, thus they are not considered alloantigens and they disappear within a short time after delivery. That the trophoblast can attach and implant in extrauterine sites such as the ovary and the bowel indicates that the decidua may not be required for pregnancy. However, implantation in the uterus is clearly advantageous over other sites in providing the trophic support that is required for embryonal development and maintaining trophoblast invasivity in check.

The neoplastic-like features of the trophoblast include adhesion to the host, cell proliferation, invasion, angiogenesis, metastasis, immune evasion, expression of tumour markers, and activation of carcinogens. On the other hand, features distinguishing trophoblast from neoplasia include preferential differentiation of CT to ST, expression of local and trophoblast-derived inhibitors of invasion, maintained maternal immune surveillance (mostly beyond the uterus), maternal environment-controlled characteristics of trophoblast cells, inactivation of mutagens/carcinogens, the presence of an embryo, and an overall trophic effect on the maternal host. These two opposing forces are necessary for maintaining this temporary but powerful balance. Our knowledge of each of these features' pro and anti-neoplasticity is still fragmentary, and the following discussion is aimed to provide the general principles rather than all the details, which are discussed, among other places, in a number of other chapters in this book.

The factors involved in these processes may have multiple roles at the same time, have different roles with advancing gestation, or have site-specific roles. The presence of growth factors (GF) or cytokines does not necessarily mean that they have a locally produced ligand, therefore both paracrine and autocrine loops may be envisaged. In addition, in some instances observations made *in vitro* may not fully correspond to those present in *in vivo* conditions. For example, epidermal growth factor (EGF) may promote proliferation and differentiation at the same time (a practically opposite effect). A further example is the notion that proliferation and invasion may not necessarily be linked (Lysiak *et al.* 1994). Overall, there is a very complex interaction between uterine, decidual, and trophoblast elements which actually changes continuously during gestation.

Facilitators and inhibitors of implantation

These are involved during the attachment of the trophoblast to the uterine surface. During the early secretory phase, the endometrium is a good host, facilitating implantation through major changes as evidenced by changes in hydrolysis of collagen IV by the blastocyst, the laminin coating of decidual cells, the presence of lymphoid-suppressor cells, and expression of integrins (Hustin and Franchimont 1992; see Chapter 7). It is believed that E-cadherin may also have an important role. The involvement of oncofetal fibronectin in this context has been reported as well. That CT cells attach to types I and IV collagen, fibronectin, and laminin suggests that these cells have specific receptors to extracellular matrix (ECM) proteins (Kliman and Feinberg 1992).

Proliferation and its promoters

In early pregnancy, the rate of trophoblast proliferation is very rapid and is much faster than in cells of adult individuals or any malignant growth. Experiments using proliferating cell nuclear antigen (PCNA) have shown that in histological sections, as expected, the staining of the ST layer was always negative, while both villous and extravillous CT maintained an elevated proliferative index practically until term (Wolf and Michalopolous 1992). It is estimated that from fertilization until the eighth week of gestation two billion cells are formed (10^9, or approximately 2 g) at a very rapid doubling rate. The cell cycle time is estimated to be 15 h (Gerbie *et al.* 1968). Later, however, the rate of proliferation drops markedly, since at term the placenta weighs less than 500 g, a 20-fold increase within an additional 32-week period. Some highly proliferative CT cells have nevertheless been reported also at term. Trophoblastic invasion in humans continues until about the fourth month of gestation (Boyd and Hamilton 1970).

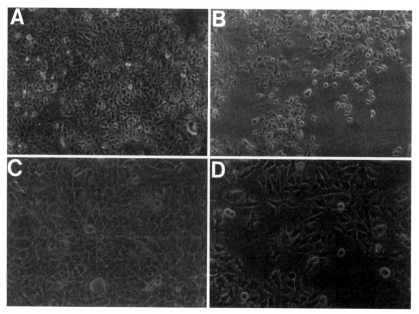

Fig. 15.1   Microphotographs of the inhibitory of EDF-B on MCF-7 cell proliferation after four days in culture. A,B, Control (buffer treated) dishes at ×100 and ×200 fold magnifications, respevtively. C,D: ×100 and ×200 fold magnifications following addition of EDF-B.

Both EGF and transforming growth factor α (TGFα), small glycoproteins with a 30 per cent homology to each other, are present in the trophoblast; both bind to locally present EGF receptors. These factors have been found to promote the proliferation of CT cells *in vitro* as evidenced by tritiated (^{3}H-TdR) incorporation (Lysiak *et al.* 1994). According to Maruo *et al.* (1992*a*) this is most evident in the 4–5 weeks of gestation but not after.

There are changes in the expression of EGF and its receptor across gestation. Very early, both are present in the CT, but in the second trimester, EGF is detected in CT but its receptor is localized in the ST (Hoffman *et al.* 1992). *In situ* hybridization studies reveal that in the cytoplasmic domain of the EGF receptor, *erb*-B mRNA is more abundant in early placenta than at term (Maruo *et al.* 1992*b*). That a specific TGFα antibody added to the culture had no effect while the EGF antibody decreased proliferation, indicates that endogenous EGF, but not TGFα, may have an important local proliferative role. The involvement of other endogenous ligands such as amphiregulin, which bind to the EGF receptor, was suggested as well (Lysiak *et al.* 1994).

The involvement of the β chain of platelet-derived growth factor (PDGF) through binding to the PDGF receptor in CT proliferation and activating the expression of the *myc* proto-oncogene has been reported (Franklin *et al.* 1993). The highest level of expression of PDGFα was found in the CT at the base of the growing villi, though no specific receptors were detected. Therefore, it is believed that the PDGFα chain stimulates the proliferation of PDGFα receptor-positive endothelial cells in a paracrine manner, while PDGFβ (a c-*sis* proto-oncogene homologue) has the proper receptor in the CT and acts locally. The expression of PDGFβ is limited until 10 weeks (Ohlsson *et al.* 1991).

The expression of the c-*fms* oncogene by the human ST has been demonstrated as well; however, whether the granulocyte macrophage-colony stimulating factor (GM-CSF) receptor/c-*fms* protein product is expressed locally is unclear (Kenton *et al.* 1991). This and other cytokines are believed in general to be derived from macrophages (Wood 1994). This also suggests that the placenta is unusually active in proto-oncogene expression, which may be more prominent in early pregnancy.

Insulin-like growth factor 2 (IGF2) is widely distributed in the CT and ST as well as in other uterine structures, may have a limited proliferative effect, and is dependent on the local receptor which is not expressed in the ST (Ohlsson *et al.* 1989).

Differentiative and antiproliferative factors

The control of CT proliferative can be achieved by either inhibiting cell proliferation or by promoting the transformation of CT to ST. In general, the transforming growth factor β (TGFβ) family exerts an antiproliferative effect. The messenger ribonucleic acid (mRNA) for TGFβ is expressed by the ST, by extravillous trophoblast, and by the decidua, as *in situ* hybridization experiments have revealed. The inactive TGFβ that accumulates in the extracellular matrix may be activated or blocked by trophoblast-derived proteases (Lala and Lysiak 1996). As for TGFα, it binds the same receptor (Bissonnette *et al.* 1992). The presence of both the ligand and biologically active receptor in the CT, ST, and other uterine cells argues for a local regulatory role for both GFs. Binding proteins (BP) for IGF2 have been described in the decidua and trophoblast, but the actual production of this BP may occur in the decidua. Thus IGF-BP may serve also as a limiting factor in GF-induced proliferation.

According to Rodway and Rao (1995), hCG has a time-dependent differentiative effect on CT cells as evidenced by the fusion of membranes and expression of specific biochemical parameters. This effect was mimicked by addition of dibutyryl cyclic adenosine monophosphate (cAMP) and was blocked by antibodies to hCG. In contrast, choriocarcinoma cells are not affected by exogenous hCG and remain mostly mononuclear cells (Licht *et al.* 1994).

Promoters of invasion

Trophoblast invasion in humans continues until about the fourth month of gestation (Boyd and Hamilton 1970). The lower invasivity appears to be caused by the microenvironment since T cells maintain their invasivity in extrauterine locations irrespective of the gestational age. This invasivity is higher in non-pregnant subjects. Additionally, expression of appropriate adhesion phenotypes are critical during the invasion process. This is evidenced by villous CT anchored to the basement membrane stained for the α_6 and β_4 subunits of integrin and for multiple forms of laminin.

In contrast, non-polarized CT in columns primarily express the α_5 and β_1 integrins and a fibronectin-rich matrix (Bass *et al.* 1993; Irving and Lala 1994).

The trophoblast secretes several proteinases that aid in degrading the ECM. These include metalloproteases (MTP) (92 kDa and 72 kDa), which are the major forms, as well as, perhaps, serine proteases. Recently, a higher expression of both MTPs was found when comparing the first-trimester and term trophoblast (Shimonovitz *et al.* 1994). The role of the trophoblast-specific class I molecule, HLA-G in evading the maternal immune response was also suggested (see below). Very recently, interleukin 1β (IL-1β) was found to be produced by the CT and affect local expression of adhesion molecules and of MTP9 (Librach *et al.* 1994). In addition, IGF-BP1 has been shown to stimulate cell migration without affecting cell proliferation (Lysiak *et al.* 1994). As recently shown, an altered expression of p53, the tumour suppressor/oncoprotein, is associated with the malignant phenotype of trophoblast (Aboagye-Mathiesen *et al.* 1996).

Inhibitors of invasion

The decidua appears to have a major role in controlling first-trimester trophoblast invasivity as shown by testing decidua-conditioned media on first-trimester trophoblast cultures (Graham *et al.* 1994). Several local factors are operative to control trophoblast invasion. Metalloproteinase activity can be blocked through the action of local decidual TGFβ which requires activation by proteases, while the GF secreted by the T does not require activation. The expression of TGFβ may also limit trophoblast invasiveness by reducing cell migration and plasmin production, which in turn controls MTP activation. An additional mechanism may be through the upregulation of tissue MTP inhibitors (TIMP-1). Finally, as recently suggested, corticosteroids may have an inhibitory role as well (Librach *et al.* 1994).

However, it appears that in spite of the antiproliferative and anti-invasive properties of the endometrium, this layer is not effective in controlling invasive mole and choriocarcinoma progression. hCG may also decrease the invasion of intermediate CT cells by directly inhibiting the proteolytic enzymes (Yagel *et al.* 1993).

Tumour markers

In a wider context, several GFs and cytokines are expressed in tumours where they have both paracrine and autocrine functions. Expression of high levels of hCG, a major tumour marker, is short lived due to the lowering in the expression of the hCGβ gene, which coincides with the completion of embryogenesis. The expression of human placental lactogen (hPL) and schwangershaftsprotein 1 (SP$_1$) was also found in several tumours (Malkin 1992).

Immune modulation and evasion

Overall, the pregnant woman does not appear to be immunosuppressed (Jones *et al.* 1992). There is evidence that numerous placenta-derived products have immunosuppressive properties. These include both steroids and proteins. For example, progesterone is believed to be an important immunosuppressor while the role of oestradiol is more limited. With respect to proteins, although claims have been made for numerous compounds, there is only positive evidence for very few of them to indicate an important role in immunosuppression (Chard and Grudzinskas 1992). In more general terms, trophoblastic cells secrete several immunosuppressive products (many of them remain unknown) that cause inhibition of rosette formation and the mixed lymphocyte culture (MLC) reaction (Barnea *et al.* 1986; Sanyal *et al.* 1989; Nahhas and Barnea 1990; Silver *et al.* 1990); this was not observed in choriocarcinoma cells (see also Chapter 4). Very recently, the role of hCG in controlling lymphocyte proliferation was described (Rodway and Rao 1995). The placenta can immunoabsorb antibodies directed at major histocompatibility complex (MHC) antigens, protecting the fetus from humoral assault. On the other hand, there is a passage of maternal immunoglobulins into the fetal circulation, and actually most immunoglobulin G (IgG) is maternally derived; thus the trophoblast does not serve as a physical barrier.

The expression of histocompatibility antigens (HLA) by the trophoblast has been investigated. The classical HLAs (A and B) are not expressed by the trophoblast, but they are expressed by fetal villous mesenchymal cells, thus the trophoblast does create a barrier between the mother and the fetus. This inability to induce expression of HLAs is likely to be due to irreversible hypermethylation. More recently, the expression of HLA-G, a unique type of MHC different from the classic types, has been described. The expression of this non-canonical HLA in the extravillous trophoblast in the proximity of the maternal tissue suggests that it may help in the invasion process (Kovats *et al.* 1990). The role of HLA-G has not yet been established. It is hypothesized that it does not stimulate MHC-restricted rejection by maternal effector cells. This is supported by the finding that the expression of the HLA-Gα chain on HLA-A, -B, and -C null-line lymphocyte cell lines reduced their susceptibility to lysis by non-MHC-restricted natural killer (NK) and $\gamma \delta$ T-cell clones (Kovats *et al.* 1991). The expression of HLA-G appears to be limited to differentiated CT (McMaster *et al.* 1995). In addition, local production of interleukin-10 (IL-10) was shown to exert immunosuppressive effects. The placenta also contains Fcγ receptors which are present on trophoblast microvilli and may serve as a filter to sequester soluble immune complexes (Johnson 1992). Potential immunomodulators in the first-trimester trophoblast are interferons which are present at five-fold higher concentrations than at term and have antiviral, antiproliferative, and activated natural killer cell activity (Aboagye-Mathiesen *et al.* 1995). Embryo-derived signals (e.g. pre-implantation factor (PIF)) may have an immunomodulatory role allowing for successful implantation (Barnea *et al.* 1994; see Chapter 4).

Angiogenesis

The development of functional blood vessels in the trophoblast is gradual, thereby protecting the embryo from excess blood flow at high pressure and elevated oxygen tension. There is evidence that the trophoblast acquires effective circulation allowing exchange between mother and fetus only towards the end of the first trimester

(Hustin 1992). The factors involved in angiogenesis have been recently described, among which the vascular endothelial growth factor (VEGF) appears to be of importance (Wheeler *et al.* 1995). Additional angiogenic factors present locally are fibroblast growth factor (FGF) and platelet-derived growth factor (PDGF) (Holmgren *et al.* 1991; Cross and Dexter 1991). The role of hCG in this respect has been addressed (Rodway and Rao 1995). In addition, prorenin expression in the first trimester is 300-fold higher than that found at term (Downing *et al.* 1995). All these findings suggest that an intensive process of angiogenesis occurs in the first trimester which is accelerated by the appearance of mesenchymal cells leading to functional blood vessels; this process markedly slows down at term.

Promotion of and protection against mutagenesis/carcinogenesis

There is evidence that the trophoblast has the capacity to activate carcinogens through the action of P450-dependent monooxygenases (Barnea and Avigdor 1990, 1991; see Chapter 23) and peroxidases (Barnea *et al.* 1995a). This leads to metabolic and hormonal changes, as well as the breakdown of deoxyribonucleic acid (DNA) leading to the formation of DNA adducts. On the other hand, the trophoblast appears to be well equipped to inactivate mutagens/carcinogens through various phase II enzymes and glutathione (Barnea and Avigdor 1990; Avigdor *et al.* 1992; Barnea 1992; Sanyal *et al.* 1993; Barnea *et al.* 1995b). The balance between these opposing forces makes the trophoblast a metabolic filter, protecting the embryo from the adverse environment, which when combined with low oxygen tension, decreases the likelihood of formation of oxygen radicals (Barnea 1996). Although during pregnancy the trophoblast does not develop neoplastic features, such exposure may contribute to a postnatal development of malignancy, i.e. childhood leukaemia; this is supported by ample experimental evidence. A single injection of 3-methylcholanthrene during early pregnancy has been shown to cause high rates of postnatal cancers in the offspring (Anderson *et al.* 1989).

THE PROPERTIES OF NEOPLASTIC CELLS

Cancer development is the result of a failure of the immune surveillance to identify, neutralize, and eliminate abnormal cell proliferation. Consequently, cell proliferation becomes uncontrolled, immature, invasive, develops new blood vessels, suppresses the immune system, secretes antitrophic elements damaging the host, and leads to metastasis. If it remains unchecked, such a process will ultimately lead to the death of the host unless it is identified early and effective therapy is available. The following describes the salient features of cancer.

Proliferative potential

Tumour cell proliferation is not a model of unrestrained growth, but rather a type of rapid cell proliferation in which cell mortality is low. Up to 75–90 per cent of tumour cells die in the process of tumour growth (Tannock 1992). Therefore, instead of the doubling time of clinically visible tumours being 5–20 days, it is actually much slower, 2–3 months (Tannock 1983). However, tumours have a long latent period; from a single clonal cell, 10^9 cells will be formed only after 5–7 years (approximately 30 doubling times) (Tannock 1983). One of the critical factors for tumour expansion is angiogenesis which makes the tumour much more aggressive and likely to metastasize.

Oncogenes and growth factors

Proto-oncogenes are cellular DNA products which are expressed in normal cells but do not cause the development of malignancy. In addition, more than 20 viral onco-genes have been identified. Some of those are GFs, others are GF receptors, tyrosine kinases, G proteins, serine–threonine kinases, and nuclear proteins. Malignancy may result through mutation, amplification, or translocation of these gene products (Cross and Dexter 1991; Buick and Tannock 1992). These changes can be major or simply due to point mutations. The GF products act through paracrine/autocrine mechanisms by binding to specific cell membrane receptors acting through tyrosine kinase-dependent phosphorylation. Consequently Na^+ and H^+ ion exchange is promoted through the cell membrane, cAMP increases, and phosphoinositides are degraded. These stimulate the release of Ca^{2+} ions and promote the activation of protein kinase C (Ullrich and Schlessinger 1990).

Receptors with tyrosine kinase activity include several GFs: PDGF, EGF/TGFα, IGF1 and IGF2, FGF1 and FGF2, and TGFβ. One or more mechanisms of GF-induced proliferation may take place:

(1)   local production of GFs and auto-stimulation;

(2)   modification or overexpression of the GF receptor; and

(3)   constitutive activation of the receptor (Cross and Dexter 1991).

The mechanisms by which GFs stimulate malignant cell proliferation are complex and are unique for each GF. Another viral product v-*erb* is homologous to EGF and has an intrinsic tyrosine kinase activity—not needing the ligand (Minden and Pawson 1992).

Invasion and metastasis

The formation of new blood vessels is an important prerequisite for cancer to spread beyond a certain size (Folkman 1990), since specific inhibitors of angiogenesis (compounds or antibodies) have been recently reported to block the spread of cancer in mice (Chen *et al.* 1995). Tumour invasion occurs through binding to endothelial cells and accessing the basement membrane, thereby binding to membrane components (laminin, fibronectin, vitronectin, MTPs, proteoglycans, and cathepsins) (Nicholson 1988). The inhibitors of these enzymes are TIMP-1 and 2 and stefin A. Downregulation of these inhibitors increases invasivity (Testa and Quigley 1991). In some cases, TGFβ inhibits while in other cases it may actually stimulate cancer cell proliferation.

The mode of tumour spread is individual and occurs along tissue planes, and through the circulation and lymphatic vessels. There is a preferential spread to different organs, which is dependent on where first tumour cells are trapped and the role of local GF action. Metastatic efficiency is rather low and represents only 1 per cent of the tumour load. This is believed to mainly be a random process, since the properties of metastatic cells are similar to those of the primary tumour. Tumour cell detachment may be related to a decrease in the expression of cell adhesion molecules and an increase in protease activity and motility factors (Liotta 1990). More than 95 per cent of metastatic cells die due to poor local conditions and immune reaction, mainly but not exclusively through the action of NK cells. Locally, tumour cells may cause platelet aggregation and prostaglandin release. Taken together, metastatic cells may be different in membrane properties, surface receptor expression, permeability, adhesivity, antigenicity, and glycoprotein expression. More recently, the metastatic potential of cells has been associated with mutation of oncogenes and loss of various tumour suppressor genes, such as *p53*, *BRCA1*, and *DCC* (Oliner *et al.* 1992).

Tumour markers

There are practically no true tumour markers since all are also expressed, albeit at lower levels, by normal tissues. Oncofetal proteins are mainly expressed during pregnancy but do not completely disappear in the adult. It is rather obvious that most tumour markers are of embryo origin, since the trophoblast is eliminated following delivery. For example, the carcinoembryonal antigen, a large glycoprotein, is found in the gastrointestinal tract of the embryo. Its levels are elevated in several epithelial tumours, but it is not tumour-specific since it is also detected in patients with liver cirrhosis (Malkin 1992). The high expression may be due to a process of derepression or alternatively to the prevalence of clones of cells that have a high expression. Another marker is α-fetoprotein (AFP) which is an α1-globulin produced by the fetal gastrointestinal tract and yolk sac. This marker is elevated in liver cancer, testicular tumours, and liver cirrhosis.

Among hormones, hCG is of major importance. The level of this glycoprotein is very high in trophoblast malignancies including choriocarcinoma and testicular tumours, and some cases of breast and bowel malignancies. Almost all cancer cell lines studied express some form of hCG, making this hormone an almost obligatory marker of cancer (Acevedo *et al.* 1995). An alkaline phosphatase isoenzyme is a tumour marker for bone and liver cancers. In addition, hPL expression has been found in many tumours. With respect to sex steroids, the expression of both oestrogen and progesterene receptors in breast and endometrial cancers is strongly associated with response to hormonal therapy and prognosis.

Evasion of immune surveillance

It is recognized that a decrease in immunological surveillance leads in many instances to tumour development. This can be caused by viruses, chemicals, ageing, and other aetiologies. On the other hand, tumours only occasionally have an altered antigenicity and therefore are frequently recognized as 'self'. When a tumour is immunogenic, it can be recognized by receptors on T-cells and/ or B cells. An additional immunity is conferred by NK cells and macrophages. Recognition of such an immune reaction may be associated with the expression of MHC molecules. More recently, it has been demonstrated that tumorus release immunosuppressive compounds which facilitate their survival in spite of the presence of adequate immune surveillance mechanisms.

A COMPARISON OF TROPHOBLASTIC AND CANCER CELLS

In spite of several analogies between trophoblast and cancer cells, major differences are present which completely change the outcomes, i.e. birth of a new individual as opposed to death of the host; Table 15.1 shows such a comparison. During implantation, coordination and cross-signalling between endometrium and the trophoblast takes place. Adhesion of the trophoblast to the endometrium is of primary importance. In contrast, in cancer, decreased cell adhesiveness aids in the tumour spread required for metastasis. Most tumours derive from a single clone of transformed cells which, from the start, acquires a growth advantage. The trophoblast is biclonal and, in the case of twins, triplets, or even higher order, although the clonality of the T cells is multiple, no clear dominance of one clone over an other is apparent. trophoblast proliferation is more rapid than that of cancer cells, but CT cells are benign stem cells which proliferate to create other CT cells with a similar degree of differentiation, or are transformed into ST cells, a permanent non-proliferative state.

Cancer may therefore be viewed as an aberrant stem cell renewal, in which subsequent generations of cells are malignant and become progressively immature. However, in culture, malignant cells can under certain circumstances differentiate, losing their malignant nature, thereby resembling CT cells. Factors involved in proliferation and invasion are similar for cancer and the trophoblast and involve a large number of autocrine/paracrine loops of GFs and cytokines. In the trophoblast, protooncogenes may promote proliferation, but the presence of effective inhibitors (tumour-suppressor gene products) and BPs locally and in the decidua makes proliferation controlled. In cancer, oncogenes have a major role in expressing GFs, their receptors, and cellular mediators, frequently acting constitutively—perhaps the major difference from what occurs in the trophoblast. In the trophoblast and surrounding tissues, the expression of ligands, their receptors, and specific second messengers is required for function.

With advancing gestation, trophoblast proliferation slows down and becomes mostly directed towards ST formation, decreasing both its invasivity and proliferation. In contrast, with advancing cancer, the tumour becomes progressively more virulent and the cells become anaplastic. Proliferation, however, becomes limited by the chaotic proliferation of the vascular tree, hypoxia, and associated cell death and necrosis. A tumour can not grow beyond a certain size without the formation of associated new vessels. In contrast, angiogenesis occurs rather late when trophoblast size is rather large, hCG level has reached a plateau, and cell differentiation accelerates, consequently limiting the neoplastic potential of the trophoblast. The absence of significant angiogenesis in a hydatidiform mole may actually represent a protective phenomenon.

Table 15.1 Comparative aspects of trophoblastic and embryonal cell properties in early and late gestation and malignant cell properties in early and advanced cancer

Cell properties	Trophoblast		Embryo		Cancer	
	First trimester	Term	First trimester	Term	Early	Advanced
Cellular properties						
Clonality	bi	bi	bi	bi	mono	mono
Proliferation rate	+++	++	++++	+++	++	+++
Differentiation	++	+++	++	++++	+	−
Apoptosis	++	+	++++	++	++	+
Cell immortality	++	=	++	=	+	++
Senescence						
(telomerase)	?	++	?	++	+	−
Mechanisms of proliferation						
Proto-oncogene						
activation	++	+	++	+	+	+++
Autocrine effect of GFs	+	+++	+	+++	+	=
GF *trans*-activation	=	=	=	=	+	+++
Tumour-suppressor						
gene(s)	+	++	+	+++	++	−
Proliferation blockers	+	++	+++	++	+	−
Invasivity						
Invasivity	++	=	N/A	N/A	+	+++
Adhesiveness	+	++	N/A	N/A	+	−
MTP/TIMP ratio	+++	+	N/A	N/A	+	+++
Metastatic efficiency	+++	+	N/A	N/A	=	+
Cellular features						
Angiogenesis	+	+++	++	++++	=	+++
Oxygen tension	+	++	+	+++	+++	+
Phase II/I enzyme ratio	+	+	+	+++	++	+
Trophic effect on host	+	+++	+	+++	+	−
Tumour markers	+	+++	+	+++	+	+++
Immunological aspects						
Surface antigenicity	=	=	=	+	=	=
Immunosuppressor						
secretion	+	+++	+	+++	+	++
Repair of DNA damage	++	+++	+++	++++	+	−

+, low; ++, moderate; +++, large; ++++, marked.
= not present
− decrease

Mechanisms for cancer and trophoblast invasion appear to be similar: a balance between the MTPs/TIMPs that control degradation of the ECM. In this respect, the trophoblast may be more invasive early on, since CT cells penetrate deep, reaching the uterine circulation. In cancer, in many instances it takes a long time before basement membrane is penetrated (the rate-limiting step in tumour development). Once, however, the tumour is advanced, it becomes invasive and metastasizes, although with only a low efficiency, similarly to the trophoblast. On the other hand, the trophoblast metastasizes relatively easily but without the associated consequences that are seen in cancer.

High levels of circulating hCG are the hallmark of the aggressive phase of trophoblast development. This marker is also elevated in several cancers. The expression of similar other markers has also been reported (proteins, GFs, and steroids). With respect to immune function, both the trophoblast and cancer cells secrete immunosuppressive compounds and are recognized as 'self'—in cancer by not changing cell surface antigenicity, and in the T by not expressing classical HLA antigens but only a special HLA-G type. Overall, the specific properties of the trophoblast make it unique and necessary for pregnancy.

In conclusion, pregnancy may be paralleled to a state of 'controlled cancer'. However, the conceptus, unlike cancer, can be rejected at any stage, i.e. earlier by spontaneous abortion or later by delivery. Perhaps an effective surveillance mechanism makes elimination of an abnormal embryo almost obligatory through embryo self-policing. The ultimate result is that only a low number of malformations are compatible with life and embryo that end up developing into fetuses and reaching delivery are more likely to have mosaic-type than pure chromosomal anomalies. Moreover, it appears that pregnancies that are not compatible with life cannot be rescued. This is seen, for example, in cases of habitual abortion where treatment does not lead to an increase in the malformation rate.

On the other hand, cancer development following embryogenesis might actually represent an incomplete regression to the embryo stage when cell proliferation is maximal, cell differentiation is minimal, apoptosis is reduced, and expression of embryo-specific markers is prevalent, but with the difference that the body's ability to control cell proliferation is impaired, having lost the protective control mechanisms that are operative during embryogenesis.

EMBRYO–TROPHOBLASTIC DEPENDENCE IN MAMMALS

The function of the embryo is to carry the genome and lead to its successful expression; it can be considered a 'parasite' which harnesses the maternal and trophoblast resources for its advantage, survival, and development. The highest rate of cell proliferation in mammals occurs during embryogenesis, where cell replication proceeds with high fidelity and apparently with very few errors. This is plausible since the presence of even a few abnormal cells early on would be greatly magnified, leading almost inevitably to embryonal demise, because of its incompatibility with life. This is true for both the embryo and the trophoblast. Thus, when major development errors occur during embryogenesis, spontaneous abortion almost always occurs.

Early trimester loss is approximately 15 per cent, which is rather low, considering the high probability for errors in cell proliferation/migration/differentiation/apoptosis. Thus, very precise and powerful control mechanisms must exist, allowing differentiation into specific organs, while maintaining in check the abnormal cells formed, perhaps by eliminating them. This checks-and-balances system appears to be extremely well developed in the embryo, while if such control mechanisms exist in the trophoblast, they would be more rudimentary since they would only be required to transform highly proliferative CT cells through intermediate stages into ST cells.

Experiments using transgenic mice have helped, in recent years, to determine which genes are needed for which particular function and whether the embryo can survive in their absence (see Chapter 24). Thus, it appears that the close proximity of embryo to the trophoblast may have an important role in allowing the exertion of the supportive role of the trophoblast to the embryo. On the other hand, as recent studies suggest, the embryo modulates trophoblast function according to its needs while advancing its own development.

The most compelling evidence for this argument is that in mice in whom the embryo is removed surgically at 10 days of gestation, the trophoblast in culture becomes spontaneously cancerous (choriocarcinoma) (Teshima *et al.* 1983); this was confirmed by subsequent work (Faria *et al.* 1990). In fetectomy experiments in primates, Panigel and Myers (1972) reported that the trophoblast that remains *in situ* does not appear to undergo malignant transformation during the period of observation. This would suggest that the pregnant animal is capable of preventing cell transformation locally and is not immunosuppressed. In a certain respect, malignancy and teratocarcinomas may be regarded as developmental defects in gene expression (Mintz and Fleischman 1981).

Cells from normal embryos' neural crest transplanted into adult mouse testes lead to the development of teratocarcinoma, the transformation being due to the abnormal environment (Pierce and Speers 1988). In contrast, the injection of teratocarcinoma cells into mouse blastocysts leads to the development of normal mouse offspring that are mosaic, containing cells derived from both parents and from the tumour (Brinster 1974). This would suggest that the embryo is capable of transforming cancerous cells into differentiated elements enabling their integration into the fetus. Pregnancy has also been shown to protect against transplantation of lymphoma cells in rats. The injections of serum from pregnant rats also conferred some protection against cancer in non-pregnant rats compared to serum from non-pregnant animals (Ioachim and Moroson 1986).

Recent data have shown that the hCGβ subunit and whole hCG exert an inhibitory effect on Kaposi's sarcoma cell line proliferation and prevented the development of tumours in nude mice. In certain mice, becoming pregnant alone conferred protection, and in others it caused regression of the tumour. However, more importantly, early inoculation of the tumour during the first 10 days of gestation caused complete protection against Kaposi's sarcoma development while later inoculation caused a small tumour development (Lunardi-Iskandar *et al.* 1995).

It is of note that mice do not express a chorionic gonadotrophin (CG) gene, and therefore the antitumour effect seen must have been exerted by different factors. This, again, confirms the uniqueness of early pregnancy with respect to the control of cell proliferation. Another example for embryo-derived protection against damage is the expression of quinone reductase, a major anticarcinogenic and mutagenic enzyme that is already expressed by the embryo (Barnea *et al.* 1995*a*).

EMBRYO–TROPHOBLASTIC DEPENDENCE IN HUMANS

In vivo evidence

Trophoblastic hormone secretion is controlled by several factors (see Chapter 10), and is under autocrine, paracrine, and endocrine influences from the decidua and ovary. One facet of the control of hCG secretion by the embryo has not been addressed until recently. This may be the case because of earlier observations on the feto-placental unit (present later in pregnancy) which are based mainly on steroid hormone metabolism. A subsequent study has shown that the placenta *in situ* can continue to function following fetal demise in the early second trimester (Davies and Glasser 1967). We suggest, on the other hand, that the critical period for which embryo/trophoblast interaction and interdependence is important is during embryogenesis and shortly thereafter. This has implications not only for that period of gestation but much beyond it as well.

Several facts support such a control, and this has previously been discussed in detail (Barnea and Shurtz-Swirski 1992). In brief, trophoblast cultures grow poorly *in vitro* following very recent embryonal death. Ectopic pregnancies with a demonstrable embryo have higher levels of hCG than anembryonic pregnancies. Henderson *et al.* (1992) have shown that in anembryonic pregnancies, the decrease in circulating hCG in early trimesters is not only due to decreased placentation but also to downregulation of the hCGα and hCGβ genes in the trophoblast. It was recently shown that coelomic fluid derived from anembryonic pregnancies has lower levels of hCG as well as several other proteins, thus suggesting that following embryonal demise, trophoblast function is maintained only for a short time (Jauniaux *et al.* 1995; see Chapter 13/19). In addition, surgical embryo reduction for high-order pregnancy, which is done without affecting the trophoblast, leads to a decrease in hCG secretion (Fischer and Wapner 1992; Johnson *et al.* 1994). In patients with Down syndrome, hCG levels do not reach a plateau and the levels tend to be higher in the second trimester due to overexpression of the hCG subunits (Eldar-Geva *et al.* 1995). Finally, in molar pregnancies in which the embryo is present, hCG levels are lower than in those in which the embryo is absent. It has also been shown that the relationship between embryo and trophoblast is altered *in vitro* following maternal exposure *in vivo* to neuroleptics (Shurtz-Swirski *et al.* 1992). This indicates that embryo/trophoblast interaction through secretory products can be affected by maternal exposure.

In vitro evidence

Previously described observations indicate that the embryo contains regulatory compounds that help its own development and are also involved in controlling trophoblast function. Indeed, we have reported that embryo-derived factors (EDF) control hCG and progesterone secretion by placental explants in a dose-, time-, and gestational-age dependent manner. The gestational age-dependent effects noted reflect parallel changes in both neural and visceral tissue extracts. These hCG modulators were found to be of low molecular weight and secreted by embryo tissue explants as well (Barnea *et al.* 1989; Shurtz-Swirski *et al.* 1991). The topic has been reviewed in detail (Barnea 1994). In further studies, we found that EDF affect mammalian embryo survival, development, and implantation *in vitro*. The effect was cross-species effective, i.e. EDF affected mouse blastocysts, a fact which may point to the universality of the phenomenon in mammals (Barnea, unpublished observations).

The role of the embryo in controlling neoplastic proliferation

We have shown that trophoblast hormone secretion is modulated by EDF (Barnea *et al.* 1989). These observations suggest that preferentially maternal genome imprinting-dependent elements derived from the embryo are preferentially capable of controlling paternal genome-derived (trophoblast) hormone expression (Goshen *et al.* 1994). We reason that since the trophoblast has malignant potential, EDF might also control cancer cell proliferation. Evidence to this effect has been reported recently (Barnea *et al.* 1996).

We have found that EDF, separated by high-pressure liquid chromatography (HPLC), contains two active fractions of ~4.5 kDa (EDF-A) and ~10.7 kDa (EDF-B), which decreased MCF-7 human breast cancer cell counts by up to 70 per cent after four days of incubation when compared to buffer or total extract used as controls. The antiproliferative effect was also evidenced by decreased [^{3}H]thymidine incorporation. In addition, significant inhibition of proliferation was obtained of rat osteosarcoma cell line ROS clone 17/2.8; Rat-1, an established SV40-transformed rat embryo fibrosarcoma cell line (Pines *et al.* 1986); and a Balb/c 3T3 immortalized mouse cell line (Table 15.2). These results confirm observations made on other malignant cell lines including sarcomas, ovary malignancies, kidney malignancies, and osteosarcomas (Barnea, unpublished observations). The EDF-induced inhibition of both mouse and rat cell lines, in addition to their effect on humans, indicates a cross-species effectivity. In contrast, certain fractions significantly enhanced cell proliferation.

The antiproliferative effect of EDF was time-dependent, non-toxic, and cells remained viable at the end of culture as shown by trypan blue staining. Following

Table 15.2   Inhibitory effect of EDF on the proliferation of transformed cell lines following four days of incubation as compared to controls (100 per cent)

Cell line	EDF-A	EDF-B
MCF-7	65%	68%
ROS	10%	30%
Rat-1	38%	40%
Balb/c 3T3	48%	40%

exposure, cell morphology appeared to be changed: cells tended not to aggregate, and frequently had a fusiform or stellate appearance. The SDS-PAGE analysis of EDF-B revealed two major (~14 kDa) and a few minor (< 30 kDa) bands while EDF-A only had a few faint low molecular weight bands using Coomassie blue staining.

Preliminary data suggest that EDF may prevent tumour development in X-ray irradiated mice (Barnea, unpublished observations). The EDF appear to be potent low molecular weight proteins whose effect is not organ- or epithelial tumour-specific. Even though EDFs are of neural origin, they affect epithelial and mesenchymal proliferation, indicating that in addition to their local effect, they may also have a multi-targeted role during embryonal development. Indeed, kidney morphogenesis, for example, is dependent on the expression of nerve GF receptors (Sariola *et al.* 1991). Overall, the gestational age-dependent expression of EDF might reflect a transition from a cell proliferation and differentiation stage to an organ development stage.

The identity and the mechanisms of action of EDF are currently under investigation. We suggest that these factors may limit GF action. Binding to specific sites which embryonal cells may share with neoplastic cells is also a possibility, since these factors also suppress mice blastocyst development *in vitro* (p. 00). Based on our data, TGFβ, a 25 kDa homodimer, does not appear responsible for the antiproliferative effect noted since

(1)   the 23–30 kDa region fractions, used as control, did not affect malignant cell proliferation;

(2)   the size of the ~4.5 kDa fraction was very small;

(3)   inhibition was observed on Rat-1 cell proliferation, on which, in contrast, TGFβ has a stimulatory effect (Barnard *et al.* 1990); and

(4)   the embryonal spinal cord does not express TGFβ1, 2, or 3 (Millan *et al.* 1991).

Therefore, embryonal tissues contain both inhibitors and promoters that maintain the delicate balance between these two opposing but vital forces necessary for embryonal development.

The previous adds to the body of information on the apparent paradox between pregnancy and cancer (as discussed in detail where pregnancy appears to protect against a large number of cancers; Fernandez *et al.* 1994). This is quite remarkable considering the massive cell proliferation and altered immune response that is present during that period.

CONCLUDING REMARKS

We have provided a theoretical discussion followed by supportive experimental data on the existence and function of the embryo/trophoblast unit in early pregnancy. On one hand, the embryo and trophoblast are a paradox since they derive from the same zygote but develop in completely different directions. In addition, the trophoblast has certain neoplastic features but is actually profoundly different from cancer cells; as trophoblast development progresses, it loses most of its neoplastic-like properties. At least part of the control of the trophoblast is provided by the embryo, as supported by *in vivo* and *in vitro* data. Our *in vitro* data also show that embryo-derived compounds are capable of controlling trophoblast hormonal indexes, as well as cancer cell proliferation, perhaps because of similarities existing between trophoblast and cancer cells and major differences between embryo and cancer cells; the mechanisms involved remain to be determined. We suggest that the identification of these compounds and elucidation of their mechanisms of action may lead to important diagnostic and therapeutic implications for pregnancy in particular and control of proliferation in general.

REFERENCES

Aboagye-Mathiesen, G., Tóth, F.D., Zdravkovic, M., and Ebbesen, P. (1995). Human trophoblast interferons: production and possible roles in early pregnancy. *Early Pregnancy: Biology and Medicine*, 1, 41–52.

Aboagye-Mathiesen, G., Zdravkovic, M., Tóth, F.D., Graham, C.H., Lala, P.K., and Ebbesen, P. (1996). Altered expression of the tumor suppressor/oncoprotein p53 in SV40 Tag-transformed human placental trophoblast and malignant trophoblast cell lines. *Early Pregnancy: Biology and Medicine*, 2, 102–12.

Acevedo, H.F., Tong, J.Y., and Hartsock, R.J. (1995). Human chorionic gonadotropin-beta subunit gene expression in cultured human fetal and cancer cells of different types and origins. *Cancer*, 76, 1467–75.

Anderson, L.M., Jones, A.B., Riggs, C.W., and Kovatch, R.M. (1989). Modification of transplacental tumorigenesis by 3-methylcholanthrene in mice by genotype and the Ah locus in pretreatment with β-naphthoflavone. *Cancer Research*, 49, 1676–81.

Avigdor, S., Zakheim, D., and Barnea, E.R. (1992). Quinone reductase activity in the first trimester placenta: effect of cigarette smoking and polycyclic aromatic hydrocarbons. *Reproductive Toxicology*, 6, 363–6.

Barnard, J.A., Lyons, R.M., and Moses, H.L. (1990). The cell biology of transforming growth factor β. *Biochimica Biophysica Acta*, 1032, 79–87.

Barnea, E.R. (1992). Placental biochemistry. In *The first twelve weeks of gestation*, (ed. E.R. Barnea, J. Hustin, and E. Jauniaux), pp. 111–27. Springer, Berlin.

Barnea, E.R. (1994). Dual effects of embryo-derived factors on hCG secretion by placental explants. In *Implantation and early pregnancy in humans*, (ed. E.R. Barnea, J.H. Check, J.G. Grudzinskas, and T. Maruo), pp. 271–82. Parthenon, Carnforth.

Barnea, E.R. and Challier, J.P. (1997). Prevention of environmentally-induced damage to the embryo: novel perspectives. *Gynécologie, Fertility and Reproduction*. (In press.)

Barnea, E.R. and Avigdor, S. (1990). Coordinated induction of estrogen hydroxylase and catechol-O-methyl transferase by xenobiotics in first trimester human placental explants. *Journal of Steroid Biochemistry*, 35, 327–31.

Barnea, E.R. and Avigdor, S. (1991). Aryl hydrocarbon hydroxylase activity in the first trimester placenta: induction by carcinogens and chemoprotectors. *Gynecological and Obstetrical Investigation*, 32, 4–9.

Barnea, E.R. and Shurtz-Swirski (1992). Endocrinology of the placenta and embryo–placental interaction. In *The first twelve weeks of gestation*, (ed. E.R. Barnea, J. Hustin, and E. Jauniaux), pp. 128–53. Springer, Berlin.

Barnea, E.R., Sanyal, M.K., Brami, C., and Bischof, P. (1986). *In vitro* production of pregnancy-associated plasma protein-A (PAPP-A) by trophoblastic cells. *Archives of Gynecology*, 237, 187–90.

Barnea, E.R., Simon, R.J., and Kol, S. (1989). Human embryonal extracts modulate placental function in the first trimester: effects of visceral tissues upon chorionic gonadotropin and progesterone secretion. *Placenta*, **10**, 331–44.

Barnea, E.R., Lahijani, K.I., Roussev, R., Barnea, J.D., Coulam, C.B. (1994). Use of lymphocyte platelet binding assay for detecting a preimplantation factor: a quantitative assay. *American Journal of Reproductive Immunology*, **32**, 105–8.

Barnea, E.R., Shklyar, B., Moskowitz, A., Barnea, J.D., Sheth, K., and Rose, F.V. (1995*a*). Expression of quinone reductase activity in embryonal and adult porcine tissues. *Biology of Reproduction*, **51**, 433–7.

Barnea, E.R., Sorkin, M., and Barnea, J.D. (1995*b*). Peroxidase activity and gluthatione content in the first trimester placenta and decidua. *Early Pregnancy: Biology and Medicine*, **1**, 141–7.

Barnea, E.R., Barnea, J.D., and Pines, M. (1996). Control of cell proliferation by embryonal-origin factors. *American Journal of Reproductive Immunology*, **35**, 318–24.

Bass, K.E., Roth, I., Damsky, C.H., and Fisher, S.J. (1993). Regulation of human cytotrophoblast invasion. In *In vitro fertilization and embryo transfer in primates*, (ed. D.P. Wolf, R.L. Stouffer, and R.M. Brenner), pp. 182–94. Springer, New York.

Bissonnette, F., Cook, C., Geoghegan, T., Steffen, M., Henry, J., Yussman, M.A., *et al.* (1992). Transforming growth factor-α and epidermal growth factor messenger ribonucleic acid and protein levels in human placentas from early, mid, and late gestation. *American Journal of Obstetrics and Gynecology*, **166**, 192–9.

Boyd, J.D. and Hamilton, W.J. (ed.) (1970). *The human placenta*. MacMillan, London.

Brinster, R.L. (1974). Effect of cells transferred into the mouse blastocyst on subsequent development. *Journal of Experimental Medicine*, **140**, 1049–56.

Buick, R.N. and Tannock, I.F. (1992). Properties of malignant cells. In *The basic science of oncology*, 2nd edn, (ed. I.F. Tannock and R.P. Hill), pp. 139–53. McGraw Hill, New York.

Chard, T. and Grudzinskas, J.G. (1992). Placental proteins and steroids and the immune relationship between mother and fetus. In *Immunological obstetrics*, (ed. C.B. Coulam, W.P. Faulk, and J.A. McIntyre), pp. 282–9. W.W. Norton, New York.

Chen, C., Parangi, S., Tolentino, M.J., and Folkman, J. (1995). A strategy to discover circulating angiogenesis inhibitors generated by human tumors. *Cancer Research*, **55**, 4230–3.

Cross, M. and Dexter, M.T. (1991). Growth factors in development, transformation, and tumorigenesis. *Cell*, **64**, 271–80.

Davies, J. and Glasser, S.R. (1967). Light and electron microscopic observations on a human placenta two weeks after fetal death. *American Journal of Obstetrics and Gynecology*, **98**, 1111–2.

Downing, J., Poisner, A.M., and Barnea, E.R. (1995). First trimester villous placenta has high prorenin and active renin concentrations. *American Journal of Obstetrics and Gynecology*, **172**, 864–7.

Eldar-Geva, T., Hochberg, A., de Groot, N., and Weinstein, D. (1995). High maternal serum chorionic gonadotropin level in Downs' syndrome pregnancies is caused by elevation of both subunits messenger ribonucleic acid level in trophoblasts. *The Journal of Clinical Endocrinology and Metabolism*, **80**, 3528–31.

Faria, T.N., Deb, S., Kwok, S.C.M., Vandeputte, M., Talamantes, F., and Soares, M.J. (1990). Transplantable rat choriocarcinoma cells express placenta lactogen: identification of placental lactogen-I immunoreactive protein and messenger ribonucleic acid. *Endocrinology*, **127**, 3131–7.

Fernandez, E., Goldberg, J., Johnson, E., Rutherford, T., and Barnea, E.R. (1994). In *Implantation and early pregnancy in humans*, (ed. E.R. Barnea, J.H. Check, J.G. Grudzinskas, and T. Maruo), pp. 355–78. Parthenon, Carnforth.

Fischer, R.L. and Wapner, R.J. (1992). Surgical therapy. In *The first twelve weeks of gestation*, (ed. E.R. Barnea, J. Hustin, and E. Jauniaux), pp. 434–50. Springer, Berlin.

Folkman, J. (1990). Introduction—endothelial cells and angiogenic growth factors in cancer growth and metastasis. *Cancer Metastasis Review*, **9**, 171–4.

Franklin, G.C., Holmgren, L., Donovan, M., Adam, G.I.R., Walsh, C., Pfeifer-Ohlsson, S., *et al.* (1993). Expression and control of PDGF stimulatory loops in the developing placenta. In *Trophoblast research*, Vol. 7, (ed. H. Schneider, P. Bischof, and R. Leiser), pp. 287–303. University of Rochester Press.

Gerbie, A.B., Hathaway, H.H., and Brewer, J.L. (1968) Autoradiographic analysis of normal trophoblastic proliferation. *American Journal of Obstetrics and Gynecology*, **100**, 640–8.

Goshen, R., Tannos, V., Ben-Rafael, Z., de Groot, N., Gonik, B., Hochberg, A.A., *et al.* (1994). The role of genomic imprinting in implantation. *Fertility and Sterility*, **62**, 903–10.

Graham, C.H., Connelly, I., MacDougall, J.R., Kerbel, R.S., Stetler-Stevenson, W.G., and Lala, P.K. (1994). Resistance of malignant trophoblast cells to both antiproliferative and antiinvasive effects of transforming growth factor-β. *Experimental Cell Research*, **214**, 93–9.

Hamilton, W.J. (ed.) (1987). *Human embryology*. Heinemann, London.

Henderson, D.J., Bennett, P.R., and Moore, G.E. (1992). Expression of human chorionic gonadotrophin α and β subunits is depressed in trophoblast from pregnancies with early pregnancy failure. *Human Reproduction*, **7**, 1474–8.

Hoffman, G.E., Drews, M.R., Scott, R.T., Navot, D., Heller, D., and Deligdish, L. (1992). Epidermal growth factor and its receptor in human implantation trophoblast: immunohistochemical evidence for autocrine/paracrine function. *The Journal of Clinical Endocrinology and Metabolism*, **74**, 981–8.

Holmgren, L., Glaser, A., Pfeifer-Ohlsson, S., and Ohlsson, R. (1991). Angiogenesis of human extraembryonic tissue involves the spatiotemporal control of PDGF ligand and receptor genes. *Development*, **113**, 749–54.

Hustin, J. (1992). The maternotrophoblastic interface: uteroplacental blood flow. In *The first twelve weeks of gestation*, (ed. E.R. Barnea, J. Hustin, and E. Jauniaux), pp. 97–110. Springer, Berlin.

Hustin, J. and Franchimont, P. (1992). The endometrium and implantation. In *The first twelve weeks of gestation*, (ed. E.R. Barnea, J. Hustin, and E. Jauniaux), pp. 26–42. Springer, Berlin.

Ioachim, H.L. and Moroson, H. (1986). Protective effect of pregnancy against transplantation of lymphoma in rats. *Journal of the National Cancer Institute*, **77**, 809–14.

Irving, J.A. and Lala, P.K. (1994). Insulin-like growth factor binding protein (IGFBP)-1 stimulates the migration of first trimester human trophoblast *in vitro*. *Clinical and Experimental Metastasis*, **12**, 58.

Jauniaux, E., Gulbis, B., Nagy, A.M., Jurkovic, D., Campbell, S., and Meuris, S. (1995). Coelomic fluid chorionic gonadotrophin protein concentrations in normal and complicated first trimester human pregnancies. *Human Reproduction*, **10**, 214–20.

Johnson, P.M. (1992). Immunology of human extraembryonic fetal membranes. In *Immunological obstetrics*, (ed. C.B. Coulam, W.P. Faulk, and J.A. McIntyre), pp. 177–88. W.W. Norton, New York.

Johnson, M.R., Abbas, A., and Nicolaides, K.H. (1994). Maternal plasma levels of human chorionic gonadotropin, oestradiol and progesterone in multifetal pregnancies before and after fetal reduction. *Journal of Endocrinology*, **143**, 309–12.

Jones, M.C., MacLeod, A.M., Dillon, D.M., and Catto, G.R. (1992). The maternal immune response. In *Immunological obstetrics*, (ed. C.B. Coulam, W.P. Faulk, and J.A. McIntyre), pp. 227–44. W.W. Norton, New York.

Karin, M. (1990). Too many transcription factors: positive and negative interactions. *New Biology*, **2**, 126–31.

Kauffman, S.A. (1992). *Origins of order: self-organization and selection in evolution*. Oxford University Press.

Kenton, P., Webb, P.D., Lister, R.K., and Johnson, P.M. (1991). Does human syncytiotro-phoblast express the M-CSF receptor/c-*fms* protein product? In *Uterine and embryonic factors in early pregnancy*, (ed. J.F. Strauss and C.R. Lyttle), pp. 195–204. Plenum, New York.

Kessel, M. and Gruss, P. (1990). Murine developmental genes. *Science*, **249**, 374–9.

Kliman, H.J. and Feinberg, R.F. (1992). Differentiation of the trophoblast. In *The first twelve weeks of gestation*, (ed. E.R. Barnea, J. Hustin, and E. Jauniaux), pp. 3–25. Springer, Berlin.

Kovats, S., Main, E.K., Libeck, C., Stubbine, M., Fisher, S.J., and DeMars, R. (1990). A class I antigen, HLA G, expressed in human trophoblasts. *Science*, **248**, 220–3.

Kovats, S., Librach, C., Fisch, P., Main, E.K., Sondel, P.M., Fisher, S., *et al.* (1991). Expression and possible function of the HLA-G alpha chain in human cytotrophoblasts. In *Cellular and molecular biology of the materno-fetal relationship*, Vol. 212, (ed. J. Chauat and J. Mowray), pp. 21–9. John Libbey Eurotext Ltd, New York.

Lala, P.K. and Lysiak, J.J. (1996). Autocrine–paracrine regulation of human placental growth and invasion by locally-active growth factors. In *Immunology of human reproduction*, (ed. M. Kurpicz and N. Fernandez). Bios Scientific Publishers, Oxford. (In press.)

Librach, C.L., Feigenbaum, S.L., Bass, K.E., Cui, T., Verastas, N., Sadovsky, Y., *et al.* (1994). Interleukin-1 β regulates human cytotrophoblast metalloproteinase activity and invasion *in vitro*. *The Journal of Biological Chemistry*, **269**, 17125–31.

Licht, P., Cao, H., Zuo, J., Lei, Z.M., Rao, Ch.V., Merz, W.E., *et al.* (1994). Lack of self-regulation of human chorionic gonadotropin biosynthesis in human choriocarcinoma cells. *The Journal of Clinical Endocrinology and Metabolism*, **78**, 1188–94.

Liotta, L.A. (1990). Introductory overview: the role of cellular proteases and their inhibitors in invasion and metastasis. *Cancer Metastasis Review*, **9**, 285–87.

Loke, Y.W. (1983). Human trophoblast in culture. In *Biology of trophoblast*, (ed. Y.W. Loke and A. Whyte), pp. 663–701. Elsevier, North Holland.

Lunardi-Iskandar, Y., Bryant, J.L., Zeman, R.A., Ham, V.H., Samaniego, F., Benier, J.M., *et al.* (1995). Tumorigenesis and metastasis of neoplastic Kaposi's sarcoma cell line in immuno-deficient mice blocked by a human pregnancy hormone. *Nature*, **375**, 64–8.

Lysiak, J.L., Connelly, I.H., Khoo, N.K.S., Stetler-Stevenson, W., and Lala, P.K. (1994). Role of transforming growth factor-α (TGF-α) and epidermal growth factor (EGF) on prolifera-tion and invasion by first trimester human trophoblast. In *Trophoblast research*, Vol. 8, (ed. R.K. Miller and H.A. Thiede), pp. 455–68. University of Rochester Press.

McMaster, M.T., Librach, C.L., Zhou, Y., Lim, Y.K.-H., Janatpour, M.J., DeMars, R., *et al.* (1995). Human placental HLA-G expression is limited to differentiated cytotrophoblasts. *Journal of Immunology*, **154**, 3771–8.

Malkin, A. (1992). Tumor markers. In *The basic science of oncology*, 2nd edn, (ed. I.F. Tannock and R.P. Hill), pp. 196–206. McGraw-Hill, New York.

Maruo, T. and Mochizuki, M. (1994). Molecular endocrine aspects in the diagnosis of gesta-tional trophoblastic diseases. In *Implantation and early pregnancy in humans* (ed E.R. Barnea, J.H. Check, J.G. Grudzinskas, and T. Maruo), pp. 485–504, Porthenon, Carnforth.

Maruo, T., Ladines-Llave, C.A., Matsuo, H., Manalo, A.S., and Mochizuki, M. (1992*a*). A novel change in cytologic localization of human chorionic gonadotropin and human placen-tal lactogen in first trimester placenta in the course of gestation. *American Journal of Obstetrics and Gynecology*, **167**, 217–22.

Maruo, T., Matsuo, H., Katayama, K., Ladines-Llave, C.A., Manalo, A.S., and Mochizuki, M. (1992*b*). In *Trophoblast research*, Vol. 7, (ed. H. Schneider, P. Bischof, and R. Leiser), pp. 251–63. University of Rochester Press.

Millan, F.A., Kondaiah, P., Denhez, F., and Akhurst, R.J. (1991). Embryonic gene expression pattern of TGF-β 1,2,3 suggest different developmental functions *in vivo*. *Development*, **111**, 131–44.

Minden, M.D. and Pawson, A.J. (1992). Oncogenes. In *The basic science of oncology*, 2nd edn, (ed. I.F. Tannock and R.P. Hill), pp. 61–87. McGraw-Hill, New York.

Mintz, B. and Fleischman, R.A. (1981). Teratocarcinomas and other neoplasms as developmental defects in gene expression. *Advances in Cancer Research*, **34**, 211–78.

Nahhas, F. and Barnea, E.R. (1990). Human embryonic origin early pregnancy factor before and after implantation. *American Journal of Reproductive Immunology*, **22**, 105–8.

Nicholson, G.L. (1988). Organ specificity of tumor metastasis: role of preferential adhesion, invasion and growth of malignant cells at specific secondary sites. *Cancer Metastasis Review*, **7**, 143–88.

Ohlsson, R., Holmgren, L., Glaser, A., Szpecht, A., and Pfeifer-Ohlsson, S. (1989). Insulin-like growth factor 2 and short-range stimulatory loops in control of human placental growth. *European Molecular Biology Organization Journal*, **8**, 1993–9.

Ohlsson, R., Franklin, G., Donovan, M., Glaser, A., Adam, G., Pfeifer-Ohlsson, S., *et al.* (1991). The molecular and cellular biology of growth stimulatory pathways during human placental development. In *Uterine and embryonic factors in early pregnancy*, (ed. J.F. Strauss and C.R. Lyttle), pp. 219–33. Plenum, New York.

Oliner, J.D., Kinzler, K.W., Meltzer, P.S., George, D.L., and Vogelstein, B. (1992). Amplification of a gene encoding a p53-associated protein in human sarcomas. *Nature*, **358**, 80–3.

Panigel, M. and Myers, R.E. (1972). Histological and ultrastructural changes in Rhesus monkey placenta following interruption of fetal placental circulation by fetectomy or interplacental umbilical vessel ligation. *Acta Anatomica*, **81**, 481–506.

Pierce, G.B. and Speers, W.C. (1988). Tumors as caricatures of the process of tissue renewal: prospects for therapy by directing differentiation. *Cancer Research*, **48**, 1996–2004.

Pines, M., Santora, A., and Spiegel, A. (1986). Effect of phorbol esters and pertussis toxin on agonist stimulated cyclic-AMP production in rat osteosarcoma cells. *Biochemical Pharmacology*, **35**, 3639–41.

Rodway, M.R. and Rao, Ch. V. (1995). A novel perspective on the role of human chorionic gonadotropin during pregnancy and in gestational trophoblastic disease. *Early Pregnancy: Biology and Medicine*, **1**, 176–87.

Sanyal, M.K., Brami, C.J., Bischof, P., Simmons, E., Barnea, E.R., Dwyer, J.M., *et al.* (1989). Immunoregulatory activity in supernatants from cultures of normal human trophoblast cells of the first trimester. *American Journal of Obstetrics and Gynecology*, **161**, 446–53.

Sanyal, M.K., Li, Y.L., Biggers, W.J., Satish, J., and Barnea, E.R. (1993). Augmentation of polynuclear aromatic hydrocarbon metabolism potential of human placental tissues of the first trimester pregnancy by cigarette smoke exposure. *American Journal of Obstetrics and Gynecology*, **168**, 1587–97.

Sariola, H., Saarma, M., Sainio, K., Arumäe, U., Palgi, J., Vaahtokari, A., *et al.* (1991). Dependence of kidney morphogenesis on the expression of nerve growth factor receptor. *Science*, **254**, 571–3.

Shimonovitz, S., Hurwitz, A., Dushnik, M., Anteby, E., Geva-Eldar, T., and Yagel, S. (1994). Developmental regulation of the expression of 72 and 92 kDa type IV collagenases in human trophoblasts: A possible mechanism for control of trophoblast invasion. *American Journal of Obstetrics and Gynecology*, **171**, 832–8.

Shurtz-Swirski, R., Simon, R.J., Cohen, Y., and Barnea, E.R. (1991). Human embryo modulates placental function in the first trimester: effects of neural tissues upon chorionic gonadotropin and progesterone secretion. *Placenta*, **12**, 521–31.

Shurtz-Swirski, R., Cohen, Y., and Barnea, E.R. (1992). Patterns of secretion of human chorionic gonadotropin by superfused placental explants and the embryo–placental relationship following maternal use of medications. *Human Reproduction*, **7**, 300–4.

Silver, R.K., Turbov, J.M., Beaird, J.A., and Golbus, J. (1990). Soluble factors produced by isolated first trimester chorionic villi directly inhibit proliferation of T cells. *American Journal of Obstetrics and Gynecology*, **163**, 1914–9.

Strowitzki, T., Rettig, I., Runkel, C., von Eye Corleta, H., and Häring, H.U. (1994). Role and regulation of growth factors in secretory endometrium: *in vitro* studies and review. In *Implantation and early pregnancy in humans*, (ed. E.R. Barnea, J.H. Check, J.G. Grudzinskas, and T. Maruo), pp. 9–28. Parthenon, Carnforth.

Szulman, A.E. (1992). Gestational trophoblastic disease: the biology of hydatidiform moles. In *Immunological obstetrics*, (ed. C.B. Coulam, W.P. Faulk, and J.A. McIntyre), pp. 479–91. W.W. Norton, New York.

Tannock, I.F. (1983). Biology of tumor growth. *Hospital Practices*, **18**, 81–93.

Tannock, I.F. (1992). Cell proliferation. In *The basic science of oncology*, 2nd edn, (ed. I.F. Tannock and R.P. Hill), pp. 154–77. McGraw-Hill, New York.

Teshima, S., Shimosato, Y., Koide, T., Kuroki, M., Kikuchi, Y., and Aizawa, M. (1983). Transplantable choriocarcinoma of rats induced by fetectomy and its biological activities. *Gann*, **74**, 205–12.

Testa, J.E. and Quigley, J.P. (1991). Reversal of misfortune: TIMP-2 inhibits tumor cell invasion. *Journal of the National Cancer Institute*, **83**, 740–2.

Ullrich, A. and Schlessinger, J. (1990). Signal transduction by receptors with tyrosine kinase activity. *Cell*, **61**, 203–12.

Wheeler, T., Elcock, C., and Anthony, F. (1995). Hypoxia increases the transcription and translation of vascular endothelial growth factor (VEGF) in cultured placental fibroblasts. *Early Pregnancy: Biology and Medicine*, **1**, 236–7.

Wolf, H.K. and Michalopolous, G.K. (1992). Proliferating cell nuclear antigen in human placenta and trophoblastic disease. *Pediatric Pathology*, **12**, 147–54.

Wood, G.A. (1994). Role of uterine cytokines in pregnancy. In *Trophoblast research*, Vol. 8, (ed. R.K. Miller and H.A. Thiede), pp. 485–501. University of Rochester Press.

Yagel, S., Eldar-Geva, T., and Solomon, H. (1993). High levels of hCG retard first trimester trophoblast invasion *in-vitro* by decreasing uPA and collagenase activities. *The Journal of Clinical Endocrinology and Metabolism*, **77**, 1506–11.

16 | *Ultrasound features of normal early pregnancy*

Katharina Gruboeck, Carolyn Paul, and Davor Jurković

INTRODUCTION

The assessment of embryonic anatomy *in vivo* has been hampered by the complexity of early development and the limited resolution of ultrasound equipment (DeCrespigny *et al.* 1988; Timor-Tritsch *et al.* 1988). The increased quality of ultrasound images has recently enabled definition of standard anatomical features of early embryonic development. The examination of the first trimester embryo is thus becoming similar to the routine 20 weeks' anomaly scan. This may open the possibility of screening for congenital anomalies in early pregnancy when termination is associated with less physical and psychological trauma to the mother (Timor-Tritsch *et al.* 1990).

The aim of this chapter is to compare embryological development with the corresponing ultrasound features, to describe normal findings and to outline the advantages and limitations of first trimester ultrasound examination.

GESTATIONAL SAC

The earliest reliable sign of pregnancy is the visualization of the gestational sac which is first seen as a ring-like structure with an echogenic rim at 4^{+3} weeks (i.e. four weeks and three days) gestation (post-menstrual age) (Yeh *et al.* 1986). (Fig. 16.1) The term 'gestational sac' refers to the chorionic cavity. The rim represents invading chorionic villi and the underlying decidual reaction. It is usually located eccentrically in the upper part of the uterine cavity. The shape of an early gestational sac is usually round up to the size of 1 cm, but as it enlarges, it acquires a more elliptic outline. A healthy gestational sac grows approximately 1 mm in diameter per day (Rossavik *et al.* 1988).

The early gestational sac contains two separate fluid-filled compartments: the amniotic and the exocoelomic (chorionic) cavity. In very early pregnancy the exocoelomic cavity predominates (Fig. 16.2). Its mean volume doubles between six and eight weeks to reach a maximum of 5–6 ml at nine weeks and then starts to decrease gradually.

Amniotic fluid is initially a dermal transudate which is gradually supplemented by fetal urine. Urine becomes the predominant component once the skin is cornified. The amniotic fluid cannot be measured before six weeks' gestational age as the amniotic

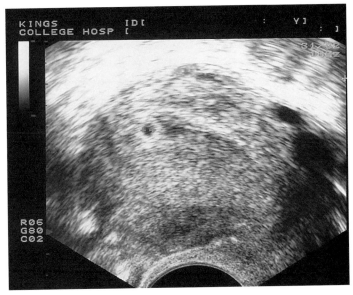

Fig. 16.1 A four week intrauterine gestational sac is shown implanted into the upper right side of the uterine cavity.

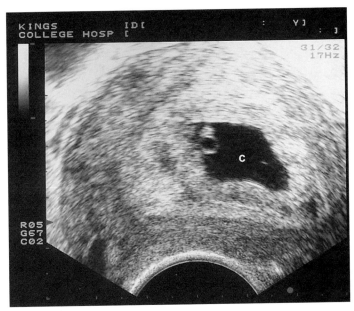

Fig. 16.2 An early pregnancy at five weeks and three days. The embryo is seen lying on top of the yolk sac. The amniotic cavity cannot be seen at this stage and the gestational sac is nearly completely taken up by the chorionic cavity (c).

cavity is not visible until seven weeks' gestation. At that time it can be visualized as a clear space alongside the fetal body. It starts to expand rapidly after that and from nine weeks onwards the amniotic sac occupies most of the gestational sac volume (Fig. 16.3). Fast expansion continues until the end of the first trimester when amniotic and chorionic membranes eventually become fused thus completely obliterating the exocoelomic cavity (Jurkovic *et al.* 1993).

Recent papers have established a normal range for gestational and amniotic sac size in early pregnancy (Grisolia *et al.* 1993; Zimmer *et al.* 1994). A linear correlation was noted between the mean diameter of both gestational and amniotic sacs and gestational age. It has been documented that an enlarged amniotic cavity in early pregnancy may indicate embryonic death (Horrow 1992). On the other hand oligohydramnios in early pregnancy is often associated with fetal malformations (Bronshtein and Blumenfeld 1991). This was confirmed by Christodoulou *et al.* (1995) who found that abnormally small gestational sacs are associated with subsequent spontaneous miscarriage in 57 per cent of cases even if fetal heart action is demonstrated.

Several studies have shown that, with modern sonographic equipment and transvaginal transducers, a gestational sac of 2–3 mm can be detected as early as four weeks and three days menstrual age (Yeh *et al.* 1986). The diagnostic value of sonographic findings can be enhanced by correlation with serum βhCG levels. The secretion of βhCG by the cells of the syncytiotrophoblast begins very early in pregnancy, before nidation is completed, and can first be detected in maternal blood eight days

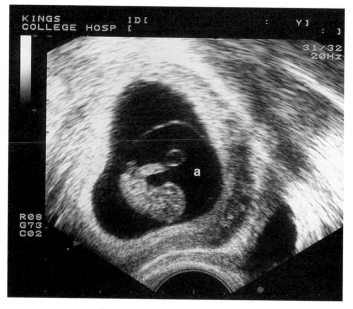

Fig. 16.3   A transverse section through an eight-week-old gestational sac showing the embryo and amniotic cavity (a) which occupies most of the gestational sac.

after ovulation. Radioimmunoassays used for the determination of βhCG levels can be calibrated against two different preparations, either the First International Reference Preparation or the Second International Standard (Bernaschek *et al.* 1988), and 1 IU/l of βhCG calibrated against the Second International Standard equals 2.2 IU/l calibrated against the First International Reference Preparation.

Knowledge of the threshold level of βhCG above which an intrauterine gestational sac should be seen is particularly important for the distinction between normal pregnancies and various forms of early pregnancy failure, including ectopic pregnancies. The level above which an intrauterine pregnancy can consistently be detected with ultrasound is called the 'discriminatory level' (Kadar *et al.* 1981). Originally this level was around 6500 IU/l but since the advent of high resolution transvaginal ultrasound examination the discriminatory zone has been defined at a new lower level. Most authors agree that a discriminatory βhCG level should be equal to or more than 1000 IU/l (First International Reference Preparation) when modern transvaginal ultrasound equipment is used (Bernaschek *et al.* 1988).

The mean doubling time of βhCG is a useful additional feature to discriminate between normal and abnormal early pregnancy. In normal pregnancies this period is approximately two days when the initial level is less than 1200 IU/l and three days between 1200 and 6000 IU/l (Speroff *et al.* 1989). In abnormal pregnancies the doubling time is prolonged (Goldstein *et al.* 1988; Bree *et al.* 1989). Falling levels of βhCG are also useful indicators, and it has been shown that the diagnosis of miscarriage is likely when its half-life is shorter than 1.4 days (Kadar and Romero 1988). The absolute level of βhCG is also useful in prediction of pregnancy outcome. Inappropriately low βhCG level in relation to the gestational sac size and embryonic crown–rump length was shown to be highly predictive of spontaneous miscarriage in pregnancies with demonstrable heart action (Christodoulou *et al.* 1995).

SECONDARY YOLK SAC

With the formation of the extraembryonic coelomic cavity at the end of SYS fourth week, the primary yolk sac is pinched off and the secondary yolk sac is formed. During organogenesis and before the placental circulation is established, the SYS is the primary source of exchange between the mother and the embryo. It has nutritive, metabolic, endocrine, immunologic, excretory, and haematopoietic functions (see Chapter 11).

At the beginning of the sixth week it becomes visible as the first structure inside the chorionic cavity. It is a circular, well defined, echo-free area, that measures 3–4 mm in diameter (Fig. 16.4). At that time the gestational sac diameter is 8–10 mm. The SYS grows slowly until it reaches a maximum diameter of approximately 6 mm at 10 weeks (Jauniaux *et al.* 1991). The vitelline duct can be followed from its origin all the way to the cord insertion (Fig. 16.5). As the gestational sac grows and the amniotic cavity expands, the SYS as an extraembryonic structure is gradually separated from the embryo. Different theories exist about the fate of the SYS. Until recently it was assumed that it disappears by the end of the 12th week due to compression by the rapidly expanding amniotic cavity. In a recent study it has been shown that the SYS

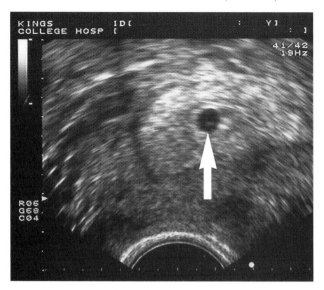

Fig. 16.4   A five week gestational sac which contains a very small yolk sac (arrow).

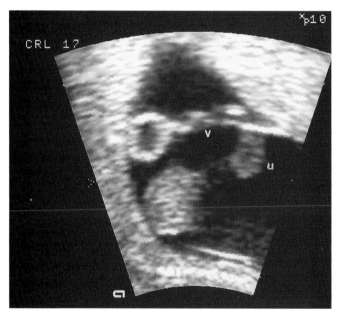

Fig. 16.5   A section through a seven week gestational sac demonstrating a yolk sac and the full length of the vitelline duct (v) and umbilical cord (u).

degenerates first and then disappears as a result of involution rather then mechanical pressure (Jauniaux *et al.* 1991). Colour Doppler studies have shown a decrease in SYS vascularity after nine weeks of gestation (Kurjak *et al.* 1994). At that time the exocoelomic cavity is still relatively large and the decrease in blood flow is unlikely to be caused by its compression.

Following the original ultrasonic descriptions of the SYS (Mantoni and Pederson 1979), it was generally considered that its appearance has little significance for the outcome of pregnancy (Crooji *et al.* 1982). An absent yolk sac in the presence of an embryo is thought to indicate an abnormal pregnancy and is usually followed by embryonic death (Levi *et al.* 1990; Lindsay *et al.* 1992). In cases of missed abortion with a visible embryo, the SYS tends to be larger and its wall is thinner than in normal pregnancies. The reason for the relatively large size of the yolk sac is not clear but it may be due to the accumulation of nutritive secretions, which are not utilized by the embryo (Ferazzi *et al.* 1988). Most studies did not show any significant correlation between size and shape of the yolk sac and pregnancy outcome (Reece *et al.* 1988; (Jauniaux *et al.* 1991); Kurtz *et al.* 1992).

EMBRYO

At four weeks the embryo consists of a bilaminar germ disc and prechordial plate. At around day 30 menstrual age the intraembryonic mesoderm starts to develop and the three layers give rise to the organs. At the beginning of the sixth week the embryo measures around 2 mm and can be demonstrated on transvaginal ultrasound (Bree *et al.* 1989). The embryonic pole is seen as a straight echogenic line, adjacent to the yolk sac and close to the connecting stalk (Fig. 16.6). Sometimes it cannot be seen clearly and the pulsation of the embryonic heart can be used as a sign of its presence.

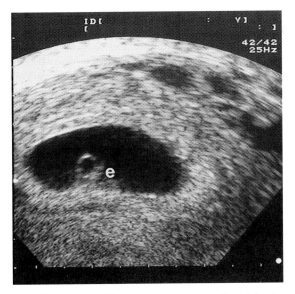

Fig. 16.6 A five-week-old embryo (e) is seen as an echogenic thickening at the periphery of the yolk sac.

The cardiac activity begins approximately at day 37 ($5^{+2}/40$) menstrual age. This corresponds to a crown–rump length of 1.5–3 mm. When the embryo reaches 5 mm in length it can be seen consistently separate from the yolk sac and all embryos of that size should have visible cardiac activity. This corresponds to a gestational age of 6^{+3} weeks gestation and a sac diameter of 15–20 mm (Goldstein *et al.* 1988).

The detection of embryonic echo is associated with normal pregnancy outcome in most patients. Goldstein (1994) has shown that when embryonic cardiac activity was visualized, subsequent pregnancy loss occurred in 7.2 per cent of patients with an embryo up to 5 mm, 3.3 per cent for an embryo between 6 and 10 mm, and only in 0.5 per cent for embryos larger than 10 mm. Therefore, the presence of a well developed embryo may be taken as a reassuring finding in all patients who are at risk of first trimester miscarriage.

Normal ranges for fetal heart rate in pregnancy have been described (Tezuka *et al.* 1991). From six to nine weeks gestation there is a rapid increase of the mean heart rate from 113 to 167 beats per minute (Van Heeswijk *et al.* 1990). After 10 weeks menstrual age the heart rate starts to decline slightly. Comparison between normally developing pregnancies and pregnancies that resulted in early miscarriage showed a late onset of cardiac activity in the latter group. Another interesting observation was a decreased heart rate in all cases that ended in spontaneous abortion (Schaats *et al.* 1990; Tezuka *et al.* 1991). Therefore fetal bradycardia in the first trimester should be considered as an indicator of poor outcome.

The embryo grows around 1 mm per day. When it reaches a crown–rump length of 12 mm at the age of 7^{+3} weeks the head can be discriminated from the torso (Fig. 16.7). The differentiation of the nervous system is the dominant phenomenon in the

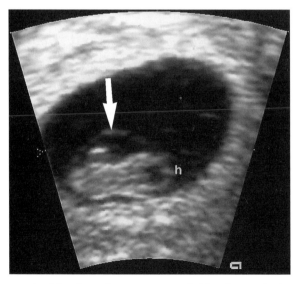

Fig. 16.7 A seven-week-old embryo is seen surrounded by the amniotic membrane (arrow). The head (h) is seen on the right and torso on the left.

early development of the embryo. With the closure of the caudal neuropore the ventricular system starts to develop. In very early pregnancy it is difficult to analyse intracranial anatomy (Cullen *et al.* 1990). Usually before seven weeks there is only one cavity recognizable on ultrasound, which used to be called the 'single ventricle' (Siedler and Filly 1987). This is the rhombencephalic cavity which is the dominant brain structure during the embryonic period (Fig. 16.8(a),(b)). In a longitudinal study of 29 patients Blaas *et al.* (1994/1995) demonstrated the development of embryonic hindbrain from seven to 12 weeks of gestation. The rhombencephalon was always visible from exactly seven weeks onwards. In embryos up to 16 mm crown–rump length, the increase in length of the rhombencephalic cavity was much faster than that of the crown–rump length. However, between 16 and 24 mm the crown–rump length grew more rapidly than the rhombencephalon, leading to a relative but not actual decrease in its size.

The cerebellum could be demonstrated for the first time at nine weeks gestation, and was visible in all embryos only after 10 weeks and 3 days (Blaas *et al.* 1995*b*) (Fig. 16.9(a), (b)) The other intracranial structures visible from seven weeks gestation are the diencephalon with its cavity, the third ventricle, the hemispheres with their

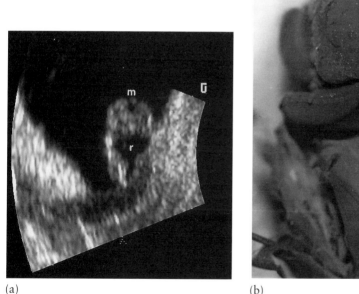

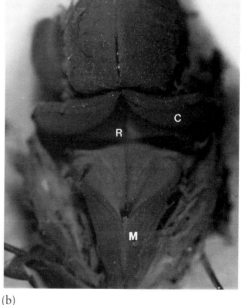

(a)   (b)

Fig. 16.8   (a) An oblique section through the embryonic head at seven weeks showing the prominent rhombencephalic cavity (r) and the mesencephalon anteriorly and above it (m). (b) A histological specimen at the same gestational age shows a large rhombencephalic cavity (R). The cavity is closed by the cerebellar lobes (c) on the top and medulla oblongata (M) at its bottom end. (Courtesy of Dr G. Moscoso, King's College Hospital, UK.)

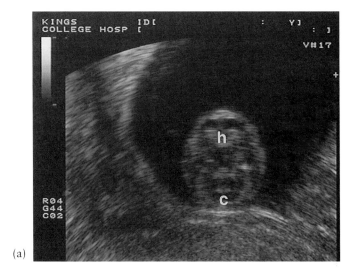

(a)

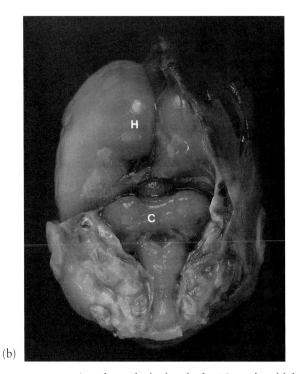

(b)

Fig. 16.9   (a) A transverse section through the head of a 10 weeks old fetus. The cerebellar lobes (c) are visualized as two bright echoes in the posterior cranial fossa. (h = hemispheres.) (b) A histological specimen at the same gestational age clearly demonstrates the cerebellum (c) and hemispheres (H) anteriorly and above it. (Courtesy of Dr G. Moscoso, King's College Hospital, UK.)

cavities, the lateral ventricles, and the mesencephalon with the aqueduct of Sylvius (Blaas *et al.* 1994/1995; Timor-Tritsch *et al.* 1992) (Fig. 16.10). At nine weeks gestation all these structures are seen in every case and can be measured. Blaas *et al.* have produced reference ranges for the size of intracranial structures in the first trimester which is the first serious attempt to standardize the morphological assessment of first trimester embryos. This opens the possibility to diagnose conditions such as holoprosencephaly or Dandy–Walker malformation which might be expected to cause sufficient distortion of intracranial anatomy to make early diagnosis possible.

During the ninth week the crown–rump length reaches approximately 2 cm and rapid changes begin in the appearance of the embryo. The upper and lower limb buds are now seen more clearly (Fig. 16.11(a), (b)). In a dorsal coronal section of the embryo the spinal canal can be seen as two parallel lines. Prolonged observation will detect the earliest embryonic movements at that time. The site of the definitive placenta is distinguishable and the umbilical cord can be traced to both its placental and embryonic attachments (Fig. 16.12). A recent study has shown that there is a relationship between the first trimester umbilical cord length and menstrual age in normal fetuses. The length of the umbilical cord is roughly equivalent to the crown–rump length. The vessels of the umbilical cord can now be seen, but not accurately counted, up to around 11 weeks. The amnion which is still closely wrapped around the embryo is now seen as an echogenic line. When the head is visualized in a sagittal plane the typical convoluted arrangement of the fetal brain becomes evident and the cavities can be imaged more clearly.

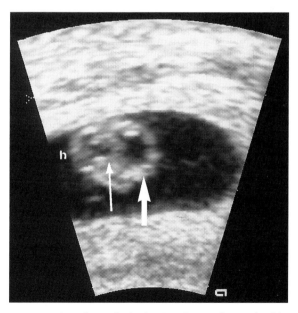

Fig. 16.10   A transverse section through the brain of an eight week old embryo showing the fourth ventricle (thick arrow), the third ventricle (thin arrow), and the hemispheres (h) anterior to it.

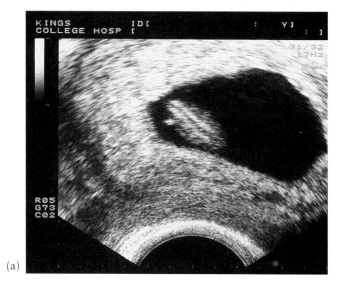

(a)

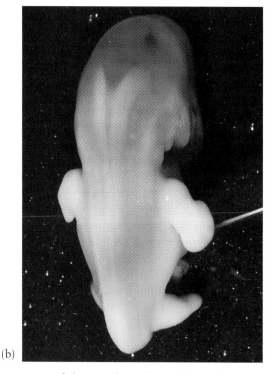

(b)

Fig. 16.11 (a) A sonogram of the spinal canal at eight weeks' gestation. (b) The spine and limbs can be identified clearly on a macroscopic specimen at similar gestational age. (Courtesy of Dr G. Moscoso, King's College Hospital, UK.)

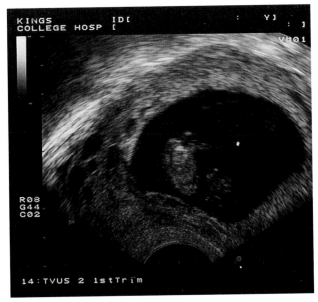

Fig. 16.12   A demonstration of the full length of the umbilical cord at 9 weeks.

At nine weeks, when the embryo measures more than 2 cm, the anterior and posterior contours can be evaluated and slight deviations from normal shape, such as nuchal thickening, is apparent (Timor-Tritsch *et al.* 1992). The assessment of the anterior contour is more important after 12 weeks. During its development the midgut rotates and grows to such an extent that it can no longer be contained in the abdominal cavity. Room is temporarily found within the umbilical cord which forms a physiological hernia of the midgut. This is visible during the 10th week as a widening of the visibly pulsating umbilical cord close to its abdominal insertion (Fig. 16.13). By the end of the 13th week the capacity of the abdomen has increased substantially thus allowing the intestine to slide back. From that time on abdominal wall defects can be detected.

At 10 weeks the development of the brain is characterized by the partition of the ventricles and their rapid and progressive growth. The lateral ventricles contain the prominently echogenic choroid plexus which are obvious features within the embryonic head during the 11th week. On the sagittal section of the head, the falx cerebri can be seen dividing the hemispheres (Achiron and Achiron 1991) (Fig. 16.14).

During weeks 10 and 11 the embryo reaches a crown–rump length of 40 mm and develops a 'human appearance'. Limb movements are apparent at this stage. The long bones, initially femur then humerus and finally tibia, fibula, radius, and ulna can consistently be visualized by the 12th week (Fig. 16.15). Stomach and urinary bladder and occasionally kidneys may also be seen at that stage. Within the brain the choroid plexi occupy around one-third of the lateral ventricle and are imaged above the level of the thalami. The foramen magnum is demonstrable close to the base of the skull (Takeuchi 1992).

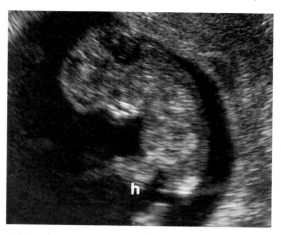

Fig. 16.13   A physiological hernia (h) at 10 weeks' gestation.

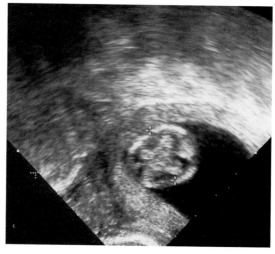

Fig. 16.14   Typical prominent appearance of the choroid plexi after 10 weeks' gestation on a transverse section.

Maxilla and mandibula are now seen in every fetus. The palate becomes visible after the closure of the posterior part is completed which occurs between weeks 12 and 14. Other additional features visible at 12 weeks are the digits of the hands and sometimes of the feet (Timor-Tritsch *et al.* 1991). Their demonstration requires patience as they are often obscured by active movement of the limbs. At the end of the 12th week, the brachiocephalic and carotid arteries are readily seen in every fetus. Intracranially the cerebellum, the thalami, and the eyes are better defined than before. Nuchal translucency measurements are more easily performed at this stage abdominally and may be used as a screening test for chromosomal defects.

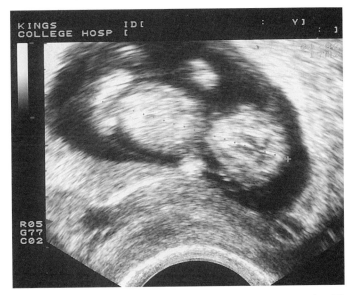

Fig. 16.15 A demonstration of all four extremities on a scan at 11 weeks. The technique of the crown–rump measurement is also demonstrated.

At 13 weeks there is only a small amount of additional information compared to 12 weeks: the toes are now more clearly seen; inside the brain the falx cerebri can be demonstrated, the frontal and the sagittal sinuses are visible, and the choroid plexus retracts from the frontal horn (Timor-Tritsch *et al.* 1989).

At 14 weeks the four-chamber view of the fetal heart can be analysed. This opens up the possibility for early detection of congenital heart defects (Gembruch *et al.* 1993).

Between weeks 12 and 14 complete ossification of the vertebrae is achieved and each vertebra can be seen separately. A sign suggestive of abnormal development of the spine in the first trimester is a widening of the echogenic lines of the vertebrae and divergence from a parallel configuration. Splitting of the vertebral column as a failure of fusion of vertebral arches can be recognized.

From that time onwards the fetus approaches a size at which most parts are lying out of range of the vaginal probe and further assessment is achieved more easily by transabdominal ultrasound examination.

MULTIPLE PREGNANCY

Multiple pregnancies are relatively uncommon in humans. The incidence of twins world-wide is one in 80 pregnancies (Benirschke and Kim 1973). However, the incidence and also the number of fetuses in multiple pregnancies has increased over the past 30 years mostly due to the increased use of stimulation of ovulation. Another factor influencing the rising rate is that more women delay their pregnancies into their thirties when the natural frequency of multifetal pregnancies is higher.

There are two different types of multiple pregnancies: dizygotic and monozygotic. Of all multiple pregnancies, 75 per cent are dizygotic. The cause of this is the shedding of two or more ova at the same time in one ovarian cycle and their fertilization by two different spermatozoa. In twins the two zygotes implant separately and two separate placentas may form with two chorions and two amnions; but in some cases the placentae may fuse to form a joint single placenta.

Monozygotic twin pregnancies occur when one fertilized ovum splits to form, eventually, two or more fetuses which will be identical. Most of the divisions occur post-implantation, usually between days four and eight, which is before the development of the amniotic cavity. This results in a monochorionic-diamniotic pregnancy. If the zygote divides between days 8 and 13, after the amniotic cavity has developed, the pregnancy will be monochorionic-monoamniotic. A zygote which divides between days 13 and 16 will result in conjoined twins, which is reported in 1 in 33 000 to 1 in 165 000 births.

Although the incidence of twin deliveries is known, it is difficult to estimate the true rate of multiple pregnancies. Ultrasound studies have shown that the frequency of twin gestations is much higher than the incidence of twin deliveries. The fact that the accurate assessment of true first trimester pregnancy loss is very difficult makes the estimation of the correct number of multiple pregnancies more arduous.

Considerably fewer twins are observed at delivery than are identified by ultrasound in the first trimester. Studies have shown that up to 50 per cent of multiple pregnancies are either reduced or lost completely during the first trimester of pregnancy, which usually presents with the symptom of vaginal bleeding (Landy *et al.* 1986).

Multifetal pregnancies are associated with significantly higher mortality and morbidity than singleton pregnancies. The perinatal mortality rate is 3–5 times higher than that of singletons and early diagnosis is therefore important for optimal antenatal management (McCarthy *et al.* 1981).

With transvaginal ultrasound the diagnosis of multiple pregnancy can be made as early as five weeks' gestation (Fig. 16.16). At that time the number of gestational sacs can be counted. The number of fetuses can be assessed at approximately six weeks, when the fetal heart starts to beat. It is not recommended to determine the number of fetuses by counting the number of yolk sacs. This may be misleading, when the cleavage of the zygote occurs late, and a single yolk sac is seen with two or more fetuses (Monteagudo *et al.* 1996).

Whilst determining chorionicity and amnionicity in the second and third trimesters can at times be quite difficult, this is relatively easy in the first trimester. If each sac contains only one fetus, the pregnancy is dichorionic and diamniotic. This diagnosis can be made as early as five weeks. If two fetuses are seen within the same gestational sac (Fig. 16.17), amnionicity cannot be determined until the eighth week of gestation. Before that time the amnion is difficult to see and the number of amniotic sacs impossible to count. At seven to eight weeks the amniotic cavity expands, which facilitates its clear identification (Monteagudo *et al.* 1996).

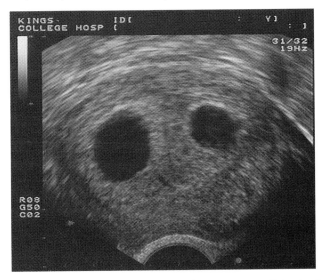

Fig. 16.16 A transverse section through the uterus demonstrates a dichorionic twin pregnancy at five weeks.

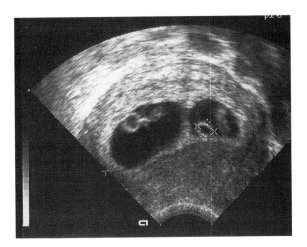

Fig. 16.17 A case of dichorionic diamniotic twins at 6 weeks. Two yolk sacs are also shown.

In monochorionic-diamniotic pregnancies a single gestational sac with amniotic cavities can be seen at seven to eight weeks. In the case of a monochorionic-monoamniotic gestation, two or more fetuses are seen within a single amniotic cavity (Fig. 16.18).

Documentation of early fetal loss in multiple gestations was difficult before the use of ultrasound. As discussed above, multiple gestational sacs can be identified by transvaginal ultrasound as early as in singleton pregnancies. However, the diagnosis of multiple pregnancy in early gestation should be made with caution. With the use of

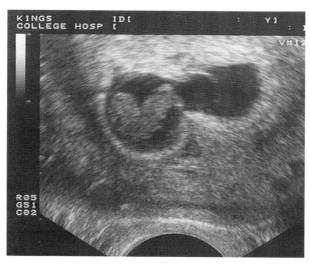

Fig. 16.18 A monoamniotic monochorionic twin pregnancy. The embryos were firmly attached to each other at the pelvic level which enabled the diagnosis of conjoined twins.

sonography in the first trimester the phenomenon of the 'vanishing twin' has been reported. It implies the disappearance of one or more gestational sacs with or without an embryo, in viable pregnancies, which have been confirmed on earlier ultrasound scans, and are not detectable on a subsequent scan. The phenomenon of the 'vanishing twin' is often associated with bleeding. However, the prognosis for the remaining fetus(es) is very good (Landy *et al.* 1986).

A few physiological conditions associated with pregnancy have a similar ultrasound appearance as multiple pregnancies and the phenomenon of the 'vanishing twin': retroplacental collection of blood, hydropic changes in chorionic villi, or decidual reaction in the second horn of a bicornuate uterus are ultrasound features which may simulate multiple gestational sacs. In doubtful cases a repeat ultrasound scan to confirm the findings is indicated to avoid false diagnosis.

BIOMETRY IN THE FIRST TRIMESTER

In embryology the gestational age is measured from the day of conception. In obstetrics, however, calculations are made from the first day of the last menstrual period, assuming a 'normal' menstrual cycle of 28 days. As less than 50 per cent of women are certain about their dates this calculation is not always accurate. Fetal growth can be monitored accurately later in pregnancy only if the exact information about gestational age is available. Therefore, every effort should be made to estimate fetal age early in pregnancy when biological variability is minimal.

The first sonographic structure that can be used for the estimation of age is the gestational sac. When the gestational sac is seen first, it measures approximately 2–3 mm in size. Due to the oval shape of the sac and the fact that it can be distorted by uterine contractions, fibroids, full bladder, or the pressure of the probe, it is best to estimate the size of the sac by measuring the mean sac diameter. The mean sac diameter is calculated by adding its longitudinal, transverse, and antero-posterior diameters and dividing them by three. The interface between the chorion and the exocoelomic fluid demonstrates the margin of the sac. Gestational sac measurements are less reliable for the assessment of gestational age than the crown–rump length. However, the sac size may be used for dating of very early pregnancies before the embryo becomes visible. Later in gestation the measurement of the gestational sac diameter allows an estimate of gestational age with a variability of ± 12–14 days (Kohorn and Kaufmann 1974).

As soon as the embryo becomes visible the gestational age can be estimated by measuring the crown–rump length. This ultrasound-based measurement was first introduced by Robinson in 1973 and although sonography has been developing rapidly ever since, the original data based on transabdominal measurements are still accepted as being very accurate (Nelson 1981). Through the advances in *in vitro* fertilization programmes it is now possible to study fetal growth without the uncertainties caused by the irregularities of menstrual cycle. However, there is still a number of factors which can affect the size of an early embryo and may cause inaccuracies in the estimation of gestational age. These are measurement errors, differences in growth rates between individuals, and the growth starting time. It has also been shown that the conventional curves constructed using optimal menstrual history tend to underestimate the gestational age by 2–3 days compared to the reference ranges constructed with a known date of conception (MacGregor *et al.* 1987).

The biological variability of the crown–rump length is small. According to some authors female fetuses might be smaller than male (Pederson 1980), and other features that can reduce the crown–rump length include diabetic pregnancies (Pederson and Molsted-Pederson 1979) and threatened abortion (Pederson and Molsted-Pederson 1989). Up to seven weeks the crown–rump length measurements are not very accurate, mainly because it is difficult to define the upper and lower ends of the embryo which lies very close to the yolk sac and the wall of the gestational sac. The ultrasound measurement of crown–rump length can therefore underestimate the true size of the embryo at early stages of pregnancy. From the end of the seventh week the crown–rump length increases by approximately 8–11 mm per week and this measurement becomes the most accurate parameter for pregnancy dating in the first trimester. Taking into account the features of early embryonic development the term 'crown–rump length' is not entirely appropriate before eight weeks of gestation. Until the embryo reaches a length of 3–4 mm it is straight and we are in fact measuring the 'greatest length'. At the embryo grows it flexes and becomes almost C-shaped. At that time the greatest length is achieved by measuring the neck–rump length. It is not until the greatest long-axis measurement reaches 18–22 mm that we approach the true crown–rump length (Goldstein 1991). To achieve accurate data it is advisable to use the average crown–rump-length (CRL) measurement from three satisfactory images. By taking only a single CRL measurement fetal age can be estimated with a 95 per cent confidence interval of 2.3–11.4 days and 95 per cent prediction interval of 9.3–15.7 days (Wisser *et al.* 1994). Some authors have shown that repeated measurements can increase the accuracy of gestational age prediction (Robinson 1993).

Although the crown–rump length is the most used parameter in the first trimester, other parameters, such as biparietal diameter, femur length, abdominal circumference, and foot length can also be used for monitoring growth. An interesting finding is that all these biometric measurements correlate better with the crown–rump length than with gestational age. This can be demonstrated even in women with certain menstrual dates. This suggests that either a wide range in the day of conception also occurs in women with certain dates, or that genetic or environmental factors already modulate growth in the first trimester. Since all these parameters correlate with the CRL, the latter measurement may be used as an index of growth as well as of gestational age.

The crown–rump length can be measured as long as the fetus can be visualized in its full length on the screen. With transvaginal probes this is up to approximately 12 weeks. From that time on other diameters such as the biparietal diameter, the femur length, or the abdominal circumference are preferable for the estimation of gestational age and growth monitoring.

CONCLUDING REMARKS

Recent improvements in ultrasound diagnosis have enabled more detailed *in vivo* studies to be made of early embryonic development. This will enable the diagnosis of many major structural defects in the first trimester of pregnancy. The detection of more subtle pathological changes such as abnormalities in placentation or embryonic growth may improve our understanding of the natural history of various pregnancy complications and help to develop new and more effective treatment strategies in the future.

REFERENCES

Achiron, R. and Achiron, A. (1991). Transvaginal ultrasonic assessment of the early fetal brain. *Ultrasound in Obstetrics and Gynecology*, **1**, 336–44.

Benirschke, K. and Kim, C.K. (1973). Multiple pregnancy (second of two parts). *New England Journal of Medicine*, **282** (25), 1329–36.

Bernaschek, G., Rudelsdorfer, R., and Csaicsich, P. (1988). Vaginal sonography versus serum human chorionic gonadotropin in early detection of pregnancy. *American Journal of Obstetrics and Gynecology*, **158**, 608–11.

Blaas, H.G., Eik-Nes, S.H., and Kiserud, D. (1994). Early development of the forebrain and midbrain: a longitudinal ultrasound study from 7 to 12 weeks of gestation. *Ultrasound in Obstetrics and Gynecology*, **4**, 183–9.

Blaas, H.G., Eik-Nes, S.H., Kiserud, T., and Hellevik, L.R. (1995). Early development of the hindbrain: a longitudinal ultrasound study from 7 to 12 weeks of gestation. *Ultrasound in Obstetrics and Gynecology*, **5**, 151–8.

Bree, R., Edwards, M., and Boehm-Velez, M. (1989). Transvaginal sonography in the evaluation of normal early pregnancy: correlation with hCG level. *American Journal of Radiology*, **153**, 75–9.

Bronshtein, M. and Blumenfeld, Z. (1991). First and early second trimester oligohydramnios—prediction of poor fetal outcome except in iatrogenic oligohydramnios post chorionic villus biopsy. *Ultrasound in Obstetrics and Gynecology*, 1, 245–7.

Christodoulou, C., Zonas, C., Lukaides, T., Maniatias, A., Giannikos, L., Giannakopoilos, C., and Fassoula, M. (1995). Low βhCG is associated with poor prognosis in association with an embryo with positive cardiac activity. *Ultrasound in Obstetrics and Gynecology*, 5, 267–9.

Crooji, M.J., Westhuis, M., and Shoemaker, J. (1982). Ultrasonographic measurement of the yolk sac. *British Journal of Obstetrics and Gynaecology*, 89, 931–4.

Cullen, M.T., Green, J., and Whetham, J. (1990). Transvaginal ultrasonographic detection of congenital anomalies in the first trimester. *American Journal of Obstetrics and Gynecology*, 163, 466–70.

DeCrespigny, L., Cooper, D., and McKenna, M. (1988). Early detection of intrauterine pregnancy with ultrasound. *Journal of Ultrasound Medicine*, 7, 7–11.

Ferrazzi, E., Brambati, B., and Lanzani, A. (1988). The yolk sac in early pregnancy failure. *American Journal of Obstetrics and Gynecology*, 158, 137–41.

Gembruch, U., Knoepfle, G., Bald, R., and Hansmann, M. (1993). Early diagnosis of fetal congenital heart disease by transvaginal echocardiography. *Ultrasound in Obstetrics and Gynecology*, 3, 310–17.

Goldstein, S. (1991). Embryonic ultrasonographic measurements: crown–rump length revisited. *American Journal of Obstetrics and Gynecology*, 165, 497–9.

Goldstein, S. (1994). Embryonic death in early pregnancy: a new look at the first trimester. *Obstetrics and Gynecology*, 84, 294–9.

Goldstein, S., Synder, J., Watson, C., and Danon, M. (1988). Very early pregnancy detection with endovaginal ultrasound. *Obstetrics and Gynecology*, 72, 200–4.

Grisolia, G., Milano, V., and Pilu, G. (1993). Biometry of early pregnancy with transvaginal sonography. *Ultrasound in Obstetrics and Gynecology*, 3, 403–11.

Horrow, M. (1992). Enlarged amniotic cavity: a new sonographic sign of early embryonic death. *American Journal of Radiology*, 158, 359–62.

Jauniaux, E., Jurkovic, D., Henriet, Y., Rodesch, F. and Hustin, I. (1991). Development of the secondary human yolk sac: correlation of sonographic and anatomical features. *Human Reproduction*, 6, 1160–5.

Jurkovic, D., Jauniaux, E., Campbell, S., Pandya, P., Cardy, D., and Nicolaides, K. (1993). Coelocentesis: a new technique for early prenatal diagnosis. *Lancet*, 341, 1623–4.

Kadar, N. and Romero, R. (1988). Further observation on serial hCG patterns in ectopic pregnancy and abortions. *Fertility and Sterility*, 50, 367–71.

Kadar, N., DeVore, G., and Romero, R. (1981). Discriminatory hCG zone: its use in the sonographic evaluation of ectopic pregnancy. *Obstetrics and Gynecology*, 58, 156–60.

Kohorn, E.I. and Kaufman, M. (1974). Sonar in the first trimester of pregnancy. *Obstetrics and Gynecology*, 44, 473–9.

Kurjak, A., Kupesic, S., and Kostovic, L. (1994). Vascularization of yolk sac and vitteline duct in normal pregnancies studied by transvaginal colour and pulsed Doppler. *Journal of Perinatal Medicine*, 22, 433–40.

Kurtz, A.B., Needleman, L., and Pennell, R.G. (1992). Can detection of the yolk sac in the first trimester be used to predict the outcome of pregnancy? A prospective sonographic study. 158, 843–6.

Landy, H.J., Weiner, S., Corson, S.L., Batzer, F.R., and Bolgonese, R.J. (1986). The 'vanishing twin': ultrasonographic assessment of fetal disappearance in the first trimester. *American Journal of Obstetrics and Gynecology*, 155, 14–19.

Levi, C.S., Lyons, E.A., and Lindsay, D.J. (1988). Early diagnosis of non-viable pregnancy with endovaginal ultrasound. *Radiology*, 167, 383–7.

Levi, C.S., Lyons, E.A., and Zheng, X.H. (1990). Endovaginal US: demonstration of cardiac activity in embryos of less than 5 mm in crown–rump length. *Radiology*, 176, 71–6.

Lindsay, D.J., Lovett, I.S., and Lyons, E.A. (1992). Yolk sac diameter and shape at endovaginal ultrasound: predictors of pregnancy outcome in the first trimester. *Radiology*, **183**, 115–19.

McCarthy, B.J., Sachs, B.P., Layde, P.M., Burton, A., Terry, J.S., and Rochat, R. (1981). The epidemiology of neonatal death in twins. *American Journal of Obstetrics and Gynecology*, **141**, 252–6.

MacGregor, S.N., Tamure, R.K., Sabbagha, R.E., Minogue, J.P., Gibson, M.E., and Hoffman, D.I. (1987). Underestimation of gestational age by conventional crown–rump length dating curves. *Obstetrics and Gynecology*, **70**, 344–8.

Mantoni, M. and Pederson, J.F. (1979). Ultrasound visualization of the human yolk sac. *Journal of Clinical Ultrasound*, **7**, 459–64.

Monteagudo, A., Haberman, S., and Timor-Tritsch, I. (1996). The diagnosis of multiple pregnancy in the first trimester. In *Ultrasound and early pregnancy*, (ed. D. Jurkovic, and E. Jauniaux, pp. 19–30. Parthenon, London.

Nelson, L.H. (1981). Comparison of methods for determining crown–rump measurement by real-time ultrasound. *Journal of Clinical Ultrasound*, **9**, 67–70.

Pederson, J.F. (1980). Ultrasound evidence of sexual difference in fetal size in first trimester. *British Medical Journal*, **281**, 1253–4.

Pederson, J.F. and Molsted-Pederson, L. (1979). Early growth retardation in diabetic pregnancy. *British Medical Journal*, **1**, 18–21.

Pederson, J.F. and Molsted-Pederson, L. (1981). Early fetal growth delay detected by ultrasound marks increased risk of congenital malformation in diabetic pregnancy. *British Medical Journal*, **283**, 269–72.

Reece, E.A., Scioscia, A.L., and Pinter, E. (1988). Prognostic significance of the human yolk sac assessed by ultrasonography. *American Journal of Obstetrics and Gynecology*, **159**, 1191–4.

Robinson, H.P. (1973). Sonar measurement of the fetal crown–rump length as a means of assessing maturity in the first trimester of pregnancy. *British Medical Journal*, **4**, 28–30.

Robinson, H.P. (1993). Gestational age determination: first trimester. In *Ultrasound in obstetrics and gynecology*, (ed. F.A. Chervenak, G.L. Isaacson, and S. Campbell), pp. 295–304. Little, Brown and Co., Boston.

Rossavik, I., Torjusen, G., and Gibbons, W. (1988). Conceptual age and ultrasound measurements of gestational sac and crown–rump length in *in vitro* fertilization pregnancies. *Fertility and Sterility*, **49**, 1012–15.

Schats, R., Jansen, C., and Wladimiroff, J. (1990). Embryonic heart activity: appearance and development in early human pregnancy. *British Journal of Obstetrics and Gynaecology*, **97**, 989–93.

Siedler, D. and Filly, R. (1987). Relative growth of the higher fetal brain structures. *Journal of Ultrasound Medicine*, **6**, 573–8.

Speroff, L., Gloss, R., and Kase, N. (1989). *Clinical gynaecologic endocrinology and infertility*, pp. 329–45. Williams and Wilkins, Baltimore.

Takeuchi, H. (1992). Transvaginal ultrasound in the first trimester of pregnancy. *Early Human Development*, **29**, 381–7.

Tezuka, N., Satoshi, S., Kanasugi, H., and Hiroi, M. (1991). Embryonic heart rates: development in early first trimester and clinical evaluation. *Gynecological and Obstetrical Investigation*, **32**, 210–15.

Timor-Tritsch, I., Farine, D., and Rosen, M. (1988). A close look at early embryonic development with the high-frequency transvaginal transducer. *American Journal of Obstetrics and Gynecology*, **159**, 676–82.

Timor-Tritsch, I.E., Warren, W.B., and Preisner, D.B. (1989). First trimester midgut-herniation: a high-frequency transvaginal sonographic study. *American Journal of Obstetrics and Gynecology*, **161**, 831–5.

Timor-Tritsch, I., Peiner, D., and Raju, S. (1990). Sonoembryology: an organ-orientated approach using a high frequency vaginal probe. *Journal of Clinical Ultrasound*, **18**, 286–90.

Timor-Tritsch, I.E., Monteagudo, A., and Warren, W.B. (1991). Transvaginal ultrasonographic definition of the central nervous system in the first and early second trimesters. *American Journal of Obstetrics and Gynecology*, **164**, 497–503.

Timor-Tritsch, I.E., Monteagudo, A., and Peisner, D.B. (1992). High-frequency transvaginal sonographic examination for the potential malformation assessment of the 9-week to 14-week fetus. *Journal of Clinical Ultrasound*, **20**, 231–5.

Van Heeswijk, M., Nijhuis, J., and Hollanders, H. (1990). Fetal heart rate in early pregnancy. *Early Human Development*, **22**, 151–4.

Wisser, J., Dirschedl, P., and Krone, S. (1994). Estimation of gestational age by transvaginal sonographic measurement of greatest embryonic length in dated human embryos. *Ultrasound in Obstetrics and Gynecology*, **4**, 457–62.

Yeh, H., Godman, J., Carr, L., and Rabinowitz, J. (1986). Intradecidual sign: A US criterion of early intrauterine pregnancy. *Radiology*, **161**, 463–7.

Zimmer, E., Chao, C., and Santos, R. (1994). Amniotic sac, fetal heart area, fetal curvature and other morphometrics using first trimester vaginal ultrasonography and color Doppler imaging. *Journal of Ultrasound Medicine*, **13**, 685–91.

17 | Embryo reduction: new model to study early pregnancy endocrinology

A. Abbas, N.J. Sebire, and K.H. Nicolaides

INTRODUCTION

In the past two decades with the increasing availability of assisted reproductive technologies the rate of triplet and other higher order multiple pregnancies has risen dramatically. Such multifetal pregnancies are associated with a high risk of perinatal death, mainly due to preterm delivery, and therefore iatrogenic embryo reduction has become one of the options in their management.

In multifetal pregnancies undergoing embryo reduction there is a procedure-related risk of spontaneous abortion, which usually occurs within two weeks of the intervention and with a frequency of about 1–2 per cent; this is similar to that of amniocentesis or chorion villus sampling. However, there is a persisting risk of spontaneous abortion or severe preterm delivery which is much higher than in spontaneously conceived twins. For example, the prevalence of preterm delivery before 32 weeks of gestation is about 1 per cent in singleton pregnancies, 10 per cent in twins, and 30 per cent in triplets (DOH 1993); in multifetal pregnancies reduced to twins the prevalence is about 15 per cent (Evans *et al.* 1994).

A possible explanation for spontaneous miscarriage or severe preterm delivery several months after embryo reduction is the development of an inflammatory response to the resorbing dead feto-placental tissue with release of cytokines and stimulation of prostaglandins. Alternatively, in the human the maximum capacity of the endometrium/decidua to maintain a pregnancy is achieved with twins; in multifetal pregnancies there is crowding and each fetal–placental–endometrial unit has less potential for growth and development than in twin pregnancies. After embryo reduction the surviving twins remain at a disadvantage compared with natural twins and this is manifested as spontaneous abortion or severely preterm delivery.

This chapter investigates these concepts by examining the effects of multifetal pregnancy on the levels of fetal, placental, deciduo-endometrial, and ovarian products in the maternal circulation, before and after embryo reduction.

EMBRYO REDUCTION

The most commonly used technique for embryo reduction is ultrasound-guided intracardiac injection of potassium chloride, which results in immediate cessation of cardiac activity. This procedure, which is carried out at 8–12 weeks of gestation, usually aims to reduce the pregnancy to twins. During the three to four months following reduction there is resorption of the dead fetuses and their placentas.

ENDOMETRIAL PRODUCTS

The major protein products of the endometrium/decidua of early pregnancy are placental protein 14 (PP14) and placental protein 12 or insulin-like growth factor binding protein 1 (IGF-BP1). These proteins were originally isolated by Bohn (1985) from extracts of whole placentae and were therefore called placental proteins. However, it is now clear that they arise from the maternal endometrium rather than the fetal trophoblast. The biological functions of PP14 are uncertain but it may play a role in the immunomodulation of early pregnancy. IGF-BP1 may be a paracrine regulator of placental growth. The amniotic fluid levels of these proteins are about 100 times higher than those in maternal blood, but the highest levels are observed in the extraembryonic coelom (See Chapter 13).

Singleton pregnancies

In singleton pregnancies plasma levels of PP14 and IGF-BP1 rise with gestation to reach a peak at about 10 and 20 weeks respectively. Subsequently, the levels of PP14 decline with gestation, whereas the levels of IGF-BP1 do not change (Figs 17.1 and 17.2). The differences between the two glycoproteins reflect the fact that PP14 is synthesized exclusively by the decidua (Julkumen et al. 1986) and therefore the levels reflect the functional decline of this tissue in the second trimester. In contrast, IGF-BP1 is also secreted by extrauterine tissues and high levels are maintained throughout pregnancy (Chard and Grudzinskas 1992).

Multiple pregnancies

Maternal plasma IGF-BP1 and PP14 in twin pregnancies are higher than those in singletons (Figs 17.1 and 17.2), but the levels are not further increased with larger numbers of fetuses (Abbas et al. 1994a). These findings suggest that the maximum secretory capacity of the endometrium is achieved with twin pregnancies.

Multifetal pregnancies after embryo reduction

In multifetal pregnancies that are reduced to twins, maternal plasma PP14 and IGF-BP1 concentrations decrease to levels characteristic of singleton rather than twin pregnancies (Figs 17.3 and 17.4).

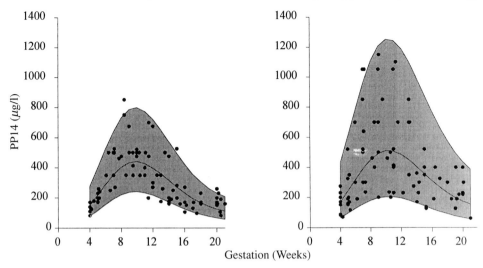

Fig. 17.1 Maternal plasma PP14 in singleton (left) and twin (right) pregnancies with gestation (mean, 5th, and 95th centiles).

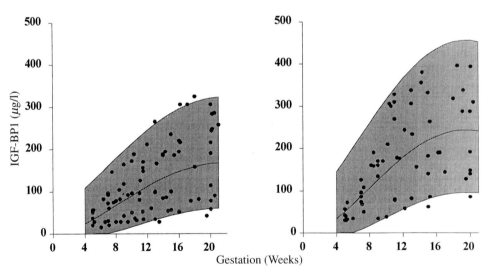

Fig. 17.2 Maternal plasma IGF-BP1 in singleton (left) and twin (right) pregnancies with gestation (mean, 5th, and 95th centiles).

The most likely explanation for these findings is that following reduction, there is degeneration of decidua adjacent to the dead feto-placental units making the plasma levels dependent on the surface area of remaining decidua. An alternative explanation is that decidual secretory function is dependent on other pregnancy hormones, such as oestradiol and progesterone, and the decrease in decidual products is secondary to the decrease in placental steroids observed after fetal reduction (see later).

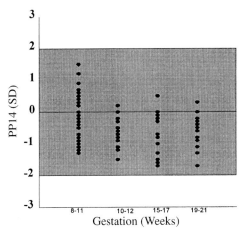

Fig. 17.3 Maternal plasma PP14 in multifetal pregnancies immediately before embryo reduction to twins at 8–11 weeks and subsequent visits at 10–12 weeks, 15–17 weeks, and 19–21 weeks. Individual values are expressed as standard deviations (SD) from normal mean for gestation.

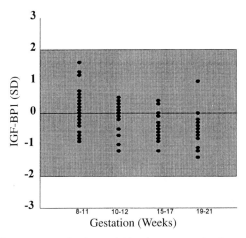

Fig. 17.4 Maternal plasma IGF-BP1 in multifetal pregnancies immediately before embryo reduction to twins at 8–11 weeks and subsequent visits at 10–12 weeks, 15–17 weeks, and 19–21 weeks. Individual values are expressed as standard deviations (SD) from normal mean for gestation of twin pregnancies.

PLACENTAL PRODUCTS

Pregnancy associated plasma protein A (PAPP-A)

This is a glycoprotein which is both placental and decidual in origin and the maximum secretory capacity is determined by both sources (Lin *et al.* 1976; Schindler *et al.* 1984; Roseu 1986). Circulating levels of PAPP-A are detected from 28 days after conception and increase throughout pregnancy (Bischof 1989). The biological functions of PAPP-A are thought to be immunomodulatory and control of haematological events such as haemostatic mechanisms in pregnancy.

Pregnancy-specific β1-glycoprotein (SP1)

This belongs to a large family of glycoproteins that are closely related to the carcinoembryonic antigen family (Chou and Plouzek 1991). SP1 is produced by the syncytiotrophoblast and it is detectable in maternal blood from as early as six days after ovulation (Gordon *et al.* 1977). Levels increase with gestation but reach a plateau at around the 35th week, corresponding to the period in gestation when there is a diminishing rate of placental growth.

Human chorionic gonadotrophin (hCG)

This is a glycoprotein produced by syncytiotrophoblast and is detectable in maternal blood from 10 days after fertilization. The levels then rise to a peak at around 10 weeks and subsequently decline to until 18 weeks, remaining fairly constant thereafter until term.

Oestradiol

This is one of the classical ovarian oestrogens (oestrone, oestradiol, and oestriol). During the normal menstrual cycle the principal sources of oestradiol are the granulosa cells and the corpus luteum. In pregnancy oestradiol is primarily produced by the corpus luteum during the first six weeks of gestation, by both the corpus luteum and placenta at 7–10 weeks and by the placenta only after this. The androgen compounds utilized for oestrogen synthesis in human pregnancy are, in the early months of gestation, derived from the maternal blood stream but near term, about 50 per cent of oestradiol produced in placenta arises from the utilization of maternal plasma dehydroepiandrosterone (DHEA) sulphate and 50 per cent arises from fetal plasma DHEA sulphate. The maternal plasma concentration rises progressively throughout gestation and the rate limiting step in determining the level of oestradiol is conversion of its precursors in the placenta (Madden *et al.* 1976).

Progesterone

In the non-pregnant female, progesterone is synthesized mainly by the adrenals and ovaries. As with oestradiol, during pregnancy, the placenta is the major source of progesterone after a transition period of shared function between it and the corpus luteum at the 7–10th weeks of gestation (Csapo *et al.* 1973). The placenta utilizes precursors from mother or fetus but the massive amount of progesterone produced in pregnancy depends mainly on maternal–placental cooperation. The maternal plasma progesterone concentration increases with gestational age and reaches a plateau at 36 weeks gestation. The biological effects of progesterone are to prepare the reproductive system for the support of pregnancy and to provide nourishment to the conceptus, suppression of the maternal immunological response to fetal antigens, and may have a role in control of parturition.

Singleton and multiple pregnancies

In twin pregnancies the circulating maternal serum concentrations of PAPP-A, SP1, hCG, oestradiol, and progesterone are higher than in singleton pregnancies (Figs 17.5–17.9) and in all, except PAPP-A, the levels increase with number of fetuses present. However, the relationship between the maternal concentrations and fetal number is not linear, suggesting that either the supply of substrate for the synthesis of these placental products cannot increase in proportion to the number of fetuses, or steroid metabolism by the liver is correspondingly increased leading to increased clearance. Unlike the other hormones that are mainly placental in origin, PAPP-A is a deciduo-placental product and the maximum maternal serum levels are reached with twins, suggesting that the maximum secretory capacity of the decidua is reached in twin pregnancies.

Multifetal pregnancies after embryo reduction

Maternal serum levels of PAPP-A, SP1, hCG, oestradiol, and progesterone in multi-fetal pregnancies after embryo reduction to twins are compared with levels in control twin pregnancies in Figs 17.10–17.14.

During a 10–12 week period following multifetal pregnancy reduction to twins there is a relative decrease in the maternal levels of all hormones. However, there are

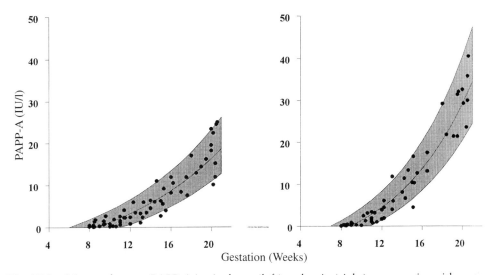

Fig. 17.5 Maternal serum PAPP-A in singleton (left) and twin (right) pregnancies with gestation (mean, 5th, and 95th centiles).

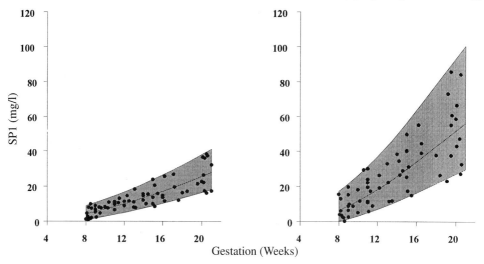

Fig. 17.6 Maternal serum SP1 in singleton (left) and twin (right) pregnancies with gestation (mean, 5th, and 95th centiles).

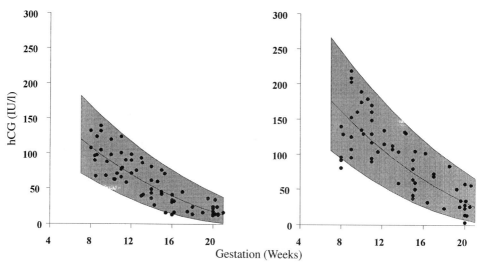

Fig. 17.7 Maternal plasma hCG in singleton (left) and twin (right) pregnancies with gestation (mean, 5th, and 95th centiles).

differences in the pattern of this decrease. Thus, compared to mean values obtained with control twins the levels of PAPP-A remained higher, SP1 and hCG decreased to similar levels, whereas progesterone and oestradiol fell to below normal values (Johnson *et al.* 1994a; Abbas *et al.* 1995).

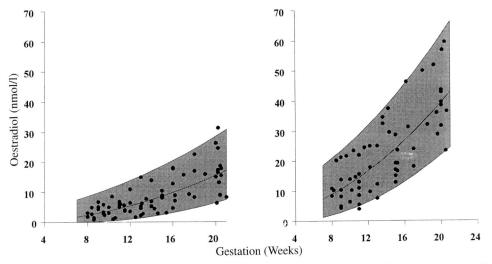

Fig. 17.8 Maternal plasma oestradiol in singleton (left) and twin (right) pregnancies with gestation (mean, 5th, and 95th centiles).

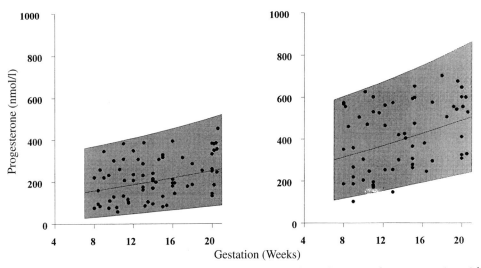

Fig. 17.9 Maternal plasma progesterone in singleton (left) and twin (right) pregnancies with gestation (mean, 5th, and 95th centiles).

The pattern of change in SP1 and hCG (both pure placental products) suggests that after multifetal pregnancy reduction the residual placental function is similar to that in normal twins. The persistence of high levels of PAPP-A during the 12 week period following reduction may be the consequence of its longer half-life compared

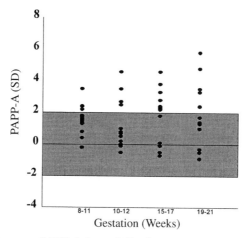

Fig. 17.10 Maternal serum PAPP-A in multifetal pregnancies immediately before embryo reduction to twins at 8–11 weeks and subsequent visits at 10–12 weeks, 15–17 weeks, and 19–21 weeks. Individual values are expressed as standard deviations (SD) from normal mean for gestation of twin pregnancies.

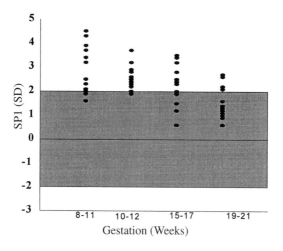

Fig. 17.11 Maternal serum SP1 in multifetal pregnancies immediately before embryo reduction to twins at 8–11 weeks and subsequent visits at 10–12 weeks, 15–17 weeks, and 19–21 weeks. Individual values are expressed as standard deviations (SD) from normal mean for gestation of twin pregnancies.

to SP1 (Bohn 1974; Lim *et al.* 1976), or continuing production from extraplacental sources.

The fall in circulating progesterone and oestradiol concentrations to levels below those of control twins suggests that placental function in the residual twins is less

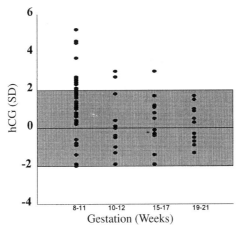

Fig. 17.12 Maternal plasma hCG in multifetal pregnancies immediately before embryo reduction to twins at 8–11 weeks and subsequent visits at 10–12 weeks, 15–17 weeks, and 19–21 weeks. Individual values are expressed as standard deviations (SD) from normal mean for gestation of twin pregnancies.

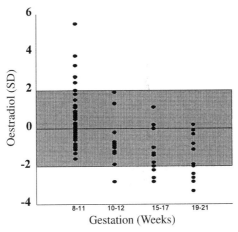

Fig. 17.13 Maternal plasma oestradiol in multifetal pregnancies immediately before embryo reduction to twins at 8–11 weeks and subsequent visits at 10–12 weeks, 15–17 weeks, and 19–21 weeks. Individual values are expressed as standard deviations (SD) from normal mean for gestation of twin pregnancies.

than in normal twins; but this impairment would have to be limited to steroid synthesis by the placenta as the levels of SP1 and hCG following reduction are equivalent to those of normal twins. Alternatively, fetal reduction reduces the rate of release of progesterone and oestradiol to that of normal twins, but the circulating levels may be further decreased because of increased metabolism by the maternal liver; in multifetal

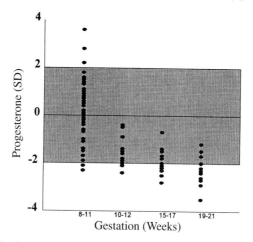

Fig. 17.14 Maternal plasma progesterone in multifetal pregnancies immediately before embryo reduction to twins at 8–11 weeks and subsequent visits at 10–12 weeks, 15–17 weeks, and 19–21 weeks. Individual values are expressed as standard deviations (SD) from normal mean for gestation of twin pregnancies.

pregnancies maternal steroid metabolism is increased and this increase persists following fetal reduction. Such an increase in hepatic enzyme activity has indeed been described in response to oestrogens (Song and Kappas 1968).

PURE OVARIAN PRODUCTS

Relaxin

This is a polypeptide hormone produced primarily by the human corpus luteum of pregnancy, although it has also been identified in placenta, decidua, and chorion (Weiss *et al.* 1978; Fields and Larkin 1981; Lopez-Bernal *et al.* 1987). The maternal serum concentration rises during the first trimester and although levels decline in the second trimester, appreciable relaxin secretion continues throughout pregnancy (quagliareuo *et al.* 1979; Eddic *et al.* 1986). In the human the function of relaxin is not known but there is some evidence suggesting that it may influence the time of onset and progression of labour possibly via its ability to promote cervical ripening (MacLennan *et al.* 1986), modulate myometrial contractility (Johnson *et al.* 1992), and initiate the release of collagenases from the fetal membranes (Koay *et al.* 1983).

Singleton and multiple pregnancies

The pattern of change in maternal serum concentration of relaxin with gestation is similar to that of hCG (Johnson *et al.* 1994*b*) and the levels increase with the number of fetuses (Fig. 17.15).

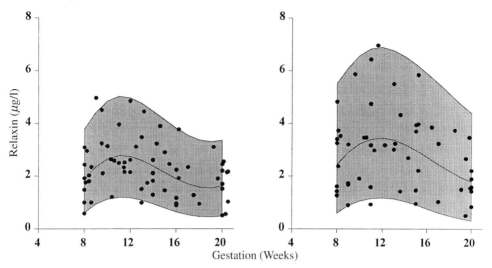

Fig. 17.15 Maternal plasma relaxin in singleton (left) and twin (right) pregnancies with gestation (mean, 5th, and 95th centiles).

Changes following multifetal pregnancy reduction

Fetal reduction does not affect plasma relaxin levels (Fig. 17.16). This finding suggests that although the fetus has a luteotrophic influence on the synthesis of relaxin this effect is imprinted during the first few weeks of pregnancy and is subsequently not affected by iatrogenic death of some of the fetuses (Johnson *et al.* 1992) Persistence of high levels of relaxin may offer an explanation for the increased risk of severe preterm delivery of multifetal pregnancies despite reduction to twins, which is higher than in normal twins.

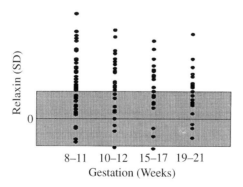

Fig. 17.16 Maternal plasma relaxin in multifetal pregnancies immediately before embryo reduction to twins at 8–11 weeks and subsequent visits at 10–12 weeks, 15–17 weeks, and 19–21 weeks. Individual values are expressed as standard deviations (SD) from normal mean for gestation of twin pregnancies.

PURE FETAL PRODUCTS

Alpha-fetoprotein

Alpha-fetoprotein (AFP) is an albumin-like polypeptide originally produced in the yolk sac and subsequently in the fetal liver and gastrointestinal tract (Gitlin 1975). The mechanisms which control the synthesis of AFP remain unknown but in the fetus, AFP serves an oncotic function similar to that of albumin in the adult. The concentration of AFP in fetal serum rises rapidly with gestation to a peak at 12–14 weeks and falls thereafter; the fall continues in the neonatal period reaching adult levels at eight months of age. The amniotic fluid concentration of AFP decreases with gestation from a peak in the first trimester. Transfer of AFP to the maternal circulation is achieved either directly from the fetal circulation across the placenta, or by absorption from the amniotic fluid. Maternal AFP levels rise with gestation to peak at 32 weeks and then decrease towards term.

Singleton and multiple pregnancies

At 8–20 weeks, maternal serum AFP levels rise with gestation and are proportional to the number of fetuses (Fig. 17.17).

Changes following multifetal pregnancy reduction

Following the iatrogenic death of fetuses in multifetal pregnancies there is an increase in maternal serum AFP (Fig. 17.18) which persisted for at least eight weeks (Abbas

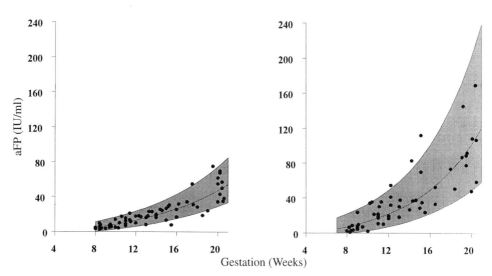

Fig. 17.17 Maternal serum AFP in singleton (left) and twin (right) pregnancies with gestation (mean, 5th, and 95th centiles).

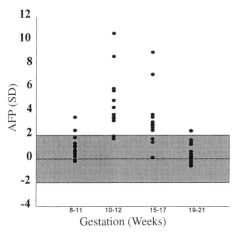

Fig. 17.18 Maternal serum AFP in multifetal pregnancies immediately before embryo reduction to twins at 8–11 weeks and subsequent visits at 10–12 weeks, 15–17 weeks, and 19–21 weeks. Individual values are expressed as standard deviations (SD) from normal mean for gestation of twin pregnancies.

et al. 1994*b*). Subsequently, maternal serum AFP levels decreased and by 12 weeks following reduction the levels were within the normal range for twins. Previous reports have also documented high levels of AFP in the amniotic fluid of twin pregnancies after the spontaneous death of one of the fetuses (Bass *et al.* 1986; Streit *et al.* 1989) and in multifetal pregnancies after reduction (Grau *et al.* 1990). Similarly, spontaneous fetal death (Seppälä and Ruoslahti 1973) and disruption in the feto-placental barrier (Blackmore *et al.* 1986) are associated with high maternal serum AFP levels.

The temporary rise in maternal serum AFP following reduction is unlikely to be purely the consequence of disruption in the feto-maternal barrier and chronic leakage from the live fetuses to the mother across the placenta because the half life of AFP in the maternal circulation is only 4–5 days (Seppälä and Ruoslahti 1973). Additionally, there was a significant association between maternal serum AFP and the number of dead fetuses. Therefore the most likely explanation is increased concentration of AFP in the amniotic fluid due to tissue breakdown from the dead fetuses which is slowly absorbed systemically. Maternal serum AFP returns to the normal range 8–12 weeks after the reduction because, by this time, there has been complete resorption of the dead fetuses.

CONCLUDING REMARKS

Changes in the maternal blood levels of the various hormones following multifetal pregnancy reduction can be explained according to the site of production and control of the products. The maximum secretory capacity of the endometrium may be achieved with twin pregnancies; therefore in multifetal pregnancies reduced to twins, levels of the endometrial products IGF-BP1 and PP14 decrease to levels characteristic of singleton rather than normal twin pregnancies. The persistence of high levels of PAPP-A, a placental–decidual product, following reduction may be the consequence of its long half-life or continuing production from extraplacental sources. The maternal levels of the placental products hCG and SP-1, which are initially related to the number of fetuses, fall to those of twin pregnancies after reduction. Oestrogen and progesterone are also placental products but decrease in maternal levels following reduction to levels lower than in normal twins, may be the consequence of persistent increase in their metabolism. Levels of relaxin, an ovarian product, increase with the number of fetuses, but following reduction to twins the levels do not change, presumably because relaxin is a product of the corpus luteum whose function is unaffected by feto-placental death. In the case of AFP, fetal reduction was associated with an increase in maternal levels which persisted for at least eight weeks; the most likely explanation for this is that AFP, which is stored in fetal tissues, is released into the amniotic fluid during tissue breakdown, from where it is absorbed into the maternal circulation.

REFERENCES

Abbas, A., Johnson, M.R., Chard, T., and Nicolaides, K.H. (1994*a*). Maternal plasma concentrations of insulin-like growth factor binding protein-1 and placental protein 14 in multifetal pregnancies before and after fetal reduction. *Human Reproduction*, **10**, 207.

Abbas, A., Johnson, M.R., Bersinger, N., and Nicolaides, K.H. (1994*b*). Maternal serum alpha-fetoprotein in multifetal pregnancies before and after fetal reduction. *British Journal of Obstetrics and Gynaecology*, **101**, 156.

Abbas, A., Sebire, N.J., Johnson, M., Bersinger, N., and Nicolaides, K.H. (1996). Maternal serum concentrations of pregnancy-associated placental protein-A and pregnancy-specific B-1-glycoprotein in multiform pregnancy before and after fetal reaction. *Human reproduction* 1996: 11:4: 900–02.

Bass, H.N., Oliver, J.B., and Srinivasan, M. (1986). Persistently elevated AFP and AChE in amniotic fluid from a normal fetus following the demise of its twin. *Prenatal Diagnosis*, **6**, 33.

Bischof, P. (1989). Three pregnancy proteins (PP12, PP14 and PAPP-A): their biological and clinical relevance. *American Journal of Perinatology*, **6**, 110.

Blackmore, K., Baumgarten, A., Schoenfeld-Dimaio, M., Hobbins, J.C., Mason, E.A., and Mahoney, M.J. (1986). Rise in maternal serum α-fetoprotein concentration after chorionic villus sampling and the possibility of isoimmunization. *American Journal of Obstetrics and Gynecology*, **155**, 988.

Bohn, H. (1974). Untersuchungen uber das Schwangerschafts-spezifische B1-Glykoprotein (SP1). *Archiv für Gynakologie*, **216**, 347.

Bohn, H. (1985). Biochemistry of placental proteins. In *Proteins of the placenta*, (ed. P. Bischof and A. Klopper), pp. 1–25. Karger, Basel.

Chard, T. and Grudzinskas, J.G. (1992). Pregnancy protein secretion. *Seminars on Reproductive Endocrinology*, **10**, 61.

Chou, J.Y. and Plouzek, C.A. (1991). Pregnancy-specific β1-glycoprotein. *Seminars on Reproductive Endocrinology*, **10**, 116.

Csapo, A.I., Pulkkinen, M., and Wiest, W.G. (1973). Effect of luteectomy and progesterone replacement therapy in early pregnancy patients. *American Journal of Obstetrics and Gynecology*, **115**, 759.

DOH (Department of Health Statistics and Research) (1993). SR28, Annual summaries of LHS 27/1 returns. United States Annual Vital Statistics Reports. Vol. I. Natality, 1989. Department of Health, Washington DC.

Eddie, L.W., Bell, R.J., Lester, A., Geier, M., Bennett, G., Johnston, P.D., and Niall, H.D., (1986). Radioimmunoassay of relaxin in pregnancy with an analogue of human relaxin. *Lancet*, **i**, 1344.

Evans, M., Dommergues, M., Timor-Tritsch, I., Zador, I.E., Wapner, R.J., Lynch, L., *et al.* (1994). Transabdominal versus transcervical and transvaginal multifetal pregnancy reduction: International collaborative experience of more than one thousand cases. The induction of ovulation. *American Journal of Obstetrics and Gynecology*, **170**, 902.

Fields, P.A. and Larkin, L.H. (1981). Purification and immunohistochemical localization of relaxin in human term placenta. *Journal of Clinical Endocrinology and Metabolism*, **52**, 79.

Gitlin D. (1975). Normal biology of α-fetoprotein *Annals of the New York Academy of Sciences*, **259**, 7.

Gordon, Y.B., Grudzinskas, J.G., Jeffrey, D. and Chard, T. (1977). Concentrations of pregnancy-specific β1-glycoprotein in maternal blood in normal pregnancy and intrauterine growth retardation. *Lancet*, **i**, 331

Grau, P., Robinson, L., Tabsh, K., and Crandall, B.F. (1990). Elevated maternal serum alpha-fetoprotein and amniotic fluid alpha-fetoprotein after multifetal pregnancy reduction. *Obstetrics and Gynecology*, **76**, 1042.

Johnson, M.R., Allman, A.C.J., Steer, P.J., and Lightman S.L. (1992). Circulating levels of relaxin may influence the time of onset and progression of labour. *Journal of Endocrinology*, (Suppl.), **135**, 31.

Johnson, M.R., Abbas, A., and Nicolaides, K.H. (1994*a*). Maternal plasma levels of human chorionic gonadotropin, oestradiol and progesterone before and after fetal reduction. *Journal of Endocrinology*, **143**, 309–12.

Johnson, M.R., Abbas, A., Nicolaides, K.H., and Lightman, S.L. (1994*b*). The regulation of plasma relaxin levels during human pregnancy. *Journal of Endocrinology*, **142**, 261.

Julkunen, M., Koistinen, R., Sjoberg, J., Rutanen, E.M., Wahlstrom, T., and Seppälä, M. (1986). Secretory endometrium synthesizes placental protein 14. *Endocrinology*, **118**, 1782.

Koay, E.S.C., Too, C.L., Greenwood, F.C., and Bryant-Greenwood, G.D. (1983). Relaxin stimulates collagenase and plasminogen activator secretion from dispersed chorion cells 'in vitro' *Journal of Clinical Endocrinology and Metabolism*, **56**, 1332.

Lin, T.M., Halbert, S.P., Spellacy, W., and Gall, S. (1976). Human pregnancy-associated proteins during the postpartum period. *American Journal of Obstetrics and Gynecology*, **124**, 382.

Lopez-Bernal, A., Bryant-Greenwood, G.D., Hansell, D.J., Hicks, B.R., Greenwood, F.C., and Turnbull, A.C. (1987). Effect of relaxin and prostaglandin E production by the human amnion: changes in relation to the onset of labour. *British Journal of Obstetrics and Gynaecology*, **94**, 1045.

MacLennan, A.H., Green, R.C., Grant, P., and Nicholson, R. (1986). Ripening of the human cervix and induction of labour with intracervical purified porcine relaxin. *Obstetrics and Gynecology*, **68**, 598.

Madden, J.D., Siiteri, P.K., MacDonald, P.C., and Grant, N.F. (1976). The pattern and rates of metabolism of maternal dehydroisoandrosterone sulphate in human pregnancy. *American Journal of Obstetrics and Gynecology*, **125**, 915.

Quagliarello, J., Steinetz, B.G., and Weiss, G. (1979). Relaxin secretion in early pregnancy. *Obstetrics and Gynaecology*, **53**, 62.

Rosen, S.W. (1986). New placental proteins: chemistry, physiology and clinical use. *Placenta*, 7, 575.

Schindler, A.M., Bordington, P., and Bischof, P. (1984). Immunohistochemical localisation of pregnancy-associated plasma protein A (PAPP-A) in decidua and trophoblast. Comparison with hCG and fibrin. *Placenta*, 5, 227.

Seppälä, M. and Ruoslahti, E. (1973). Alpha fetoprotein: physiology and pathology during pregnancy and application to antenatal diagnosis. *Journal of Perinatal Medicine*, 1, 104.

Song, C.S. and Kappas, A. (1968). The influence of estrogens, progestogens and pregnancy on the liver. *Vitamins and Hormones*, 26, 147.

Streit, J.A., Penick, G.D., Williamson, R.A., Weiner, C.P., and Benda, J.A. (1989). Prolonged elevation of alphafetoprotein and detectable acetylcholinesterase after death of an anomalous twin fetus. *Prenatal Diagnosis*, 9, 1.

Weiss, G., O'Byrne, E.M., Hochman, J., Steinetz, B.G., Goldsmith, L., and Flitcraft, J.G. (1978). Distribution of relaxin in women during pregnancy. *Obstetrics and Gynecology*, 52, 569.

IV | *Medicine of the embryo and early fetus*

18 | *Epidemiology of early pregnancy failure*

Joe Leigh Simpson

Of clinically recognized pregnancies, 10–15 per cent are lost. Of married women in the United States, 4 per cent have experienced two recognized losses and 3 per cent have experienced three or more losses (US Department of Health and Human Services 1982). This chapter will enumerate the relative likelihood of loss in various circumstances and the causes of early pregnancy failure. We shall restrict our comments to clinically recognized losses because preclinical losses are covered by other authors in this volume.

FREQUENCY AND TIMING OF PREGNANCY LOSSES

Clinically recognized first trimester fetal loss rates of 10–12 per cent are now well documented in both retrospective and prospective cohort studies (Simpson and Carson 1993). This rate contrasts with the 22 per cent preclinical loss rate derived by Wilcox *et al.* (1988) in a cohort study involving urinary hCGβ assays serially performed from 20 days' gestation; the clinical loss rate in that study was 9 per cent. Higher clinical loss rates reported in certain older studies may have reflected misclassification, namely unwitting inclusion of surreptitious illicit abortions. The latter was common during the era in which legal termination was proscribed, and not often appreciated by physicians.

Absolute loss rates reflect the many factors to be discussed in this chapter, but two associations are worth emphasizing in the present context. First, maternal age greatly increases risk of pregnancy loss, a 40 year old woman carrying twice the risk of a 20 year old woman. Second, prior pregnancy history is important. Among nulliparous women who have never experienced a loss (Regan 1988), the rate is 6 per cent. This increases to 25–30 per cent for women with three or more losses. These risks apply not only to women whose losses were recognized of 9–12 weeks' gestation, but to those whose pregnancies were ascertained in the fifth week of gestation (Simpson *et al.* 1994). In couples with prior losses abortion rates seem *lowest* when conception occurred in mid-cycle (Gray *et al.* 1995). Mid-cycle fertilization should not involve oocytes or sperm aged *in vivo* before fertilization, although this is not necessarily the explanation for the effect.

Fetal demise occurs prior to the time overt clinical signs become manifested, a deduction made on the basis of cohort studies showing that only 3 per cent of viable pregnancies are lost after eight weeks' gestation (Simpson *et al.* 1987). Given a clinical loss rate of 10–12 per cent, fetal demise must have occurred weeks before maternal symptoms appear; thus, fetuses aborting clinically at 9–12 weeks will usually have died weeks previously. Loss of viability after eight weeks will most likely occur in the third and fourth gestational months, given that loss rates are only 1 per cent in women confirmed by ultrasound to have viable pregnancies at 16 weeks (see Chapter 19). Because almost all losses are retained *in utero* prior to expulsion, 'missed abortions' are actually physiologic.

The converse of these recurrence risk figures should be kept in mind, namely the likelihood of maintaining pregnancy being 70 per cent despite two or three prior losses (Table 18.1). Indeed, Vlaanderen and Treffers (1987) reported successful pregnancies in each of 21 women having unexplained prior repetitive losses but subjected to no intervention. Other groups reached similar conclusions (Houwert-de Jong *et al.* 1989; Liddell *et al.* 1991). To be judged efficacious, therapeutic regimens must therefore demonstrate success rates greater than 70 per cent, corrected for maternal age and other confounding variables.

AETIOLOGIES OF EARLY PREGNANCY FAILURE

Chromosomal abnormalities

The major cause of clinically recognized pregnancy losses is chromosomal abnormalities. At least 50 per cent of clinically recognized pregnancy losses result from a chromosomal abnormality (Boué *et al.* 1975; Hassold 1980; Simpson and Bombard 1987). If one analyses chorionic villi after ultrasound diagnosis of fetal demise, rather than relying upon recovery of spontaneously expelled products, the frequency of chromosomal abnormalities is 75–90 per cent (Sorokin *et al.* 1991; Strom *et al.* 1992). Overall, first trimester frequencies closer to 70 per cent are probably closer to reality.

Table 18.1   Approximate recurrence risk figures useful for counselling women with repeated spontaneous abortions

	Prior abortions	Risk (%)
Women with live-born infants	0	5–10
	1	20–25
	2	25
	3	30
	4	30–40
Women without live-born infants	≥ 3	40–45

Based on data from Warburton and Fraser (1964), Poland *et al.* (1977), and Regan (1988). Recurrence risks are slightly higher in older women and those who smoke cigarettes or drink alcohol, and for those exposed to high levels of selected chemical toxins.

Autosomal trisomy

Autosomal trisomies comprise the largest (approximately 50 per cent) single class of chromosomal complements in cytogenetically abnormal spontaneous abortions (Table 18.2). Trisomy for every chromosome except No 1 has been reported, with that trisomy observed only in an 8-cell embryo (Watt *et al.* 1987). The most common trisomy is No 16.

Table 18.2 Chromosomal complements in spontaneous abortions recognized clinically in the first trimester

Complement	Frequency	(%)
Normal		
46, XX or 46, XY		54.1
Triploidy		
		7.7
69, XXX	2.7	
69, XYX	0.2	
69, XXY	4.0	
Other	0.8	
Tetraploidy		2.6
92, XXX	1.5	
92, XXYY	0.55	
Not stated	0.55	
Monosomy X		8.6
Structural abnormalities		1.5
Sex chromosomal polysomy		0.2
47, XXX	0.05	
47, XXY	0.15	
Autosomal monosomy (G)		0.1
Autosomal trisomy		22.3

	Chromosome	
	No 1	0
	No 2	0.11
	No 3	0.25
	No 4	0.64
	No 5	0.04
	No 6	0.14
	No 7	0.89
	No 8	0.79
	No 9	0.72
	No 10	0.36

Table 18.2 (*contd*)   Chromosomal complements in spontaneous abortions
recognized clinically in the first trimester

	Chromosome (*contd*)	
	No 11	0.04
	No 12	0.18
	No 13	1.07
	No 14	0.82
	No 15	1.68
	No 16	7.27
	No 17	0.18
	No 18	1.15
	No 19	0.01
	No 20	0.61
	No 21	2.11
	No 22	2.26
Double trisomy		0.7
Mosaic trisomy		1.3
Other abnormalities or not specified		0.9
		100.0

Pooled data from several series, as referenced elsewhere by Simpson and Bombard A.T. (1987).

Most trisomies show a maternal age effect, but the effect varies among chromosomes. The maternal age effect is especially impressive for double trisomies. Given the maternal age effect, autosomal trisomies are predictably more likely to arise cytologically in maternal meiosis than in paternal meiosis. Most (90 per cent) trisomies arise during maternal meiosis, usually maternal meiosis I. This holds for trisomy 21 and for all the acrocentric chromosomes (Zaragoza *et al.* 1994). Trisomy 16 is virtually exclusively attributable to errors in maternal meiosis I (Warburton *et al.* 1987a). However, trisomy 18 usually arises at maternal meiosis II (Delhanty and Handyside 1995; Fisher *et al.* 1995).

In accordance with expectations predicted from a maternal age effect, Hassold *et al.* (1995) showed decreased maternal recombination in trisomy 16. It follows that periconceptional events (exposure to toxins or fertilization involving gametes aged *in vivo* by delayed fertilization) are unlikely to play an aetiologic role in most trisomies because errors in maternal meiosis I would have originated years before. In turn this is consistent with our failing to find increased Down syndrome in pregnancies conceived by natural family planning users, women whose practice of periodic abstinence theoretically places them at increased risk for conceptions involving ageing gametes (Castilla *et al.* 1995; Simpson *et al.* 1988).

Polyploidy

Triploidy (3*n* = 69) and tetraploidy (4*n* = 92) occur often in abortuses. Triploid abortuses are usually 69,XXY or 69,XXX, the result of dispermy. An association exists between triploidy and hydatidiform mole, a 'partial mole' said to exist if molar tissue and fetal parts coexist (see Chapter 12). 'Complete' hydatidiform moles are 46,XX, of androgenetic origin (Beatty 1978).

Tetraploidy is uncommon, rarely progressing beyond 4–5 weeks of gestation.

Monosomy X

Monosomy X is the single most common chromosomal abnormality among spontaneous abortions, accounting for 15–20 per cent of abnormal specimens (Fig. 18.1).

Monosomy X usually (80 per cent) occurs as result of paternal sex chromosome loss (Chandley 1981; Hassold *et al.* 1985). The mean maternal age if the remaining X is paternal in origin (45, X^p) is 23.8 ± 6.1; the mean maternal age if the remaining X is maternal (45, X^m) is 29.6 ± 5.5 (Hassold *et al.* 1985).

Structural chromosomal rearrangement

An important cause of *repetitive* spontaneous abortions, structural chromosomal rearrangements account for only 1.5 per cent of abortuses in the general population (Table 18.2). Rearrangements (e.g. translocation) may either arise *de novo* during gametogenesis or be inherited from a parent carrying a 'balanced' translocation or

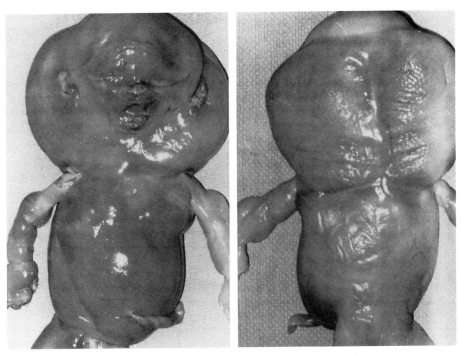

Fig. 18.1 A 45, X abortus. The cystic hygroma and generalized oedema are evident. From Simpson and Bombard (1987).

inversion. Phenotypic consequences depend upon the specific duplicated or deficient chromosomal segments.

Sex chromosomal polysomy

The complements 47,XXY and 47,XYY each occur about 1 per 800 live-born male births; 47,XXX occurs in 1 per 800 female births. X and Y polysomies are only slightly more common in abortuses than in live-born infants. The cytologic origin in 47,XXX is 59 per cent for maternal meiosis I, 16 per cent for maternal meiosis II, 6 per cent paternal meiosis I or II, and the remainder postzygotic (Macdonald *et al.* 1994). In 47,XXY, the distribution shows more paternal origin (46 per cent); maternal origin is usually meiosis I (Macdonald *et al.* 1994).

Recurrent aneuploidy

Numerical chromosomal abnormalities (aneuploidy) may be responsible for both recurrent as well as sporadic losses. This reasoning is based on observations that the complements of successive abortuses in a given family are more likely to be either recurrently normal or recurrently abnormal (Table 18.3). If the complement of the first abortus is abnormal, the likelihood is 80 per cent that the complement of the second abortus also will be abnormal (Warburton *et al.* 1987b). The recurrent abnormality usually is trisomy.

It can be argued that corrections for maternal age render the ostensible non-random distribution marginally non-significant (Warburton *et al.* 1987b). However, it seems more likely that couples are predisposed towards chromosomally abnormal conceptions. If recurrent aneuploidy is a true phenomenon, couples might logically be at increased risk not only for aneuploid abortuses but also for aneuploid live-born infants. The trisomic autosome in a subsequent pregnancy might not always confer lethality, but rather might be compatible with life (e.g. trisomy 21). Indeed, the risk of live-born trisomy 21 following an aneuploid abortus is about 1 per cent (Alberman 1981).

Table 18.3 Recurrent aneuploidy: the relationship between karyotypes of successive abortuses

Complement of first abortus	Complement of second abortus					
	Normal	Trisomy	Monosomy	Triploidy	Tetraploidy	*De novo* rearrangement
Normal	142	18	5	7	3	2
Trisomy	31	30	1	4	3	1
Monosomy X	7	5	3	3	0	0
Triploidy	7	4	1	4	0	0
Tetraploidy	3	1	0	2	0	0
De novo rearrangement	1	3	0	0	0	0

Tabulation by Warburton *et al.* (1987a).

Novel cytogenetic mechanisms

Several novel cytogenetic aberrations in the placenta and fetus could contribute to pregnancy loss. These would not be appreciated by conventional cytogenetic studies because the fetus would be characterized by a normal diploid number of chromosomes. None the less, aetiology reflects chromosomal perturbations.

One mechanism is mosaicism restricted to the placenta, the embryo *per se* being normal. This phenomenon is termed confined placental mosaicism (CPM). Actually, losses due to this mechanism may already have been reflected in existing data (e.g. Table 18.2) because cytogenetic studies of abortuses usually involve analysis of villous material. Irrespective, loss rates with CPM are not greatly increased compared to pregnancies undergoing chorionic villus sampling (CVS) that do not show CPM—3 per cent v. 1 per cent (Wapner *et al.* 1992). A relationship between CPM and intrauterine growth retardation is being explored.

Another novel mechanism is uniparental disomy. Both homologues for a given chromosome may be derived from a single parent, probably as a result of expulsion of a chromosome from a trisomic zygote. If the extruded chromosome were from the parent contributing only one chromosome, the karyotype would appear normal (46,XX or 46,XY) but the genome of the embryo would lack a contribution from that parent. Uniparental disomy has been confirmed in an abortus for chromosome 21 (Henderson *et al.* 1994), and other chromosomes are surely also involved. This phenomenon has also been claimed to exist in placentas of pregnancies showing intrauterine growth retardation.

Chromosomal translocations

The most common structural rearrangement encountered in abortions is a translocation, observed in about 5 per cent of couples experiencing repeated losses (Simpson *et al.* 1981, 1989; De Braekeleer and Dao 1990). Individuals with balanced translocations are phenotypically normal, but abortuses or abnormal live-born infants may show chromosomal duplications or deficiencies as result of normal meiotic segregation (Fig. 18.2). About 60 per cent of the translocations detected are reciprocal; 40 per cent are Robertsonian. Females are about twice as likely as males to show a balanced translocation (Simpson *et al.* 1981).

If a child has Down syndrome as result of a translocation, the rearrangement will proved to have originated *de novo* in 50–75 per cent of cases. That is, neither parent will have a balanced translocation. The likelihood of Down syndrome offspring recurring in such a couple is thus minimal. On the other hand, the risk is substantive in the 25–50 per cent of families in which individuals have Down syndrome as result of a balanced parental translocation [e.g. 45,XX, −14, −21, + (14q;21q)]. The theoretical risk of such a woman having a child with Down syndrome is 33 per cent, but empirical risks are fortunately less. The likelihood is only 10 per cent if the mother carries the translocation, 2 per cent if the father carries the translocation (Boué and Gallano 1984; Daniel *et al.* 1989). If Robertsonian (centric-fusion) translocations involve chromosomes other than numbers 14 and 21, empiric risks are lower. In t(13q;14q), the risk for live-born trisomy 13 is 1 per cent or less.

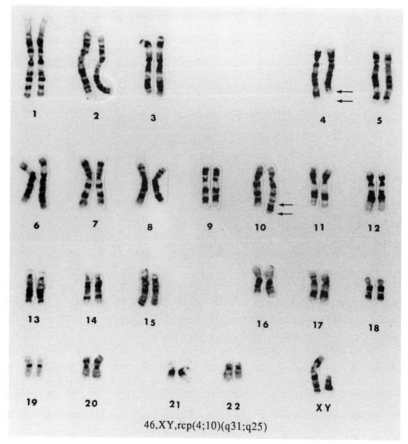

46,XY,rcp(4;10)(q31;q25)

Fig. 18.2 Balanced reciprocal between chromosomes 4 and 10 (long arms), translocation detected in a woman experiencing multiple abortions. From Simpson and Tharapel (1991).

Reciprocal translocations do not involve centromeric fusion. Empirical data for specific translocations are usually not available, but a few generalizations can be made on the basis of data pooled from many different translocations. Theoretical risks for abnormal offspring (unbalanced reciprocal translocations) are far greater than empiric risks. The risk is 12 per cent for offspring of either female heterozygotes or male heterozygotes (Boué and Gallano 1984; Daniel *et al.* 1989). Antenatal cytogenetic studies should be offered in subsequent pregnancies. The frequency of unbalanced fetuses is lower if the parental balanced translocation was ascertained through repetitive abortions (3 per cent) than through an anomalous live-born infant (nearly 20 per cent) (Boué and Gallano 1984). Segregation studies utilizing sperm chromosomes or fluorescent *in situ* hybridization (FISH) with chromosome-specific probes might provide data relevant for a translocation in a specific family, but these data are currently available only on an investigational basis.

Occasionally a translocation precludes the possibility of a normal live-born infant. This occurs when translocations involve homologous chromosomes [e.g. t(13q13q) or t(21q21q)]. If the father carries such a structural rearrangement, artificial insemination may be appropriate. If the mother carries the rearrangement, donor oocytes or donor embryos (assisted reproductive technologies) should be considered.

Chromosomal inversions

Less often responsible for repetitive pregnancy losses than translocations is an inversion, a rearrangement in which the order of the genes is reversed. Individuals heterozygous for an inversion would generally be clinically normal if their genes were merely rearranged, but they could suffer adverse reproductive consequences as result of normal meiotic phenomena, namely crossing over in their gametes to yield unbalanced gametes. Pericentric inversions exist in perhaps 0.1 per cent of females and 0.1 per cent of males experiencing repeated spontaneous abortions.

Counselling a couple having an inversion is complex. Inversions involving either a small portion of the total chromosomal length or paradoxically a very large portion are of least significance clinically because the large duplications or large deficiencies that follow crossing over usually prove lethal. By contrast, inversions involving 30–60 per cent of the total chromosomal length are relatively more likely to be characterized by duplications or deficiencies compatible with survival (Sutherland *et al.* 1976). Females with a pericentric inversion carry a 7 per cent risk of abnormal live-born infants; males carry a 5 per cent risk. Pericentric inversions ascertained through phenotypically normal probands are less likely to result in abnormal live-born infants.

Few recurrent data are available for *paracentric* inversions. Compared with paracentric inversions, there should be less risk for unbalanced products at CVS or amniocentesis because paracentric recombinants should more often be lethal. On the other hand, abortions and abnormal live-born infant have been observed within the same kindred, and the risk for unbalanced viable offspring has been tabulated at 4 per cent (Pettanati *et al.* 1995). Antenatal cytogenetic studies should be offered.

Luteal phase defects

Implantation in a inhospitable endometrium is a plausible explanation for spontaneous abortion. Progesterone deficiency in particular is said to result in the oestrogen-primed endometrium being unable to sustain implantation. Luteal phase deficiency (LPD) is the term used to describe the endometrium manifesting an inadequate progesterone effect. Progesterone secreted by the corpus luteum is necessary to support the endometrium until the trophoblast produces sufficient progesterone to maintain pregnancy, an event occurring around seven gestational (menstrual) weeks or five weeks after conception. Given this luteal–placental shift, various pathogenic mechanisms could be postulated as explanations for LPD: decreased gonadotrophin-releasing hormone (GnRH), decreased follicle-stimulating hormone (FSH), decreased luteinizing hormone (LH), inadequate ovarian steroidogenesis, or endometrial receptor defects.

Once almost universally accepted as a common cause for fetal wastage, LPD is now generally considered an uncommon cause. Although quite plausible, there are still no randomized studies that validate the disorder as a genuine entity. Efficacy of treatment is unproved. Moreover, histology identical to that observed with luteal phase 'defects' exists in fertile women. When regularly menstruating fertile women with no history of abortions underwent endometrial biopsies in serial cycles, the frequency of LPD was 51.4 per cent in any single cycle and 26.7 per cent in sequential cycles (Davis *et al.* 1989). Interobserver variation in reading endometrial biopsies is also considerable. Biopsies read by five different pathologists resulted in marked differences of interpretation sufficient to have altered management in one-third of patients (Scott *et al.* 1988). In another study pathologists reading coded endometrial biopsy slides a second time agreed in only 25 per cent of samples with their initial diagnosis of LPD (Li *et al.* 1989). Hormone levels offer no improvement in sensitivity and specificity, a low serum progesterone in the luteal phase being only 71 per cent predictive of a luteal phase defect as defined on the basis of an abnormal endometrial biopsy (Daya *et al.* 1988). Abnormalities of endometrial receptors might be more reproducibly determined were this to prove an explanation; however, molecular studies have not yet been reported.

No study has been robust enough to demonstrate efficacy of progesterone or progestin therapy. Studies by Tho *et al.* (1979) and Daya and Ward (1988) are often cited as evidence of efficacy, but the experimental designs can be criticized (Simpson 1996) because valid control groups were not recruited. A meta-analysis by Karamardian and Grimes (1992) showed no beneficial effect after progesterone treatment. The consensus remains that LPD is either an arguable entity or cannot be proved to be treated successfully with progesterone or progestational therapy.

Of recent interest are observations that have suggested a relationship between fetal loss and either oligomenorrhoea (Quenby and Farquharson 1993) or polycystic ovary disease (PCO) (Sagle *et al.* 1988), either of which could reflect endometrial dysynchrony. However, again, the diagnostic criteria are contentious. In one study, PCO was diagnosed only by ultrasound (Sagle *et al.* 1988), but Regan *et al.* (1990) reported elevated serum LH in women experiencing pregnancy loss. Additional data are necessary.

Thyroid abnormalities

Decreased conception rates and increased fetal losses are associated with overt hypothyroidism or hyperthyroidism, but subclinical thyroid dysfunction is probably not an explanation for repeated losses (Montoro *et al.* 1981). One study observed an increased frequency of anti-thyroid antibodies among couples experiencing repeated losses (Pratt *et al.* 1994).

Diabetes mellitus

Women with poorly controlled diabetes mellitus clearly show increased risk for fetal loss (Mills *et al.* 1988). In one cohort study, women whose glycosylated haemoglobin was greater than four standard deviations above the mean showed higher pregnancy loss rates than either diabetic women showing lower glycosylated haemoglobin levels or euglycaemic controls. Similar findings were observed in retrospective studies (Miodovnik *et al.* 1986). Poorly controlled diabetes mellitus should be considered one cause for early pregnancy loss, but subclinical or gestational diabetes are probably not causes. Moreover, the number of insulin-dependent diabetic women who experience pregnancy loss because of poor control is too few to exert a large effect in the general population.

Intrauterine adhesions (synechiae)

Intrauterine adhesions could interfere with implantation or with early embryonic development. Most often these adhesions arise after overzealous uterine curettage during the puerperium, intrauterine surgery (e.g. myomectomy), or endometritis. Adhesions are most likely to develop if curettage is performed three or four weeks postpartum. Individuals with uterine synechiae usually manifest hypomenorrhoea or amenorrhoea, but 15–30 per cent show repeated abortions. Adhesions are a genuine cause of early pregnancy failure, but the incidence is very low.

Incomplete Mullerian fusion

Mullerian fusion defects (Fig. 18.3) are well accepted causes of *second* trimester losses and pregnancy complications. Low birth weight, breech presentation, and uterine

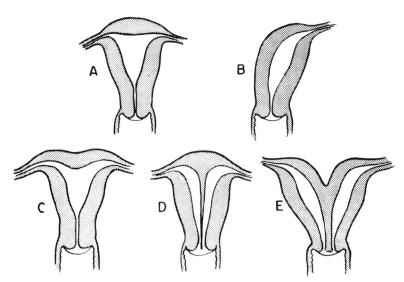

Fig. 18.3 Diagrammatic representation of selected Mullerian fusion anomalies: A, normal uterus, Fallopian tubes, and cervix; B, uterus unicornis (absence of one uterine horn); C, uterus arcuatus (broadening and medial depression of a portion of the uterine septum); D, uterus septus (persistence of a complete uterine septum; and E, uterus bicornis unicollis (two hemiuteri, each leading to same cervix). From Simpson (1976).

bleeding are other abnormalities associated with these anomalies. Ben Rafael *et al.* (1991) confirmed these conclusions by comparison to women with hysterosalpingogram (HSG)—proven normal uteri, but most reports lack controls (Stampe-Sorensen 1988; Candiani *et al.* 1990; Stein and March 1990; Makino *et al.* 1991; Michalas 1991; Golan *et al.* 1992; Moutos *et al.* 1992). Some studies claim poorer outcomes with septate uteri (Moutos *et al.* 1992) or T-shaped uteri (Makino *et al.* 1991), but others show no discernible differences among various anomalies (Stein and March 1990).

One major problem in attributing cause and effect for second trimester complications and uterine anomalies is that the latter occur so frequently that observed adverse outcomes could be coincidental. For example, Stampe-Soresen (1988) found unsuspected bicornuate uteri in two of 167 (1.2 per cent) women undergoing laparoscopic sterilization; 3.6 per cent had a septate uterus and 15.3 per cent fundal anomalies. Simon *et al.* (1991) found Mullerian defects in 3.2 per cent (22/679) of fertile women; 20 of the 22 defects were septate.

Attribution is even more of a problem in *first* trimester losses. Septate uteri plausibly might increase the risk of pregnancy loss if implantation occurs on an inhospitable surface. If this were the mechanism underlying early losses, there should be no increased losses with bicornuate uteri or T-shaped uteri. One should probably attribute abortions to uterine fusion defects only if they occur after ultrasonographic confirmation of a viable pregnancy at eight or nine weeks. Losses having no confirmation of fetal viability at that time are statistically more likely to represent missed abortions in which fetal demise occurred prior to eight weeks. Overall, quantitative estimates of the role rate of uterine anomalies in first trimester losses cannot be cited with confidence.

Leiomyomas

Leiomyomas occur frequently, but relatively few women with leiomyomas develop symptoms requiring medical or surgical therapy. That leiomyomas cause early pregnancy failure rather than obstetric complications like prematurity is plausible, but probably rare. Analogous to uterine anomalies, the coexistence of uterine leiomyomas and reproductive losses need not necessarily imply a causal relationship. Location of leiomyomas is probably more important than size, submucous leiomyomas being most likely to cause abortion. Plausible mechanisms that lead to pregnancy could loss include thinning of the endometrium over the surface of a submucous leiomyoma, predisposing to implantation in a poorly decidualized site, or rapid growth due to the hormonal milieu of pregnancy, compromising blood supply of the leiomyoma and resulting in necrosis ('red degeneration') which in turn leads to uterine contractions or infections that eventually lead to fetal expulsion. One should initially assume clinically and epidemiologically that leiomyomata have no aetiologic relationship to pregnancy loss. Surgery should be reserved for women whose abortuses were both phenotypically and karyotypically normal and in whom fetal viability until at least 9–10 weeks was documented.

Incompetent internal cervical os

A functionally intact cervix and lower uterine cavity are obvious prerequisites for a successful intrauterine pregnancy. Characterized by painless dilation and effacement, cervical incompetence usually occurs during the mid-second or early third trimester. This condition frequently follows traumatic events like cervical amputation, cervical lacerations, forceful cervical dilatation, or conization. There is less reason to postulate a relationship to early pregnancy failure than to second trimester losses.

Infections

Infections are accepted causes of late fetal wastage, and logically could be responsible for early fetal loss as well. Among the many microorganisms reported to have been associated with spontaneous abortion are *Variola, Vaccinia, Salmonella typhi, Vibrio fetus, Malaria, Cytomegalovirus, Brucella, Toxoplasmosis, Mycoplasma hominis, Chlamydia trachomatis,* and *Ureaplasma urealyticum*. Transplacental infection doubtless occurs with each of these microorganisms, and sporadic losses could logically be caused by any.

Verification of these logical deductions has not, however, been forthcoming. One line of support is that *Ureaplasma* and *Mycoplasma hominis* have been isolated in mid-trimester placentas and abortuses, but only rarely from *induced* (control) mid-trimester abortions (Sompolinsky *et al.* 1975). Other support includes studies in which empiric antibiotic therapy ostensibly benefits couples experiencing repeated losses. Among repetitive aborters treated for four weeks while not pregnant with tetracycline, Toth *et al.* (1986) reported recurrent fetal losses in only 10 per cent of aborters who chose not to take tetracycline, 38 per cent experienced another loss. However, the two groups in that study were not randomized and therefore were not necessarily comparable. Moreover, other studies have found no difference in outcome between women treated and not treated with antibiotics (Van Iddelinge and Hofmeyr 1991). Of the organisms implicated in *repetitive* abortion, *Ureaplasma* and *Chlamydia* seem most plausible because they fulfil two prerequisites: (1) their existence in an asymptomatic state, and (2) virulence is not always severe enough to cause infertility from Fallopian tube occlusion. From 46 women with histories of three or more consecutive losses of unknown aetiology, Stray-Pedersen *et al.* (1978) recovered *Ureaplasma* significantly more often among women with repetitive abortions (28 per cent) than among controls (7 per cent). Infected women and their husbands ($n = 43$) were then treated with doxycycline, with subsequent cultures confirming eradication of *Ureaplasma*. Nineteen of the 43 women became pregnant; of the 19, three experienced another spontaneous abortion, whereas 16 had normal full-term infants. Among 18 women with untreated *Ureaplasma*, there were only five full-term pregnancies. Data are less compelling for other organisms. Based on the presence of chlamydial antibodies in the sera of women who experienced repeated losses, an association has been claimed on the basis of presence of high titres (Quinn *et al.* 1987; Witkin and Ledger 1992). However, other data show no relationship (Olliaro *et al.* 1991; Rae *et al.* 1994). Toxoplasmosis antibodies have been observed in Mexican and in Egyptian women having repetitive losses (Zavala-Vlazquez *et al.* 1989; el Ridi *et al.* 1991), but given the ubiquitous nature of the organism antibody frequencies are not necessarily higher than in the general Mexican or Egyptian populations.

A key question is whether any implicated infectious agents are causative with respect to fetal losses or merely arose following fetal demise due to a non-infectious aetiology. Surveillance of infections beginning early in pregnancy is thus required to determine the true role of infections in pregnancy loss. To this end we have prospectively determined the frequency of infections in pregnant women who were subjects in our multi-centre United States NICHD 'Diabetes in early pregnancy' study (Simpson *et al.* 1995). Data were collected prospectively on clinical infections in 386 diabetic subjects and 432 control subjects seen frequently during the first trimester. There was no clinical evidence that infection occurred more often in the 112 subjects experiencing pregnancy loss compared to the 706 having successful pregnancies. This held both for the two-week interval in which a given loss was recognized clinically as well as in the prior two-week interval. Similar findings were observed for both control as well as diabetic subjects, and further held when data were stratified by genital infection only or by systemic infection only. These prospective data suggest that the attributable risk of infection in first trimester spontaneous abortion is small; however, a role for a specific organism (e.g. ureaplasma) could still exist in selective women with repetitive abortions.

Anti-fetal antibodies and embryotoxic antibodies

An otherwise normal mother may produce antibodies against her fetus on the basis of genetic dissimilarities. The most well known example is fetal loss due to rhesus-negative (RhD–) women having anti-D antibodies. Usually rhesus-isoimmunization exerts its effect in the late second or third trimester. More relevant for early pregnancy loss is isoimmunization due to anti-P antibodies. Most individuals are genotype Pp or PP, but homozygosity for p (pp) occurs. If a woman of genotype pp has a Pp or PP mate, resulting offspring may or must be Pp. If the mother develops anti-P antibodies, Pp fetuses will be rejected (aborted) early in gestation. This cause is very rare but established.

Hill and colleagues (Hill *et al.* 1995) have proposed that embryotoxic antibodies can cause repetitive abortions in women with specific T-helper cell perturbations. Progesterone therapy is said to ameliorate against the deleterious effects. The experiments of Hill *et al.* (1995) have been carefully conducted and interpreted. That these antibodies exist prior to fetal loss has not been conclusively established, nor has it been possible to conduct prospective, population-based studies in women who have no prior history of abnormal outcomes. The contribution of this phenomenon to pregnancy loss in the general population thus remains uncertain, in my addition.

Autoimmune disease and anti-sperm antibodies

An association between second trimester pregnancy loss and autoimmune disease is generally accepted (Branch and Ward 1989; Cowchock 1991). The types of antibodies found in women with pregnancy losses are diverse, ranging from non-specific antinuclear antibodies (ANA) to antibodies against cellular components like phospholipids, histones, double-, or single-stranded DNA. Individuals having antiphospholipid antibodies, a broad category that includes lupus anticoagulant (LAC) antibodies and anticardiolipin antibodies (aCL), constitute the group most often implicated with fetal wastage. Most investigators (Scott *et al.* 1987) agree that mid-trimester fetal death is increased in women with LAC or anti-cardiolipin antibodies, perhaps dramatically so. Lupus anticoagulant (LAC) in particular has been associated with subplacental clotting and fetal losses (Elias and Eldor 1984), thus 'lupus anticoagulant antibody' is a misnomer; the abortifacient mechanism is presumably decidual.

Despite the established relationship between antiphospholipid antibodies and losses in the *second* and third trimester, data are far less clear for *first* trimester pregnancy losses. Initially, studies seemed to show also increased anti-cardiolipin antibodies in women with such losses. More recent studies show frequencies of various antiphospholipid antibodies (LAC, aCL, aPL) to be similar in women who experience and do not experience first trimester abortions (Petri *et al.* 1987; Carp *et al.* 1993; Mishell 1993; Ergolu and Scopelitis 1994). A major pitfall in assessing significance of antibodies in first trimester losses is the unavoidable selection bias inherent in studying couples only after they have presented with losses. That antibodies could have arisen only after the pregnancy loss can not be excluded in such an experimental design. Again, using the multi-centre NICHD collaborative study cohort (Diabetes in early pregnancy study), in which we prospectively obtained sera from insulin-dependent and non-diabetic women within 21 days of conception, 93 women who later experienced pregnancy loss (48 diabetic; 45 non-diabetic) were matched 2:1 with 190 controls (93 diabetic and 97 non-diabetic) who subsequently had a normal live-born offspring (Carson *et al.* 1996). No association was observed between pregnancy loss and presence of either aPL or aCL. Neither aCL nor aPL would seem to contribute greatly, if at all, to first trimester pregnancy loss in the general population.

Another group of antibodies in which a relationship to fetal loss has been claimed is anti-sperm antibodies (ASA) which arise in approximately 50 per cent of males after vasectomy. These antibodies adversely affect the ability to conceive even when vasectomy reversal is surgically successful. Women may also manifest anti-sperm antibodies, which plausibly could adversely affect fertilization. Some studies show an increased frequency of anti-sperm antibodies among women experiencing repeated abortions (Hass *et al.* 1986; Witkin and Chaudhry 1989; Erguven *et al.* 1990; Zhang 1990), but others do not (Yan 1990; Clarke and Baker 1993). If an association does exist, the biologic basis might reflect antibody cross-reaction with paternally derived whole-body antigens needed for embryonic survival.

In order to obtain prospective data on the relationship between presence of anti-sperm antibodies (ASA) in maternal sera and first trimester pregnancy losses, our group studied first trimester sera obtained from the NICHD cohort described as having been recruited within 21 days of conception. For this particular study, 111 women who experienced pregnancy loss (55 diabetic; 56 non-diabetic) were matched 2:1 with 104 diabetic and 116 non-diabetic women (controls) who subsequently had a normal live-born infant (Simpson *et al.* 1996). No differences were observed with respect to IgG, IgA, and IgM binding when a positive ASA test was defined as 50 per cent of sperm showing antibody binding. No association was found for IgG and IgM ASA antibodies at 20 per cent binding, although a significant difference was observed for IgA ASA at 20 per cent binding. This one positive finding probably reflects multiple comparisons. Anti-sperm antibodies contribute little to pregnancy loss in the general population; a role in selective couples experiencing repeated losses is not excluded.

Alloimmune disease (shared parental antigens) and embryonic antibodies

Logically the fetus should be rejected by its mother on the grounds of having foreign (paternal) antigens. The maternal immune system apparently mitigates against fetal rejection through blocking or suppressive factors.

Parental (and, hence, maternal–fetal) histo*in*compatibility has been proposed as salutary for pregnancy maintenance. Conversely, shared parental HLA between mother and father could result in maternal–fetal homozygosity for a given allele, exerting a deleterious effect. Support for a beneficial effect of maternal–fetal incompatibility in animals can be cited:

1. Increased placental size in mice results from matings in which paternal and maternal histocompatibility antigens differ.
2. Higher implantation frequencies occur in histoincompatible (H2) murine zygotes.

Whether increased human HLA sharing *per se* constitutes an analogous mechanism underlying lack of parental differences in humans thus began to be studied. A few couples sharing HLA-DR antigens may experience no spontaneous abortions despite ten or more pregnancies (Ober *et al.* 1983), but about half the reported studies (Coulam 1992; Laitinen *et al.* 1993) show increased parental HLA sharing when couples experiencing abortions were compared to controls. The most rigorous population-based studies are those of Ober *et al.* (1992), who observe an association between losses and parental HLA-B sharing in the Hutterites, a highly inbred population.

If fetal rejection occurs as a result of diminished fetal–maternal immunologic interaction (alloimmune factors), immunotherapy to stimulate beneficial blocking antibodies generated at the few potentially differing loci is not unreasonable. This rationale was originally based on observations that blood transfusions *prior to* kidney transplantation decreased allograft rejection (Norman *et al.* 1986). Women lacking blocking antibodies but sharing HLA antigens with their spouse have been immunized with paternal leucocytes, third party leucocytes, or trophoblast membranes. Efficacy of immunotherapy remains highly controversial. The first prospective randomized trial was very impressive (Mowbray *et al.* 1985), but later studies less so. At present the consensus is that any benefit is more limited. A multi-centre effort toward pooling the results of immunotherapy by injection of paternal leucocytes showed an 11 per cent increased pregnancy rate in the immunized group. A meta-analysis by Fraser *et al.* (1993) found an odds ratio of only 1.3 in favour of a beneficial effect.

Alternative genetic explanations can be proposed as explanations for some but not all couples who share HLA antigens and have untoward outcomes. The ostensible effect could indeed be due to maternal–fetal histo*in*compatibility, but not for HLA. Instead, the locus could be closely linked, specifically to HLA-B. Such a hypothesis would be consistent with HLA-G being the only HLA antigen expressed on trophoblasts.

Deleterious effects of shared parental alleles may not be immunologically mediated at all. A lethal recessive gene, again perhaps closely linked to HLA, could exist. Murine embryos homozygous for certain alleles at the T/t locus die at early stages of embryogenesis. The existence of a T/t-like complex exists in humans could help to explain kindreds in which multiple family members have repeated losses (Christiansen *et al.* 1990). However, postulating the same mutant gene in heterozygous form in multiple unrelated spouses makes a recessive genetic basis less appealing. Moreover, if only homozygous offspring were lethal, the abortus to live-born ratio should be 1:3 (25:75 per cent) if both parents were heterozygous for the same mutant allele; however, a 1:0 ratio (100 per cent: 0) for consecutive abortuses is often observed.

In summary, sharing of parental antigens leading to fetal rejection is an attractive hypothesis, but it has not yet been shown to play a numerically large role in the general population. This phenomenon could be, but is not necessarily, related to the observations of Hill *et al.* (1995) on embryotoxic antibodies.

Drugs, chemicals, and noxious agents

Many exogenous agents have been implicated in fetal losses but relatively few can be indicted with confidence. The difficulty is that pregnant women are exposed frequently to relatively low doses of almost ubiquitous agents.

Outcomes are usually assessed by case control studies conducted after exposure to exogenous agents. Although having great power to detect any associations present, case control studies suffer the inherent bias of control women having less incentive to recall antecedent events than women experiencing an abnormal outcome (recall bias). Another experimental difficulty is that exposure to potentially dangerous chemicals is usually unwitting and, hence, poorly documented. When exposure unequivocally occurs (e.g. industrial accidents or proximity to toxic waste sites), quantitation of exposure may be difficult or impossible. Moreover, pregnant women usually are exposed to many agents concurrently, further making it difficult to attribute adverse effects to a single agent.

Given these caveats, physicians should be cautious about attributing pregnancy loss to exogenous agents. On the other hand, common sense dictates that exposure to potentially noxious agents be minimized.

Environmental chemicals

Limiting exposure to potential toxins is recognized as prudent for pregnant women in the work place. Many chemical agents have been claimed to be associated with fetal losses (Barlow and Sullivan 1982; Fija-Talamanaca and Settimi 1984), but consensus seems to be settling around a selected few (Savitz *et al.* 1994). These include anaesthetic gases, arsenic, aniline dyes, benzene, solvents, ethylene oxide, formaldehyde, pesticides, and certain divalent cations (lead, mercury, cadmium). Among workers at greatest risk are those in rubber industries, battery factories, and chemical production plants. As mentioned earlier, the difficulty lies in defining the precise effect of lower exposures and in attributing a quantitative risk.

One study has shown no increased risk for pregnant laboratory workers (Taskinen *et al.* 1986).

X-irradiation

External irradiation and internal radionuclides in high doses are proven abortifacients. Of course, therapeutic X-rays or chemotherapeutic drugs are administered during pregnancy only to seriously ill women whose pregnancies often must be terminated for maternal indications. Pelvic X-ray exposure of up to perhaps 0.1 Gy places a woman's fetus at little to no increased risk. Exposure doses are usually far smaller (0.01–0.02 Gy). The attributable contribution of X-irradiation to clinically recognized losses is thus small.

Chemotherapeutic agents

Similar to X-irradiation, exposures in high doses are abortifacients, but are administered only in dire circumstances. A potential for deleterious effects on hospital personnel handling chemotherapeutic agents exists; thus, it is prudent for pregnant hospital workers to minimize exposure.

Caffeine

The consensus has long been that no deleterious effects exist with caffeine; however, most studies have been retrospective. Recent data gathered in cohort fashion by the author and colleagues (Mills *et al.* 1993) are thus of interest. The odds ratio for an association between caffeine (coffee and other dietary forms) was only 1.15 (95 per cent CI of 0.89–1.49) (Mills *et al.* 1993). Additional data on women exposed to higher levels (> 300 mg) of daily caffeine would be useful, but in general reassurance can be given concerning moderate caffeine exposure and pregnancy loss.

Cigarette smoking

An association between smoking and spontaneous abortion is commonly accepted. Kline *et al.* (1980) found increased abortion rates in smokers, independent of maternal age and independent of alcohol consumption. A modest dose–response curve was found by Alberman *et al.* (1976).

Alcohol

An association between alcohol consumption and fetal loss was once fully accepted, but more recently seems less certain. In one early study (Kline *et al.* 1980), 616 women experiencing spontaneous abortions were compared with 632 women delivering at ≥ 28 gestational weeks or more. Among women whose pregnancies ended in spontaneous abortion, 17 per cent drank alcohol at least twice per week; 8.1 per cent of controls drank similar quantities. Harlap and Shiono (1980) also found increased risk for abortion in women who drank in the first trimester, but Halmesmärki *et al.* (1989) found that alcohol consumption was nearly identical in women who did and did not experience an abortion. In the latter study 13 per cent of aborters and 11 per cent of control women drank on average 3–4 drinks per week. Other investigations have recently reached similar conclusions (Parazzini *et al.* 1990).

Alcohol consumption should be avoided or minimized during pregnancy for many reasons, but alcohol may increase the pregnancy loss rate relatively little. Given the high frequency of alcohol ingestion in the general population, however, even a small effect could have great epidemiologic significance.

Contraceptive agents

Conception with an intrauterine device in place clearly increases the risk of fetal loss. However, if the device is removed prior to pregnancy, there is no increased risk of spontaneous abortions. Use of oral contraceptives before or during pregnancy is not associated with fetal loss, nor is spermicide exposure prior to or after conception (Simpson 1985).

Trauma

Women commonly attribute pregnancy losses to trauma like a fall or blow to the abdomen. However, fetuses are actually well protected from external trauma by intervening maternal structures and amniotic fluid. The contribution of this aetiology to early pregnancy loss can be considered quite small.

Psychological factors

Impaired psychological well-being has been claimed to predispose to early fetal losses. Investigations cited as proving a benefit to psychological well-being are those of Stray-Pederson and Stray-Pederson (1984). Those pregnant women previously experiencing repetitive abortions received increased attention but no specific medical therapy ('tender loving care'). These women ($n = 16$) proved more likely (85 per cent) to complete their pregnancies than 42 women not provided with such close attention (36 per cent successful outcome). One pitfall was that only women living 'close' to the university were eligible to be placed in the increased attention group. Women living further away served as 'controls', although they may have differed from the experimental group in ways other than geographic proximity. A few other studies have also been cited as consistent with a beneficial effect of psychological well-being (Houwert-de Jong *et al.* 1989; Liddell *et al.* 1991; Rai and Regan 1995). However, any ostensible positive effect of psychological well-being could be either more apparent than real or secondary to other factors. Neurotic or mentally ill women experience losses just like other women, but the loss rate in the former is not necessarily increased.

Severe maternal illness

Symptomatic maternal diseases causing *early* pregnancy loss include Wilson's disease, maternal phenylketonuria, cyanotic heart disease, haemoglobinopathies, and inflammatory bowel disease. Many other debilitating maternal diseases have been implicated in early abortion. Pathogenesis presumably involves one or more of the mechanisms discussed previously, probably endocrinologic or immunologic. Overall, relatively few fetal losses will prove the result of severe maternal disease.

Mendelian and polygenic factors

Consecutive abortuses in a given family show a non-random distribution with respect to chromosomal complements (Hassold 1980). If the complement of the first abortus is abnormal, the likelihood is about 80 per cent that the complement of the second abortus also will be abnormal (Warburton *et al.* 1987). The recurrent chromosomal abnormality is usually trisomy, but it may be monosomy or polyploidy. These data suggest that certain couples are predisposed toward chromosomally abnormal conceptions, most of which naturally result in a spontaneous abortion. Conversely, recurrence also applies for chromosomally normal abortuses. In the past there has been a tendency to assume that if no laboratory tests confirm the presence of a genetic disorder, one should search for non-genetic causes. With almost weekly elucidation of the genetic basis for many given conditions, investigators should no longer display such naïvety.

In spontaneous abortions not showing chromosomal abnormalities, Mendelian mutations could play key roles. The potential extent can be envisioned by recalling that 1.0 per cent of live-born infants have an abnormality due to a single-gene (Mendelian) mutation and that 1.0 per cent have a polygenic/multifactorial condition. In contrast, only 0.6 per cent have a chromosomal abnormality. Thus, the 40–50 per cent of abortuses with normal chromosomes need not necessarily require explanation on a non-genetic basis like infections, luteal phase insufficiency, or uterine anomalies. Such losses could be caused by a mutant gene. The scientific task over the next decade is to enumerate genes whose perturbations result in pregnancy loss. A host of mechanisms readily come to mind, for example genes necessary for placental transport of key nutrients. The role of developmental genes like *PAX* or *HOX* will be of special interest.

REFERENCES

Alberman, E.D. (1981). The abortus as a predictor of future trisomy 21. In *Trisomy 21 (Down Syndrome)*, (ed. F.F. De la Cruz and P.S. Gerald) pp. 69–? University Park Press, Baltimore.
Alberman, E.D., Creasy, M., Elliott, M., and Spicer, C. (1976). Maternal effects associated with fetal chromosomal anomalies in spontaneous abortions. *British Journal of Obstetrics and Gynaecology*, 83, 621–27.
Barlow, S. and Sullivan, F.M. (1982). *Reproductive hazards of industrial chemicals: an evaluation of animal and human data*. Academic Press, New York.
Beatty, R.A. (1978). The origin of human triploidy: an integration of qualitative and quantitative evidence. *Annals of Human Genetics*, 41, 299–314.
Ben Rafael, Z., Seidman, D.S., and Recabi, K. (1991). Uterine anomalies. A retrospective, matched control study. *Journal of Reproductive Medicine*, 36, 723–7.

Boué, A. and Gallano, P. (1984). A collaborative study of the segregation of inherited chromo-some structural arrangements in 1356 prenatal diagnoses. *Prenatal Diagnosis*, 4, 45–67.

Boué, J., Boué, A., and Lazar, P. (1975). Retrospective and prospective epidemiological studies of 1500 karyotyped spontaneous human abortions. *Teratology*, 12, 11–26.

Branch, D.W. and Ward, K. (1989). Autoimmunity and pregnancy loss. *Seminars on Reproductive Endocrinology*, 7, 168–79.

Candiani, G.B., Fedele, L., Parazzini, F., and Zamberletti, D. (1990). Reproductive prognosis after abdominal metroplasty in bicornuate or septate uterus: a life table analysis. *British Journal of Obstetrics and Gynaecology*, 97, 613–17.

Carp, H.J., Menashe, Y., Frenkel, Y., Many, A., Nebel, L., Toder, V., and Masiach, S. (1993). Lupus anticoagulant. Significance in habitual first-trimester abortion. *Journal of Reproductive Medicine*, 38, 549–52.

Carson, S.A., Simpson, J.L., Chesney, C., Conley, M.R., Metzger, B., and Aarons, J. (1996). Anti-phospholipid antibodies and first trimester spontaneous abortion: prospective study of possible pregnancies detected within 21 days of conception [Abstract]. *Journal of the Society for Gynecological Investigation*, 3(25), 198 A.

Castilla, E.E., Simpson, J.L., and Queenan, J.T. (1995). Down syndrome is not increased in off-spring of natural family planning users (case control analysis) (Letter). *American Journal of Medical Genetics*, 59, 525.

Chandley, A.C. (1981). The origin of chromosome aberrations in man and their potential for survival and reproduction in the adult human populations. *Annals of Genetics*, 24, 5–11.

Christiansen, O.B., Mathiesen, O., Lauritsen, J.G., and Grunnet, N. (1990). Idiopathic recur-rent spontaneous abortion: evidence of familial predisposition. *Acta Obstetrica et Gynecologia Scandinavica*, 69, 597–601.

Clarke, G.N. and Baker, H.W. (1993). Lack of association between sperm antibodies and recurrent spontaneous abortion. *Fertility and Sterility*, 59, 463–4.

Coulam, C.B. (1992). Immunologic tests in the evaluation of reproductive disorders: a critical review. *American Journal of Obstetrics and Gynecology*, 167, 1844–51.

Cowchock, S. (1991). Autoantibodies and pregnancy wastage. *American Journal of Reproductive Immunology*, 26, 38–41.

Daniel, A., Hook, E.B., and Wulf, G. (1989). Risks of unbalanced progeny at amniocentesis to carriers of chromosome rearrangements: data from United States and Canadian Laboratories. *American Journal of Medical Genetics*, 31, 14–53.

Davis, O.K., Berkley, A.S., Naus, G.J., Cholst, I.N., and Freedman, K.S. (1989). The incidence of luteal phase defect in normal, fertile women, determined by serial endometrial biopsy. *Fertility and Sterility*, 51, 582–6.

Daya, S. and Ward, S. (1988). Diagnostic test properties of serum progesterone in the evalua-tion of luteal phase defects. *Fertility and Sterility*, 49, 168–70.

Daya, S., Ward, S., and Burrows, E. (1988). Progesterone profiles in luteal phase defect cycles and outcome of progesterone treatment in patients with recurrent spontaneous abortions. *American Journal of Obstetrics and Gynecology*, 158, 225–32.

De Braekeleer, M. and Dao, T.N. (1990). Cytogenetic studies in couples experiencing repeated pregnancy losses. *Human Reproduction*, 5, 519–28.

Delhanty, J.D.A. and Handiside, A.H. (1995). The origin of genetic defects in the human and their detection in the preimplantation embryo. *Human Reproduction Update*, 1, 201–15.

el Ridi, A.M., Nada, S.M., Aly, A.S., Ramadan, M.E., Hagar, E.G., and Taha, T.A. (1991). Toxoplasmosis and pregnancy: an analytical study in Zagazig, *Journal of the Egyptian Society of Parasitology*, 21, 81–5.

Elias, M. and Eldor, A. (1984). Thromboembolism in patients with 'lupus' type circulating anticoagulant. *Archives of Internal Medicine*, 144, 510–15.

Ergolu, G.E. and Scopelitis, E. (1994). Antinuclear and antiphospholipid antibodies in healthy women with recurrent spontaneous abortion. *American Journal of Reproductive Immunology*, **31**, 1–6.

Erguven, S., Asar, G., Gulmezoglu, A.M., and Yergok, Y.Z. (1990). Antisperm and anticardiolipin antibodies in recurrent abortions. *Mikrobiyol Bulgaria*, **24**, 1–7.

Fija-Talamanaca, I. and Settimi, L. (1984). Occupational factors and reproductive outcome. In *Spontaneous abortion*, (ed. E.S.E. Hafez), pp. 61–80. MTP Press, Lancaster.

Fisher, J.M., Harvey, J.F., Morton, N.E., and Jacobs, P.A. (1995). Trisomy 18: studies of the parent and cell division of origin and the effect of aberrant recombination on nondisjunction. *American Journal of Human Genetics*, **56**, 669–75.

Fraser, E.J., Grimes, D.A., and Schultz, K.F. (1993). Immunization as therapy for recurrent spontaneous abortion: a review and meta-analysis. *Obstetrics and Gynecology*, **82**, 854–9.

Golan, A., Langer, R., Keuman, M., Wexler, S., Sege, V.E., and David, M.P. (1992). Obstetric outcome in women with congenital uterine malformations. *Journal of Reproductive Medicine*, **37**, 233–6.

Gray, R.H., Simpson, J.L., Kambic, R.T., Queenan, J.T., Barbato, M., and Perez, A. (1995). Timing of conception and the risk of spontaneous abortion among pregnancies occurring during the use of natural family planning. *American Journal of Obstetrics and Gynecology*, **172**, 1567–72.

Halmesmärki, E., Valimaki, M., Roine, R., Ylikahri, R., and Ylikorkala, O. (1989). Maternal and paternal alcohol consumption and miscarriage. *British Journal of Obstetrics and Gynaecology*, **96**, 188–91.

Harlap, S. and Shiono, P.H. (1980). Alcohol, smoking and incidence of spontaneous abortions in the first and second trimester. *Lancet*, **ii**, 173–6.

Hass, G.G.J., Kubota, K., Quebbeman, J.F., Jijon, A., Menge, A.D., and Beer, A. (1986). Circulating antisperm antibodies in recurrent aborting women. *Fertility and Sterility*, **45**, 209–15.

Hassold, T. (1980). A cytogenetic study of repeated spontaneous abortions. *American Journal of Human Genetics*, **32**, 723–30.

Hassold, T., Benham, F., and Leppert, M. (1985). Cytogenetic and molecular analysis of sex-chromosome monosomy. *American Journal of Human Genetics*, **42**, 534–41.

Hassold, T., Merrill, M., Adkins, K., Freeman, S., and Sherman, S. (1995). Recombination and maternal age-dependent nondisjunction: molecular studies of trisomy 16. *American Journal of Human Genetics*, **57**, 867–74.

Henderson, D.J., Sherman, L.S., Loughna, S.C., Bennett, P.R., and Moore, G.E. (1994). Early embryonic failure associated with uniparental disomy for human chromosome 21. *Human Molecular Genetics*, **3**, 1373–6.

Hill, J.A., Polgar, K., and Anderson, D.J. (1995). T-helper 1-type immunity to trophoblast in women with recurrent spontaneous abortion. *Journal of the American Medical Association*, **273**, 1958–9.

Houwert-de Jong, M.H., Termijtelen, A., Eskes, T.K., Manting, L.A., and Bruinse, H.W. (1989). The natural course of habitual abortion. *European Journal of Obstetrics Gynecology and Reproductive Biology*, **33**, 221–8.

Karamardian, L.M. and Grimes, D.A. (1992). Luteal phase deficiency: effect of treatment on pregnancy rates. *American Journal of Obstetrics and Gynecology*, **167**, 1391–8.

Kline, J., Shrout, P., Stein, Z.A., Susser, M., and Warburton, D. (1980). Drinking during pregnancy and spontaneous abortion. *Lancet*, **ii**, 176–80.

Laitinen, T., Koskimies, S., and Westman, P. (1993). Foeto-maternal compatibility in HLA-DR, -DQ, and -DP loci in Finnish couples suffering from recurrent spontaneous abortions. *European Journal of Immunology*, **20**, 249–58.

Li, T.C., Dockery, P., Rogers, A.W., and Cooke, I.D. (1989). How precise is histologic dating of endometrium using the standard dating criteria? *Fertility and Sterility*, **51**, 759–63.

Liddell, H.S., Pattison, N.S., and Zanderigo, A. (1991). Recurrent miscarriage—outcome after supportive care in early pregnancy. *Australian and New Zealand Journal of Obstetrics and Gynecology*, 31, 320–21.

Macdonald, M., Hassold, T., Harvey, J., Wang, L.H., Morton, N.E., and Jacobs, P. (1994). The origin of 47, XXY and 47, XXX aneuploidy: heterogeneous mechanisms and role of aberrant recombination. *Human Molecular Genetics*, 3, 1365–71.

Makino, T., Sakai, A., Sugi, T., Toyoshima, K., Iwasaki, K., and Maruyama, T. (1991). Current comprehensive therapy of habitual abortion. *Annals of the New York Academy of Science*, 626, 597–604.

Michalas, S.P. (1991). Outcome of pregnancy in women with uterine malformation: evaluation of 62 cases. *International Journal of Gynecology and Obstetrics*, 35, 215–19.

Mills, J.L., Simpson, J.L., Driscoll, S.G., Jovanovic-Peterson, L., Van Allen, M., Aarons, J.H., et al. (1988). Incidence of spontaneous abortion among normal women and insulin-dependent diabetic women whose pregnancies were identified within 21 days of conception. *New England Journal of Medicine*, 319, 1617–23.

Mills, J.L., Holmes, L., Aarons, J.H., Simpson, J.L., Brown, Z.A., Jovanovic-Peterson, L.G., et al. (1993). Moderate caffeine use and the risk of spontaneous abortion and intrauterine growth retardation. *Journal of the American Medical Association*, 269, 593–7.

Miodovnik, M., Mimouni, F., Tsang, R.C., Ammar, E., Kaplan, L., and Siddiqi, T.A. (1986). Glycemic control and spontaneous abortion in insulin dependent diabetic women. *Obstetrics and Gynecology*, 68, 366–9.

Mishell, D.J. (1993). Recurrent abortion. *Journal of Reproductive Medicine*, 38, 250–9.

Montoro, M., Collea, J.V., Frasiers, D., and Mestman, J.H. (1981). Successful outcome of pregnancy in women with hypothyroidism. *Annals of Internal Medicine*, 94, 31–4.

Moutos, D.M., Damewood, M.D., Schlaff, W.D., and Rock, J.A. (1992). A comparison of the reproductive outcome between women with a unicornuate uterus and women with a didelphic uterus. *Fertility and Sterility*, 58, 88–93.

Mowbray, J.F., Gibbings, C., Liddell, H., Reginald, P.W., and Underwood, J.W. (1985). Controlled trial of treatment of recurrent spontaneous abortion by immunization with paternal cells. *Lancet*, 1, 941–3.

Norman, D.J., Barry, J.M., and Fischer, S. (1986). The beneficial effect of pretransplant third-party blood transfusions on allograft rejection in HLA identical sibling kidney transplants. *Transplantation*, 41, 125–6.

Ober, C.L., Simpson, J.L., Hauck, W.W., Amos, D.B., Kostyu, D.D., Fotino, M., and Allen, F.H.J. (1983). Shared HLA antigens and reproductive performance among Hutterites. *American Journal of Human Genetics*, 35, 994–1004.

Ober, C., Elias, S., Kostyu, D.D., and Hauck, W.W. (1992). Decreased fecundability in hutterite couples sharing HLA-DR. *American Journal of Human Genetics*, 50, 6–14.

Olliaro, P., Regazzetti, A., Gorini, G., Milano, F., Marchetti, A., and Rondanelli, E.G. (1991). Chlamydia trachomatis infection in 'sine causa' recurrent abortion. *Bollettino dell Istituto Sierolerapico Milanese*, 70, 467–70.

Parazzini, F., Bocciolone, L., LaVecchia, C., Negri, E., and Fedele, L. (1990). Maternal and paternal moderate daily alcohol consumption and unexplained miscarriages. *British Journal of Obstetrics and Gynaecology*, 97, 618–22.

Petri, M., Golbus, M., Anderson, R., Whiting-O'Keefe, Q., Corash, L., and Hellmann, D. (1987). Lupus anticoagulant. Significance in habitual first-trimester abortion. *Arthritis and Rheumatism*, 30, 601–6.

Pettanati, M.J., Rao, P.N., Phelan, M.C., Grass, F., Rao, K.W., and Cosper, P. (1995). Paracentric inversions in humans: a review of 446 paracentric inversions with presentation of 120 new cases. *American Journal of Medical Genetics*, 55, 171–87.

Poland, B.J., Miller, J.R., Jones, D.C., and Trimble, B.K. (1977). Reproductive counseling in patients who have had a spontaneous abortion. *American Journal of Obstetrics and Gynecology*, 127, 685–91.

Pratt, D., Novotny, M., Kaberlein, G., Didkiewicz, A., and Gleicher, N. (1994). Antithyroid antibodies and the association with non-organ-specific antibodies in recurrent pregnancy loss (Comments). *American Journal of Obstetrics and Gynecology*, 170, 956–7.

Quenby, S.M. and Farquharson, R.G. (1993). Predicting recurring miscarriage: what is important? *Obstetrics and Gynecology*, 82, 132–8.

Quinn, P.A., Petric, M., Barkin, M., Butany, J., Derzko, C., and Gysler, M. (1987). Prevalence of antibody to *Chlamydia trachomatis* in spontaneous abortion and infertility. *American Journal of Obstetrics and Gynecology*, 156, 291–6.

Rae, R., Smith, I.W., Liston, W.A., and Kilpatrick, D.C. (1994). Chlamydial serologic studies and recurrent spontaneous abortion. *American Journal of Obstetrics and Gynecology*, 170, 782–5.

Rai, C.K. and Regan, L. (1995). Future pregnancy outcome in women with unexplained recurrent miscarriage. *Human Reproduction*, 10, 19–20.

Regan, L. (1988). A prospective study on spontaneous abortion. In *Early pregnancy loss: mechanisms and treatment*, (ed. R.W. Beard and F. Sharp), pp. 23–37. The Royal College of Obstetricians and Gynaecologists, London.

Regan, L., Owen, E.J., and Jacobs, H.S. (1990). Hypersecretion of lutenising hormone, infertility, and miscarriage. *Lancet*, 336, 1141–3.

Sagle, M., Bishop, K., Ridley, N., Alexander, I.M., Michel, M., and Bonney, R.C. (1988). Recurrent early miscarriage and polycystic ovaries. *British Medical Journal*, 297, 1027–8.

Savitz, D.A., Sonnenfeld, N.L., and Olshan, A.F. (1994). Review of epidemiologic studies of paternal occupational exposure and spontaneous abortion. *American Journal of Ind Medicine*, 25, 361–83.

Scott, J.R., Rote, N.S., and Branch, D.W. (1987). Immunologic aspects of recurrent abortions and fetal death. *Obstetrics and Gynecology*, 70, 645–56.

Scott, R.T., Synder, R.R., Strickland, D.M., Tybinski, C.C., Bagnall, J.A., and Reed, K.R. (1988). The effect of interobserver variation in dating endometrial history on the diagnosis of luteal phase defects. *Fertility and Sterility*, 50, 888–92.

Simon, C., Martinez, L., Pardo, F., Tortajada, M., and Pellicer, A. (1991). Mullerian defects in women with normal reproductive outcome. *Fertility and Sterility*, 56, 1192–3.

Simpson, J.L. (1976). *Disorders of sexual differentiation, etiology and clinical delineation*. Academic Press, New York.

Simpson, J.L. (1985). Relationship between congenital anomalies and contraception. *Advances in Contraception*, 1, 3–30.

Simpson, J.L. (1996). Fetal wastage. In *Obstetrics: normal and abnormal pregnancies*, (3rd edn), (ed. S.G. Gabbe, J.R. Niebyl, and J.L. Simpson). Churchill Livingstone, New York.

Simpson, J.L. and Bombard, A.T. (1987). Chromosomal abnormalities in spontaneous abortion: Frequency, pathology and genetic counselling. In *Spontaneous abortion*, (ed. K. Edmonds and M.J. Bennett), pp. 51–76. Blackwell, London.

Simpson, J.L. and Carson, S. (1993). Causes of fetal loss. In *Symposium on biological and demographic determinants of human reproduction*, (ed. R. Gray, L. Leridon, and F. Spira), pp. 287–315. Oxford University Press, Oxford.

Simpson, J.L. and Tharapel, A.T. (1991). Principles of cytogenetics. In *Scientific foundations of obstetrics and gynaecology*, (4th edn), (ed. E. Philip and J. Barnes), pp. 27–50. Heinemann, London.

Simpson, J.L., Elias, S., and Martin, A.O. (1981). Parental chromosomal rearrangements associated with repetitive spontaneous abortion. *Fertility and Sterility*, 36, 584–90.

Simpson, J.L., Mills, J.L., Holmes, L.B., Ober, C.L., Aarons, J., Jovanovic, L. and Knopp, R.H. (1987). Low fetal loss rates after demonstration of a live fetus in the first trimester. *Journal of the American Medical Association*, 258, 2555–7.

Simpson, J.L., Gray, R.H., Queenan, J.T., Mena, P., Perez, A., and Kambic, R.T. (1988). Pregnancy outcome associated with natural family planning (NFP): scientific basis and experimental design for an international cohort study. *Advances in Contraception*, 4, 247–64.

Simpson, J.L., Meyers, C.M., Martin, A.O., Elias, S., and Ober, C. (1989). Translocations are infrequent among couples having repeated spontaneous abortions but no other abnormal pregnancies. *Fertility and Sterility*, **51**, 811–14.

Simpson, J.L., Gray, R.H., Queenan, J.T., Barbato, M., Perez, A., and Mena, P. (1994). Risk of recurrent spontaneous abortion for pregnancies discovered in the fifth week of gestation (Letter). *Lancet*, **344**, 964.

Simpson, J.L., Mills, J.L., Lee, J., Holmes, J.B., Kim, H., Metzger, B., *et al.* (1996). Infectious processes: an infrequent cause of first trimester spontaneous abortions. *Human Reproduction*, **11**, 618–72.

Simpson, J.L., Carson, S.A., Mills, J.L., Conley, M.R., Aarons, J., and Holmes, L.B. (1996). Prospective study showing that antisperm antibodies are not associated with pregnancy loss. *Fertility and Sterility*, **66**(1), 36–42.

Sompolinsky, D., Solomon, F., Elkina, L., Weinraub, Z., Bukovsky, I., and Caspi, E. (1975). Infections with mycoplasma and bacteria in induced midtrimester abortion and fetal loss. *American Journal of Obstetrics and Gynecology*, **121**, 610–16.

Sorokin, Y., Johnson, M.P., Uhlman, W.R., Zador, I.E., Drugan, A., and Koppitch, F.C. (1991). Postmortem chorionic villus sampling: correlation of cytogenetic and ultrasound findings. *American Journal of Medical Genetics*, **39**, 314–16.

Stampe-Sorensen, S. (1988). Estimated prevalence of mullerian anomalies. *Acta Obstetrica et Gynecologia Scandinavica*, **67**, 441–5.

Stein, A.L. and March, C.M. (1990). Pregnancy outcome in women with mullerian duct anomalies. *Journal of Reproductive Medicine*, **35**, 411–14.

Stray-Pedersen, B. and Stray-Pedersen, S. (1984). Etiologic factors and subsequent reproductive performance in 195 couples with a prior history of habitual abortion. *American Journal of Obstetrics and Gynecology*, **148**, 140–6.

Stray-Pedersen, B., Eng, J., and Reikvam, T.M. (1978). Uterine T-mycoplasma colonization in reproductive failure. *American Journal of Obstetrics and Gynecology*, **130**, 307–11.

Strom, C., Ginsberg, N., Applebaum, M., Bozorgi, N., White, M., Caffarelli, M., and Verlinsky, Y. (1992). Analyses of 95 first trimester spontaneous abortions by chorionic villus sampling and karyotpye. *Journal of Assisted Reproductive Genetics*, **9**, 458–61.

Sutherland, G.R., Gardiner, A.J., and Carter, R.F. (1976). Familial pericentric inversion of chromosome 19 inv (19) (p13q13) with a note on genetic counseling of pericentric inversion carriers. *Clinical Genetics*, **10**, 54–9.

Taskinen, H., Lindbohm, M.-L., and Hemninki, K. (1986). Spontaneous abortions among women working in the pharmaceutical industry. *British Journal of Industrial Medicine*, **43**, 199–205.

Tho, P.T., Byrd, J.R., and McDonough, P.C. (1979). Etiologies and subsequent reproductive performance of 100 couples with recurrent abortions. *Fertility and Sterility*, **32**, 389–95.

Toth, A., Lesser, M.L., Brooks-Toth, C.W., and Feiner, C. (1986). Outcome of subsequent pregnancies following antibiotic therapy after primary or multiple spontaneous abortions. *Surgery, Gynecology and Obstetrics*, **163**, 243–50.

US Department of Health and Human Services (1982). Reproductive impairments among married couples. In *US Vital and Health Statistics Series 23*, Vol. 11, p. 5. National Center of Health Statistics, Hyattsville, MD.

Van Iddelinge, B. and Hofmeyr, G.J. (1991). Recurrent spontaneous abortion—aetiological factors and subsequent reproductive performance in 76 couples. *South African Medical Journal*, **80**, 223–6.

Vlaanderen, W. and Treffers, P.E. (1987). Prognosis of subsequent pregnancies after recurrent spontaneous abortion in first trimester. *British Medical Journal of Clinical Research*, **295**, 92–3.

Wapner, R., Simpson, J.L., Golbus, M.S., Desnick, R.J., Jackson, L., and Lubs, H.A. (1992). Confirmed chorionic mosaicism: association with fetal loss but not with adverse perinatal outcome. *Prenatal Diagnosis*, **12**, 347–56.

Warburton, D. and Fraser, F.C. (1964). Spontaneous abortion risks in man: data from reproductive histories collected in a medical genetics unit. *American Journal of Human Genetics*,
16, 1–25.

Warburton, D., Kline, J., Stein, Z., Hutzler, M., Chin, A., and Hassold, T. (1987). Does the
karyotype of a spontaneous abortion predict the karyotype of a subsequent abortion?
Evidence from 273 women with two karyotyped spontaneous abortions. *American Journal
of Human Genetics*, 41, 465–83.

Watt, J.L., Templeton, A.A., Messinis, I., Bell, L., Cunningham, P., and Duncan, R.O. (1987).
Trisomy I in an eight cell human pre-embryo. *Journal of Medical Genetics*, 24, 60–4.

Wilcox, A.J., Weinberg, C.R., O'Connor, J.F., Baird, D.D., Schlatterer, J.P., and Canfield, R.E.
(1988). Incidence of early loss of pregnancy. *New England Journal of Medicine*, 319,
189–94.

Witkin, S.S. and Chaudhry, A. (1989). Association between recurrent spontaneous abortions
and circulating IgG antibodies to sperm tails in women. *Journal of Reproductive
Immunology*, 15, 151–8.

Witkin, S.S. and Ledger, W.J. (1992). Antibodies to *Chlamydia trachomatis* in sera of women
with recurrent spontaneous abortions. *American Journal of Obstetrics and Gynecology*, 167,
135–9.

Yan, J.H. (1990). Evaluation of circulating antisperm antibodies and seminal immunosupres-
sive material in repeatedly aborting couples. *Chung Hua Fu Chan Ko Tsa Chih*, 25, 343–4.

Zaragoza, M.V., Jacobs, P.A., and James, R.S. (1994). Nondisjunction of human acrocentric
chromosomes: studies of 432 trisomic fetuses and liveborns. *Human Genetics*, 64, 411–17.

Zavala-Vlazquez, J., Guzman-Marin, E., Barrera-Perez, M., and Rodriguez-Feliz, M.E. (1989).
Toxoplasmosis and abortion in patients at the O'Horon Hospital of Merida, Yucatan. *Salud
publica de Mexico*, 31, 664–8.

Zhang, X.C. (1990). Clinical study on circulating antisperm antibodies in women with recurrent abortion. *Chung Hua Fu Chan Ko Tsa Chih*, 25, 21–3.

19 | *Assessment of embryonic and early fetal viability*

Eric Jauniaux and Richard Jaffe

INTRODUCTION

The advent of high resolution ultrasound imaging moved prenatal diagnosis initially from the third to the second trimester of pregnancy and more recently into the first trimester within a few weeks of conception. This has changed our perception of human development *in utero* and the embryo is more easily perceived as an individual by its parents than was the mid-pregnancy fetus of 20 years ago. Some of the new methods of prenatal testing are now available to parents from three weeks after implantation. Thus, demand for early prenatal diagnosis is increasing continually, especially among women of advanced maternal age with higher education and socio-economic levels. Numerous ethical, social, financial, and medical questions have been raised by the rapid development of these new procedures. In particular, the potential long-term risk to the developing fetus associated with some of these techniques is a matter of permanent debate. In the present chapter, we review the various non-invasive and invasive techniques recently developed for prenatal screening and diagnosis in early pregnancy.

NON-INVASIVE TECHNIQUES

Spontaneous abortion is the most common complication of pregnancy in humans. It has been shown that about 30–40 per cent of all conceptions are lost within the first few weeks after implantation (Miller *et al.* 1980; Zinaman *et al.* 1996) and about 15 per cent are lost before the end of the second month of gestation (Goldstein 1994). At least 80 per cent of miscarriages are associated with disturbed embryonic development diagnosable on ultrasound scanning before the end of the first trimester. At 10–13 weeks of gestation when dating scans are being performed in the general population, the prevalence of pregnancy failure drops to 2–3 per cent (Goldstein 1994; Pandya *et al.* 1996). Non-invasive tests have been used for both low and high risk pregnancies to assess embryonic viability and screen for chromosomal abnormalities. They are becoming widely available and should be a prerequisite to genetic counselling and be performed before an invasive procedure is offered to a couple with a fetus at increased risk of chromosomal or genetic disorders.

Maternal biochemistry

Threatened abortions

Endocrinology has been used extensively in the diagnosis of ectopic pregnancy and the evaluation of molar pregnancy but there is little convincing evidence that maternal endocrinology is clinically useful in predicting pregnancy failure. Indeed, the correlations of ultrasound and circulating placental protein measurements indicate that the diagnostic value of ultrasound in threatened abortion is often better than that of most biochemical tests (Stabile 1992). Before the appearance of any clinical symptoms, some forms of early pregnancy failure may be associated with abnormal serum levels of specific placental protein, but this is still a matter of some debate (Johnson *et al.* 1993). A recent prospective controlled study has demonstrated that a single serum measurement of free human chorionic gonadotropin β (hCGβ) taken in early pregnancy is valuable in the immediate diagnosis of early pregnancy failure and the long-term prognosis of viability (Al-Sebai *et al.* 1996).

Missed abortions

Anembryonic pregnancies are probably the earliest form of missed abortion in which the embryo died a considerable time prior to the first ultrasound examination (Jauniaux *et al.* 1994a, 1995a). In about one-third of these cases, maternal circulating levels of placental specific proteins remain within the normal range and it has been suggested that the production of these proteins by the trophoblast is independent, to some extent, of normal embryonic development (Stabile 1992). Measurements of alpha-fetoprotein (AFP) levels in maternal serum (MS) have been widely used to predict early pregnancy complications chromosomal abnormalities, and various fetal malformations. In a recent study, comparing AFP levels inside the gestational sac with those of MS, seven out of the nine patients with an empty gestational sac on ultrasound had high MS-AFP levels whereas these levels were low in six of the corresponding coelomic fluid samples. These findings suggest that elevated MS-AFP in these abnormal early pregnancies is the result of an increased AFP transfer through the placenta, probably due to a breakdown of the trophoblastic barrier rather than an abnormally high production of AFP inside the gestational sac. In these cases, AFP in both coelomic fluid and MS from the gestational sac is predominantly of secondary yolk sac origin, indicating that most pregnancies traditionally classified as anembryonic result from early embryonic demise, the embryo having developed for at least 14 days after ovulation, corresponding to the stage of embryonic life when the secondary yolk sac starts to form.

Aneuploidies with a viable fetus

The frequency of associated chromosomal abnormalities in first trimester clinical spontaneous abortion is as high as 50 per cent and includes 31 per cent trisomy, 30 per cent triploidy, and 25 per cent monosomy X (Jauniaux *et al.* 1996a). Most cases of triploidy and monosomy X are lost before the end of the second month of gestation whereas at least one-third of trisomies and, in particular, cases of trisomy 21 survive into the second or third trimester of pregnancy without major obstetrical complications and/or detectable fetal abnormalities. Maternal serum biochemistry has therefore been the focus of a lot of interest for the screening of fetuses for Down syndrome and other aneuploidies. The relationship between abnormal MS-hCG and MS-AFP levels with second trimester fetal trisomy has been described in numerous published reports. More recent reports have suggested that free hCGβ and various other specific placental markers such as pregnancy-associated plasma protein A (PAPP-A) may be more efficient for the screening of trisomy in early pregnancy (Brambati *et al.* 1994; Jauniaux *et al.* 1996*b*; Wald *et al.* 1996). There is no obvious physiopathological explanation for the pattern of changes in maternal serum levels of placental and fetal proteins found in trisomies. The relative immaturity of the feto-placental function or a change in the balance of placental versus fetal protein secretion are the two main theories proposed to explain the second trimester findings of high MS-hCG and low MS-AFP in pregnancies presenting with trisomy 21 (Chard 1991). The absence of a change in the expression of the α and β subunits of hCG in samples of placental tissue from pregnancies presenting with trisomy 21 between 11 and 15 weeks of gestation suggest that the mechanism involved in the increased serum level of free hCGβ in trisomy 21 occurs during the post-translational phase of hCG biosynthesis (Brizot *et al.* 1995). By contrast, in trisomy 18 the decrease in MS-hCG subunits results from an impairment in the transcription of the corresponding gene (Fig. 19.1) which affects to a greater extent the β subunit than the α subunit (Brizot *et al.* 1996).

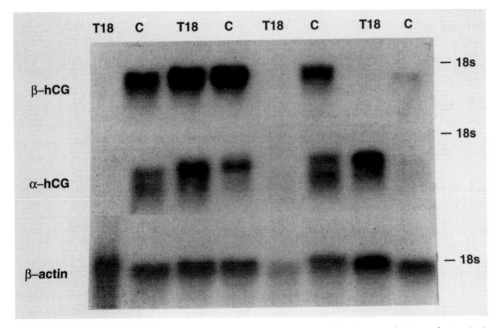

Fig. 19.1   Representative Northern blot showing expression of β-hCG, α-hCG and β-actin in 4 series of placental samples from normal and trisomic pregnancies matched for gestational age. (From Brizot *et al.* 1996.)

Sonography

The early gestational sac

The deciduo-placental interface and the exocoelomic cavity are the first sonographic evidence of a pregnancy (Fig. 19.2) and can be visualized with transvaginal ultrasound around 4.4–4.6 menstrual weeks (32–34 days) when they reach together a size of 2–4 mm (see Chapter 16). In normal pregnancies between the fifth and sixth weeks, the gestational sac grows at a rate of 1 mm/day in mean diameter. Once a gestational sac has been documented ultrasonographically, subsequent loss of viability in the embryonic period is still 11.5 per cent (Goldstein 1994). A smaller than expected gestational sac is a predictor of poor pregnancy outcome (Table 19.1), even in the presence of embryonic cardiac activity (Bromley *et al.* 1991; Dickey *et al.* 1994). Triploidy and trisomy 16 are more often associated with a small chorionic sac before nine weeks of gestation than other chromosomal abnormalities (Dickey *et al.* 1994).

The first structure to be seen inside the gestational sac (inside the exocoelomic cavity) before the embryo itself is the secondary yolk sac (SYS). The earliest SYS structures should be observed from the beginning of the fifth week of gestation or when the gestational sac reaches 10 mm in diameter (Jauniaux *et al.* 1991). The SYS diameter increases slightly between 5 and 10 weeks (Fig. 19.2) of gestation and then decreases. The predictive value of SYS measurements in determining the outcome of an early pregnancy is limited (Table 19.1). Most pregnancies which abort during the third month have normal SYS measurements at their initial scan before eight weeks of gestation (Jauniaux *et al.* 1991). Furthermore, it is usually the yolk sac which is found to persist inside the gestational sac after the embryo has disappeared (Jauniaux *et al.*

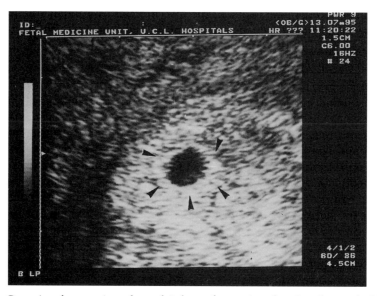

Fig. 19.2   Gestational sac at 4 weeks and 5 days of gestation showing the trophoblastic ring surrounding the exocoelomic cavity.

Table 19.1 Significance of sonographic measurements in early pregnancy and their individual predictive value in determining pregnancy outcome

Variable	Decreased	Increased	Predictive value
Gestational sac size	SA Tris 16/Trip	Twin Early conception	High
Yolk sac size	SA	SA	Low
Crown–rump length	SA Tris 18/Trip	Early conception	High
Fetal heart rate	SA Tris 18/13/16	Tris 21	High
Uterine Doppler PI	GTD	SA PIH	Low
Umbilical Doppler PI	N/A	Tris 18/Trip	Low
Intervillous flow	N/A	SA/pre-eclampsia	High

SA = spontaneous abortion; Tris = trisomy; Trip = triploidy; GTD = gestational trophoblastic disorders; PIH = pregnancy-induced hypertension; PI = pulsatility index; N/A = not available.

1995a). Thus variations of SYS size and sonographic appearance in most abnormal pregnancies are probably the consequence of poor embryonic development or embryonic death rather than being the primary cause of early pregnancy failure (Jauniaux et al. 1995a).

The embryo and early fetus

Precise determination of gestational age and embryonic or fetal size is a prerequisite for diagnosis of deviations from normality. If an embryo has developed up to 5 mm, subsequent loss of viability occurs in 7.2 per cent (Goldstein 1994). Loss rates drop to 3.3 per cent for embryos of 6–10 mm and to 0.5 per cent for embryos over 10 mm. Fetal growth can start to slow down at the end of the first trimester in ongoing pregnancies presenting with a chromosomal abnormality (Table 19.1) and in particular, in cases of trisomy 18 and triploidy (Kuhn et al. 1995). A comparison of crown–rump length (CRL) measurements with gestational ages calculated from the last menstrual period indicates that a CRL smaller than expected from dates is associated with a significant risk of chromosomal anomalies (Drugan et al. 1992). The larger the discrepancy, the higher the possibility that the aneuploidy affecting the pregnancy is of the severe or lethal type.

First trimester placenta

After 9–10 weeks of gestation, when the definitive placenta is formed, the relationship of the internal os to the lower edge of the placenta can be evaluated by transvaginal sonography (Hill et al. 1995). Approximately 6 per cent of patients will have a placenta praevia between 9 and 13 weeks of gestation. The likelihood that a placenta praevia will persist until later in pregnancy increases if the placenta covers the internal cervical os by 1.6 cm.

Gestational trophoblastic tumours can be routinely diagnosed by ultrasound during the second half of the first trimester (Jauniaux *et al.* 1995*b*). The distinction between complete and partial mole is based on clinical, endocrinological, and ultrasound criteria. Complete or classical hydatidiform mole (CHM) may coexist with a normal fetus and placenta in cases of molar transformation of one ovum in a dizygotic twin pregnancy (Fig. 19.3). This condition has often been wrongly incorporated in the partial hydatidiform mole (PHM) category, in particular when discovered in the first trimester of pregnancy. In these cases, ultrasound and pathologic investigations will demonstrate a CHM together with a distinct normal placenta. With advancing gestation, the diagnosis may be more difficult as the CHM may grow, partially covering the normal placental mass (Jauniaux and Nicolaides 1997). PHM are usually triploid, having two sets of chromosomes of paternal origin and one of maternal origin. Diploid PHM, confined placental triploid mosaicism, placental changes associated with Beckwith–Wiedemann syndrome, and a recently described placental vascular malformation associated with mesenchymal dysplasia of the villi can appear as PHM on a scan (Jauniaux *et al.* 1995*b*). In these cases, the fetus is usually anatomically normal and has a diploid karyotype. Following uterine evacuation, 10 per cent of patients with complete moles develop persistent gestational trophoblastic disease. It has been demonstrated recently that patients with partial moles may also develop (1–11 per cent) clinical residual trophoblastic tumours and should, therefore, be offered a follow-up similar to that of women with complete mole (Jauniaux *et al.* 1996*a*).

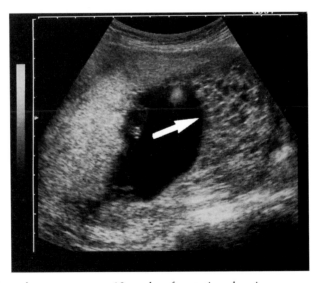

Fig. 19.3   Twin molar pregnancy at 12 weeks of gestation showing a normal placenta opposite to a classical mole (arrow).

Doppler ultrasound

Embryonic and fetal heart rate

Heart action is the earliest proof of a viable fetus and any pregnancy ultimately ending in a normal outcome has cardiac activity present in the early embryonic stages (Goldstein 1992). Fetal cardiac activity can be observed by sonography as early as six weeks of gestation, approximately at the time when the heart tube starts to beat (Fig. 19.4). Between six and nine weeks' gestation, there is a rapid increase in the mean heart rate from 125 to 175 beats per minute (bpm), followed by a gradual decrease to around 160 bpm at 14 weeks (Wisser and Dirschedl 1994). The rise in the heart rate parallels the increase in crown–rump length and is maximal when the morphological development of the embryonic heart is completed (Wisser and Dirschedl 1994).

Abnormal fetal heart rate patterns have been observed in pregnancies which subsequently abort (Table 19.1). A single observation of an abnormally slow heart rate does not necessarily indicate subsequent fetal death but a continuous decline in heart activity is inevitably associated with abortion (Merchiers *et al.* 1991). The incidence of pregnancy loss after confirmation of early cardiac activity is substantially greater in patients ≥ 36 years old (Smith and Buyalos 1996), probably because of the higher prevalence of chromosomal defects in that population. Sporadic cases of fetuses with Down syndrome presenting with an abnormally low heart rate in the first trimester of pregnancy have been previously reported (Laboda *et al.* 1989; Schats *et al.* 1990).

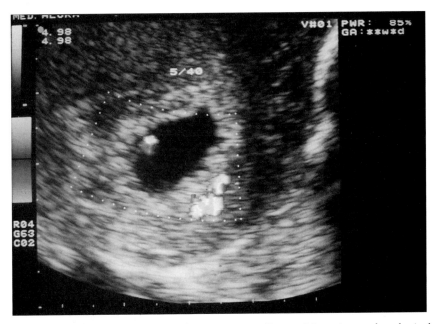

Fig. 19.4   Heart action of a 3.5 mm embryo corresponding to 25 somites embryological stage (5 weeks and 6 days postmenstruation). Note the absence of Doppler signal inside the placenta. *In colour*

However, Van Lith *et al.* (1992), in a study of 10 chromosomally abnormal fetuses between 6 and 16 weeks, including five with trisomy 21, found no difference in the fetal heart rate compared to normal fetuses. In contrast, we recently found that some trisomy 21 fetuses have a stable and significant increase in their mean fetal heart rate (Table 19.2) during the first trimester (Jauniaux *et al.* 1996c). Cardiac septal defects often found in fetuses with Down syndrome could be associated with a delay in the development of the conductive pathways between the upper and lower halves of the heart. The relationship in early pregnancy between congenital heart defects, fetal tachycardia, and fetal hydrops needs further exploration.

The placental circulations

The ability of Doppler ultrasound to detect flow velocity waveforms within the different branches of the uterine and feto-placental circulations has aroused much enthusiasm from clinicians interested in predicting early and late pregnancy complications related to an abnormal placentation (Jauniaux *et al.* 1995c, 1996c).

Flow resistance indices obtained from the umbilical artery remain high in early pregnancy, suggesting minor changes in vascular resistance until the beginning of the second trimester (Jauniaux *et al.* 1995a,b,c). Umbilical artery end-diastolic flow starts to appear after 10 weeks of gestation but is often incomplete and/or inconsistently present in normal fetuses between 11 and 13 weeks. In some fetuses with trisomy 18 or triploidy, an increased resistance to blood flow in the umbilical artery can already be found in early pregnancy (Table 19.2). The abnormal development of the placental tissue with poor vascularization of the villous trees can explain the increased resistance to flow observed in the umbilical artery of these cases (Jauniaux *et al.* 1996c).

An increased impedance to flow in the utero-placental circulation at 18–22 weeks and persistent notching predict the development of pregnancy—induced hyper-

Table 19.2 Comparison between fetal heart rate and umbilical Doppler ultrasound features in trisomy 21 and trisomy 18 with matched controls for gestational age (from Jauniaux *et al.* 1996c).

Variables	T_{21}	Controls	t p	T_{18}	Controls	t p
Heart rate (bpm)	170 ± 11 ($n = 21$)	162 ± 8 ($n = 63$)	10.1 (< 0.005)	160 ± 10 ($n = 13$)	163 ± 8 ($n = 39$)	1.1 NS
Variability 1 (bpm)	2.9 ± 2.4 ($n = 21$)	3.3 ± 2.5 ($n = 63$)	0.1 NS	2.0 ± 1.7 ($n = 13$)	3.0 ± 2.8 ($n = 39$)	2.0 NS
Variability 2 (bpm)	1.7 ± 1.5 ($n = 21$)	2.5 ± 1.9 ($n = 63$)	0.06 NS	1.8 ± 1.1 ($n = 13$)	2.3 ± 1.6 ($n = 39$)	0.41 NS
Umbilical PI	2.03 ± 0.43 ($n = 11$)	2.29 ± 0.43 ($n = 33$)	1.7 NS	2.58 ± 0.45 ($n = 10$)	2.32 ± 0.46 ($n = 30$)	2.0 NS

Data are presented as mean ± SD. t = rank test; NS = not significant; PI = pulsatility index.

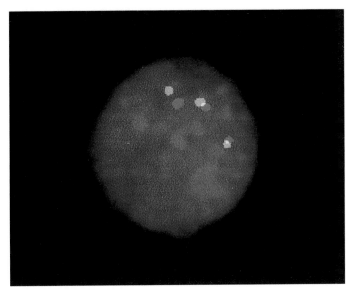

Fig. 2.4 Interphase nucleus from an 8-cell embryo showing three copies of chromosome 21, detected with two specific DNA probes, red, and green.

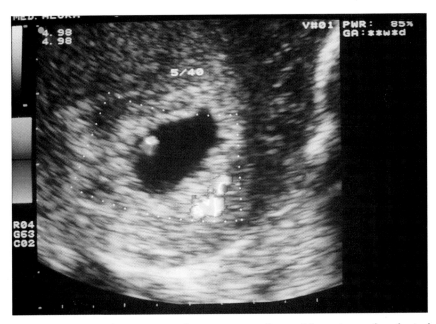

Fig. 19.4 Heart action of a 3.5 mm embryo corresponding to 25 somites embryological stage (5 weeks and 6 days postmenstruation). Note the absence of Doppler signal inside the placenta.

tension and/or intrauterine growth retardation later in gestation. Abnormal Doppler values in these cases have been associated with defective placentation and, in particular, with inadequate trophoblastic invasion and transformation of the spiral arteries of the placental bed. Similar histological features have been described in cases of spontaneous abortions (Hustin *et al.* 1990), suggesting that abnormal Doppler features may also be observed in these cases. However, transvaginal colour Doppler studies have shown that in first trimester missed abortions the resistance to flow in the uterine circulation does not differ significantly from that of normal pregnancies (Jaffe and Warsof 1992; Jauniaux *et al.* 1994*b*). Unlike in normal pregnancies, an intervillous flow is often detected in complicated early pregnancies (Fig. 19.5). This abnormal flow pattern may have a predictive value in a high risk population (Jaffe *et al.* 1995) and could be used to screen for early pregnancy failure or complication (Table 19.3).

Trophoblastic infiltration of the placental bed is probably not the only factor regulating the transformation of the spiral arteries. It is possible that even in cases of missed abortion or anembryonic pregnancies where the trophoblastic infiltration is significantly reduced, sufficient placental biochemical activity is maintained to allow, to a certain extent, some transformation of utero-placental circulation. In these cases the trophoblastic shell is thinner and discontinuous and the intervillous space and the

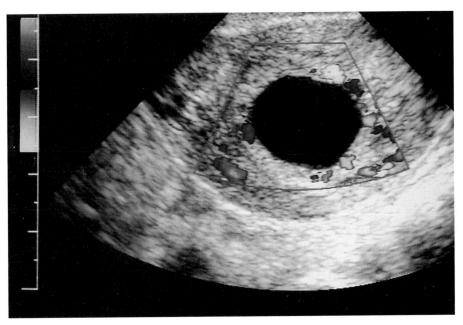

Fig. 19.5 Transvaginal color Doppler mapping of an 8 weeks anembryonic pregnancy. Colour mapping shows hypervascular areas in direct contact with the exocoelomic cavity corresponding to intense and diffuse intervillous blood flow pattern (From Jauniaux *et al.* 1994*b*). *In colour.*

Table 19.3   Distribution of pregnancy complications in relation to first trimester colour flow mapping of the placenta (modified from Jaffe *et al.* 1995).

Outcome	Colour flow mapping		
	Normal (n = 72)	Abnormal (n = 28)	*p*
Spontaneous abortion	1	12	< 0.001
PIH diabetes	1	5	< 0.001
Normal	70	11	< 0.001

PIH = pregnancy-induced hypertension.

endometrium are massively infiltrated by maternal blood (Jauniaux *et al.* 1994*b*). These findings suggest that one of the functions of trophoblastic plugging of the spiral arteries is to restrict maternal blood flow into the intervillous space in early pregnancy (see Chapter 13). Thus, the premature entry of maternal blood into the intervillous space at this stage of gestation disrupts the materno-embryonic interface and is probably the final mechanism causing abortion (Fig. 19.6).

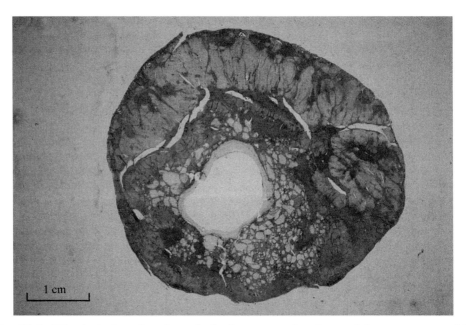

1 cm

Fig. 19.6   Histological section through the intact gestational sac of the case presented in Figure 5 (H&E ×350). No embryonic remnant was found inside the amniotic cavity. The placenta and the decidua are dislocated by a massive entry of maternal blood (From Jauniaux *et al.* 1994*b*). *In colour.*

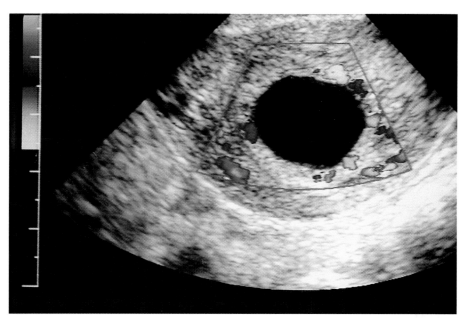

Fig. 19.5 Transvaginal color Doppler mapping of an 8 weeks anembryonic pregnancy. Colour mapping shows hypervascular areas in direct contact with the exocoelomic cavity corresponding to intense and diffuse intervillous blood flow pattern (From Jauniaux *et al.* 1994*b*).

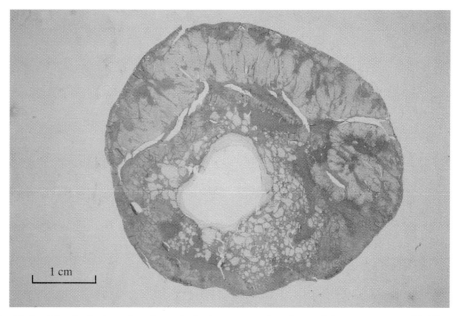

Fig. 19.6 Histological section through the intact gestational sac of the case presented in Figure 5 (H&E ×350). No embryonic remnant was found inside the amniotic cavity. The placenta and the decidua are dislocated by a massive entry of maternal blood (From Jauniaux *et al.* 1994*b*).

Isolation of fetal cells from maternal peripheral tissues

The fact that fetal cells are present in maternal peripheral tissues has generated a lot of interest over the past decade. Three types of fetal cells have been identified and isolated in maternal blood or cervical mucus: fetal lymphocytes, trophoblastic cells, and fetal erythroblasts. These cells are found in small amounts, among maternal cells, in particular their number in peripheral blood is extremely low, they do not divide readily in conventional *in vitro* culture, and samples sorted with monoclonal antibodies often remain heavily contaminated with maternal cells (Adinolfi 1995). Theoretically, trophoblastic cells appear to be the best targets since they are normally not found in the blood of healthy women. An enrichment process is often required, utilizing techniques such as fluorescence-activated cell sorting (FACS) together with techniques enhancing fetal genetic material such as fluorescent *in situ* hybridization (FISH). However, overall isolation of fetal cells from the maternal circulation is still hampered by many technical difficulties and requires complex and expensive equipment.

Cervical mucus obtained by flushing, aspiration, or simply taken with cotton swabs is a simple alternative to maternal blood investigation and to amniocentesis for first trimester prenatal diagnosis (Rodeck *et al.* 1995). Transcervical mucus sampling is extremely easy to perform and relatively inexpensive. As with maternal blood, concerns persist about contamination of the cervical sample by maternal cells and about the still difficult task of obtaining a fetal karyotype from a few isolated trophoblastic cells. Even though mucus aspiration seems not to be associated with an increased risk of pregnancy loss, some variations of the transcervical sampling technique, i.e. flushing or endocervical aspiration, are more invasive and there is a need to evaluate the risks of these procedures to large groups of continuing pregnancies. Transcervical collection of fetal cells is marginally invasive and can be considered as a 'minimally' invasive technique for prenatal diagnosis.

INVASIVE TECHNIQUES

Fetal karyotyping is the most common indication for an invasive procedure at any stage of pregnancy and is mainly used for high risk pregnancies. Ultrasound guidance of the needle has undoubtedly improved the safety and accuracy of the two most commonly used invasive techniques—chorionic villus sampling (CVS) and amniocentesis—and enabled the development of new techniques.

Early amniocentesis

Early amniocentesis (10–14 weeks) has, theoretically, most of the practical advantages of late amniocentesis (Elejade *et al.* 1990) and, therefore, has the potential of becoming an attractive alternative for fetal karyotyping and DNA analysis. Biochemical investigation of mid-gestation amniotic fluid provides more data about the function of different fetal organs than placental samples and allows the detection of structural fetal abnormalities including neural tube defects, ventral wall defects or urinary tract obstruction (Crandall and Chua 1995). However, the value of most amniotic fluid biochemical analyses before 12 weeks is limited because the corresponding fetal organs are not always functionally mature at this stage.

The amniotic space is obviously narrower in the first trimester and the risk of fetal injury during early amniocentesis should be higher than with second trimester amniocentesis. The earlier the procedure is performed, the higher the risk of subsequent complication. Potential hazards are probably related to the operator's experience in performing invasive procedures under ultrasound guidance and with well trained teams, no differences are apparently observed between early and late amniocentesis with respect to maternal complications, or pregnancy outcome (Jauniaux and Rodeck 1995a). However, fetal loss rates are difficult to evaluate from the data presented in these studies because of crucial drawbacks such as small sample numbers and unbalanced gestational age distribution with an excess of cases over 12 weeks of gestation. The rate of spontaneous abortion is 'naturally' high before 10 weeks of gestation and is directly influenced by maternal age, making these results difficult to evaluate.

The rates of short and medium term complications secondary to early amniocentesis such as intrauterine bleeding, and amniotic fluid leakage are higher than (1.9 versus 0.2 percent and 2.9 versus 0.2 percent, respectively) those reported for late amniocentesis (Brumfield *et al.* 1996). During an early amniocentesis a greater proportion of the amniotic fluid is withdrawn and the damage this may induce, for fetal organs such as the developing lungs, may be less reversible than later in pregnancy. This classically described long-term complication of mid-trimester amniocentesis, i.e. oligohydramnios and pulmonary hypoplasia with secondary birth respiratory distress syndrome and pneumonia (Hislop and Fairweather 1982), has been investigated in fetuses born after early aminiocentesis (Greenough and Nicolaides, 1997) and indicate that a greater proportion of the corresponding infants require admission to a neonatal intensive-care unit because of respiratory problems.

Chorionic villus sampling (CVS)

Chorion villous tissue can be successfully obtained after six weeks of gestation transabdominally using the free-hand ultrasound-guided needle aspiration technique or forceps inserted through the cervical canal under abdominal ultrasound guidance (Jauniaux and Rodeck 1995d). There are no medical contraindications to invasive procedures with the transabdominal method whereas an active vaginal infection is a contraindication for a transvaginal or transcervical invasive procedure. In early series, up to 30 per cent of the catheters used for the procedure were reported to be colonized by bacteria and there was some concern about secondary intrauterine infection (Silverman *et al.* 1994). However, the rate of fetal loss is not directly associated with bacterial colonization of the cervix and life-threatening infections have not been encountered since the use of single catheters for repeated insertions has been abandoned.

Villous samples are suitable for DNA analysis and biochemical investigation. Cytogenetic results from CVS may be obscured by contamination of the sample by maternal tissue and chromosomal mosaicism and pseudomosaicism which occur in 1 and 0.4 per cent of cases, respectively (Smidt-Jensen *et al.* 1993). Overall, early amniotic fluid samples are about 10 times less often altered by inherent mosaicism problems than villous samples but CVS produces larger samples which are convenient when direct cell preparation and DNA analysis are planned. Early amniocentesis and CVS after 10 weeks of gestation have theoretically similar success rates in obtaining cell culture and chromosomal analysis and similar harvest time (Byrne *et al.* 1991). However, before 10 weeks of gestation, amniotic fluid samples contain fewer cells and compared to very early villous samples, they require longer harvest times (up to 40 days more) and their success rate in culture is only about 50 per cent (Kennerknecht *et al.* 1992).

Vaginal spotting or bleeding is the most common (1–4 per cent) immediate complication of a CVS procedure and is mainly (up to 20 per cent of cases) observed after transcervical sampling (Jauniaux and Rodeck 1995). Direct vascular injury of small branches of the utero-placental or umbilico-placental circulations may also lead to a retro-placental haematoma and/or a subchorionic haemorrhage and subsequently to a miscarriage. The procedure-related accident is obviously related to the operator's experience and, in particular, to the number of attempts needed to obtain a sufficient villous sample (Jauniaux and Rodeck 1995*d*). Intrauterine infection and chronic amniotic fluid leakage are two possible but very rare medium-term complications of CVS, occurring within a few days to three weeks after the procedure. Very early CVS has also been associated with an overall 10-fold increase in the incidence of limb reduction defects and oromandibular–limb hypogenesis (Firth *et al.* 1994; Hsieh *et al.* 1995). This pattern and the much higher (two to three times) incidence in limb reduction deformities before nine weeks compared with sampling after nine weeks suggest a causal relationship (Rodeck 1993). The spectrum of limb defects after CVS is more severe than limb defects seen in the general population and directly related to the timing of CVS during pregnancy, but it must be stressed that the larger the series, the lower the risk of limb defects. About 50 per cent of CVS-exposed infants with limb disruption defects also present at birth with one or more haemangiomas (Burton *et al.* 1995). Embryoscopic demonstration of cutaneous haemorrhagic lesions in human pregnancies being terminated after intentionally vigorous CVS support the concept that placental trauma may cause fetal damage (Quintero *et al.* 1993). Hypoperfusion and peripheral hypoxia due to excessive feto-maternal haemorrhage, or vasoconstriction or emboli are the possible pathophysiologic mechanisms that may lead to arrested development or distal necrosis (Jauniaux and Rodeck 1995*d*). However, recent large studies have failed to show any differences in infants exposed to CVS from the background population in the overall frequency or pattern distribution of limb deficiencies (Froster and Jackson 1996; Kuliev *et al.* 1996).

Embryoscopy

With the considerable improvements in fibre-optic equipment, endoscopic visualization of the embryo is now possible. The first modern embryoscopes were rigid endoscopes passed transabdominally or transcervically into the exocoelomic cavity under ultrasonographic guidance. New, flexible microfibrescopes with a 0.5 mm outer diameter can be introduced successfully into the amniotic sac through a 21-gauge needle under ultrasound guidance, in patients undergoing pregnancy termination (Reece *et al.* 1993). With this technique, visualization of the embryo is successful in > 95 per cent of cases and small structural abnormalities are expected to be diagnosable, enabling the early prenatal diagnosis of specific genetic syndromes in pregnancies at risk. Embryoscopy also permits direct organ biopsy, and embryonic blood sampling appears feasible. If the concept of human gene therapy becomes a reality, embryoscopy may also open new possibilities for early fetal therapy.

Coelocentesis

The extraembryonic coelomic cavity can be visualized from the end of the fifth week of gestation and sufficient coelomic fluid can be aspirated (Fig. 19.7) to allow the analysis of various biochemical constituents (see Chapter 13) and genetic studies (Jurkovic *et al.* 1993, 1995). Coelocentesis has a success rate of more than 95 per cent between 6 and 10 weeks of gestation and in theory, it is the ideal alternative for early amniocentesis and CVS because the risk of directly injuring the growing embryo or damaging its placenta is almost non-existent. Furthermore, the procedure is easy to learn, induces only minimal discomfort to the mother, and is associated with a very low rate of contamination of the sample by maternal cells (Jurkovic *et al.* 1995).

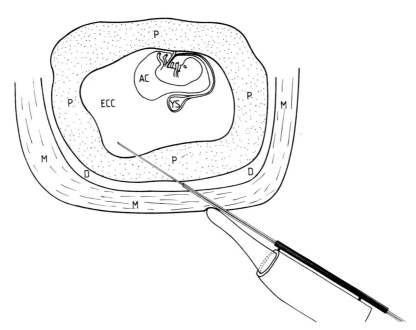

Fig. 19.7   Diagrammatic representation of exocoelomic cavity (ECC) puncture under transvaginal ultrasound guidance. The 18G needle guide attached to the shaft of the probe is introduced inside the uterine wall. Exocoelomic fluid is first aspirated through a 20G needle and subsequently another 20G needle can be subsequently introduced inside the Amniotic Cavity (AC) or the Placenta (P). M = Myometrium; D = Decidua; YS = Yolk Sac; E = Embryo.

Although there are still no data about the relative risks of coelocentesis, the rate of fetal loss should be similar or lower than that associated with early amniocentesis. The high failure rate of cell culture from coelomic samples limits at the moment the applications of coelocentesis to DNA analysis. The use of coelocentesis also clearly provides a very early means of injecting haematopoietic and other stem cells into the gestational sac of embryos known to carry specific forms of inherited haematopoietic disease. The chance of these cells being incorporated into the embryo proper could be high, either via the chorionic circulation or the secondary yolk sac (Edwards *et al.* 1995), without associated direct fetal puncture.

REFERENCES

Adinolfi, M. (1995). Non- or minimally invasive prenatal diagnostic tests on the maternal blood samples or transcervical cells. *Prenatal Diagnosis*, **15**, 889–96.

Al-Sebai *et al.* (1996).

Al-Sebai, M.A.H., Diver, M., and Hipkin, L.J. (1996). The role of a single free b-human chorionic gonadotropin measurement in the diagnosis of early pregnancy failure and the prognosis of fetal viability. *Human Reproduction*, **11**, 991–8.

Brambati, B., Tului, L., Bonacchi, I., Shrimanker, K., Suzuki, Y., and Grudzinskas, J.G. (1994). Serum PAPP-A and free βhCG are first-trimester screening markers for Down syndrome. *Prenatal Diagnosis*, **14**, 1043–7.

Brizot, M.L., Jauniaux, E., Mckie, A.T., Farzaneh, F., and Nicolaides, K.H. (1995). Placental expression of α and β subunits of human chorionic gonadotropin in early pregnancies with Down syndrome. *Molecular Human Reproduction*, **1**, 2506–9.

Brizot, M.L., Jauniaux, E., Mckie, A.T., Farzaneh, F., and Nicolaides, K.H. (1996). Placental mRNA expression of α and β human chorionic gonadotropin in early trisomy 18 pregnancies. *Molecular Human Reproduction*, **2**, 463–5.

Bromley, B., Harlow, B.L., Laboda, L.A., and Benacerraf, B.R. (1991). Small sac size in the first trimester: a predictor of poor fetal outcome. *Radiology*, **178**, 375–7.

Brumfield, C.G., Lin, S., Conner, W., Cosper, P., Davis, R.O., and Owen, J. (1996). Prenancy outcome following genetic amniocentesis at 11–14 versus 16–19 weeks' gestation. *Obstetric and Gynecology*, **88**, 114–18.

Burton, B.K., Schulz, C.J., Angle, B., and Burd, L.I. (1995). An increased incidence of haemangiomas in infants born following chorionic villus sampling (CVS). *Prenatal Diagnosis*, **15**, 209–14.

Byrne, D., Marks, K., Azar, G., and Nicolaides, K. (1991). Randomized study of early amniocentesis versus chorionic villus sampling: a technical and cytogenetic comparison of 650 patients. *Ultrasound in Obstetrics and Gynecology*, **1**, 235–40.

Chard, T. (1991). Biochemistry and endocrinology of the Down's syndrome pregnancy. *Annals of the New York Academy of Sciences*, **626**, 580–96.

Crandall, B.F. and Chua, C. (1995). Detecting neural tube defects by amniocentesis between 11 and 15 weeks' gestation. *Prenatal Diagnosis*, **15**, 339–43.

Dickey, R.P., Gasser, R., Olar, T.T., Taylor, S.N., Curole, D.N., Rye, P.H., and Matulich, E.M. (1994). Relationship of initial chorionic sac diameter to abortion and abortus karyotype based on new growth curves for the 16th to 49th post-ovulation day. *Human Reproduction*, **9**, 559–65.

Drugan, A., Johnson, M.P., and Isada, N.B. (1992). The smaller than expected first-timester fetus is at risk for chromosome anomalies. *American Journal of Obstetrics and Gynecology*, **167**, 1525–8.

Edwards, R., Jauniaux, E., Bins, R.M., Layton, M., Jurkovic, D., Grillo, T.A.I., and Campbell, S. (1995). Induced tolerance in human fetuses using coelocentesis: a medical opportunity? Human Reproduction Update, **1**, 419–27.

Elejade, B.R., de Elejade, M.M., Acuna, J.M., Thelen, D., Trujillo, C., and Karrmann, M. (1990). Prospective study of amniocentesis performed between weeks 9 and 16 of gestation: its feasibility, risks, complications and use in early prenatal diagnosis. *American Journal of Medical Genetics*, **35**, 188–96.

Firth, H.V., Boyd, P.A., Chamberlain, P., Mackenzie, I.Z., Morriss-Kay, G.M., and Huson, S.M. (1994). Analysis of limb reduction defects in babies exposed to chorionic villus sampling. *Lancet*, **343**, 1069–71.

Froster, U.G. and Jackson, L. (1996). Limb defects and chorionic villus sampling: results from an international registry, 1992–94. *Lancet*, **347**, 489–94.

Goldstein, S.R. (1992). Significance of cardiac activity on endovaginal ultrasound in very early embryos. *Obstetrics and Gynecology*, **80**, 670–2.

Goldstein, S.R. (1994). Embryonic death in early pregnancy: a new look at the first trimester. *Obstetrics and Gynecology*, **84**, 294–7.

Greenough, A. and Nicolaides, K.H. (1997). Chorionic villus sampling and early amniocentesis for prenatal diagnosis. *Lancet*, **349**, 1395–6.

Hill, L.M., DiNofrio, D.M., and Chenevey, P. (1995). Transvaginal sonographic evaluation of first-trimester placenta previa. *Ultrasound in Obstetrics and Gynecology*, **5**, 301–3.

Hislop, A. and Fairweather, I. (1982). Amniocentesis and lung growth: an animal experiment with clinical implications. *Lancet*, **ii**, 1340–1.

Hsieh, F.J., Shyu, M.K., Sheu, B.C., Lin, S.P., Chen, C.P., and Huang, F.Y. (1995). Limb defects after chorionic villus sampling. *Obstetrics and Gynecology*, **85**, 84–8.

Hustin, J., Jauniaux, E., and Schaaps, J.P. (1990). Histological study of the materno-embryonic interface in spontaneous abortion. *Placenta*, **11**, 477–86.

Jaffe, R. and Warsof, S.L. (1992). Color doppler imaging in the assessment of uteroplacental blood flow in abnormal first trimester intrauterine pregnancies: an attempt to define etiologic mechanisms. *Journal of Ultrasound Medicine*, **11**, 41–4.

Jaffe, R., Dorgan, A., and Abramowicz, A. (1995). Color Doppler imaging of uteroplacental circulation in the first trimester: value in predicting pregnancy failure or complication. *American Journal of Reproduction*, **164**, 1255–8.

Jauniaux and Nicolaides, K.H. (1997). Early ultrasound diagnosis and follow-up of molar pregnancies. *Ultrasound in Obstetrics and Gynecology* (In press.)

Jauniaux, E., Jurkovic, D., Henriet, Y., Rodesch, F., and Hustin, J. (1991). Development of the secondary human yolk sac: correlation of sonographic and anatomic features. *Human Reproduction*, **6**, 1160–6.

Jauniaux, E., Jurkovic, D., Gulbis, B., Zaidi, J., Meuris, S., and Campbell, S. (1994a). Biochemical composition of the coelomic fluid in anembryonic pregnancy. *American Journal of Obstetrics and Gynecology*, **171**, 849–53.

Jauniaux, E., Zaidi, J., Jurkovic, D., Campbell, S., and Hustin, J. (1994b). Comparison of color Doppler features and pathologic findings in complicated early pregnancy. *Human Reproduction*, **9**, 2432–7.

Jauniaux, E., Gulbis, B., Jurkovic, D., Gavriil, P., and Campbell, S. (1995a). The origin of alpha-fetoprotein in first trimester anembryonic pregnancies. *American Journal of Obstetrics and Gynecology*, **173**, 1749–53.

Jauniaux, E., Gavriil, P., and Nicolaides, K.H. (1995b). Ultrasonographic assessment of early pregnancy complications. In *Ultrasound and early pregnancy*, (ed. D. Jurkovic and E. Jauniaux), pp. 53–64. Parthenon, Carnforth.

Jauniaux, E., Jurkovic, D., and Campbell, S. (1995c). *In vivo* investigation of the placental circulations by Doppler echography. *Placenta*, **16**, 323–31.

Jauniaux, E. and Rodeck, C. (1995*d*). Use, risks and complications of amniocentesis and chorion villous sampling for prenatal diagnosis in early pregnancy. *Early Pregnancy Biology and Medicine*, **1**, 245–52.

Jauniaux, E., Kadri, R., and Hustin, J. (1996*a*). Partial mole and triploidy: screening in patients with first trimester spontaneous abortion. *Obstetrics and Gynecology*, **88**, 616–19.

Jauniaux, E., Nicolaides, K.H., Nagy, A.M., Brizot, M., and Meuris, S. (1996*b*). Total amount of circulating human chorionic gonadotropin α and β subunits in first trimester trisomies 21 and 18. *Journal of Endocrinology*, **148**, 27–31.

Jauniaux, E., Gavriil, P., Khun, P., Kurdi, W., Hyett, J., and Nicolaides, K.H. (1996*c*) Fetal heart rate and umbilicoplacental doppler flow velocity waveforms in early pregnancies with a chromosomal abnormality and/or increased nuchal translucency thickness. *Human Reproduction*, **11**, 435–9.

Johnson, M.R., Riddle, A.F., Grudzinskas, J.G., Sharma, V., Collins, W.P., and Nicolaides, K.H. (1993). The role of trophoblast dysfunction in the aetiology of miscarriage. *British Journal of Obstetrics and Gynaecology*, **100**, 353–9.

Jurkovic, D., Jauniaux, E., Campbell, S., Pandya, P., Cardy, D.L., and Nicolaides, K.H. (1993). Coelocentesis: a new technique for early prenatal diagnosis. *Lancet*, **341**, 1623–4.

Jurkovic, D., Jauniaux, E., Campbell, S., Mitchell, M., Lees, C., and Layton, M. (1995). Detection of sickle gene by coelocentesis in early pregnancy: a new approach to prenatal diagnosis of single gene disorders. *Human Reproduction*, **10**, 1287–9.

Kennerknecht, I., Baur-Aubele, S., Grab, D., and Terinde, R. (1992). First trimester amniocentesis between the seventh and 13th weeks: evaluation of the earliest possible genetic diagnosis. *Prenatal Diagnosis*, **12**, 595–601.

Kuhn, P., Brizot, M.L., Pandya, P.P., Snijders, R.J., and Nicolaides, K.H. (1995). Crown–rump length in chromosomally abnormal fetuses at 10–13 weeks' gestation. *American Journal of Obstetrics and Gynecology*, **172**, 32–5.

Kuliev, A., Jackson, L., Froster, U., Brambati, B., Simpson, J.L., Verlinsky, Y., *et al.* (1996). Chorionic villus sampling safety. *American Journal of Obstetrics and Gynecology*, **174**, 870–1.

Laboda, L.A., Estroff, J.A., and Benacerraf, B.R. (1989). First trimester bradycardia. A sign of impending fetal loss. *Journal of Ultrasound Medicines*, **8**, 561–3.

Merchiers, E.H., Dhont, M., De Sutter, P.A., Beghin, C.J., and Vandekerckhove, D.A. (1991). Predictive value of early embryonic cardiac activity for pregnancy outcome. *American Journal of Obstetrics and Gynecology*, **165**, 11–14.

Miller, J.F., Williamson, E., Glue, J., Gordon, Y.B., Grudzinskas, J.G., and Sykes, A. (1980). Fetal loss after implantation. *Lancet*, **i**, 554–6.

Pandya, P., Snijders, R.J.M., Psara, N., Hibert, L., and Nicolaides, K.H. (1996). The prevalence of non-viable pregnancy at 10–13 weeks of gestation. *Ultrasound Obstetrics and Gynecology*, **7**, 170–3.

Quintero, R.A., Romero, R., Mahoney, M.J., and Hobbins, J. (1993). Embryoscopic demonstration of hemorrhagic lesions on the human embryo after placental trauma. *American Journal of Obstetrics and Gynecology*, **168**, 756–9.

Reece, E.A., Whetham, J., Rotmensch, S., and Wiznitzer, A. (1993). Gaining access to the embryonic–fetal circulation via first-trimester endoscoy: a step into the future. *Obstetrics and Gynecology*, **82**, 876–9.

Rodeck, C.H. (1993). Fetal development after chorionic villus sampling. *Lancet*, **341**, 468–9.

Rodeck, C., Tutschek, B., Sherlock, J., and Kingdom, J. (1995). Methods for the transcervical collection of fetal cells during the first trimester of pregnancy. *Prenatal Diagnosis*, **15**, 933–42.

Schats, R., Jansen, C.A.M., and Wladimiroff, J.W. (1990). Abnormal embryonic heart rate pattern in early pregnancy associated with Down's syndrome. *Human Reproduction*, **7**, 877–9.

Silverman, N.S., Sullivan, M.W., Jungkind, D.L., Weinblatt, V., Beavis, K., and Wapner, R.J. (1994). Incidence of bacteremia associated with chorionic villus sampling. *Obstetrics and Gynecology*, **84**, 1021–4.

Smidt-Jensen, S., Lind, A.M., Permin, M., Zachary, J.M., Lundsteen, C., and Philip, J. (1993). Cytogenetic analysis of 2928 CVS samples and 1075 amniocentesis from randomized studies. *Prenatal Diagnosis*, **13**, 723–40.

Smith, K.E. and Buyalos, R.P. (1996). The profound impact of patient age on pregnancy outcome after early detection of fetal cardiac activity. *Fertility and Sterility*, **65**, 35–40.

Stabile, I. (1992). Anembryonic pregnancy. In *The embryo: normal and abnormal development and growth*, (ed. M. Chapman, G. Grudzinskas and T. Chard), pp. 35–43. Springer, London.

Van Lith, J.M.M., Visser, G.H.A., Mantingh, A., and Beekhuis, J.R. (1992). Fetal heart rate in early pregnancy and chromosomal disorders. *British Journal of Obstetrics and Gynaecology*, **99**, 741–4.

Wald, N.J., George, L., Smith, D., and Densen, J.W. (1996). Serum screening for Down's syndrome between 8 and 14 weeks of pregnancy. *British Journal of Obstetrics and Gynaecology*, **103**, 407–12.

Wisser, J. and Dirschedl, P. (1994). Embryonic heart rate in dated human embryos. *Early Human Development*, **37**, 107–15.

Zinaman, M.J., Clegg, E.D., Brown, C.C., O'Connor, J., and Selevan, S.G. (1996). Estimates of human fertility and pregnancy loss. *Fertility and Sterility*, **65**, 503–9.

20 | *Spontaneous evolution of fetal malformations detected in the first trimester*

M. Bronshtein and Z. Blumenfeld

INTRODUCTION

Recent technological advances in ultrasound have benefited many areas of obstetric practice, including gestational dating, first-trimester detection of abnormalities, and evaluation of the severity and significance of specific malformations. The recent improvements in sonographic technology and in particular the use of 5–7.5 MHz transvaginal sonographic (TVS) probes has allowed a more detailed study of the first trimester fetus. Moving prenatal diagnosis from mid-gestation to the end of the first trimester has obvious benefits which, along with logistic, economic, and other human advantages, have opened up the possibility of fetal therapy at a time in development when the tissues of the embryo or early fetus have less risk of inducing a 'graft–host' rejection reaction. Therefore, our goal must now be to detect severe and, in particular, lethal malformations as early as possible after conception. Furthermore, early ultrasound examination increases the detection rate of chromosomal abnormalities. There is now mounting evidence that transient anomalies like fetal nuchal oedema, echogenic bowel, and pyelectasis may serve as markers of possible aneuploidies in early pregnancy (Benacerraf *et al.* 1990; Nicolaides *et al.* 1992; Nyberg *et al.* 1993).

The early detection of fetal anomalies has several obvious advantages—in particular, it enables early termination of pregnancy to be made when indicated, before psychologic and sentimental maternal fetal bonding occurs, avoiding also the necessity to explain to relatives and others who will not yet have been told of the pregnancy. Early prenatal diagnosis in general keeps the decision making process for chorionic villus biopsy, amniocentesis, or selective abortion when indicated, while minimizing parental grief, as it frequently occurs in the late mid-trimester. In this chapter, summarize the various aspects and potentials of ultrasound for the prenatal diagnosis of fetal anatomical malformations before twelve weeks of gestation.

EARLY DETECTION OF HUMAN MALFORMATIONS

It is estimated that about 3–5 per cent of all new-born infants have a congenital anomaly (Oakley 1986). The introduction of ultrasound has enabled the prenatal diagnosis of many of these anomalies. In most cases, the diagnosis used only to be performed at an advanced stage of gestation. Because of the limited resolution of ultrasound machines, patients were routinely scheduled for ultrasound examination at about 20 weeks' gestation. However, both embryological and sonographic data have demonstrated that many abnormalities occur at a much earlier stage of gestation (Cullen *et al.* 1990; Rottem and Bronshtein 1990). Overall, about 80 per cent of fetal anomalies appear in the first trimester and are now detectable using modern ultrasound equipment. An additional 15 per cent of fetal anomalies can be identified at 15–16 weeks' gestation, including most cases of hydrocephaly, club feet, intestinal obstruction, and several common cardiac anomalies. The remaining 5 per cent of fetal abnormalities will appear after 24 weeks of gestation. A particular emphasis must be put on chromosomal defects which are identifiable due to associated structural anomalies in about 65 per cent of cases by the end of the first trimester (Brambati *et al.* 1995; Rottem 1995).

The early detection of gestational uterus contents by transvaginal sonography (TVS) has also enabled the *in vivo* study of normal embryologic development or 'sonoembryology' (Timor-Tritsch *et al.* 1989). This *in vivo* embryology differs notably from the previously used speculations on embryology and teratology based upon on post-abortion *in vitro* examination of expelled uterine contents. The technique of vaginal scanning is not difficult. However, a good knowledge of basic embryology is required because the structures observed can only be understood in the light of their embryonic development (see Chapter 6). For example, it is important to know that ossification of the calvarium takes place at the end of the first trimester and, therefore, a diagnosis of anencephaly before 9 weeks' gestation is almost impossible (Fig. 20.1). Likewise, herniation of the midgut into the umbilical cord is a normal process until 11 weeks and should not mistaken for exomphalos during the third month of gestation (Timor-Tritsch *et al.* 1989).

Overall, it is desirable to use mechanical, high frequency transvaginal probes for better results, since the electronic high frequency instruments have a resolution limitation in the *z* axis. Therefore, moving objects such as the fetal heart and valves are difficult to examine using these electronic instruments. We use a 7.5 MHz annular array mechanical transvaginal transducer with a focal range of 5 cm. We believe that the ultrasound manufacturing companies should be urged to develop high frequency instruments with higher resolutions. We also think that a new era of non-invasive diagnosis will arrive when we will use our equipments and high resolution probes as an *in vivo* 'sonographic microscope' whereby critical phenomena could be followed in real time. For example, we hope that the normal embryonic folding occurring soon after conception will be evidenced *in utero*, thus enabling us to detect unknown aspects of ontogeny, possibly shedding new light on early physiologic and pathologic phenomena of early embryogenesis.

We review below some sonographic criteria for the diagnosis of human abnormalities during the first trimester of pregnancy.

Anomalies of the head and central nervous system

The 'cranial vesicle' is detectable by TVS at 7 to 8 weeks of gestation and the normal ossification of the cranial vault occurs only afterwards (Blaas *et al.* 1995). It seems therefore wise to suggest that a definitive diagnosis of anecephaly should not be attempted before 10 weeks of gestation (Fig. 20.1). In some cases, however, when severe kyphoscoliosis, due to body wall complex anomaly, is also present it may be possible to detect an anencephalic fetus around nine weeks of gestation (Bronshtein and Ornoy 1991; Bar-Hava *et al.* 1993). Midline induction starts at about 9–11 weeks of gestation and from 12 weeks it is possible to clearly visualize the fetal cerebellum. Thus it is not surprising to find prenatal descriptions of malformations such as spina bifida, severe scoliosis, holoprosencephaly, exencephaly, cranioschisis or Dandy–Walker malformation, which are all potentially diagnosable at this stage of pregnancy (Hamada *et al.* 1992; Achiron *et al.*, 1993; Nishi and Nakano, 1994; Grange *et al.*, 1994).

The fetal eyes are detectable as early as 11–12 weeks of gestation. We have observed a case where the fetal orbits were clearly visualized by TVS at the end of the first trimester but subsequently the fetus was delivered with bilateral anophthalmia. Thus, it is not yet clear whether fetal anophthalmia is a primary or secondary anomaly (Bronshtein *et al.* 1991*a*; Zimmer *et al.* 1993). Similarly, the fetal ears are detectable around 12 weeks and, therefore, micro-ottia should also be identifiable in early pregnancy. Fetal proboscis and cleft lip (Fig. 20.2) have been formally identified by TVS as early as 11 weeks of gestation (Bronshtein *et al.* 1991*b* 1994*a*).

Anomalies of the respiratory and cardiovascular systems

Fetal hydrothorax has been identified by TVS in a 10 week fetus subsequently diagnosed to have Turner syndrome (Klare *et al.* 1992).

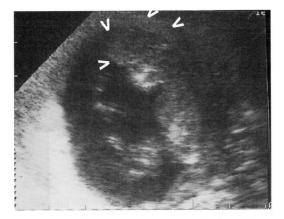

Fig. 20.1 Transvaginal sonography of an 11 weeks and 2-day-old fetus showing an apparently normal fetal head (arrowheads). This fetus was found to be anencephalic at 15 weeks of gestation. Note the irregular shape of the head.

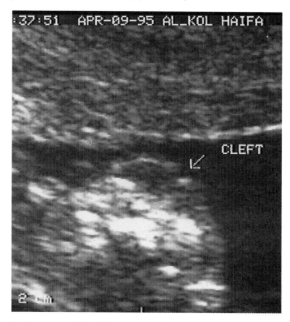

Fig. 20.2 Transvaginal sonography of an 11-week-old fetus showing a cleft lip appearing on a tangential coronal sonographic view of the face through the upper lip.

The two separate fetal parts of the heart, left and right, are identifiable as early as 9 to 10 weeks of gestation. Accordingly, cardiac anomalies such as asymmetry (hypoplasia of the right or left side of the heart), dextrocardia, ectopic cordis (unpublished case), and cardiac arrhythmias have been diagnosed as early as 10–12 weeks (Achiron *et al.* 1994; Hyett *et al.* 1995). From 11 to 12 weeks, using modern TVS probes it is possible to see the classical four-chamber view of the heart in about 50 per cent of cases and, less frequently, the location of the cardiac valves and the great vessels. Fetal anomalies already detected at this gestational age include common atrioventricular canal, ectopic cordis, hypoplastic left heart, single cardiac trunk, and tetralogy of Fallot. We believe that anomalies of the aortic arch are also diagnosable during the first trimester, as well as transposition of the great vessels, absence of inferior vena cava, and fetal arrhythmias. Actually, with increasing experience about 70 per cent of congenital heart defects could be detected as early as the end of the first trimester (Bronshtein *et al.* 1992*a*, 1993*a*).

Anomalies of the gastrointestinal system and abdominal wall

Severe cases of exomphalos (Fig. 20.3) or gastroschisis have been detected as early as 11 weeks of gestation. Accordingly, bladder exstrophy has also been detected during the first trimester, and diaphragmatic hernia from 13 weeks (Bulas *et al.* 1992). There have been cases of duodenal stenosis and oesophageal atresia described at 12 weeks of gestation (Tsukerman *et al.* 1993).

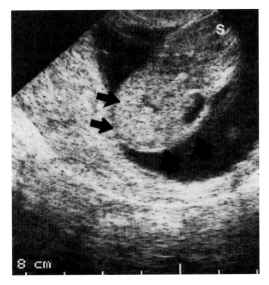

Fig. 20.3 Massive abdominal wall defect and exomphalos visualized by TVS of an 11 week old fetus. The herniated liver and stomach are marked by arrows (S = fetal spine.)

Anomalies of the urinary tract system

The fetal kidneys and urinary bladder are detectable as early as 10 weeks of gestation. Several major urinary tract malformations have been identified during the first trimester including posterior urethral valve, Potter syndrome, and prune-belly syndrome—multicystic dysplastic (infantile type) kidneys (Bronshtein *et al.* 1990, 1992*b*, 1993*b*, 1994*b*).

Anomalies of the skeletal system

The fetal limb buds can be visualized between 9 and 11 weeks and it is possible to rule out the absence of long bones at this stage. The fetal fingers can be seen around 12 weeks and toes around 13 weeks of gestation. Most finger malformations have been described by the beginning of the second trimester (Fig. 20.4). Although we have observed a case of club foot at 12 weeks, most are seen on ultrasound around 15–16 weeks of gestation (Bronshtein *et al.* 1993*c*). Major skeletal dysplasia such as osteogenesis imperfecta and rhizomelic chondrodysplasia punctuata have also been described by ultrasound at the end of the first trimester (Sastrowijoto *et al.* 1994; Berge *et al.* 1995).

SPONTANEOUS EVOLUTION OF SOME EMBRYONIC ABNORMALITIES

The technological breakthrough generated by high frequency TVS has revealed transient phenomena in fetal morphologic development which disappear subsequently in

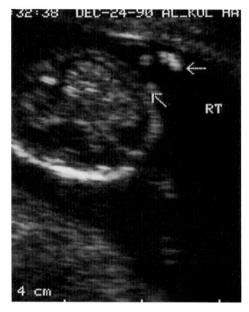

Fig. 20.4   Simple syndactyly in an 11-week-old fetus detected by TVS. The upper arrow points towards the conjoined three fingers (third, fourth, and fifth), whereas the lower arrow points towards the fetal thumb adjacent to the skull. The second finger is visualized between them. (RT = right)

fetal life. The term 'transient anomalies' has been used in many cases where a structural anomaly is evident at the end of the first trimester or at the beginning of the second trimester and disappears as pregnancy advances, including cases of major fetal abnormality (Rottem and Bronshtein 1990). Had the ultrasound examination been postponed from this period until 20 weeks, most of these transient malformations would not have been detected. Unusual transient sonographic findings of fetal anomalies such as cysts of the choroid plexus, abdominal cysts, or bizarre calcifications in the fetal liver, heart, or other locations have been observed during the first trimester. Most, if not all, of these fetal anomalies disappear by term, and if not associated with other malformations, have no influence on the fetal outcome (Bronshtein and Blazer 1995). The exact interpretation of some of them is unknown at present.

In vivo follow-up of abnormal fetuses permits the discovery of completely new aspects of human teratogenesis and, in particular, enables us to study the 'natural' evolution of some fetal malformations. Three representative examples are described below.

Anencephaly

According to classical embryology literature, this is a malformation which causes the non-closure of the anterior neuropore which should normally occur between 5 and 7 weeks of gestation (Lemire 1988). Typically, these fetuses have no cerebral hemispheres and lack the cranial vault. Acrania is now a relatively well-known pathological entity which can be diagnosed by ultrasound in early pregnancy. It is characterized by the absence of a cranial vault but with brain tissue which seems initially to be complete (Cullen *et al.* 1990; Bronshtein and Ornoy 1991; Yand *et al.* 1992). On TVS, the brain, which is surrounded by a thin and uncalcified membrane, may appear to be floppy and its shape may change according to the fetal position, probably due to gravity and/or because of external pressure exerted on the uterus during the examination (Fig. 20.1). There have been case reports of fetuses with a sonographic diagnosis of acrania who ultimately turned out to be anencephalic when the pregnancy was terminated, suggesting that anencephaly results from a secondary re-opening of a normally closed neural tube. This hypothesis is supported by the fact that a very dense and viscid amniotic fluid is commonly found on scan in anencephalic fetuses. In the absence of the cranial vault, a process of mechanical or chemical damage or trauma may lead to shedding of cerebral tissue into the amniotic fluid and the damaged neural tissue will appear on ultrasound as small floating flakes with a low level, 'milky' echogenicity (Bronshtein and Ornoy 1991; Bar-Hava *et al.* 1993).

Pilonidal sinus

This is a relatively common anomaly, traditionally believed to be generated by inward growing of hair follicle (s) in the sacral region, instead of the normally externally directed growth. In our preliminary experience of several cases, this malformation follows the remaining of the fetal 'tail', which then interferes with the normal closure of the fetal skin, a process which usually takes place after the normal disappearance of the embryonic 'tail' in the human fetus (unpublished observation).

Nuchal thickening or oedema

This is a transient fetal anomaly which has been reported very frequently since the early nineties (Nicolaides *et al.* 1992; Shulman *et al.* 1992; van Zalen-Sprock *et al.* 1992; Wilson *et al.* 1992; Bronshtein *et al.* 1993*d*; Johnson *et al.* 1993; Nadel *et al.* 1993). Various types of cystic lesions of the fetal neck have also been reported. Definite sonographic criteria are not yet available to differentiate between the different lesions occurring in early gestation. The terms 'nuchal fold thickening' or 'nuchal translucency' are often used, sometimes interchangeably, to describe small lesions, whereas 'cystic hygroma' is used for larger lesions. However, it is possible that all these lesions are different variants of a spectrum of lesions resulting from a lymphatic malformation. During organogenesis, the lymphatic vessels initially drain into large sacs lateral to the jugular veins and, eventually, at about 40 days of gestation, connect to the venous system as the terminal portion of the right lymphatic duct and the thoracic duct. Failure of canalization and development of this communication results in jugular lymphatic obstruction and lymphatic fluid accumulation in the cervical tissues. If some of the cystic lesions resolve as pregnancy advances, others may continue to grow, giving place to large cystic hygromas (Shulman *et al.* 1992; van Zalen-Sprock *et al.* 1992; Wilson *et al.* 1992; Bronshtein *et al.* 1993*a*; Johnson *et al.* 1993; Nadel *et al.* 1993). Even in these cases, ultimately most of the lesion is transient and disappears following reabsorption before 16–18 weeks and the fetal outcome is good. However, the presence of thicker than normal nuchal space, even if transient, is associated with an increased risk of fetal aneuploidy and chorionic villus sampling or amniocentesis should be offered to determine the fetal karyotype.

REFERENCES

Achiron, R., Achiron, A., and Yagel, S. (1993). First trimester transvaginal sonographic diagnosis of Dandy–Walker malformation. *Journal of Clinical Ultrasound*, 21, 62–4.

Achiron, R., Rotstein, Z., Lipitz, S., Mashiach, S., and Hegesh, J. (1994). First trimester diagnosis of fetal congenital heart disease by transvaginal ultrasonography. *Obstetrics and Gynecology*, 84, 69–72.

Bar-Hava, I., Bronshtein, M., Ornoy, A., and Ben-Rafael, Z. (1993). First trimester sonographic diagnosis of acrania. *Harefuah.*, 124, 685–7.

Blaas, H.G., Eik-Nes, S.H., Kiserud, T., and Hellevik, L.R. (1995). Early development of the hindbrain: a longitudinal ultrasound study from 7 to 12 weeks of gestation. *Ultrasound in Obstetrics and Gynecology*, 5, 148–50.

Benacerraf, B.R., Mandell, J., Estroff, J.A., Harlow, B.L., and Frigoletto, F.D. (1990). Fetal pyelectasis: a possible association with Down syndrome. *Obstetrics and Gynecology*, 76, 58–60.

Berge, L.N., Marton, V., Tranebjaerg, L., Kearney, M.S., Kiserud, T., and Oian, P. (1995). Prenatal diagnosis of osteogenesis imperfecta. *Acta Obstetrica Gynecologica Scandinavica*, 74, 321–3.

Brambati, B., Cislaghi, C., Tului, L., Alberti, E., Amidani, M., Colombo, U., and Zuliani, G. (1995). First trimester Down's syndrome screening using nuchal translucency: a prospective study in patients undergoing chorionic villus sampling. *Ultrasound in Obstetrics and Gynecology*, 5, 9–14.

Bronshtein, M. and Blazer, S. (1995). Prenatal diagnosis of liver calcifications. *Obstetrics and Gynecology*, 86, 739–43.

Bronshtein, M. and Ornoy, A. (1991). Acrania: anencephaly resulting from secondary degeneration of a closed neural tube: two cases in the same family. *Journal of Clinical Ultrasound*, 19, 230–4.

Bronshtein, M., Yoffe, N., Brandes, J.M., and Blumenfeld, Z. (1990). First and early second trimester diagnosis of fetal urinary tract anomalies using transvaginal sonography. *Prenatal Diagnosis*, 10, 653–66.

Bronshtein, M., Zimmer, E., Gershoni-Baruch, R., Yoffe, N., Meyer, H., and Blumenfeld, Z. (1991a). First and second trimester diagnosis of fetal ocular defects and associated anomalies: report of eight cases. *Obstetrics and Gynecology*, 77, 443–9.

Bronshtein, M., Mashiah, N., Blumenfeld, I., and Blumenfeld, Z. (1991b). Pseudoprognathism—an auxiliary ultrasonographic sign for transvaginal ultrasonographic diagnosis of cleft lip and palate in the early second trimester. *American Journal of Obstetrics and Gynecology*, 165, 1314–16.

Bronshtein, M., Siegler, E., Eshcoli, Z., and Zimmer, E.Z. (1992a). Transvaginal ultrasound measurements of the fetal heart at 11 to 17 weeks of gestation. *American Journal of Perinatology*, 9, 38–42.

Bronshtein, M., Bar-Hava, I., and Blumenfeld, Z. (1992b). Clues and pitfalls in the early prenatal diagnosis of 'late onset' infantile polycystic kidney. *Prenatal Diagnosis*, 12, 293–8.

Bronshtein, M., Zimmer, E.Z., Gerlis, L.M., Lorber, A., and Drugan, A. (1993a). Early ultrasound diagnosis of fetal congenital heart defects in high risk and low risk pregnancies. *Obstetrics and Gynecology*, 82, 1–5.

Bronshtein, M., Bar-Hava, I., and Blumenfeld, Z. (1993*b*). Differential diagnosis of the non-visualized fetal urinary bladder by transvaginal sonography in the early second trimester. *Obstetrics and Gynecology*, **82**, 490–3.

Bronshtein, M., Keret, D., Deutsch, M., Liberson, A., and Bar-Hava, I. (1993*c*). Transvaginal sonographic detection of skeletal anomalies in the first and early second trimester. *Prenatal Diagnosis*, **13**, 597–601.

Bronshtein, M., Bar-Chava, I., Blumenfeld, I., Bejar, J., Toder, V., and Blumenfeld, Z. (1993*d*). The difference between septated and nonseptated nuchal cystic hygroma in the early second trimester. *Obstetrics and Gynecology*, **81**, 683–7.

Bronshtein, M., Blumenfeld, I., Kohn, J., and Blumenfeld, Z. (1994*a*). Detection of cleft lip and palate by early second trimester transvaginal sonography. *Obstetrics and Gynecology*, **84**, 73–6.

Bronshtein, M., Amit, A., Achiron, R., Noy, I., and Blumenfeld, Z. (1994*b*). The early prenatal sonographic diagnosis of renal agenesis: technique and possible pitfalls. *Prenatal Diagnosis*, **14**, 291–7.

Bulas, D.I., Saal, H.M., Allen, J.F., Kapur, S., Nies, B.M., and Newman, K. (1992). Cystic hygroma and congenital diaphragmatic hernia: early prenatal sonographic evaluation of Fryns' syndrome. *Prenatal Diagnosis*, **12**, 867–75.

Cullen, M.T., Green, J., Whetham, J., Salafia, C., Gabrielli, S., and Hobbins, J.C. (1990). Transvaginal ultrasonographic detection of congenital anomalies in the first trimester. *American Journal of Obstetrics and Gynecology*, **163**, 466–76.

Grange, G., Favre, R., and Gasser, B. (1994). Endovaginal sonographic diagnosis of craniorachischisis at 13 weeks of gestation. *Fetal Diagnosis and Therapy*, **9**, 391–4.

Hamada, H., Oki, A., Tsunoda, H., and Kubo, T. (1992). Prenatal diagnosis of holoprosencephaly by transvaginal ultrasonography in the first trimester. *Asia and Oceania Journal of Obstetrics and Gynaecology*, **18**, 125–9.

Hyett, J.A., Moscoso, G., and Nicolaides, K.H. (1995). First trimester nuchal translucency and cardiac septal defects in fetuses with trisomy 21. *American Journal of Obstetrics and Gynecology*, **172**, 1411–13.

Johnson, M.P., Johnson, A., Holzgreve, W., Isada, N.B., Wapner, R.J., Treadwell, M.C., *et al.* (1993). First trimester simple hygroma: cause and outcome. *American Journal of Obstetrics and Gynecology*, **168**, 156–61.

Klare, P., Sydow, P., and Korner, H. (1992). Severe hydrops fetalis in a first trimester pregnancy with Ulrich–Turner syndrome. *Zentralblatt für Gynaekologie*, **114**, 141–2.

Lemire, R.J. (1988). Neural tube defects. *Journal of the American Medical Association*, **259**, 558–62.

Nadel, A., Bromley, B., and Benacerraf, B.R. (1993). Nuchal thickening or cystic hygromas in first and early second trimester fetuses: progress and outcome. *Obstetrics and Gynecology*, **82**, 43–8.

Nicolaides, K.H., Azar, G., Byrne, D., Mansur, C., and Marks, K. (1992). Fetal nuchal translucency: ultrasound screening for chromosomal defects in first trimester of pregnancy. *British Medical Journal*, **304**, 867–9.

Nishi, T. and Nakano, R. (1994). First trimester diagnosis of exencephaly by transvaginal ultrasonography. *Journal of Ultrasound Medicine*, **13**, 149–51.

Nyberg, D.A., Dubinsky, T., Resta, R.G., Mahoney, B.S., Hickok, D.E., and Luthy, D.A. (1993). Echogenic fetal bowel during the second trimester: clinical importance. *Radiology*, **188**, 527–31.

Oakley, G.P. (1986). Frequency of human congenital malformations. *Clinical Perinatology*, **13**, 545–9.

Rottem, S. (1995). Early detection of structural anomalies and markers of chromosomal aberrations by transvaginal ultrasonography. *Current Opinion in Obstetrics and Gynecology*, **7**, 122–5.

Rottem, S. and Bronshtein, M. (1990). Transvaginal sonographic diagnosis of congenital anomalies between 9 weeks and 16 weeks menstrual age. *Journal of Clinical Ultrasound*, **18**, 307–14.

Sastrowijoto, S.H., Vandenberghe, K., Moerman, P., Lauweryns, J.M., and Fryns, J.P. (1994). Prenatal ultrasound diagnosis of rhizomelic chondrodysplasia punctata in a primigravida. *Prenatal Diagnosis*, **14**, 770–6.

Shepard, T.H. (1986). Human teratogenicity. *Advances in Pediatrics*, **33**, 225–9.

Shulman, L.P., Emerson, D.S., Felker, R.E., Phillips, O.P., Simpson, J.L., and Elias, S. (1992). High frequency of cytogenetic abnormalities in fetuses with cystic hygroma diagnosed in first trimester. *Obstetrics and Gynecology*, **80**, 80–2.

Timor-Tritsch, I.E., Warren, W.B., Peisner, D.B., and Pirrone, E. (1989). First trimester midgut herniation: a high frequency transvaginal sonographic study. *American Journal of Obstetrics and Gynecology*, **161**, 831–3.

Tsukerman, G.L., Krapiva, G.A., and Kirillova, I.A. (1993). First trimester diagnosis of duodenal stenosis associated with oesophageal atresia. *Prenatal Diagnosis*, **13**, 371–6.

van Zalen-Sprock, R.M., van Vugt, J., and van Geijn, H.P. (1992). First trimester diagnosis of cystic hygroma, course and outcome. *American Journal of Obstetrics and Gynecology*, **67**, 94–8.

Wilson, R.D., Venir, N., and Farquharson, D.F. (1992). Fetal nuchal fluid-physiological or pathological in pregnancies less than 17 menstrual weeks. *Prenatal Diagnosis*, **12**, 755–63.

Yand, Y.C., Wu, C.H., Chang, F.M., Liu, C.H., and Chein, C.H. (1992). Early prenatal diagnosis of acrania by transvaginal ultrasonography. *Journal of Clinical Ultrasound*, **20**, 343–5.

Zimmer, E.Z., Bronshtein, M., Ophir, E., Meizner, I., Auslander, R., Groisman, G., and Meyer, H. (1993). Sonographic diagnosis of fetal congenital cataracts. *Prenatal Diagnosis*, **13**, 503–11.

21 | *Medical therapy of early pregnancy disorders*

Carolyn B. Coulam

Recent developments in understanding early pregnancy events has made medical therapy available for several early pregnancy disorders. Such advances are most welcome since the early prenatal period holds by far the greatest risk to human life. At least 60 per cent of human embryos die before the end of the first trimester of pregnancy (Edmond *et al.* 1982). The majority of deaths occur before or at the time of implantation (Wilcox *et al.* 1988). and the remaining 15 per cent occur post-implantation (Warburton and Frazer 1964). Chromosomal abnormalities have been found in 20–50 per cent of preimplantation embryos (Zenes and Casper 1992) and 50–70 per cent of postimplantation abortuses (Boue *et al.* 1975). Little information on other causes of death *in utero* is available. Data are accumulating which suggest a role of the immune system in the success of pregnancy (King and Loke 1991; Clark *et al.* 1994). Immunologic causes of early pregnancy disorders have manifest as recurrent spontaneous abortion (McIntyre *et al.* 1989). As many as 5 per cent of all couples conceiving experience two or more consecutive abortions (Coulam 1991). Less frequent early pregnancy disorders associated with unsuccessful pregnancies include metabolic defects and structural anomalies. All unsuccessful pregnancies result in substantial physical and emotional pain. Effective treatment therefore is needed. Medical therapies for early pregnancy disorders include immunotherapy for prevention of recurrent spontaneous abortion, pharmacologic management using dexamethasone for treatment of metabolic defects manifest as congenital adrenal hyperplasia, and folic acid for prevention of structural anomalies of neural tube defects.

IMMUNOTHERAPY FOR PREVENTION OF RECURRENT SPONTANEOUS ABORTION

Various forms of immunotherapy have been introduced to treat couples suffering from recurrent spontaneous abortions (Coulam 1995; Coulam *et al.* 1994, 1995*a*). Understanding the mechanisms involved in recurrent abortion allows a more focused approach to specific treatment. At the time of implantation, human trophoblastic cells form two layers—an inner layer of cytotrophoblasts and an outer layer of fused cytotrophoblasts called syncytiotrophoblasts. Any agent that would interfere with differentiation of cytotrophoblasts to syncytiotrophoblasts could inhibit normal placentation and result in failed implantation. Antiphospholipid antibodies have been shown to inhibit differentiation of cytotrophoblasts to syncytiotrophoblasts (Rote 1992). Later in pregnancy, antiphospholipid antibodies have been associated with vasculopathy, thrombosis, and infarction in placentas of women experiencing fetal death (De Wolf *et al.* 1982).

As the cytotrophoblasts differentiate to syncytiotrophoblasts they are stimulated to proliferate and invade into the decidua. Stimulation for proliferation and invasion is mediated by cytokines produced by trophoblastic, decidual, and lymphomyeloid cells present at the site of implantation. These lymphomyeloitic cells include CD8+ lymphocytes and CD56+ natural killer (NK) cells. Trophoblastic cells are resistant to lysis of cytotoxic lymphocytes and NK cells (Head 1989), but are susceptible to activated NK cells that have the asialo-granulocytic monocytic (GM)/+ marker (lymphokine-activated killer, LAK, cells) (Clark 1991). Suppression of the activation of NK to LAK cells is necessary for successful pregnancy to occur. CD8+ cells and CD56+ CD16– NK cells secrete factors that inhibit activation of NK cells to LAK cells. These cytokines include a 34 kDa protein produced by CD8+ cells with progesterone receptors (Szekeres-Bartho *et al.* 1990) and TGFβ$_2$ produced by CD56+ CD16– cells (Clark *et al.* 1995*a*). Women with recurrent miscarriage show a deficient activation of their CD8+ cells in early pregnancy (Szekeres-Bartho *et al.* 19) and a relative loss of CD56+ CD16– cells with an excess of CD56+ CD16+ cells in placental bed biopsies of incipiently aborting women (Michel *et al.* 1989). Quantitation of CD56+ NK cells in peripheral blood of women with recurrent spontaneous abortion with a failing pregnancy has shown a significant elevation associated with spontaneous abortion of a conceptus of normal karyotype and a normal level associated with loss of embryos that are karyotypically abnormal Coulam *et al.* 1995*b*). Further, high blood NK levels in non-pregnant women have been found to predict abortive pregnancies (Aoki *et al.* 1995). Thus CD8+ and NK cells play an important role in immunologically preventable spontaneous abortion. Agents that enhance CD8+ activity and suppress NK cell activation would be expected to prevent immunologic abortions. Immunization with lymphocytes stimulates CD8+ cell activation. Intravenous immunoglobulin both enhances CD8+ cell activity (Delfraissy *et al.* 1985) and downregulates NK+ cell activity (Newman and Hines 1979), as well as providing a pool of antiantiphospholipid antibodies. Other therapies available for the treatment of women with antiphospholipid antibody syndrome include aspirin, heparin, and prednisone (Coulam 1995). Leukocyte immunization has been used to treat women experiencing unexplained recurrent spontaneous abortion who show absence of circulating antiphospholipid antibodies and maternal antipaternal lymphocytotoxic antibodies (Coulam 1995; Coulam *et al.* 1994). We have recently reported that PIF determination may also be useful in the early detection of pregnancy loss since this factor disappears prior to clinical symptoms appearing (Coulam *et al.* 1995).

Treatment of antiphospholipid antibody syndrome

Autoantibodies associated with recurrent pregnancy loss include antiphospholipid, antinuclear, and antithyroid antibodies. Although the mechanisms by which antinuclear and antithyroid antibodies cause pregnancy loss are not known, much work has been done to elucidate the activity of antiphospholipid antibodies. Phospholipids function as adhesion molecules in the formation of syncytiotrophoblasts (Sessions and Horowitz 1983). Exposure of surface phospholipids (especially phosphoethanolamine) creates an immunogenic state (Rauch and Janoff 1990). Antibodies to these phospholipids interfere with the formation of syncytiotrophoblasts from cytotrophoblasts (Rote 1992) leading to delayed syncytialization of the trophoblast. This mechanism has been proposed in the pathogenesis of recurrent spontaneous abortion (Rote 1992). Later in pregnancy, antiphospholipid antibodies have been associated with decidual vasculopathy, thrombosis, and infarction in the placentas of women experiencing fetal death (De Wolf *et al.* 1982). In a case–control study of 47 pregnancies resulting in fetal death, placentas from women with antiphospholipid antibodies had substantially more fibrosis, hypovascular villi, thrombosis, and infarction and less vasculosyncytial membranes compared with those from women without antiphospholipid (Out *et al.* 1991). In fact, 85 per cent of placentas from antiphospholipid antibody-positive women had evidence of thrombosis or infarction (Out *et al.* 1991). Immunoglobulin type IgG from women with antiphospholipid antibodies has been shown to increase the concentration of placental thromboxane (Peaceman and Rehnberg 1993). Thromboxane production by the placenta could lead to platelet aggregation and thrombosis at the uteroplacental interface.

Aspirin therapy

The finding of thrombotic lesions within the uteroplacental interface provided the rationale for the use of low dose aspirin therapy during pregnancies of women with antiphospholipid antibodies. The dosage of aspirin advocated is 80 mg/day. However, results of clinical trials have shown it to be half as effective as treatment including prednisone or heparin. In a recent prospective controlled trial of aspirin alone compared with heparin plus aspirin for the treatment of recurrent spontaneous abortion associated with antiphospholipid antibodies, heparin plus aspirin provided a significantly better outcome than aspirin alone (live birth rate 83 per cent v. 46 per cent, $p < 0.05$) (Kutteh and Webster 1993).

Prednisone and aspirin therapy

Prednisone has various immunosuppressive effects and is commonly used to treat autoimmune conditions. The rationale for this type of therapy was suppression of antiphospholipid antibodies. However, pregnancy outcome with prednisone treatment does not appear to correlate with the suppression of antiphospholipid antibodies. Thus the mechanism of action of prednisone in treatment of recurrent spontaneous abortions associated with antiphospholipid is not clear. Prednisone is usually given as a daily dose of 40–60 mg beginning at the diagnosis of pregnancy. A daily dose of aspirin 80 mg is usually started preconceptually. Early reports from non-controlled studies have been summarized by Cowchock (1991). The average live birth rate in women with at least two pregnancy losses associated with antiphospholipid antibodies after treatment with prednisone and aspirin was 70 per cent. A randomized controlled trial subsequently confirmed the efficacy of prednisone and aspirin for treatment of recurrent spontaneous abortion associated with antiphospholipid antibodies (Hasegawa *et al.* 1992). In this study, women treated with prednisone and aspirin had a live birth rate of 77 per cent compared with non-treated control women who had a live birth rate of 8 per cent. However, risks associated with the dosages of prednisone used to treat recurrent spontaneous abortion associated with antiphospholipid antibodies include signs of iatrogenic Cushing's syndrome, severe acne, increased risk of gestational diabetes, osteopenia, posterior capsular cataract, listeriosis, pneumonia, and even maternal death from miliary tuberculosis (Branch *et al.* 1985; Alarcon-Segovia *et al.* 1989; Ramsdon and Farquharson 1990; Peaceman and Rehnberg 1993). Early pre-eclampsia is more common in pregnancy in women receiving prednisone, and premature rupture of membranes and associated preterm birth are almost always observed after prednisone therapy (Ramsdon and Farquhasson 1990; Cowchock *et al.* 1992).

Heparin and aspirin therapy

Because of the significant side effects connected to the treatment of recurrent spontaneous abortion associated with antiphospholipid antibodies using prednisone, alternative treatments have been sought. Since most of the clinical conditions associated with antiphospholipid antibodies have a vascular or thrombotic origin, heparin has been investigated for the treatment of recurrent spontaneous abortion associated with antiphospholipid antibodies. In addition, heparin has been shown to inhibit binding of antiphospholipid antibodies to phospholipids (Wagenknecht and McIntyre 1993), thereby protecting the trophoblast from interference of differentiation from cytotrophoblasts to syncytiotrophoblasts (Rote 1992). Heparin is usually administered at a dose of 5000–10 000 units subcutaneously twice a day along with aspirin 80 mg each day. Side effects of heparin therapy include prolonged coagulation times, thrombocytopenia, and osteoporosis. When a controlled clinical trial compared heparin and aspirin with prednisone and aspirin for treatment of recurrent spontaneous abortion associated with antiphospholipid antibodies, live birth rates of 75 per cent were obtained in both groups. However, both maternal morbidity and the frequency of preterm delivery were significantly higher in pregnant women treated with prednisone (Cowchock *et al.* 1992). Another controlled clinical trial showed a live birth rate of 74 per cent using heparin and aspirin compared with 45 per cent using aspirin alone (Kutteh and Webster 1993). Therefore, the current recommendation for 'first attempt' treatment for recurrent spontaneous abortion associated with antiphospholipid antibodies is heparin and aspirin.

Intravenous immunoglobulin therapy

Intravenous immunoglobulin (IVIg) therapy has been used to treat antiphospholipid antibody-positive women experiencing recurrent spontaneous abortion who have failed previous treatment with aspirin and heparin or prednisone (Lubbe and Liggins 1985; Carreras *et al.* 1988; Cowchock *et al.* 1988; Francois *et al.* 1988; Scott *et al.* 1988; Parke *et al.* 1989; MacLachlan *et al.* 1990). The rationale for the use of IVIg therapy in the original studies was suppression of lupus anticoagulant in a woman being treated for severe thrombocytopenia (Wapner *et al.* 1989). More recently, IVIg preparations have been shown to contain autoanti-idiotypes and immunomodulation by IVIg has been reported to result from the passive transfer of anti-idiotypic antibodies (Brand *et al.* 1988).

The estimated live birth rate of 71 per cent for women at very high risk for failure with a history of previous treatment failures suggested the IVIg treatment was effective (Cowchock *et al.* 1992). More recently, IVIg therapy alone has been used successfully to treat women with antiphospholipid antibodies (Christiansen *et al.* 1992). This report, along with a previous report of successful treatment with IVIg in a woman who had lost 12 previous pregnancies while being treated with aspirin and heparin or prednisone (Bernstein and Crawford 1988), suggests that IVIg therapy alone is successful in treating women with recurrent spontaneous abortion associated with antiphospholipid antibodies.

Treatment of recurrent spontaneous abortion associated with elevated concentrations of circulating CD56+ cells

Recent data suggest that IVIg therapy is useful in maintaining pregnancies in women with a history of recurrent spontaneous abortion who lose karyotypically normal embryos after detection of embryonic cardiac activity on ultrasonographic examination and who demonstrate elevated levels of natural killer (CD56+) cells in maternal blood (Coulam *et al.* 1995*b*). In this study, 13 women received IVIg and none experienced a pregnancy loss. The frequency of elevated levels of circulating CD56+ cells associated with viable outcome are compared between women receiving and not receiving IVIg. A significantly higher proportion of women with CD56+ cell levels raised by more than 12 per cent and who received IVIg had viable pregnancies ($p = 0.0002$).

Treatment of unexplained recurrent spontaneous abortion

Immunologic mechanisms have been implicated in a number of otherwise unexplained recurrent spontaneous abortions and various forms of immunotherapy have been introduced to treat couples suffering from this condition (Coulam 1995; Coulam *et al.* 1994, 1995*a*). Randomized clinical trials testing the efficacy of immunotherapy for unexplained recurrent spontaneous abortion have been conducted using allogeneic leukocyte immunization (Coulam 1994) and intravenous (IV) immunoglobulin (Ig) (Coulam 1995*a*).

Allogeneic leukocyte immunization

Allogeneic leukocyte immunizations have been used to treat couples considered to have an immunologic mechanism of loss based upon historic and theoretic notions. These couples have experienced three or more consecutive unexplained early pregnancy losses, have not had more than one live birth, and have had no losses with another partner. The original rationale for this form of immunotherapy was to present an allogeneic stimulus to the maternal immune system which would evoke an appropriate response to antigens on the fetal trophoblastic cells needed to protect the pregnancy from failure. However, it was subsequently shown that the trophoblasts which envelope the fetus and form the feto-maternal interface are immunogenic lacking expression of HLA-A, -B, -C, and -DR/DQ susceptible to transplantation immunity (Clark 1991). The occurrence of successful non-abortive pregnancies in women with agammaglobulinaemia is not consistent with a need for blocking antibody, and blocking antibody is not always demonstrable in women with successful pregnancies (Sargent *et al.* 1988). Therefore the rationale for treatment of recurrent spontaneous abortion using leukocyte immunization has shifted to encompass new knowledge of the mechanism. In humans, there is evidence that CD8+ lymphocytic cells may recognize trophoblast; these lymphocytic cells carry the $\gamma\delta$-type receptor rather than the $\alpha\beta$ lymphocytic-cell receptor which requires HLA-A, -B, -C for efficient recognition and binding. In normal successful pregnancy or after T-cell activation, as occurs with immunization, CD8+ cells are activated, express progesterone receptors, and in response to the hormone, secrete a factor that inhibits NK cells (Szekeres-Bartho *et al.* 1990). Other cytokines may also be produced by activated CD8+ cells and it is hypothesized that some of these may enhance antibody responses (IL-4), inhibit macrophages (IL-10), and facilitate activation of bone-marrow-derived TGF-β-producing suppressor cells (IL-3, GM-CSF) found in the decidua (Erard *et al.* 1990; Mooere and Soderberg 1990). Women with recurrent miscarriage show a deficient activation of their CD8+ cells in early pregnancy (Szekeres-Bartho *et al.* 1989).

A rationale for immunotherapy using leukocyte immunization has been provided. However, results of clinical trials evaluating allogeneic leukocyte immunization have both supported (Mowbray *et al.* 1985; Gatenby *et al.* 1993) and refuted (Cauchi *et al.* 1991; Ho *et al.* 1991) this method for treatment of recurrent spontaneous abortion. To address the uncertainties caused by conflicting results of the effectiveness of leukocyte immunization, a world-wide collaborative observational study and meta-analysis were performed (Coulam *et al.* 1994). Fifteen collaborating centres participated in the study. Nine randomized trials (seven double-blinded) were evaluated independently by two data analysis teams to assure robust conclusions. Although the independent analyses used different definitions and statistical methods, the results were similar. The live birth ratios (ratio of live births in treatment and control groups) with 95 per cent confidence intervals were 1.16 (range 1.01–1.34; $p = 0.03$) and 1.21 (range 1.04–1.37; $p = 0.02$). The absolute differences in live birth rates between treatment and control groups were 8 per cent and 10 per cent, respectively, in the respective analyses. In this analysis women with autoantibodies and antipaternal alloantibodies or prior successful pregnancy with their partner were included. A supplementary analysis was published including only women with no prior live births and only paternal leukocytes and excluding women with autoimmunity and pre-existing antipaternal antibody as well as women who did not conceive (Daya and Gunby 1994). When women with different numbers of prior losses were considered, up to 30 per cent absolute improvement was seen for those who had had five or six prior abortions, with a lesser effect for those with less than four or greater than seven prior abortions (Daya and Gunby 1994; Clark and Coulam 1995). The prognosis for women with or without treatment declined dramatically as the number of prior abortions increased (Clark and Coulam 1995). One explanation emerged from studies being done independently on karyotypes from failing pregnancies (Stern *et al.* 1996): abnormal karyotypes were found in 60 per cent of abortions from women with a history of recurrent spontaneous abortion. By simple branching tree analysis, those aborting karyotypically abnormal concepti would have a 60–70 per cent risk of producing another abortus (Clark and Coulam 1995). The risk of repeated chromosomal abnormality suggested by this model has been confirmed by empiric data published by Warburton *et al.* (1987).

Intravenous immunoglobulin

Since the world-wide collaborative observational study and meta-analysis on allogenic leukocyte immunotherapy for recurrent spontaneous abortion showed a low treatment effect with an absolute reduction of risk of further abortion between 8 per cent and 10 per cent (the number of cases one needs to treat to achieve one additional live birth is between 9 and 13) (Coulam *et al.* 1994), alternative treatments for recurrent spontaneous abortion have been sought. Among alternative treatments reported to result in successful pregnancies is IVIg therapy (Mueller-Eckharot *et al.* 1991; Christiansen *et al.* 1992; Maruyama *et al.* 1994; Coulam *et al.* 1995a). Immuno-modulation by IVIg has been postulated to result from passively transferred blocking or anti-idiotypic antibodies (Brand *et al.* 1988), blockade of Fc receptor (Kimberly *et al.* 1987), enhancement of suppressor T-cell function (Delfraussy *et al.* 1985), downregulation of B-cell function (Nydegger 1991), and/or reduction of activation of complement components (Kulics *et al.* 1983; Zielinski *et al.* 1985), natural killer cell activity, and cytokine production (Newman and Hines 1979). Thus IVIg would be expected to both upregulate CD8+ cells and downregulate CD56+ CD16+ cells—activities that would enhance the probability of successful pregnancy. In addition, it has been suggested that IVIg might contain small amounts of a pregnancy-protective antibody (Clark and Coulam 1995).

The syncytiotrophoblast bears an antigen called R80K (80 kDa molecule) to which all women make antibody during successful pregnancy (Jalali *et al.* 1989); the antibody can be eluted from term placentae and reacts in an immunologically specific way with an antigen on the husband's B lymphocytes and monocytes, and also with his father's B lymphocytes and monocytes (Underwood *et al.* 1995). The antibody appears to inhibit NK cell activity (Jalali *et al.* 1995). A mouse monoclonal antibody directed against a framework determinant of R80K also inhibits NK cell killing (of K562 target cells) (Clark *et al.* 1995b).

Two randomized controlled trials of IVIg in recurrent miscarriage have been done (Coulam *et al.* 1995a; Muellers-Eclchardt *et al.* 1994). A European-based study showed a positive trend but did not achieve statistical significance due to too few patients for the magnitude of the benefits, but a second US-based trial did show a significant benefit. As the latter trial did not have larger numbers of patients, the positive result was due to an effect of greater magnitude; the latter could have arisen by chance or by use of a different study design wherein patients began IVIg treatment prior to conception (Coulam *et al.* 1995a). The greater putative anti-abortion effect of IVIg occurs around the time of implantation or the week after (Clark *et al.* 1992). Therefore, starting treatment after the appearance of hCG in maternal circulation would minimize the effect of IVIg and select for women who are most apt to have a successful pregnancy in both the treatment and placebo groups. Indeed, the difference in results between the two studies was not in the treatment groups but rather in the control groups. In the European study, when women were entered after a positive pregnancy test, the control patients had the same live birth rate as the treated patients (Mueller-Eckhardt *et al.* 1994).

The US study was a randomized, double-blinded, placebo-controlled trial using IVIg for treatment beginning preconceptually (Coulam *et al.* 1995*a*). The difference in live birth rates between women receiving IVIg (62 per cent) and placebo (34 per cent) was significant ($p = 0.04$) (Coulam *et al.* 1995). Based on the magnitude of effect, one needs to treat four women to achieve one additional live birth making IVIg therapy three times more effective then leukocyte immunization. It is possible that IVIg may achieve better results than leukocyte immunization in unselected women being treated for recurrent spontaneous abortion by virtue of an ability to ameliorate rather than to aggravate subclinical autoimmunity that may be causing recurrent losses or it may provide a broader spectrum of treatment in some women by mechanisms yet to be defined.

In summary, recurrent pregnancy loss is a health care concern. Safe and effective treatments are necessary. Women experiencing recurrent pregnancy loss are a heterogeneous population. Chromosomal abnormalities are evident in 60 per cent of primary recurrent abortions. Women experiencing recurrent aneuploidy in their abortuses would be expected to respond to immunotherapy. To eliminate abnormal chromosomes within concepti as a confounding variable for clinical trials testing various forms of immunotherapy, specific markers are necessary to identify those who have abnormal embryos. Currently available diagnostic markers include karyotyping the trophoblast and immunologic tests listed in Table 21.1. IVIg has been used to successfully treat women with karyotypically normal embryos with both autoimmune and other risk factors for recurrence of loss (Table 21.2).

PHARMACOLOGIC MANAGEMENT OF METABOLIC DEFECTS

The concept of fetal therapy is not new. The first thoughts of ameliorating fetal haemolytic disease came in the 1960s. Since then drugs and other agents have been administered to pregnant women for treatment of fetal disorders including prenatal treatment of genetically determined metabolic defects. Prenatal treatment of methymalonic acidaemia with cyanocobalamin and of multiple carboxylase deficiency with biotin have been administered late in pregnancy in the hope of improving postnatal

Table 21.1   Immunologic tests available for evaluation of couples experiencing recurrent spontaneous abortion

- Antiphospholipid antibodies including lupus-like anticoagulant
- Antinuclear antibodies
- Thyroid antibodies
- Reproductive immunophenotype (CD56+ cells)
- Embryotoxicity assay

Table 21.2   Treatment options for couples experiencing recurrent spontaneous abortion

Immunologic tests		Treatment
Antiphospholipid antibody, APTT Activated partial Antinuclear antibody thromboplastin time		Heparin, aspirin
Antithyroid antibody RIP Reproductive immunophenotype ETA Embryotoxicity assay LAD Leukocyte antibody detection assay		IVIg Intravenous immunoglobulin

outcome with successful results. Only congenital adrenal hyperplasia has been treated in the first trimester of pregnancy.

The fetal adrenal gland can be pharmacologically suppressed by maternal replacement doses of dexamethasone (Evans *et al.* 1985). In congenital adrenal hyperplasia (CAH) caused by 21-hydroxylase deficiency, impaired metabolism of cholesterol to cortisol creates excess 17-OH progesterone, which becomes androstenedione and androgens. Consequently, genetic females are exposed to excess androgens and can be masculinized. The abnormal differentiation can vary from clitoral hypertrophy to complete formation of a phallus and apparent scrotum.

In an attempt to prevent this birth defect, Evans and colleagues administered dexamethasone, a fluorinated steroid, to an at-risk mother beginning in the 10th week of gestation (Evans *et al.* 1985). Maternal oestriol and cortisol values indicated rapid and sustained fetal and maternal adrenal gland suppression. This fetus ultimately turned out to be a carrier.

Following the initial observation of Evans and colleagues, Forest and David used the same protocol of 0.25 mg of dexamethasone qid beginning at nine weeks to treat several fetuses and demonstrated that fetuses known to be clinically affected with the severe form of 21-hydroxylase deficiency CAH were prevented from external congenital masculinization (David and Forest 1984). To date, several infants with classic CAH, who clearly would have been masculinized, have been born with normal genitalia. In a few cases some masculinization has still been observed following this regimen beginning at nine weeks. The current recommendation, therefore, is to begin at seven weeks, although there have been too few cases to assess this modification (Pang *et al.* 1994). These events represent the first prevention of a birth defect and may serve as a model for other attempts at pharmacologic fetal therapy.

PREVENTION OF STRUCTURAL ABNORMALITIES WITH FOLIC ACID

Animal studies suggest that neural tube defects (NTDs) can arise from a variety of vital or mineral deficiencies. In humans, increased frequencies of NTDs have been observed in women with poor dietary histories or with intestinal bypasses (Elwood and Elwood 1980). Over the past two decades, the question of whether periconceptional vitamin supplementation reduces the risk of NTDs has received attention. Early tests of the hypothesis were focused primarily on prevention of recurrent NTDs because of the higher risk among women who had already given birth to an affected child (Smithells *et al.* 1983). Results of a controlled trial established that the use of a 4 mg folic acid supplement a day before and during early pregnancy reduced the risk of NTDs by 72 per cent (Smithelss *et al.* 1983). A more recent study has shown that daily periconceptual intake of 0.4 mg of folic acid reduced the risk of first (occurrent) NTDs by 60 per cent (Werler *et al.* 1993). Thus the use of folic acid supplements before and during early pregnancy reduces the risk of NTDs.

CONCLUDING REMARKS

To date, medical therapies of early pregnancy disorders have been limited. Much progress has been made in the understanding of causes of early pregnancy loss or abortion. Abortion is the most common complication of pregnancy and the most common risk of human life. Immunotherapy for prevention of abortion is successful in approximately 30 per cent of women. Sensitive and specific markers are needed to identify such women. As diagnostic techniques of early embryonic events improve, other pharmacologic and preventative therapies will become available. With the availability of a probe for the gene for enzymatic defects such as congenital adrenal hyperplasia, a nearly definitive diagnosis would be possible by DNA analysis of chorionic villi in the first trimester or by coeliocentesis even sooner. Treatment with dexamethasone could be administered to affected females preventing unwanted masculinization. The fundamental principles addressed in such attempted prevention of masculinization can be logically extended to other early pregnancy disorders.

The finding that folic acid supplements are associated with a 60 per cent reduction in the risk of occurrence of neural tube defects stimulates other considerations relevant to public policy. Half of women conceiving have not consulted a health care provider. Based upon the embryonic timing of neural tube closure, folic acid must be consumed prior to a woman knowing she is pregnant. Therefore, this or any other such interventions would have to be directed at all women of childbearing potential to achieve maximum effect.

The prevention of early pregnancy disorders will involve both individuals and populations. With the evolution of yet more sophisticated diagnostic and therapeutic techniques, medical treatment of early pregnancy disorders will become as common as that of late adult disorders. Gene therapy which requires direct entry into the pre-embryo or embryo will be an added focus for the medical treatment of early pregnancy disorders in the future.

REFERENCES

Alarcon-Segovia, D., Deleze, M., Oria, C.V., Sanchez-Guerro, J., Gomez-Pacheco, L., Cabiedas, J., *et al.* (1989). Antiphospholipid antibodies and the antiphospholipid antibody syndrome in systemic lupus erythematosus. *Medicine*, **68**, 353–65.

Aoki, K., Kajiura, S., Matsumoto, Y., Ogasawara, M., Okada, S., Yagami, Y., *et al.* (1995). Preconceptual natural killer cell activity as a predictor of miscarriage. *Lancet*, **345**, 1340–2.

Babcock, R.B., Dumper, C.W., and Scharfman, W.B. (1976). Heparin-induced immunothrombocytopenia. *New England Journal of Medicine*, **295**, 237–41.

Bernstein, R.M. and Crawford, R.J. (1988). Intravenous IgG therapy for anticardiolipin syndrome: a case report. *Clinical and Experimental Rheumatology*, **6**, 198.

Boue, J., Boue, A., and Lazar, P. (1975). Retrospective and prospective epidemiological studies of 1500 karyotyped spontaneous human abortions. *Teratology*, **12**, 11–26.

Branch, D.W., Scott, J.R., Kochenour, N.K., and Hershgold, E. (1985). Obstetric complications associated with the lupus anticoagulant. *New England Journal of Medicine*, **313**, 1322–6.

Brand, A., Witvliet, M., and Class, F.H.J. (1988). Beneficial effect of intravenous gammaglobulin in a patient with complement-mediated autoimmune thrombocytopenia due to IgM-antiplatelet antibodies. *British Journal of Haematology*, **69**, 507–11.

Carreras, L.O., Perez, G.N., Vega, H.R., and Maclouf, J. (1988). Lupus anticoagulant and recurrent fetal loss: successful treatment with gammaglobulin. *Lancet*, **ii**, 393.

Cauchi, M.N., Lim, D., Young, D.E., Kloss, M., and Pepperell, R.J. (1991). Treatment of recurrent aborters by immunization with paternal cells—controlled trial. *American Journal of Reproductive Immunology*, **25**, 16–17.

Christiansen, O.B., Mathiesen, O., Lauristen, J.G., and Grunnet, N. (1992). Intravenous immunoglobulin treatment of women with multiple miscarriages. *Human Reproduction*, **7**, 718–22.

Clark, D.A. (1991). Controversies in reproductive immunology. *Critical Review of Immunology*, **11**, 214–47.

Clark, D.A. and Coulam, C.B. (1996). Is there an immunological cause of repeated pregnancy wastage? *Advances in Obstetrics and Gynecology*, **3**, 321–6.

Clark, D.A., Lea, R.G., Flanders, K.C., Banwatt, D., and Chaouat, G. (1992). Role of a unique species of transforming growth factor beta in preventing rejection of the conceptus during pregnancy. In *Progress in immunology*, (ed. J. Gergeley, M. Benczur, A. Erdei, *et al.*), Vol. III, pp. 841–44. Springer, New York.

Clark, D.A., Vince, G., Flanders, K., Hirte, H., and Starkey, P. (1994). CD56+ lymphoid cells in human first trimester pregnancy decidua as a source of novel transforming growth factor β2 related immunosuppressive factors. *Human Reproduction*, **9**, 2270–7.

Clark, D.A., Flanders, K.C., Hirte, H., *et al.* (1995*a*). Characterization of murine pregnancy decidua TFG-β2-like molecules of unusual molecular size released in bioactive form. *Biology of Reproduction*, **52**, 1380–4.

Clark, D.A., Arck, P., Jalali, R., *et al.* (1996). Psycho-neuro-cytokine/endocrine pathways in immunoregulation during pregnancy. *American Journal of Reproductive Immunology*, **35**, 330–7.

Coulam, C.B. (1991). Epidemiology of recurrent spontaneous abortion. *American Journal of Reproductive Immunology*, **26**, 23–7.

Coulam, C.B. (1995). Immunotherapy for recurrent spontaneous abortion. *Early Pregnancy: Biology and Medicine*, **1**, 13–26.

Coulam, C.B., Clark, D.A., Collins, J.A. (The Recurrent Miscarriage Immunotherapy Trialist Group) (1994). Worldwide collaborative observational study and meta-analysis on allogeneic leukocyte immunotherapy for recurrent spontaneous abortion. *American Journal of Reproductive Immunology*, **32**, 55–72.

Coulam, C.B., Krysa, L., Stern, J.J., and Bustillo, M. (1995*a*). Intravenous immunoglobulin for the treatment of recurrent pregnancy loss. *American Journal of Reproductive Immunology*, **34**, 333–7.

Coulam, C.B., Goodman, C., Roussev, R.G., Thomason, E.J., and Beaman, K.G. (1995*b*). Systemic CD56+ cells can predict pregnancy outcome. *American Journal of Reproductive Immunology*, **33**, 40–6.

Coulam, C.B., Roussev, R.G., Thomason, E.J., and Barnea, E.R. (1995c). Preimplantation factor (PIF) predicts subsequent pregnancy loss. *American Journal of Reproductive Immunology*, **34**, 88–92.

Cowchock, S. (1991). The role of antiphospholipid antibodies in obstetric medicine. *Current Obstetrical Medicine*, **1**, 229–47.

Cowchock, F.S., Wapner, R.J., Needleman, L., and Filer, R. (1988). A comparison of pregnancy outcome after two treatments for antibodies to cardiolipin (ACA). *Clinical and Experimental Rheumatology*, **6**, 200–6.

Cowchock, F.S., Resse, E.A., Balaban, D., Branch, D.W., and Plouffe, L. (1992). Repeated fetal losses associated with antiphospholipid antibodies: a collaborative trial comparing treatment with prednisone to low dose heparin. *American Journal of Obstetrics and Gynecology*, **166**, 1318–23.

David, M. and Forest, M.G. (1984). Prenatal treatment of congenital adrenal hyperplasia resulting from 21-hydroxylase deficiency. *Journal of Pediatrics*, **105**, 799–802.

Daya, S., Gunby, J., and The Recurrent Miscarriage Immunotherapy Trialist Group (1994). The effectiveness of allogeneic leukocyte immunization in unexplained primary recurrent spontaneous abortion. *American Journal of Reproductive Immunology*, **32**, 294–302.

De Wolf, F., Carreras, L.O., Moerman, P., Yermylen P, Van Assche, A., and Renaer, M. (1982). Decidual vasculopathy and extensive placental infarction in a patient with repeated thromboembolic accidents, recurrent fetal loss, and a lupus anticoagulant. *American Journal of Obstetrics and Gynecology*, **142**, 829–34.

Delfraissy, J.F., Tchernia, G., and Laurian, Y. (1985). Suppressor cell function after intravenous gammaglobulin treatment in adult chronic idiopathic thrombocytopenia purpura. *British Journal of Haematology*, **60**, 315–22.

Edmond, K.D., Lindsay, K.S., Miller, J.F., Williamson, E., and Wood, P.J. (1982). Early embryonic mortality in women. *Fertility and Sterility*, **38**, 447–53.

Elwood, J.M. and Elwood, J.H. (1980). *Epidemiology of anencephalus and spina Bifida*. Oxford University Press, New York, NY.

Erard, R., Garcia-Sanz, J.A., and Le Gros, G. (1990). Switch of CD8 T cells of noncytolytic CD8– CD4– cells that make TH2 cytokines and help B cells. *Science*, **260**, 1802–5.

Evans, M.I., Chrousos, G.P., Mann, D.L., Larsen Jr, J.W., Green, I., McCluskey, J., et al. (1985). Pharmacologic suppression of the fetal adrenal gland in utero: attempted prevention of abnormal external genital masculinization in suspected congenital adrenal hyperplasia. *Journal of the American Medical Association*, **253**, 1015.

Francois, A., Freund, M., and Reym, P. (1988). Repeated fetal losses and the lupus anticoagulant. *Annals of Internal Medicine*, **109**, 933–4.

Gatenby, P.A., Cameron, K., Simes, R.J., Adelstein, S., Bennett, M.J., Jansen, R.P.S., et al. (1993). Treatment of recurrent spontaneous abortion by immunization with paternal lymphocytes: results of a controlled trial. *American Journal of Reproductive Immunology*, **29**, 88–94.

Hasegawa, I., Takakuwa, K., Goto, S., Yamada, K., Sekizuka, N. Kanazawa, K., and Tanaka, K. (1992). Effectiveness of prednisone/aspirin therapy for recurrent aborters with antiphospholipid antibody. *Human Reproduction*, **7**, 203–7.

Head, J.R. (1989). Can trophoblasts be killed by cytotoxic cells? *In vitro* evidence and *in vivo* possibilities. *American Journal of Reproductive Immunology*, **20**, 100–5.

Ho, H.N., Gill, T.J., Hsieh, H.J., Jiang, J.J., Lee, T.Y., and Hsieh, C.Y. (1991). Immunotherapy for recurrent spontaneous abortion in a Chinese population. *American Journal of Reproductive Immunology*, **25**, 10–15.

Hunt, J.S. and Hsi, B.-L. (1990). Evasive strategies of trophoblast cells: selective expression of membrane antigens. *American Journal of Reproductive Immunology*, **23**, 57–63.

Jalali, G.R., Underwood, J.L., and Mowbray, J.F. (1989). IgG on normal human placenta is bound both to antigen and Fc receptors. *Transplantation Proceedings*, **21**, 572–4.

Jalali, G.R., Rezai, A., Underwood, J.L., Mowbray, J.F., Surridge, S.H., Allen, W.R., and Mathias, S. (1995). An 80 kDa syncytiotrophoblast antigen bound to maternally alloantibody in term placenta. *American Journal of Reproductive Immunology*, **33**, 210–13.

Kimberly, R.P., Salmon, J.E., Bussell, J.B., *et al.* (1987). Modulation of mononuclear phagocyte function by intravenous gammaglobulin. *Journal of Immunology*, **132**, 745–50.

King, A. and Loke, Y.W. (1991). On the nature and function of human uterine granular lymphocytes. *Immunology Today*, **12**, 432–5.

Kulics, J., Rajnavolgye, E., Fust, G., and Gergely, J. (1983). Interaction of C3 and C3b with immunoglobulin. *Journal of Molecular Immunology*, **20**, 805–10.

Kutteh, W.H. and Webster, R.M. (1993). A prospective controlled trial of aspirin for the treatment of recurrent pregnancy loss associated with antiphospholipid antibodies. *Fertility and Sterility* (Suppl.), S68–69.

Lubbe, W.F. and Liggins, C.G. (1985). Lupus anticoagulant and pregnancy. *American Journal of Obstetrics and Gynecology*, **153**, 322–7.

McIntyre, J.A., Coulam, C.B., and Faulk, W.P. (1989). Recurrent spontaneous abortion. *American Journal of Reproductive Immunology*, **21**, 100–4.

MacLachlan, N.A., Letsky, E., DeSwiet, M., *et al.* (1990). The use of intravenous immunoglobulin therapy in the management of antiphospholipid antibody associated pregnancies. *Clinical and Experimental Rheumatology*, **8**, 221–4.

McVerry, B., Spearing, R., and Smith, A. (1985). SLE anticoagulant: transient inhibition by high dose immunoglobulin infusions. *British Journal of Haematology*, **61**, 579–80.

Maruyama, T., Makino, T., Iwasaki, K., Sugi, T., Saito, S., Umeuchi, M., *et al.* (1994). The influence of intravenous immunoglobulin treatment on maternal immunity in women with unexplained recurrent miscarriage. *American Journal of Reproductive Immunology*, **31**, 7–18.

Michel, M., Underwood, J., Clark, D.A., Mowbray, J., and Beard, R.W. (1989). Histologic and immunologic study of uterine biopsy tissue of incipiently aborting women. *American Journal of Obstetrics and Gynecology*, **161**, 409–14.

Moore, S.C. and Soderberg, L.S.F. (1990). Mouse bone marrow natural suppressor cells: induction and activity. *FASEB Journal*, **4**, 435.

Mowbray, J.F., Liddel, H., Underwood, J.L., Gibbins, C., Reginald, P.W., and Beard, R.W. (1985). Controlled trial of treatment of recurrent spontaneous abortion by immunization with paternal cells. *Lancet*, **i**, 941–9.

Mueller-Eckhardt, G., Huni, O., and Poltrin, B. (1991). IVIg to prevent recurrent spontaneous abortion. *Lancet*, **i**, 424.

Mueller-Eckhardt, G., Mohr-Pennert, A., Heine, O., Neppert, J., Kunzel, W., and Mueller-Eckhardt, C. (1994). Controlled trial on intravenous immunoglobulin treatment for prevention of recurrent spontaneous abortion. *British Journal of Obstetrics and Gynaecology*, **101**, 1072–7.

Newman, M.J. and Hines, H.C. (1979). Production of fetally stimulated lymphocytotoxic antibodies by primiparous cows. *Animal Blood Groups Biochemical Genetics*, **10**, 87–92.

Nydegger, U.E. (1991). Hypothetic and established action mechanisms of therapy with immunoglobulin G. In *Immunotherapy with intravenous immunoglobulins*, (ed. P. Imbach), pp. 27–36. Academic Press, London.

Out, H.J., Kooijman, C.D., Bruinse, H.W., and Derksen, R.H.W.M. (1991). Histopathological findings from patients with intrauterine fetal death and antiphospholipid antibodies. *European Journal of Obstetrics and Gynecology*, **41**, 179–86.

Pang, S., Pollack, M.S., Marshall, R.N., and Immken, L. (1984). Prenatal treatment of congenital adrenal hyperplasia due to 21-hydroxylase deficiency. *New England Journal of Medicine*, **22**, 111.

Parke, A., Maier, D., Wilson, D., Andreoli, J., and Ballow, M. (1989). Intravenous gammaglobulin, antiphospholipid antibodies, and pregnancy. *Annals of Internal Medicine*, **110**, 495–6.

Peaceman, A.M. and Rehnberg, K.A. (1993). The effect of immunoglobulin G fractions from patients with lupus anticoagulant on placental prostacyclin and thromboxane production. *American Journal of Obstetrics and Gynecology*, **169**, 1403–6.

Ramsdon, C.F. and Farquharson, R.G. (1990). A woman with twelve first trimester losses in whom lupus anticoagulant was detected and treated with steroids, sandoglobulin, and heparin. *Clinical and Experimental Rheumatology*, **8**, 221.

Rauch, J. and Janoff, A.S. (1990). Phospholipid in the hexagonal (II) phase is immunogenic: evidence for immunorecognition of nonbilayer lipid phases *in vivo*. *Proceedings of the National Academy of Sciences, USA*, **87**, 4112–4.

Rote, N.S. (1992). Antiphospholipid antibodies—lobsters or red herrings? *American Journal of Reproductive Immunology*, **28**, 31–7.

Sargent, I.L., Wilkins, T., and Redman, C.W.G. (1988). Maternal immune response to the fetus in early pregnancy and recurrent miscarriage. *Lancet*, **ii**, 1099–103.

Scott, J.R., Branch, W., Kochenour, N.K., and Ward, K. (1988). Intravenous immunoglobulin treatment of pregnant patients with recurrent pregnancy loss caused by antiphospholipid antibodies and Rh immunization. *American Journal of Obstetrics and Gynecology*, **159**, 1055–6.

Sessions, A. and Horowitz, A.F. (1983). Differentiation related differences in the plasma membrane phospholipid asymmetry of myogenic and fibrogenic cells. *Biochimica et Biophysica Acta*, **728**, 103–11.

Smithells, R.W., Nevin, N.C., Seller, M.H., *et al.* (1983). Further experience of vitamin supplementation for prevention of neural tube defects recurrences. *Lancet*, **i**, 1027–31.

Stern, J.J., Dorfmann, A., Guierrez-Najan, A.J., Cerrillo, M., and Coulam, C.B. (1996). Frequency of abnormal karyotypes among abortuses from women with and without a history of recurrent spontaneous abortion. *Fertility and Sterility*, **65**, 250–8.

Szekeres-Bartho, J., Reznikoff-Etievant, M.F., Varga, P., *et al.* (1989). Lymphocytic progesterone receptors in normal and pathological human pregnancy. *Journal of Reproductive Immunology*, **16**, 239–47.

Szekeres-Bartho, J., Kinsky, R., and Chaouat G. (1990). The effect of a progesterone-induced immunologic blocking factor on NK-mediated resorption. *American Journal of Reproductive Immunology*, **24**, 105–7.

Underwood, J.L., Rezai, A., Jalali, G.R., *et al.* (1995). Transmission ratio distortion of a paternally derived syncytiotrophoblast antigen. *American Journal of Reproductive Immunology*, **33**, 474–9.

Wagenknecht, D.R. and McIntyre, J.A. (1993). Changes in β glycoprotein 1 antigenicity induced by phospholipid binding. *Thrombosis Hemostasis*, **69**, 361–5.

Wapner, R.J., Cowchock, F.S., and Shapiro, S.S. (1989). Successful treatment in two women with antiphospholipid antibodies and refractory pregnancy losses with intravenous immunoglobulin infusions. *American Journal of Obstetrics and Gynecology*, **161**, 1271–2.

Warburton, D. and Frazer, F.C. (1964). Spontaneous abortion risks in man: data from reproductive histories collected in a medical genetics unit. *American Journal of Human Genetics*, **16**, 1–23.

Warburton, D., Kline, J., Stein, Z., Hutzler, M., Chin, A., and Hassold, T. (1997). Does the karyotype of a spontaneous abortion predict the karyotype of a subsequent abortion?— evidence from 273 women with karyotyped spontaneous abortions. *American Journal of Human Genetics*, **41**, 465–8.

Werler, M.M., Shapiro, S., and Mitchell, A.A. (1993). Periconceptual folic acid exposure and risk of occurrent neural tube defects. *Journal of the American Medical Association*, **269**, 1257–61.

Wilcox, A.J., Weinburg, C.R., O'Connor, J., *et al.* (1988). Incidence of early loss of pregnancy. *New England Journal of Medicine*, **319**, 189–94.

Zenes, M.T. and Casper, R.F. (1992). Cytogenetics of human oocytes, zygotes and embryos after *in vitro* fertilization. *Human Genetics*, 88, 367–75.

Zielinski, C.C., Pries, P., and Eibl, M.M. (1985). Effect of immunoglobulin substitution on serum immunoglobulin and complement concentration. *Nephron*, 40, 253–4.

22 | *Maternal diseases in early pregnancy*

Laura A. Magee and Michael de Swiet

INTRODUCTION

This chapter focuses on maternal diseases that existed prior to pregnancy (whether diagnosed or not) given that these are the women who come to medical attention for pre-pregnancy counselling or soon after conception. This chapter will consider issues of particular relevance to the first trimester, but those relevant to management in later pregnancy and/or labour and delivery will also be mentioned, as the first trimester is the time to develop a management strategy for the whole of pregnancy. In this way, the doctors, midwife, and patient are prepared for all eventualities.

The importance of the first trimester for the fetus is well recognized. Relevant issues are potential fetal loss, and teratogenicity of maternal disease and/or its pharmacotherapy. An accurate dating scan is an invaluable part of such an evaluation, not only to confirm fetal viability and determine the risks associated with a given drug/chemical exposure, but also to enable the obstetrician to plan with confidence a premature delivery needed because of deteriorating maternal disease and/or poor fetal status.

Perhaps what is less well recognized is the importance of the first trimester for the mother who experiences most of the eventual pregnancy-related physiological changes during this time, and who may come to medical attention specifically because of a pregnancy-related change in disease control (e.g. diabetes mellitus, autoimmune disease). Maternal physiologic changes will be related to the relevant maternal disease under discussion, and the impact of pregnancy on standard 'baseline' laboratory measures in the first trimester will also be reviewed.

This chapter is not meant to be an all-inclusive review of medical disorders in pregnancy, for the details of management can be found elsewhere. The general approach will be to evaluate the following:

- the effects (or potential effects) of pregnancy on disease activity and long-term prognosis;
- the effects of the disease and/or its treatment on the pregnancy (i.e. fetal loss, teratogenicity of drugs);
- the inheritability or vertical transmission of the maternal disease to the fetus, and whether or not prenatal diagnosis is available;
- general maternal health—pregnancy represents an ideal opportunity to promote a healthy lifestyle in terms of diet, exercise, and avoidance of substance abuse and

to address specific risk factors for adverse pregnancy outcome and long-term maternal health problems (e.g. tobacco). Populations at particular risk for infectious diseases (e.g. toxoplasmosis) would also be appropriate to screen at this stage.

Maternal diseases that predate pregnancy will be discussed first, followed by those that complicate the first trimester of pregnancy. What most women need is accurate information, and in most cases, that information will be very reassuring. Therapeutic abortion is rarely required.

PRENATAL DIAGNOSIS OF INHERITABLE MEDICAL DISORDERS

There are a few disorders for which better control of the maternal disease will lower the risk of fetal abnormalities (e.g. diabetes mellitus, PKU). However, many medical disorders have a heritable basis, and many women with medical problems delay childbearing to beyond 35 years of age which puts them at increased risk of having a baby with chromosomal abnormalities. Therefore, there are many reasons why a brief discussion of prenatal diagnosis is warranted.

First of all, prenatal diagnosis is aimed at providing an accurate reproductive risk assessment, and either providing reassurance or giving parents the option of continuing with or terminating the pregnancy following an unfavourable fetal prognosis. Although prenatal diagnosis may be perceived as encouraging termination, more often than not, families are reassured about their risk of having an affected child, and the family size of at-risk couples actually increases (Valle 1994).

Obviously the best time for prenatal diagnostic counselling is prior to conception, and all couples at increased risk for having an affected child should be referred. The availability of prenatal diagnosis depends on whether inheritance is (i) chromosomal (e.g. trisomy 21); (ii) multifactorial (i.e. the diseases that 'run in families'); or (iii) monogenic (i.e. due to a single mutant gene with either an autosomal dominant, autosomal recessive, or X-linked recessive pattern of inheritance) (Table 22.1).

Chromosomal and multifactorial aetiologies are usually associated with inheritance risks of less than 10 per cent. Risk assessment in the face of monogenic disorders is more complicated, especially for autosomal dominant disease given variable clinical penetrance and less knowledge about the underlying biochemical defect. However, molecular tests that determine parental genotype, test for the gene product, or for linked molecular markers are possible for some disorders (i.e. in informative families in which the disease cosegregates with marker alleles e.g. Marfan's syndrome).

Counselling about reproductive risk, investigations into parental genotype and/or family linkage studies (if appropriate), and risk of prenatal diagnostic procedures is in the realm of the genetic counsellor, who can provide up-to-date information. Possibilities at present are the following:

(1)   fetal sampling by CVS (at 10–12 weeks term) or amniocentesis (at 15–20 weeks) for cytogenetic, biochemical, or molecular abnormalities (see Chapter 19).

Table 22.1   Most common Mendelian disorders affecting adults

Autosomal dominant disorders	Familial hypercholesterolaemia
	Hereditary haemorrhagic telangectasia
	Marfan's syndrome
	Hereditary spherocytosis
	Adult polycystic kidney disease
	Huntington's chorea
	Acute intermittent porphyria
	Osteogenesis imperfecta tarda
	von Willebrand's disease
	Myotonic muscular dystrophy
	Hypertrophic obstructive cardiomyopathy
	Neurofibromatosis
	Tuberous sclerosis
Autosomal recessive disorders	Deafness
	Albinism
	Wilson's disease
	Haemochromatosis
	Sickle cell anemia
	β-thalassaemia
	Cystic fibrosis
	Hereditary emphysema ($\alpha 1$ antitrypsin deficiency)
	Homocystinuria
	Familial mediterranean fever
	Friedreich's ataxia
	Phenylketonuria (PKU)
X-linked disorders	Haemophilia A (factor VIII) and B (factor IX)
	Glucose-6-phosphate dehydrogenase deficiency
	Fabry's disease
	Ocular albinism
	Testicular feminization
	Hypophosphatemic rickets
	Fragile-X syndrome (mental retardation)

(2)   maternal triple screening (for AFP, βhCG, oestradiol) at 14–18 weeks for neural tube defects and aneuploidies;

(3)   fetal ultrasonography (at 12~20 weeks) which can detect most major structural abnormalities (see Chapter 20)

(4)   fetal echocardiography (at 16~20 weeks) which can detect ~85 per cent of all cardiac abnormalities (and probably more of the severe lesions) (Nora and Nora 1987); and

(5)   cordocentesis after this time for blood disorders (e.g. Rhesus isoimmunization) and cytogenetics.

DISEASES THAT PRE-DATE PREGNANCY

Hypertension

Hypertension complicates up to 10 per cent of pregnancies world-wide, though this figure includes hypertension arising in pregnancy (i.e. pre-eclampsia). Blood pressure should be measured in the sitting position, with the proper sized cuff at the level of the heart (National High Blood Pressure Education Program 1990), and using Korotkoff phase V for measurement of diastolic blood pressure (Shennan *et al.* 1996). At booking, if 140/90 mm Hg is used as the cut-off between normality and hypertension, patients with the top 2 per cent of blood pressures taken before 20 weeks will be identified (Redman 1995). By definition, such patients have 'chronic' hypertension. They will most likely report a history of long term hypertension that may or may not have been treated. However, one must entertain a full differential diagnosis that considers secondary forms of hypertension (e.g. renal parenchymal or vascular disease, co-arctation of the aorta, phaeochromocytoma) as well as 'white-coat' hypertension (i.e. hypertension detected in the office setting but not confirmed by ambulatory blood pressure monitoring in the patient's home environment). Work-up includes a complete physical examination, full blood count, electrolytes, serum urea and creatinine, urinalysis, 24 h urine collection for protein and creatinine clearance, and 24 h urine collection for urinary vanillylmandelic acid (VMA) or catecholamines.

Hypertension is a concern (and is, therefore, treated) in the non-pregnant patient because of long term cardiovascular morbidity and mortality. However, hypertension over the nine months of pregnancy does not represent such a maternal risk unless it is severe (i.e. ≥ 170/110 mm Hg). Therefore, antihypertensives are titrated to keep blood pressure at levels that are safe for the mother in the short term which many consider to be less than 160–170 mm Hg systolic and/or 100–110 mm Hg diastolic (National High Blood Pressure Education Program 1990).

Many women who were on antihypertensive medication prior to pregnancy will be able to discontinue this medication, at least during the first half of pregnancy, because of the physiological fall in blood pressure, which reaches a nadir at 20 weeks. In fact, such falls may be even more dramatic in women with pre-existent hypertension. If therapy is needed, then methyldopa is considered by most to be the agent of first choice given the long history of its use in pregnancy and information about developmental follow-up to seven years of age. With the possible exception of angiotensin-converting enzyme (ACE) inhibitors (which are also contraindicated for use later in pregnancy), there is no evidence for teratogenicity of other antihypertensives on which patients may have conceived.

Hypertension increases (by five-fold) the risk of superimposed pre-eclampsia (Butler and Bonham 1963), intrauterine growth retardation (IUGR), and possibly abruptio placenta (Williams *et al.*, 1991). With regard to prophylaxis of pre-eclampsia, evidence from randomized controlled trials indicates that the increased risk of pre-eclampsia cannot be decreased by low-dose aspirin given to all primiparous women (Sibai *et al.* 1993) or pregnant women at high risk (CLASP 1994). However, subgroup analysis within one trial (Sibai *et al.* 1993) suggested that patients with chronic hypertension may have a decreased risk of pre-eclampsia when given aspirin through-out pregnancy. This remains unproved, but if such therapy is given, one can be reas-sured that aspirin is not associated with teratogenicity, maternal or fetal bleeding complications (CLASP 1994), or developmental abnormalities at 18 months of age (CLASP 1995). However, minor maternal bleeding may be increased (McCaw-Binns *et al.* 1996)

Cardiac disease

Cardiac disease has a prevalence of < 1 per cent among women of child-bearing age. It is discussed in detail here because it is responsible for a disproportionate number of maternal deaths. A full discussion of cardiac disease is a relevant issue to address in the first trimester, not only to allow for elective termination in certain cases, but also because most pregnancy-induced physiological changes have occurred by this time (i.e. a 10 per cent increase in heart rate, 40 per cent increase in cardiac output to 5–6 l/min). Peripartum cardiomyopathy will be discussed later under 'Diseases that are pregnancy induced'.

Cardiac disease is becoming more commonly associated with pregnancy in the Western world, as women born with congenital heart disease are more commonly reaching adulthood, and given current patterns of immigration. A complete classi-fication of congenital and acquired heart disease is available from standard medical texts (Elkayam and Gleicher 1982). A pragmatic approach is to classify lesions as obstructive (e.g. aortic outflow tract obstruction, mitral stenosis) or regurgitant (e.g. ventricular septal defect, mitral regurgitation) because patients with the former are more likely to deteriorate in pregnancy, whereas patients with the latter tend to toler-ate pregnancy quite well. An important point to make is that complex (and many simple lesions) have been surgically modified, and it is imperative that both the nature of the original lesions and postoperative sequelae (e.g. presence of prostheses, residual obstruction or shunt, myocardial dysfunction, arrhythmias/conduction defects) be ascertained by correspondence with the patient's cardiologist.

The 1988–1990 Report on confidential enquiries into maternal deaths (RCEMD 1994) concluded that 'Deficiencies in history taking, clinical examination and assess-ment were common causes of substandard care ...' of cardiac patients during preg-nancy. Therefore, assessment must be meticulous. Any potential abnormalities should be referred for assessment by an obstetric physician and/or cardiologist.

Conditions for which the risk of pregnancy complications is so high that elective termination is recommended are few, but include, pulmonary arterial/ venous hyper-tension of whatever aetiology, Eisenmenger syndrome, primary pulmonary hyper-tension, pulmonary veno-occlusive disease, or severe degrees of cor pulmonale.

Women with cardiac disease are at increased risk for cardiac events. A recent retro-spective cohort study of heart disease in pregnancy demonstrated that maternal cardiac events (i.e. heart failure, symptomatic tachy- or bradyarrhythmias, throm-boembolism, or death) are associated with symptoms greater than New Tork Heart Association (NYHA) class 2, left ventricular obstructive lesions, myocardial disease (e.g. dilated cardiomyopathy), electrical heart disease, and/or previous adverse cardiac events (Siu *et al.* 1996). Special attention should be paid to development of anaemia, hypertension, and urinary tract infection as potential precipitants of cardiac deterioration. A few conditions are worthy of special mention with respect to maternal complications; these are discussed below.

Multiple gestation

Multiple gestations are associated with a further 30 per cent increase in cardiac output above that associated with normal pregnancy. Such an increase is accomplished by increasing heart rate and contractility, suggesting that cardiac reserve is being tapped (Veille *et al.* 1985) and that these patients require extra vigilance.

Marfan's syndrome

Marfan's syndrome is an autosomal dominant disorder of connective tissue which occurs in 1 in 5 of 10 000 in the general population. Pregnancy appears to increase the risk of all cardiovascular complications (but particularly aortic dissection), especially in the second and third trimesters (Pumphrey *et al.* 1986). This may be due to the hyperdynamic and hypervolaemic circulation during pregnancy, and/or to changes in arterial wall structure. The patient must undergo full baseline evaluation of aortic root size and structure, preferably by transoesophageal echocardiography (or possibly by magnetic resonance imaging). Recommendations for the non-pregnant patient have been extended to cover pregnancy (Elkayam *et al.* 1995). Patients with either an aortic root diameter ≥ 5.5 cm, progressive dilatation by serial echocardiography, or a family history of aortic dissection should undergo elective replacement of the aortic root. If pregnancy has already occurred in the presence of such aortic root dilatation, then either elective termination followed by surgery, or surgery during pregnancy have been recommended, although second trimester surgery has been associated with increased fetal loss (Becker 1983). Without surgery, Caesarean section would be advisable to minimize the haemodynamic changes associated with vaginal delivery. It is important to point out that a normal aortic root diameter does not guarantee a risk-free pregnancy (Rosenblum *et al.* 1983). As proven in children and adolescents treated for 10 years (Shores *et al.* 1994), propranolol has been recommended during pregnancy to decrease the rate of development of aortic dilatation, aortic regurgitation, aortic dissection, congestive heart failure, surgery, and death (Elkayam *et al.* 1995); propranolol probably acts by decreasing the shear stress in the aorta.

Coarctation of the aorta

Post-repair residual hypertension (related to the duration of hypertension prior to repair) (Connolly *et al.* 1996) and left ventricular hypertrophy (Krogmann *et al.* 1993) may persist after surgical repair. There may also be an associated bicuspid aortic valve. These patients are at increased risk for pregnancy-induced hypertension and aortic dissection, especially during labour. They should be evaluated using echocardiography (especially transoesophageal) and Doppler velocimetry to quantify the pressure gradient across any residual aortic narrowing. Although rupture of aneurysmal arterial dilatations of the circle of Willis is a potential problem, prophylactic cerebral arteriography is not warranted. As in Marfan's syndrome, β-blockers (especially cardioselective agents) are warranted during labour, and possibly through-out pregnancy.

Hypertrophic obstructive cardiomyopathy

Hypertrophic obstructive cardiomyopathy is of concern primarily at the time of labour and delivery, when hypovolaemia and/or hypotension cause increased obstruction to left ventricular outflow. β-blockade is reserved for patients with symptomatic obstruction.

The fetus of a woman with cardiac disease in pregnancy is at increased risk of IUGR, prematurity, and stillbirth. Serial ultrasound scans (for monitoring growth and amniotic fluid volume) and Doppler ultrasonography of the umbilical cord are recom-mended. If the maternal heart disease is congenital, then recurrence in the fetus ranges in incidence from 3 per cent (in the face of primarily right-sided maternal cardiac lesions) to 18 per cent in the face of maternal obstructive left ventricular outflow tract lesions (Nora and Nora 1987). Risk also increases with maternal (rather than pater-nal) disease suggesting cytoplasmic inheritance and/or genomic imprinting. Women at risk for having an affected child should be referred for detailed fetal echocardiogra-phy at 20–24 weeks' gestation, as discussed under prenatal diagnosis.

Management of cardiac deterioration and dysrhythmias in pregnancy is the same as in the non-pregnant patient. Of particular note is the use of β-blocker therapy in the setting of mitral stenosis, to prevent the pregnancy-associated tachycardia and decrease the time available for left ventricular filling. Balloon valvuloplasty may be safely performed for selected cases of mitral stenosis and aortic stenosis.

Acute arrhythmias should be managed with cardioversion or standard antiarrhythmic therapy; any patient with a history of Wolff–Parkinson–White syndrome should not receive digoxin or verapamil. Although the safety of adenosine has not yet been estab-lished, the very short half-life of the drug makes teratogenicity highly unlikely. Whether or not to continue chronic antiarrhythmic therapy will depend on the risk of recurrence (i.e. frequency, duration, and severity) of the underlying rhythm disturb-ance, bearing in mind that pregnancy itself may be arrhythmogenic. None of the agents in common use (e.g. digoxin, β-blockers, procainamide) are known to be teratogenic, although amiodarone may cause (reversible) neonatal hypo- or hyperthy-roidism (Magee *et al.* 1995) for which screening must be performed.

Despite biases inherent in retrospective data, case series/centre cohorts have con-vincingly described systemic thromboembolism when heparin therapy has replaced warfarin therapy during pregnancy in women with artificial heart valves. The major concern is that of warfarin embryopathy which may occur after exposures during 6–9 weeks post-LMP (last menstrual period); case series and single centre cohorts indicate the risk is 10–25 per cent (Sbarouni and Oakley 1994). 'Fetopathy' (i.e. CNS malfor-mations thought to be due to central nervous system bleeding) may result from war-farin exposure at any time during pregnancy, although this has not been reported since 1984, which may relate to the lower doses of warfarin used today. Nevertheless, rare case reports have persuaded many practitioners to avoid warfarin throughout pregnancy. However, many would use heparin IV (via a Hickman line) from 6–9 weeks post-LMP and then warfarin until 36 weeks' gestation, when subcutaneous (or

IV) heparin is reinstituted in anticipation of delivery. All agree that warfarin should not be used at the time of delivery because it crosses the placenta and would result in the fetus being anticoagulated at the time of delivery.

Asthma

Asthma has a prevalence of 3 per cent among young women of child-bearing age (Littlejohns *et al.* 1989). Dyspnoea occurs in up to 50 per cent of patients by 30 weeks (Milne *et al.* 1978), but it must be taken seriously in asthmatics. The diagnostic criteria for asthma are the same in pregnancy, because respiratory rate, airway resistance, and spirometry do not change much (Milne *et al.* 1977). What do change are arterial blood gases and p_{O_2} when supine. The increase in the depth of breathing produces a chronic respiratory alkalosis (pH 7.40–7.45, $p_{CO_2} \sim 30$ mmHg, $p_{O_2} = 100$–106 mmHg, $HCO_3 \sim 19$ meq/l) (Rosman 1992), and recumbency in the third trimester can close small airways, increase the alveolar–arterial p_{O2} gradient, and decrease p_{O_2} by 5–8 mm Hg. However, oxygen saturation is still normal.

Older literature details excess prematurity, low birth weight, and placental abnormalities associated with asthma in pregnancy, probably as a result of poorer disease control. However, recent literature indicates that less severe disease is not associated with an excess of pregnancy complications (Schatz *et al.* 1990). Therefore, asthma should be managed as aggressively during pregnancy as before pregnancy. Chronic inhaled and oral medications (including prednisolone) are not teratogenic and should be continued (Nelson-Piercy and Moore-Gillon 1995). Immunotherapy can be continued, but not started in case local/systemic reactions occur. Treatment of an acute asthmatic attack is no different from that in the non-pregnant patient.

Renal disease

Renal disease refers to disorders of native as well as transplanted kidneys, so it is becoming an increasingly common question in obstetric practice. The topic has been extensively reviewed (Lindheimer and Davison 1994). The most critical thing to do is confirm the underlying diagnosis and establish the patient's baseline by determining the following: blood pressure, plasma urea and creatinine, electrolytes, urinalysis, urine culture, 24 h urine collection for protein and creatinine clearance, and possibly renal ultrasound if not previously done.

Note that physiological changes associated with normal pregnancy bring about structural and functional changes that need to be considered when making a baseline assessment. Renal size increases by about 1 cm, due to a probable increase in renal parenchymal fluid. There is also marked dilatation of the renal calyces, pelvis, and ureter which may mimic obstruction and lead to collection errors in tests based on timed collections. Finally, in normal pregnancy, glomerular filtration rate increases by 25 per cent by four weeks post-LMP and 50 per cent by the end of the first trimester, after which it remains stable and then decreases slightly (by about 15 per cent) (Davison *et al.* 1980) close to term. The normal reference ranges for each trimester are lower than in the non-pregnant patient (Table 22.2).

Table 22.2 Changes in common indices of renal function during pregnancy (mean ± SD)

	Non-pregnant	First trimester	Second trimester	Third trimester
Effective plasma flow (ml/min)	480 ± 72	841 ± 144	891 ± 279	771 ± 175
Glomerular filtration rate (ml/min)				
Inulin clearance	105 ± 24	162 ± 19	174 ± 24	165 ± 22
24 h creatinine clearance	98 ± 8	151 ± 11	154 ± 15	129 ± 10
Plasma				
Creatinine (μmol/l)	73 ± 10	60 ± 8	54 ± 10	64 ± 9
Urea (mmol/l)	4.3 ± 0.8	3.5 ± 0.7	3.3 ± 0.8	3.1 ± 0.7
Urate (μmol/l)	246 ± 59	189 ± 48	214 ± 71	269 ± 56
Osmolality (mosmol/kg)	290 ± 2.2	280 ± 3.4	279 ± 2.9	279 ± 5.0

Estimates of pregnancy risk are based on the presence/absence of hypertension and the baseline plasma creatinine level. It is controversial as to whether or not certain renal diseases (e.g. focal glomerulosclerosis, membranoproliferative glomerulonephritis, collagen vascular diseases, IgA and reflux nephropathies) are associated with poorer prognoses. However, a general rule is that patients who have good renal function (i.e. plasma creatinine ≤ 125 μmol/l) and no hypertension (especially in the absence of proteinuria) have an excellent prognosis and one can be reassuring about maternal and fetal pregnancy outcomes, and the natural course of the maternal disease (Table 22.3). Patients with high creatinine (≥ 250 μmol/l) usually have complicated pregnancies and long-term problems, making pregnancy inadvisable; pregnancy could be considered when function is improved by dialysis or, better still, by transplantation. Data are more limited for those with moderate impairment, but outcome seem to be intermediate between the other two extremes. Nevertheless, all patients should be warned that unpredictable, and irreversible rapid renal decline may occur before or just after delivery.

Table 22.3 Pregnancy prospects for women with chronic renal disease

Renal status	Plasma creatinine (μmol/l)	Problems in pregnancy (%)	Successful obstetric outcome (%)	Problems in long term (%)
Mild	≤ 125	26	96 (85)	< 3 (9)
Moderate	≥ 125	47	89 (59)	25 (71)
Severe	≥ 250	86	46 (8)	53 (92)

Estimates based on 1902 women/2813 pregnancies (1973–1993) which attained at least 28 weeks gestation (J. Davison and C. Baylis, unpublished data). Figures in brackets refer to prospects when complications developed prior to 28 weeks gestation.

A plan should be set out for maternal and fetal monitoring (as well as timing of delivery), and the patient should understand that hypertension, a deterioration in renal function, or new/increasing protein excretion may warrant hospital admission and/or premature delivery. The patient must be closely monitored for asymptomatic bacteruria and a deterioration in creatinine clearance and protein excretion. Although aggressive control of hypertension is advocated in the non-pregnant patient with renal disease, such an approach has never been proven to improve renal prognosis. There are no guidelines for treatment of pregnancy hypertension associated with renal disease. The only firm guideline is that ACE inhibitors (used in the non-pregnant patient to decrease intraglomerular pressure) are contraindicated in pregnancy.

Renal biopsy is associated with the same risks as when it is performed in the non-pregnant population, but biopsy can be justified during pregnancy only if management during pregnancy will be altered. Such is the case when sudden deterioration in renal function is of unknown aetiology, and/or is associated with systemic disease, hypertension, and/or urinary sediment that is 'active' (i.e. shows the presence of red and white blood cells and casts).

Haematological abnormalities

Anaemia

Whereas haemoglobin (Hb) levels < 12.0 g/dl are considered abnormal in non-pregnant women, only levels < 11.0 g/dl (WHO 1972) or < 10.4 gd/l (Leeuw *et al.* 1966) are considered to be abnormal in pregnancy. Such a physiological anaemia of pregnancy occurs because the increase in plasma volume is relatively greater than that in red cell mass. These changes are particularly marked in association with multiple pregnancy.

The differential diagnosis of anaemia is wide, and includes decreased/ineffective red blood cell production, abnormal haemoglobin biosynthesis, and/or increased red blood cell destruction (by bleeding or haemolysis). Attention will be focused on the most important causes of anaemia in pregnancy: haemoglobinopathies and nutritional deficiency (of iron, folate, and B_{12}) which is covered under 'Diseases that are pregnancy induced'.

Haemoglobinopathies

Normal haemoglobin is made up of two α chains and two β chains. Haemoglobinopathies (hereditary disorders of haemoglobin) may involve abnormal chain structure (e.g. sickle cell anaemia) or number (i.e. thalassaemias). They are of particular importance among women who are black, or from the Mediterranean, Middle East, Africa, South-east Asia, India, or the South Pacific such that many metropolitan centres perform routine antenatal screening (Letsky 1995*a*).

Abnormal chain structure

This is usually due to a single amino acid substitution. The most prevalent and important type is sickle haemoglobin. Others include unstable variants, variants with high oxygen affinity, and M haemoglobins (which have abnormal binding of iron to haeme).

Sickle syndromes are classified as AS (sickle cell trait), SS (sickle cell anaemia), or compound heterozygote states, the most important being SC (sickle C disease) and sickle β-thalassaemia. The prevalence depends on the ethnicity of the population studied, and the severity of the disease depends on the composition of the haemoglobin. Sickle C disease is associated with a near normal life expectancy, as is sickle cell trait. Sickle cell anaemia (i.e. Hb SS) is common among American and African Blacks; Hb is usually between 6.0 and 9.0 g/dl, 30 per cent of such patients run a severe clinical course (Letsky 1995a), and life expectancy is shortened. Sickle β-thalassaemia is common among women from the Mediterranean and Africa; more severe forms similar to Hb SS disease are associated with no normal β-chain production (i.e. sickle β^0 disease). The variants can be distinguished from each other by Hb electrophoresis, with the possible exception of Hb SS and sickle β^0 disease (Table 22.4).

Complications in the non-pregnant patient include vaso-occlusion in multiple organ systems, especially the lung, kidney, and bone. Crises may be of four types: painful, aplastic (usually following infection or due to folic acid deficiency), haemolytic, or vaso-occlusive (micro- or macro-circulations) with infarcts (and/or secondary infection). Other problems include increased susceptibility to infection (especially pneumococcus, given hyposplenism) and propensity to form gall stones. Pregnancy may increase the risk of all of these complications.

Prenatal diagnosis of an affected fetus is available for most sickle syndromes. The defect can be detected by amplified DNA from fetal trophoblast obtained by chorionic villus sampling (CVS) in the first trimester, or from amniotic fluid cells obtained by amniocentesis in the second trimester. Unfortunately, there are no therapies (including exchange transfusion) proven to decrease the risk of sickling crises during pregnancy (Koshy et al. 1988). Treatment should include daily folic acid (5 mg/day), prophylactic penicillin, pneumococcal vaccine, avoidance of dehydration, hypoxaemia, and/or acidosis (all of which may precipitate a sickling crisis).

Abnormal chain number
The quantitative defects may be in α or β chain production (Table 22.5). α-Thalassaemia is usually caused by gene deletions. The clinical severity depends on the number of genes deleted. One deletion ($\alpha-/\alpha\alpha$) causes no clinical manifestations and two (either $\alpha-/\alpha-$, or $--/\alpha\alpha$) causes only slight microcytosis and hypochromia with no chronic haemolysis or anaemia. Three deletions produce a well compensated

Table 22.4 Haemoglobin electrophoresis and sickle syndromes

Haemoglobin	AS	SS	SC	Sickle β-thalassaemia
A	55–60%	0 (unless recently transfused)	50%	10–30% (if β-chain production present)
A_2	–	2–4%		Small amount
F	–	2–20%		10–30%
S	35–40%	76–96%	50%	60–90%

Table 22.5 Classification of the thalassaemias

Diagnosis	Hb electrophoresis
α-Thalassaemia	
(α–/αα)	Normal, <u>decreased</u> HbA$_2$
(α–/α–) or (– –/αα)	Normal, <u>decreased</u> HbA$_2$
(–/α–)	HbH (β$_4$) 10–15%
(– –/– –) Hb Barts	Hb Barts
β-Thalassaemia	
Heterozygous	<u>Increased</u> HbA$_2$ (~5%) (± increase in HbF to ~2–3%)
Homozygous	<u>Increased</u> HbF

haemolytic state with evidence of target cells and/or Heinz bodies (intracellular inclusions of HbH precipitates). Four deletions (so called Hb Barts) are incompatible with life. Prenatal diagnosis is directed towards detection of affected fetuses, particularly among families from South-east Asia where both (α–) and (– –) haplotypes are quite common.

The pathogenesis of β-thalassaemia is more complex as there are a number of potential steps that can go wrong in β-chain synthesis. Clinical manifestations occur to a lesser degree in β-thalassaemia minor seen in carriers of one defective gene; their Hb is about 15 per cent lower than normal and they are often misdiagnosed as having iron deficiency anaemia. The clinical manifestations occur to a greater degree in β-thalassaemia major seen in carriers of two defective genes and characterized by severe, transfusion-dependent anaemia which results in expansion of haematopoietic tissue in the bone marrow, liver, and spleen, and more importantly, iron overload which is the major long term problem due to multisystem organ dysfunction. Treatment of the non-pregnant patient involves transfusion to Hb ≥ 9.0 g/dl, prevention of iron overload by chelating therapy, daily folate, probably splenectomy, and eventual bone marrow transplantation. Survival into adulthood is possible but pregnancy is usually associated with less severe forms of β-thalassaemia, called 'β-thalassaemia intermedia' which is characterized by genetic defects that result in high levels of HbF production, or other associated defects that result in more balanced Hb subunit synthesis.

Prenatal diagnosis is directed at patients with β-thalassaemia minor/intermedia to prevent occurrence of β-thalassaemia major. This can usually be diagnosed by DNA amplification as described for sickle syndromes.

Hypercoagulable states/thromboembolism

The incidence of both acute deep venous thrombosis (DVT) and pulmonary embolus (PE) is less than 1 per cent of pregnancies, but thromboembolic disease is a leading cause of maternal mortality (RCEMD 1994) and long term venous insufficiency (Barbour and Pickard 1995). Pregnancy is associated with a five-fold increased risk, not only because of stasis, possible injury to the deep venous system by operative delivery, and/or placental separation, but also because of a pregnancy-induced increase in many coagulation factors which is established in the first trimester; increases in factors II (fibrinogen), VII, VIII, and X are detectable by about 12 weeks' gestation (Bonnar 1987). Other pregnancy-associated risk factors include increased age, obesity, post-phlebitic syndrome, and acquired/inherited hypercoagulable states (Nachman and Silver Stein 1993), especially deficiencies of antithrombin III (AT-III), protein C, or protein S, antiphospholipid antibody syndrome, or activated protein C resistance (i.e. factor V Leiden mutation).

A thrombophilia screen involves taking a medical history (looking for association with immobilization, injury, oral contraceptive use, other medical disorders, and family history) as well as performing laboratory screening (i.e. for AT-III, protein C, protein S, fibrinogen, lupus anticoagulant—by activated partial thromboplastin time (aPTT), dilute Russell Viper Venom time (DRVVT), Kaolin clotting time (KCT), anticardiolipin antibody, and activated protein C resistance). In non-pregnant populations, a history of a DVT/PE is associated with a detectable predisposition in < 10 per cent of cases (Pabringer *et al.* 1992); a family history of thromboembolism should lead one to believe there is a familial predisposition that cannot be detected by current assays, rather than one that does not exist at all. Note that AT-III and protein C antigen levels and activity do not change in pregnancy. However, total and (especially) free protein S levels decrease in pregnancy. Platelet count and function are normal.

Treatment of established DVT

DVT during pregnancy has a predilection for the left side. Other diagnostic criteria are the same as for the non-pregnant patient. The clinical diagnosis is insensitive and non-specific. The pitfalls of various diagnostic approaches have been reviewed recently (Douketis and Ginsberg 1995). A reasonable approach is to start with a duplex ultrasound which has sensitivities and specificities of > 90 per cent. Proximal extension of an undetected calf DVT can be ruled out by serial examination. The rare case of iliac vein thrombosis may be ruled out by impedance plethysmography, although magnetic resonance venography has been advocated as the diagnostic procedure of choice. If pulmonary embolus is suspected, then ventilation/perfusion scanning should be performed, as it involves total fetal radiation exposure of < 0.5 mGy (50 mrad), far below the 0.1 Gy (10 000 mrad) or more associated with an increased risk of malformations. The risk of childhood leukaemia is less clear given that both radiation exposure and childhood leukaemia are relatively common; the worst case scenario has been estimated to be 1/1 000 000 per mrad (10^{-5} Gy) of fetal exposure. Therefore, all pregnant women with suggestive symptoms should be investigated, as the risks of radiation are far outweighed by the benefits.

In DVT, a thrombophilia work-up should be done prior to initiating treatment which will reduce the incidence of subsequent PE from over 15 per cent to 4.5 per cent, with a mortality of 0.7 per cent (Hirsh *et al.* 1972). Intravenous heparin (in non-pregnant patients with DVT and no known underlying hypercoagulable state) is the standard, with a switch made to subcutaneous heparin when the patient is improving. However, recent evidence suggests that initial treatment with low molecular weight heparin may be as safe and as efficacious (Koopman *et al.* 1996; Levine *et al.* 1996) and anti-Xa (activated Factor X) levels do not need to be monitored. Mid-trimester warfarin is also an option. Anticoagulation should continue for three months and until six weeks postpartum (whichever is the longest).

Prophylaxis against a future event?

Whether or not to administer anticoagulant prophylaxis to patients with risk factors for DVT and/or a history of previous DVT remains controversial because it is not clear that the benefits outweigh the risks.

There is fairly wide agreement on the need for prophylaxis postnatally, as postnatal thromboembolic events are at least as common as antenatal events; either subcutaneous heparin or warfarin have been used.

There is no consensus on the need for antenatal prophylaxis, and if so, which agents should be used. Prophylactic heparin therapy, adjusted to risk, can decrease recurrent thromboembolic disease from about 12 per cent (Badaracco and Vessey 1974) to 3 per cent; patients considered to be at high risk (e.g. AT-III deficiency, Conard *et al.* 1990), or those with recurrent thromboembolism, especially on long-term warfarin) warrant full anticoagulation during pregnancy/puerperium, and patients at low risk (e.g. those with a hypercoagulable state but no clinical events) warrant lower, 'prophylactic' doses of anticoagulants. However, the risks of maternal bleeding (~5 per cent), thrombocytopenia (2.4 per cent for therapeutic and 0.3 per cent for prophylactic, Hirsh and Fuster 1994) and especially the risk of clinically significant (but reversible) osteoporosis of ~2 per cent has tempered enthusiasm for this approach (Dahlman 1993).

Heparin may be administered by either fixed dose (i.e. 5000 (Ginsberg and Hirsh 1992)–10 000 (MNHWP 1993) IU SC twice daily) throughout pregnancy, or by fixed dose in the first and second trimesters with an increase in the third trimester to 10 000 IU SC twice daily or a dose that prolongs the mid-interval aPTT to 1.5 times the control value (Colvin and Barrowcliff 1993). The latter approach is based on evidence that heparin requirements are probably increased during pregnancy given greater blood volume, increases in heparin-binding proteins, greater neutralization (by platelet factor IV), increased glomerular filtration rate, and placental degradation by heparinase. Dosage adjustment has been based upon achievement of 'subtherapeutic' but detectable anti-Xa activity of 0.08–0.15 IU/ml, but whether this is necessary remains in question. Although low molecular weight heparin may be easier to administer by once-daily injection, the risks are not substantially different than with standard heparin.

Heparin-induced osteoporosis has stimulated a renewed interest in the use of warfarin, the risks of which were reviewed under 'Cardiac disease'. Aspirin prophylaxis has also been recommended to low-risk women antenatally, followed by heparin or warfarin postnatally; this is based on aspirin's ability to provide 30 per cent protection against DVT in non-pregnant populations (ATC 1994).

Bleeding diatheses

Bleeding may result from an abnormal number or function of platelets, coagulation factors, or both (e.g. disseminated intravascular coagulation (DIC)).

Thrombocytopenia

Thrombocytopenia in the non-pregnant patient is defined as a platelet count of $< 150 \times 10^9/l$. Counts of $< 100 \times 10^9/l$ are probably abnormal in pregnancy given increased platelet turnover.

The main concern in the first trimester is to distinguish immune thrombocytopenic purpura (ITP) (which occurs in 1–2 per 10 000 women of child-bearing age) from other conditions which are associated with either fetal bleeding (i.e. alloimmune thrombocytopenia) and/or other potential maternal complications (i.e. other haematological abnormalities, infections, autoimmune conditions such as SLE or antiphospholipid antibody syndrome, drug exposures, neoplasia, etc.). This is accomplished by performing a full medical history and physical examination, as well as checking for normality of red and white cells, mean platelet volume (with an increase reflecting the presence of many young, large platelets), antinuclear antibodies (ANA), HIV serology anticardiolipin antibody, DRVVT or lupus anticoagulant (LAC), and full clotting screen to rule out DIC.

DIC is associated with thrombocytopenia, red blood cell fragmentation, prolonged clotting times, decreased fibrinogen, and elevated fibrin degradation products. It is usually associated with later pregnancy, but may present in the first trimester with death of a second twin, and theoretically, after fetal reduction therapy. There is a report of successful resolution following IV heparin therapy in the setting of an intrauterine death of one twin at 26 weeks (Romero *et al.* 1986).

Potential complications are maternal and/or fetal bleeding, both of which are infrequent. Maternal bleeding is usually associated with episiotomy/surgical incisions, rather than from the placental bed. Neither antepartum nor postpartum haemorrhage are increased, as a healthy myometrium is the most important determinant of adequate haemostasis at the time of delivery. Fetal bleeding due to fetal thrombocytopenia is presumably due to transplacental passage of antiplatelet antibodies but is uncommon and not predictable in the individual patient, even in the presence of low maternal platelet counts, presence of platelet-associated antibody, or vaginal delivery (Burrows and Kelton 1992).

In *populations* of patients with ITP, certain factors may be associated with a higher risk of fetal bleeding (i.e. a history of previously severe ITP requiring splenectomy but with persistent thrombocytopenia (Burrows and Kelton 1992), a history of previous ITP with platelet-associated IgG, and possibly a history of a previously affected child). However, bleeding is not predictable in the individual patient. Patients at high risk may occassionally undergo fetal blood sampling by transabdominal cordocentesis near term for determination of fetal platelet count. If fetal thrombocytopenia is found, then Caesarean section is recommended based on the assumption that this would be less traumatic than vaginal delivery. However, this is unproved, and obstetric management still differs widely between centres.

Maternal platelet counts should be monitored monthly, and based upon the course of pregnancy, the patient should be warned that she may need intravenous IgG or prednisolone (to increase platelet counts above 50 000 in anticipation of delivery) and/or Caesarean section, and that her baby's platelet count will be expected to fall over the two to five days after delivery, but this can be treated.

Disorders of the coagulation cascade

Only the most common disorders (each with an incidence of ~1/10 000 in the general population) will be considered (i.e. von Willebrand's disease, haemophilia A (factor VIII deficiency), and haemophilia B (factor IX deficiency)). The issue of prenatal diagnosis for families with a history of the disease was addressed under 'Prenatal diagnosis'. However, it should be noted that (rarely) acquired inhibitors of coagulation can also result in bleeding (e.g. antibody to factor VIII). Quantitative or qualitative disorders of fibrinogen are rare but important as they have been associated with spontaneous abortion and placental abruption. Factor XIII deficiency has also been associated with spontaneous abortion. For information about other rarer conditions in pregnancy, the reader is referred to other sources (Caldwell *et al.* 1985).

von Willebrand's disease (vWD)

von Willebrand's disease is an autosomal dominant disorder that results from deficiency of the von Willebrand factor (vWF) portion of the factor VIII–vWF complex. Subclinical disease is common and may present in pregnancy, especially at the time of delivery.

There are a number of forms of vWD, depending on whether the abnormality in vWF is quantitative (type I) or both quantitative and qualitative (types IIa–d). The most sensitive test (> 90 per cent) is the ristocetin cofactor assay, a functional assay for vWF in which the ability of the patient's platelet-rich plasma to facilitate ristocetin-induced platelet aggregation *in vitro* is measured. Determination of the type of disorder is important as it determines the mechanism by which therapy attempts to normalize factor VIII coagulant activity and bleeding time; type I vWD may be amenable to desamino-δ-arginine vasopressin therapy (which increases endothelial release of high molecular weight monomers of vWF), whereas this is contraindicated in type III due to the thrombotic risk.

Most affected women will experience rises in factor VIII and vWF during pregnancy and most will not need specific therapy in preparation for delivery. If vWF levels have not risen into the normal range by delivery, then heat-treated factor VIII (which does not transmit HIV) or cryoprecipitate should be used to cover delivery; neither product transmits HIV but factor VIII has the disadvantage of exposing the recipient to multiple blood donors (Letsky 1995*b*). It is felt by some experts that DDAVP will not achieve further rises in vWF and is of no benefit in pregnancy. It should be noted that vWF and factor VIII levels may fall rapidly in women with severe disease, putting them at risk for delayed postpartum haemorrhage.

Haemophilia A and B

Haemophilias A and B are X-linked recessive disorders caused by deficiencies of factors VIII and IX, respectively. In pregnancy, the obvious issues for the (heterozygous) mother are bleeding, and the risk of having an affected child (discussed under 'Prenatal diagnosis').

Most pregnant women experience rises in the deficient factor into the normal range and therefore, do not require specific treatment. Although DDAVP may benefit patients with mild haemophilia A when not pregnant, it is not likely to be effective during pregnancy, for the same reasons as stated above for vWF disease. Therefore, if the factor levels are still below normal at term (as seen in some heterozygotes in whom lionization results in very low factor activity), then cryoprecipitate or factor IX concentrates (for haemophilias A and B, respectively) should be used to cover labour and delivery.

Autoimmune disease

Connective tissue disorders (CTD) (Table 22.6) and particularly, systemic lupus erythematosus (SLE), are common among women of child-bearing age. Many patients will have had a diagnosis made prior to conception and this certainly makes counselling and management during pregnancy somewhat easier. However, other patients may report a history of symptoms suggestive of CTD which have been insufficient to fulfil the diagnostic criteria for a particular CTD, but which may do so during pregnancy or the puerperium.

Baseline assessment of all patients with a history of CTD or symptoms suggestive of a CTD must include a full history including symptoms which constitute a flare for that patient, physical examination with special attention paid to hip abduction (for vaginal delivery) and neck extension (for intubation), laboratory screen (i.e. anti-nuclear antibody (ANA), anti-double-stranded DNA (anti-dsDNA), complement C3 and C4, CH50, anticardiolipin antibody, lupus anticoagulant, anti-Ro/SS-A, anti-La/SS-B, anti-SM nuclear antigen, and antiribonucleoprotein (anti-RNP)), and tests to rule out internal organ complications (i.e. renal, pulmonary, cardiac, haematological). The results will help to establish a plan of action for the mother and fetus at risk.

There are a few points which should be highlighted. Firstly, antibodies to Ro/SS-A and La/SS-B are risk factors for development of congenital heart block (risk < 3 per cent) and (self-limited) cutaneous neonatal lupus (< 25 per cent) (Lockshin *et al.* 1988); a history of a previously affected child is associated with risks of < 20 per cent and 25 per cent, respectively, and the risk of congenital heart block is low given only an antibody to Ro/SS-A 60-kDa antigen (Buyon *et al.* 1993). Secondly, decreases in

Table 22.6   The more common connective tissue disorders

Seropositive (i.e. ANA, dsDNA, rheumatoid factor, anticardiolipin)
  Systemic lupus erythematosus (SLE)
  Antiphospholipid antibody syndrome (APS)
  Rheumatoid arthritis
  Scleroderma
  Mixed connective tissue disease
  Sjogren's syndrome

Seronegative
  Ankylosing spondylitis, reactive arthritis, undifferentiated spondyloarthropathy
  Behçet's syndrome
  Vasculitis

C3 and C4 may herald/diagnose a flare of SLE as C3 and C4 increase during normal pregnancy; a decrease in C4 alone may be indicative of pre-eclampsia (Buyon *et al.* 1986). Thirdly, erythrocyte sedimentation rate (ESR) is increased in normal pregnancy and is not a good indicator of inflammatory activity; C-reactive protein (CRP) should be normal in the absence of an inflammatory state. Finally, antiphospholipid antibody syndrome deserves special mention. It is considered 'primary' if isolated and 'secondary' if associated with another autoimmune disorder, particularly SLE. The syndrome is defined by antiphospholipid antibodies (i.e. lupus anticoagulant, DRVVT, and/or anticardiolipin antibody) *plus* at least one clinical event: recurrent miscarriage, thrombosis, or thrombocytopenia; other associated features are migraines and Raynaud's phenomenon. Both the laboratory and clinical criteria are necessary, as up to 2 per cent of normal individuals have detectable antibodies, which may be of high titre.

Patients with CTD must be followed by history, physical, and serial laboratory testing. Increased disease activity may be heralded by a change in the pattern of ANA, increasing titre of anti-dsDNA, or decreases in C3 and C4. If a patient is maintained on a disease-remitting agent (e.g. gold), then monitoring must also include monthly tests for drug toxicity (i.e. full blood count (FBC), plasma creatinine, and urinalysis).

The fact that CTDs are characterized by intermittent exacerbations makes difficult the determination of the impact of pregnancy on disease activity. Most data are on SLE in pregnancy. If maternal disease has been inactive for the six months prior to conception, then the frequency of flares during the subsequent nine months is probably not increased, although postnatal flares may be a particular risk. Most (i.e. 75 per cent) patients with rheumatoid arthritis improve during pregnancy (Hench 1938), and the course of one pregnancy usually predicts the course of the next. In contrast, patients with polymyositis usually worsen, and the course of polyarteritis nodosum (Owen and Hauth 1989) may also be unfavourable although such a statement is based on a handful of case reports.

Progressive systemic sclerosis deserves special mention. It is characterized by vasculopathy and collagen deposition. The more benign, localized cutaneous form is associated with Raynaud's phenomenon but not with organ involvement. Pregnancy outcome seems to depend on internal organ involvement, particularly renal disease. Potential complications are hypertensive crisis (which may be life threatening and may represent the only justification for use of ACE inhibitors in pregnancy), pulmonary hypertension, malabsorption when there is gastrointestinal tract involvement, difficult endotracheal intubation when there is upper airway involvement, dystocia (which may be due to cervical involvement), and perinatal death (in 5/17 reported pregnancies, Karlen and Cook 1974).

In addition to flares of maternal disease, there is the potential for other pregnancy complications such as pre-eclampsia or premature rupture of membranes which may be associated with corticosteroids. SLE patients also have up to a two-fold increased risk of fetal loss in the first and second trimesters. Although much of the risk may relate to antiphospholipid antibodies, other antibodies (e.g. lymphocytotoxic antibodies to trophoblast, Soloninka *et al.* 1989) or internal organ involvement (especially renal, Hayslett and Lynn 1980) may also play a role.

Therapy

A difficult decision to make in the first trimester is whether or not to change the patient's therapeutic regimen. The risk of a pregnancy-induced increase in disease activity must be weighed against any potential teratogenicity and/or fetotoxicity of the patient's medications. The drugs that will be considered here are anti-inflammatories (i.e. aspirin and corticosteroids), analgesics (i.e. acetaminophen, codeine), azathioprine, and disease-remitting agents (i.e. hydroxychloroquine, gold, penicillamine, methotrexate, and sulphasalazine). Additional prophylaxis against fetal loss for women with primary or secondary anti-phospholipid antibody syndrome is discussed in 'Recurrent miscarriage' under 'Diseases that are pregnancy induced'.

There is no evidence that aspirin or other non-steroidal anti-inflammatory drugs (NSAID) are teratogenic (Briggs *et al.* 1994). The real question is that of feto-toxicity (i.e. premature closure of the ductus arteriosus, pulmonary hypertension, neonatal haemorrhage) when NSAIDs are taken in high, anti-inflammatory doses in the second half of pregnancy. Therefore, women should be encouraged to try to taper off NSAID therapy and gradually increase paracetamol (±codeine) or initiate low-dose corticosteroids to minimize the risks later in pregnancy.

Chloroquine phosphate and hydroxychloroquine are used for treatment of rheumatoid arthritis, systemic and discoid lupus. Data come primarily from literature describing use of these agents for malaria prophylaxis. Although the information is reassuring about the lack of teratogenicity (Briggs *et al.* 1994), drug dosage (usually 400 mg/week of hydroxychloroquine or 500 mg/week of chloroquine phosphate) was much smaller than that used for treatment of autoimmune inflammatory disorders (i.e. hydroxychloroquine 400 mg/day initially, then 200–400 mg/day). Although there are still concerns about cumulative ocular and oto-toxicity in the fetus, the considerable risk of a disease flare upon withdrawing hydroxychloroquine (Canadian Hydroxychloroquine study group 1991) has prompted some experts to recommend continuing the therapy throughout pregnancy.

Azathioprine is often used for its steroid-sparing effects. There is a large body of transplant literature which indicates that azathioprine therapy is not associated with teratogenicity. However, there are some concerns about fetal loss (Reimers and Sluss 1978) and/or teratogenicity in the next generation. Chromosome aberrations (albeit transient) have been seen in fetal lymphocytes (Price *et al.* 1976), and there is concern that damage to the DNA of germ cells (particularly the ovaries of a female fetus) will not be repaired because new DNA is synthesized only after fertilization. Although most experts would continue azathioprine in pregnancy, follow-up of exposed children will be essential.

Gold is usually chosen to initiate remission of rheumatoid arthritis, as this drug is associated with fewer long term side-effects than penicillamine or methotrexate. Approximately 70 per cent of patients respond. Although it has been recommended that gold therapy be discontinued if unplanned pregnancy occurs, the long half-life of the drug (i.e. weeks to months) guarantees that exposure will occur for at least some time in pregnancy and certainly throughout most or all of the first trimester even if gold is stopped at conception. What may be achieved is simply low drug levels during the puerperium which is the time of highest risk of flare. Therefore, given the reassuring literature to date, one could make a case for continuing gold, especially in the face of an aggressive disease history.

Penicillamine is used for treatment of rheumatoid arthritis. However, most information from its use in pregnancy has come from treatment of Wilson's disease. Although anomalies have been described in only 8/100 published case reports, there was a pattern of connective tissue anomalies which suggested that penicillamine may be teratogenic. Therapeutic alternatives should be strongly considered for disorders other than Wilson's disease.

Methotrexate is used for rheumatoid arthritis. Analogous to another antifolate, aminopterin, methotrexate appears to be a human teratogen (Van den Hof *et al.* 1990) with dose- (> 10 mg/wk) and time- (6–8 weeks after the last menstrual period) dependent effects (Feldkamp and Carey 1993). The drug should be discontinued prior to planned pregnancy; women who have done so have had healthy infants without defects (Briggs *et al.* 1994). If unplanned pregnancy occurs, methotrexate should be stopped, and data would suggest that low doses, especially when taken outside the 'critical period' for induction of malformations, do not represent a teratogenic risk.

Sulphasalazine is a compound of 5-aminosalicylic acid (5-ASA) likened to a sulphapyridine. It is used for suppression of the inflammation of rheumatoid arthritis and seronegative arthritis. Exposure during human pregnancy is not considered to be teratogenic as no pattern of defects has been reported (Briggs *et al.* 1994). The drug may also be continued, as levels of sulphasalazine and sulphapyridine in 11 newborns infants were found to be too low to displace bilirubin from albumin (Jarnerot *et al.* 1981).

Endocrine disorders

Diabetes mellitus (DM), thyroid disease, and prolactinoma will be discussed as the most common endocrine disorders encountered in pregnancy. The reader is referred to other sources for information about more unusual endocrine disorders.

Pre-existent (types I and II) diabetes mellitus (DM)

DM has a prevalence of 1–2 per cent in the general population and is commonly encountered in obstetric clinics. DM may be insulin dependent (type I), or non-insulin dependent (type II). The ideal is to have patients counselled before pregnancy. However, given that 50 per cent of pregnancies are unplanned, the ideal cannot be achieved in the majority of cases.

Baseline assessment involves evaluation of glycaemic control and end-organ damage (microvascular and macrovascular) by history and physical and laboratory investigations. The natural history of diabetic retinopathy and nephropathy are not changed by pregnancy, unless there are retinal microaneurysms not treated by laser, or hypertension and a serum creatinine level > 125 μM (as discussed under 'Renal disease'). All patients should be assessed by an ophthalmologist in the first trimester of pregnancy. The patient should be informed of the increased risk of pre-eclampsia, as well as unexplained stillbirth, macrosomia (i.e. birth weight > 90th centile), and neonatal hypoglycaemia, hyperbilirubinaemia, hypocalcaemia, polycythemia/jaundice, and respiratory distress syndrome (RDS). However, the major issues to discuss in the first trimester will be those of fetal loss and congenital malformations.

It is well known that DM is associated with increased risks of both pregnancy loss and (by approximately three fold) congenital malformations (specifically, neural tube defects, sacral agenesis, and cardiac). However, predicting babies at risk is difficult, because although both outcomes have been associated with higher blood glucose levels, there is considerable overlap between blood glucose values and glycosylated haemoglobin of mothers who have affected and mothers who have unaffected babies.

Both fetal loss and birth defects have been decreased in incidence by pre-pregnancy clinics and improvement in glycaemic control (Fuhrmann *et al.* 1983; Dicker *et al.* 1988; steel *et al.* 1990). Given that organogenesis is complete by about 10 weeks' gestation, intensive therapy should be initiated immediately in patients with poor control, probably by admission to hospital where patients can receive advice about diabetic diet, intensive home glucose monitoring (i.e. before meals, 2 h after meals, and before bedtime) as well as multiple daily injections of short and long-acting insulins. Treatment regimens vary, but blood glucose should be as normal as possible, with pre-prandial values of 4–6 mM and post-prandial values < 7 mM. This approach may cause both retinopathy to deteriorate and the frequency of hypoglycaemia to increase (Rosenn *et al.* 1995), but there is no evidence that hypoglycaemia is harmful to the human fetus (Mills *et al.* 1988). All such women should have routine antenatal serum screening including AFP (which is lower in DM pregnancy, Wald *et al.* 1979) for neural tube defects, anomaly scanning at 20 weeks, and fetal echocardiography at 24 weeks.

Special mention should be made of the use of oral hypoglycaemic agents at conception. If unplanned pregnancy occurs whilst taking these agents, then case report/series suggest that ear and skull malformations may be more common. However, whether this is the case with newer agents (such as glyburide) is not known given that they may not cross the placenta. The risk in this case would be considered to be low but warrant a routine anomaly scan at 20 weeks. Oral hypoglycaemic agents should not be intentionally used during pregnancy, but rather, they should be discontinued, and replaced by a diabetic diet with or without insulin.

Thyroid disease

Assessment of the structure and function of the thyroid changes during pregnancy. Reduction in renal tubular absorption of iodide results in thyroid gland hypertrophy and goitre. Placental-induced stimulation of thyroid-binding globulin (TBG) synthesis raises total T_4 and results in a tendency for the (calculated) free thyroxine index (FTI) to overestimate free hormone levels in pregnancy (Burr *et al.* 1979). Free T_3 and free T_4 fall slightly below the normal non-pregnant range by the second and third trimesters. Thyroid-stimulating hormone (TSH) remains unchanged, with the possible exception of the first trimester when hCG levels may suppress TSH.

Goitre

Iodized salt has eliminated endemic goitre from the Western world, although sporadic goitre may still be found. Even in the presence of normal maternal thyroid function, fetal iodine deficiency has been associated with both (i) abnormal central nervous system development (i.e. 'neurological cretinism') despite normal thyroid function, and (ii) classical 'hypothyroid cretinism'. The distinction is important because only the latter responds to iodine supplementation at birth. Therefore, in women with goitre, adequate iodine intake should be ensured by daily use of iodized salt for use in cooking and prepared food.

Hypothyroidism

Many such patients will have been on thyroxine therapy before conception as a result of investigations for symptoms, a family history of hypothyroidism, infertility, and/or recurrent fetal loss. However, screening in pregnancy has revealed asymptomatic hypothyroidism in 3/1000 pregnant women (Long *et al.* 1985) and symptomatic hypothyroidism in 9/1000 White and 3/1000 Black pregnant women (Niswander and Gorden 1972).

Contrary to what was previously thought, thyroxine does cross the placenta in small amounts (sufficient to produce 25–50 per cent normal levels in the athyrotic fetus (Vulsma *et al.* 1989). Although associations with congenital anomalies and impairment of long-term development have not been proven by recent study (Montoro *et al.* 1981; Khoury *et al.* 1989), there does appear to be an association between maternal hypothyroidism and both early fetal loss and stillbirth (Niswander and Gordon 1972), especially in the presence of antithyroid antibodies (Stagnaro-Green *et al.* 1990). Therefore, adequate maternal thyroxine replacement should be ensured throughout pregnancy.

Some investigators have found that thyroxine requirements increase in 20 per cent of women by delivery (Mandel *et al.* 1990), with an average dosage increase that is consistent with normal weight gain in pregnancy. These data have prompted the current recommendation that thyroid function tests (TFTs) be performed once per trimester and adjustments be made in response to elevated levels of TSH.

Hyperthyroidism

Thyrotoxicosis is encountered in 2/1000 pregnant women (Hollingsworth 1989). It also has a tendency to appear at the end of the first or early second trimesters. Almost all cases are due to Grave's disease which is caused by TSH receptor stimulating antibodies; the titre of such antibodies should be measured, even in previously treated Grave's, because high titres are associated with self-limited neonatal thyrotoxicosis. Antithyroid antibodies also increase the risk of postpartum thyroiditis and warrant routine postnatal TFTs.

There has been much written about the hazards of antithyroid medication in pregnancy, but not as much written about the risks of maternal thyroid crisis at delivery (25 per cent of pregnant women), fetal loss (but not malformation), or stillbirth associated with untreated disease (Davis *et al.* 1989). Thionamide therapy (with either carbimazole or prophylthiouracil) should be administered to maintain TSH at the upper limit of normal; initial concern about carbimazole-induced scalp defects (i.e. aplasia cutis) has not been borne out and the drug is not considered to be teratogenic (Van Dijke *et al.* 1987). The smallest thionamide dose possible should be used to decrease the small risk of drug-induced, self-limited, neonatal hypothyroidism, as well as the effects on childhood IQ which have been found only with doses exceeding 400 mg/day (Burrow *et al.* 1978). A short course of β-blocker for symptomatic relief would also be appropriate.

Thyroid nodules

Thyroid nodules should be investigated and treated in the same way as in the non-pregnant patient. The caveat is that the prevalence of thyroid cancer is greater in pregnancy, and in approximately 20 per cent of patients, nodules seem to grow more quickly during pregnancy (Rosen and Walfish 1986). The second trimester is the best time for surgical excision. Thyroid cancer previously diagnosed and treated is not adversely affected by pregnancy (Hod *et al.* 1989).

Pituitary adenoma

Most women with a prolactinoma will have been diagnosed prior to pregnancy because of a history of amenorrhoea, infertility, headache, or visual symptoms. Bromocriptine should be discontinued when pregnancy is diagnosed, although the drug is not considered to be teratogenic. Recent data show that pregnancy has no adverse effect on microadenomas (having diameters < 10 mm) (Kupersmith *et al.* 1994). Prolactin levels rise dramatically in normal pregnancy and measurement has no clinical value (Whittaker *et al.* 1982). Macroadenomas (having diameters > 10 mm) may grow, and therefore, both the patient's symptoms and visual fields should be monitored routinely during pregnancy. If there is evidence of regrowth, then bromocriptine should be restarted. Transphenoidal therapy can be performed if medical therapy is unsuccessful but this almost never occurs.

Pituitary tumours that produce growth hormone behave very much like prolactinomas. The only caveat is that screening should be performed for gestational diabetes. Cushing's syndrome may be caused by an ACTH-producing pituitary adenoma. However, this syndrome is rare in pregnancy given the associated infertility. It is mentioned here to highlight the fact that although diurnal variation in cortisol levels is maintained during pregnancy, plasma free cortisol, urinary free cortisol, and ACTH values are all higher in normal pregnancy, and the appropriate reference ranges should be used if a diagnosis of Cushing's syndrome is being entertained (Galvoa-Teles and Burke 1973). ACTH levels may never suppress because of corticotropin releasing hormone (CRH) production by the feto-placental unit.

It is an appropriate time to mention that any woman with Cushing's syndrome or who is receiving corticosteroids (including those with previous Sheehan's syndrome) should receive extra corticosteroid at times of stress which include elective termination, dilatation and curettage, or labour, delivery, and the first 24 h postpartum.

Neurology

Headache and epilepsy will be discussed as the most commonly encountered disorders, and myasthenia gravis because of the importance of neonatal myasthenia. A general review of all neurological disorders that may complicate pregnancy is beyond the scope of this book. Not considered here are problems that usually present later in pregnancy (e.g. neuropathies, cerebrovascular accidents, eclampsia), and conditions rarely seen in pregnancy (e.g. central nervous system tumours, chorea gravidarum). The inheritability of any neurological disorder should be considered, and referral made for genetic counselling if appropriate.

The diagnosis of neurological disorders in pregnancy is not different from the approach in the non-pregnant patient. Pregnancy does not alter the composition of cerebrospinal fluid. There is no risk associated with radiological investigations of the head in the presence of abdominal shielding. Magnetic resonance imaging is associated with no radiation exposure at all, and is the preferred imaging technique for the lumbar and thoracic spine.

Headache

Headache is a common complaint during pregnancy. The appearance of any new headache in pregnancy should prompt a full search, by history and physical examination, for more ominous causes such as cerebral vein thrombosis. Fundoscopy is essential, as papilloedema may be the only finding in patients with benign intracranial hypertension.

The distinction between migraine and muscle contraction headache may be difficult to make. Migraine (even complex migraine with neuroischaemic auras) can appear for the first time in pregnancy (Wright and Patel 1986; Jacobson and Redman 1989) or worsen during the first trimester in patients with a history of migraine, although the vast majority of such patients subsequently improve. Benign intracranial hypertension tends to worsen in pregnancy.

Treatment for muscle contraction headache is simple analgesia, ice packs, and massage. Acute migraine may be treated in the non-pregnant patient with aspirin, paracetamol, non-steroidal anti-inflammatory drugs (NSAIDs), metoclopramide, butorphanol (an opioid agonist/antagonist), ergotamine, dihydroergotamine, or sumatriptan (a selective 5-HT$_1$ agonist). Acute attacks in pregnancy are probably best treated with simple analgesia with or without narcotic. Aspirin or NSAIDs are not teratogenic, but frequent use later in pregnancy is not advisable (as discussed in 'Autoimmune diseases'). Metoclopramide (Briggs *et al.* 1994) and sumatriptan have not been associated with birth defects (Glaxo, Canada, personal communication), although information is scant and insufficient to advocate use of these drugs. Ergot preparations are contraindicated because of the potential for intense vasoconstriction to decrease placental perfusion. However, early reports of various malformations have not been confirmed by controlled studies (Heinonen *et al.* 1977; Wainscott *et al.* 1978). Inadvertent exposure should, therefore, not be considered an indication for therapeutic abortion.

Agents used for prophylaxis against frequent, troublesome migraines include low dose aspirin, NSAIDs, β-blockers (especially propranolol, 40–160 mg/day), calcium-channel blockers, tricyclic antidepressants (e.g. imipramine, amitryptiline), and valproic acid. However, migraines usually improve with pregnancy, so it is usually possible to slowly taper prophylactic therapy. If such an attempt fails, then with the exception of valproate, any of the aforementioned drugs could be considered, although there is not extensive data about the safety of calcium-channel blockers, and both β-blockers and tricyclics have the potential to cause transient, reversible neo-natal side-effects at term. Valproic acid should be avoided during the first trimester because of its potential to cause neural tube defects (as discussed below under 'Epilepsy').

Epilepsy
Epilepsy has a prevalence of 1/200 women of child-bearing age. However, all 'epilepsy' is not epilepsy, and healthy scepticism should be maintained before history and physical examination confirm such a diagnosis. Obviously the best time to see these patients is prior to conception, especially since some anticonvulsants are anti-folates, and periconceptional folate has been proven to decrease the risk of neural tube defects in other women at high risk (Van Allen 1994).

Patients should be counselled that poor control before pregnancy (i.e. more than one seizure per month) increases the risk of deterioration during pregnancy (Knight and Rhind 1975). Otherwise, the risk of deterioration is approximately 25 per cent in the absence of a seizure in the preceding nine months. Good seizure control will avoid the hypoxaemia and lactic acidosis which cannot be good for the mother or fetus. Status epilepticus is associated with increased maternal and 50 per cent fetal mortal-ity. Fetal bradycardia may be observed for 20 min after a maternal seizure and intra-ventricular haemorrhage and subsequent cognitive dysfunction are documented outcomes (Gaily *et al.* 1990).

There are many potential reasons for the worsening of maternal seizure control during pregnancy. They include cessation of therapy because of fear of teratogenicity, changes in drug disposition, sleep deprivation with the discomfort of the third trimester, stress, and hyperventilation during labour. Therefore, therapeutic drug monitoring is essential, and levels should be monitored monthly and maintained at the pre-pregnancy levels which maintained control in the patient under consideration. Plans should be made to give vitamin K_1 during the last month of pregnancy as anti-convulsants may decrease vitamin K-dependent clotting factors in the fetus.

The major first trimester concern for the fetus is the risk of congenital malforma-tions. Women with epilepsy have a two- to three-fold increased risk of malformations even when on no anticonvulsant therapy (Bjerkedal 1982; Schardein 1985). The cause is multifactorial. Obviously, it is well known that this risk is increased by anticonvul-sant therapy.

There are a number of anti-epileptic medications that women may need to take during pregnancy. Phenytoin and carbamazepine (CBZ) are (equally) efficacious for treatment of partial and secondarily generalized seizures. Valproic acid is used for a variety of seizure disorders, especially when different types coexist in the same patient. Phenobarbital (PB) and primidone (which is metabolized to PB) cause CNS sedation and are not used commonly, but are also effective for partial and generalized seizures. Ethosuximide is the drug of choice for uncomplicated absence seizures. New adjuvant therapies include lamotrigine, felbamate, gabapentin, clobazam, and clonazepam.

There has been a considerable amount of investigation into the relative teratogenic potential of the anticonvulsants. Phenytoin has long been regarded to cause the fetal hydantoin syndrome characterized by craniofacial abnormalities (e.g. broad nasal bridge, metopic ridging, microcephaly, cleft lip/palate, and ptosis) and variable degrees of hypoplasia and ossification of the distal phalanges (Schardein 1985), in addition to associated abnormalities such as impaired physical and mental growth, and congenital heart defects. The risk has been estimated to be up to 26 per cent after first trimester exposure (Hanson and Buehler 1982). However, minor defects comparable to the pattern associated with phenytoin were recently seen after CBZ (Jones *et al.* 1989). Therefore, all anticonvulsants may have the potential to cause minor anomalies which might be referred to more appropriately as the 'fetal epilepsy syndrome'. There is very little specific information about the other anticonvulsants in pregnancy. The major therapeutic points to be highlighted are the following.

- Monotherapy is safer than polytherapy.
- Unless a drug switch is contemplated prior to pregnancy, the best drug is the drug that controls that patient's epilepsy.
- CBZ and valproic acid have been associated with risks of neural tube defects of about 1 per cent and 1–2 per cent, respectively. Therefore, maternal serum AFP and careful structural review of the spine at 18–20 weeks are recommended in all such exposed fetuses. Animal work suggests that the risk associated with valproic acid may be decreased by avoiding high valproate peaks, by changing from two to four times daily dosing. Certainly, all women taking these drugs and planning pregnancy should be taking folic acid 5 mg/day periconceptionally in an attempt to decrease the risk of neural tube defects; continuation throughout pregnancy will also prevent megaloblastic anaemia.
- For the few patients who have the option of changing therapy prior to pregnancy, there is some evidence that CBZ may be safer with respect to cognitive development. A recent prospective controlled cohort study found that phenytoin monotherapy was associated with a seven-fold increased risk for global IQ ≤ 84 (1 standard deviation lower than in the general population) (Scolnick *et al.* 1994) and the effect was independent of parental and environmental factors, type of maternal epilepsy, number of seizures, or dose of drug. No differences were seen between CBZ-treated patients and their matched controls.
- Clonazepam is a benzodiazepine and clobazam a benzodiazepine derivative. An association between benzodiazepines and facial clefts has not been established; if it exists, the risk is small.

Myasthenia gravis

Myasthenia gravis is an autoimmune disorder which affects the nicotinic acetylcholine receptors, resulting in weakness of striated (but not smooth) muscle. Approximately equal proportions of patients see no change, an increase or a decrease in their symptoms (Fennell and Ringel 1987) during pregnancy. Patients with previous thymectomy are less likely to deteriorate (Eymard and Morel 1989).

Anticholinesterases should be continued during pregnancy. Maternal issues are primarily those surrounding labour and delivery. Indeed, careful review of possible drug interactions (e.g. with $MgSO_4$, procaine local anaesthetics) should be undertaken before any drug is prescribed to patients with myasthenia taking anticholinesterases.

The risk of self-limited neonatal myasthenia should be discussed early in pregnancy. This is due to transplacental passage of maternal antibody to acetylcholine receptors, is unrelated to the severity of the underlying maternal disorder, and is related to the titre of maternal acetylcholine receptor antibody which should be assayed at booking. There are no *in utero* signs, as the maternal antibody–fetal receptor interaction appears to be inhibited *in utero* by AFP. The neonatal disorder (which can be severe) appears within a few days of delivery and may last a few weeks.

Intestinal disorders

This chapter will not cover diseases predominantly of later pregnancy (i.e. gastro-oesophageal reflux, cholestasis of pregnancy, HELLP syndrome (hemolysis, elevated liver enzymes, low platelets), acute fatty liver of pregnancy, and haemorrhoids). However, if the patient had hepatic involvement in a previous pregnancy, then baseline liver enzyme measurements (i.e. aspartate aminotransferase (AST), alanine aminotransferase (ALT), gamma glutanyl transferase (GGT), alkaline phosphatase (ALP)) and function tests (i.e. bilirubin, albumin, prothrombine time (PTT)) would be warranted in the first trimester. It should be noted that the normal ranges for AST and ALT are slightly lower in pregnancy, ALP rises by about 1.5 times by term, and albumin and total protein fall by about 10.0 g/dl in the first half of pregnancy.

Constipation may complicate early (and later stages of) pregnancy, but one series of 1000 Israeli women showed that only 1.5 per cent of women required laxatives (Levy *et al.* 1971). This highlights the point that symptoms that are unexplained or unusual with respect to their severity or duration should prompt further investigation for causes unrelated to pregnancy (e.g. malignancy). Bulk-forming laxatives and lactulose (which is not absorbed) are preferred, but there is no evidence of teratogenicity with docusate, or senna glycosides. The constipation of irritable bowel syndrome should be similarly treated.

Inflammatory bowel disease

Inflammatory bowel disease (IBD) refers to Crohn's disease and ulcerative colitis (UC). Both are familial with multifactorial inheritance and are therefore not amenable to prenatal diagnosis. The first of the bimodal peaks in incidence is in the late teens, and therefore IBD is encountered with some regularity among women of child-bearing age.

The maternal issues to be addressed in the first trimester are inflammatory disease activity, presence of extraintestinal manifestations (determined by history and physical examination), nutritional status (especially B_{12} in terminal ileitis of Crohn's disease or iron with chronic blood loss in UC), and the risk of continuing maintenance drug therapy. Flares are particularly common in the first trimester (and post-partum), although disease flares occur in 30–40 per cent of patients annually, regardless of pregnancy (Miller 1986). Intestinal obstruction may occur with progressive mechanical displacement of the bowel, although much less serious problems (e.g. local bleeding and cracked skin) are more common complications of ileal or colonic stomata.

With respect to therapy, 5-ASA compounds (marketed as a pro-drug split by colonic bacteria, e.g. salazopyrine sulfamethoxasole/5-ASA) improve maintenance of remission of UC, but there is no evidence of such an effect on Crohn's disease. If useful before pregnant, 5-ASA compounds should be continued as they have not been associated with an increased risk of birth defects (Schardein 1985). Both corticosteroids and azathioprine can be used to treat flares of Crohn's disease or UC; their safety has been discussed under 'Autoimmune diseases'. Metronidazole used for treatment of perianal Crohn's disease is also not teratogenic (Burtin *et al.* 1995).

IBD is not associated with an increase in fetal loss, with the potential exception of previous surgery and very active disease at conception (Miller 1986). Recent data indicate that pregnancy outcome is very favourable even with relapse in pregnancy or first presentation in pregnancy (Fagan 1995).

Coeliac disease

Coeliac disease is characterized by small intestinal villous atrophy that results from ingestion of gluten-containing substances in susceptible individuals. The clinical symptoms/signs may be mild and go unrecognized. It is mentioned here because many patients present with nutritional anaemias in pregnancy.

Gastroenteritis

The first trimester is the time to ensure that all pregnant women have taken on board the recommendations of the Department of Health to avoid foods considered to be high risk for *Listeria* (e.g. soft, ripened cheeses) or *Salmonella* (e.g. pre-cooked poultry).

In the absence of blood, acute diarrhoea of < 72 h duration may be managed conservatively. Otherwise, stools should be tested for the presence of faecal leucocytes, as well as culture and sensitivity, ova and parasites, and/or *Clostridium difficile* toxin and culture (if antibiotics were recently ingested). Sigmoidoscopy has the same indications in pregnancy as in the non-pregnant patient.

Outlining the management of all causes of infectious diarrhoea is beyond the scope of this book. Aside from maintenance of hydration, causes that should be treated are *Campylobacter jejuni* (with erythromycin), *Shigella* (with trimethoprim–sulfamethoxasole), *C. difficile* (with oral vancomycin), and all causes of inflammatory diarrhoea according to the most likely aetiologic agent. *Salmonella* poisoning should probably not be treated given that antibiotics other than ciprofloxacin may increase faecal shedding and duration of illness; ciprofloxacin is discussed below under 'Traveller's diarrhoea'. Special mention will be made of travellers' diarrhoea and intestinal parasitic infestation.

Travellers' diarrhoea

Most consultants do not recommend prophylaxis against travellers' diarrhoea for the non-pregnant patient but rather, they recommend prompt treatment of moderate to severe disease, with agents directed at the most common cause, enterotoxigenic *E. coli*; less common causes are *Campylobacter, Salmonella, Shigella*, viruses, and parasites. Although prophylaxis may be recommended if contracting diarrhoea would have serious social/medical implications for the patient, pregnancy is not considered to be such an indication.

The agent of choice for treatment of traveller's diarrhoea in the non-pregnant patient is a fluoroquinolone. If taken inadvertently in the first trimester, then there is reassuring data to suggest that fluoroquinolones (like ciprofloxacin) are not teratogenic (Berkovitch *et al.* 1994); however, long term effects on developing cartilage remain to be established. Alternatives are tetracyclines and trimethoprim– sulfamethoxazole. Tetracyclines do not represent a fetal risk if exposure occurs before four months' gestation when the deciduous teeth begin to calcify. Trimethoprim– sulfamethoxazole is not teratogenic, although it may not be effective in areas where drug resistance has developed. If antimotility agents must be used (e.g. for travelling home), then given its limited bioavailability, loperamide is probably safe for short-term use.

Intestinal parasites
Up to half of women from developing countries harbour one or more intestinal parasites, most commonly hookworm (D'Alauro *et al.* 1985). This is likely to be an important health issue in large urban centres with a high influx of immigrants. The most common clinical manifestation is nutritional deficiency which may manifest as iron/other deficiency anaemia(s) in pregnancy. Pregnancy outcome is not affected in the presence of adequate nutrition, which is where therapeutic efforts should be directed. Specific therapy should be delayed until after delivery, with the exception of (i) symptomatic giardiasis or amoebiasis (which may be severe in pregnancy and associated with neonatal transmission (Wig *et al.* 1984); but can be safely treated with metronidazole (Burtin *et al.* 1995); (ii) ascariasis; (iii) malaria; and/or(iv) multiple infestations (Villar *et al.* 1989).

Acute abdomen (appendicitis, obstruction)
Perhaps the most important point to emphasize here is that all nausea and vomiting in the first trimester of pregnancy is not 'nausea and vomiting of pregnancy'. All abdominal pain may not be gastrointestinal; for example, a ruptured ectopic pregnancy may not be associated with vaginal bleeding and may have an elevated serum amylase relative to the normal non-pregnant range (RCEMD 1991); a normal range for pregnancy has not been established.

The most common surgical causes of an acute abdomen in pregnancy are acute appendicitis and intestinal obstruction, with incidences approaching 1/2500–3500 deliveries (Kammerer 1979). Acute appendicitis may take a more aggressive course (e.g. a higher incidence of rupture), although this may be due to a delay and/or difficulty in diagnosis. Ultrasonography may detect higher risk patients by identifying a non-compressible aperistaltic appendix, target-like appearance in the transverse view, and a diameter ≥ 7 cm (Schwerk *et al.* 1989).

Liver disease

With the exception of rises in liver enzymes associated with severe nausea and vomiting of pregnancy, this discussion will be restricted to liver disease incidental to the first trimester of pregnancy. A wide differential diagnosis should be entertained which encompasses both congenital (e.g. Wilson's disease) and acquired causes.

Hepatitis

Viral hepatitis is the most common cause of jaundice in pregnancy world-wide. Agents most likely to be responsible are hepatitis A through E (the enterically transmitted form of 'non-A non-B hepatitis'), herpes viruses (i.e. simplex, zoster, cytomegalovirus (CMV), Epstein–Barr).

Viral hepatitis

There is controversy over whether or not pregnancy is associated with more aggressive disease, as literature from developing countries has related more severe disease to poor socioeconomic conditions. However, management of acute/chronic infection in the first trimester is no different from management in the non-pregnant patient. The following issues need to be addressed, where relevant:

- immune globulin (hepatitis A, hepatitis B, varicella zoster) ± vaccination (hepatitis B) in the face of exposure in non-immune individuals;
- risk of teratogenesis (CMV, varicella zoster only);
- risk of vertical transmission (potentially all viral hepatitides) that may be higher with higher viral loads (as seen with hepatitis B, Shiraki *et al.* 1980, and C);
- caeserean section (with active herpes simplex at the time of delivery);
- immunoprophylaxis for the neonate (hepatitis B, possibly hepatitis C);
- referral for antiviral therapy (e.g. interferon) after delivery (hepatitis B and C).

Autoimmune chronic active hepatitis

This refers to chronic active hepatitis in the presence of autoimmune features (e.g. positive ANA, hypergammaglobulinaemia, antibodies to liver-specific antigens (LSP), and/or smooth muscle) in the absence of markers of viral hepatitis. Well controlled disease before pregnancy has been associated with good disease control during pregnancy, although prematurity and low birth weight may be more common (Steven *et al.* 1979). Long term therapy (with prednisolone or azathioprine) should be continued.

Wilson's disease

Wilson's disease is not common in pregnancy. Pregnancy is unlikely to occur with untreated disease associated with cirrhosis. Lifelong therapy with D-penicillamine can prevent virtually every manifestation of the disease, and although the drug may be teratogenic (as discussed under 'Autoimmune diseases'), it should not be discontinued given that relapse is common and may be severe and irreversible. Pyridoxine should also be administered as D- penicillamine has an antipyridoxine effect in animals. Baseline screening for drug toxicity (i.e. by history, physical examination, full blood count, urinalysis) should be performed to rule out the following complications: arthralgias, SLE, myasthenia gravis, granulocytopenia, thrombocytopenia, nephrotic syndrome, and Goodpasture's syndrome. Although D-penicillamine should not be discontinued, the dose may be decreased by 25–50 per cent, possibly because of a pregnancy-associated increase in ceruloplasmin and/or copper extraction by the fetus.

Cholestasis
It should be noted that congenital disorders of bilirubin excretion (i.e. Gilbert's disease for unconjugated, and Dubin–Johnson and Rotor's syndromes for conjugated hyperbilirubinaemia) are benign, but jaundice may be precipitated by pregnancy without an effect on pregnancy outcome.

Primary biliary cirrhosis
Primary biliary cirrhosis (PBC) is characterized by cholestasis, antimitochondrial antibodies, and characteristic liver histology (i.e. fall-out of bile ductules). The prognosis is good for well-controlled disease, and non-specific therapy (e.g. bile acid binders) should be continued to control maternal symptoms.

Gall stones
Hormonal changes render bile more lithogenic in pregnancy (Van Thiel 1987). However, pregnancy is not an established risk factor for cholelithiasis. Management of the asymptomatic pregnant patient with gall stones would seem to be most appropriately conservative, given the best approach has not been established for non-pregnant patients.

Diagnosis of acute cholelithiasis in pregnancy is complicated by the fact that the gall bladder increases in size throughout gestation and the mean diameter of the common bile duct may be increased in normal pregnancy. Management differs in that endoscopic retrograde cholangiopathy (ERCP) may be associated with excessive radiation if the fetus cannot be shielded, and lithotrypsy is contraindicated during pregnancy. Therefore, abdominal cholecystectomy may be the best option.

Liver transplantation
Limited experience with liver transplantation in pregnancy indicates that the long term prognosis appears to be unchanged, and perinatal outcome is good (Laifer *et al.* 1990). Immunosuppressants do not represent a major fetal risk (as discussed under 'Renal diseases').

Infectious diseases

Diagnosis and management of infectious diseases is similar to that in the non-pregnant patient. The field is vast. Highlighted here are some of the major points to remember:

* In the setting of fever, special attention should be paid to urine and genital tract cultures.
  Five per cent of pregnant women have asymptomatic bacteruria (i.e. $> 10^5$ organisms/ml of urine). Progesterone-induced dilatation of the ureters and urinary stasis, and/or increased concentrations of amino acids and lactose may be responsible for the fact that 40 per cent of women with asymptomatic bacteruria

develop urinary tract infection at some point during pregnancy. Therefore, asymptomatic bacteruria should be treated during pregnancy, usually with a week's course of antimicrobials chosen on the basis of the most likely pathogen, with subsequent reassessment when culture and sensitivity results become available. Investigations for structural abnormalities of the renal tract are warranted if there is a history of recurrent infection, slow resolution on antimicrobial therapy, or failure to clear the offending organism on repeat culture.

Sexually transmitted diseases should be diagnosed and treated as in the non-pregnant patient, with the exception that alternatives to tetracycline should be used. Congenital syphilis and ophthalmia neonatorum (related to gonorrhoea) can be prevented. Preliminary evidence suggests that screening for (and treating) genital mycoplasmas, *Chlamydia trachomatis*, or *Trichomonas vaginalis* will decrease the risk of preterm labour and/or premature rupture of membranes, but this cannot be recommended until the results of ongoing trials become available. Previous herpes simplex infection is not a contraindication to vaginal delivery at term; Caesarean section is recommended only in the presence of active maternal lesions, especially if the infection is primary.

- Leuckocytosis (between 10 and $15\,000 \times 10^9/1$) is normal.

- Septic abortion and related maternal death still occur, after both elective and spontaneous termination of pregnancy (RCEMD 1994). Septic abortion should be considered in any woman with fever and bleeding in the first trimester, and antimicrobial treatment should cover Gram positive, Gram negative, and anaerobic organisms.

- Mantoux skin testing should be assessed using the same diagnostic criteria and prophylactic therapy (e.g. isoniazid for tuberculous infection, or antimalarials for malaria) should be continued in most cases as the risk of infection is not lower, and may be higher, in pregnancy.

- Some antimicrobial agents may be teratogenic or fetotoxic.
The reader is referred to other sources for drugs of choice for various infectious diseases. What follows are some general rules about safety. Agents not associated with teratogenecity are penicillins, cephalosporins, erythromycin/other macrolides, metronidazole, isoniazid, rifampicin, sulphonamides, trimethoprim, zidovudine (AZT) (De Santis *et al.* 1995), acyclovir (Andrews *et al.* 1992), or chloroquine. Agents that are probably safe based on limited data and their pharmacology are low-dose aminoglycosides, oral vancomycin (which is not absorbed), pyrizinamide (derived from niacin), and mefloquine. Agents for which there is some concern about toxicity (to relevant fetal tissue) include ciprofloxacin (cartilage), ethambutol (retina), and aminoglycosides (inner ear). Tetracyclines are contraindicated after 16 weeks' gestation due to calcification of primary teeth. There is little data on β-lactamase inhibitors, intravenous vancomycin, or antifungals.

- Some infections may be teratogenic or fetotoxic.
Teratogenic infections share many features in common, perhaps most importantly the fact that subclinical infection occurs in at least half of maternal cases. Therefore, the physician or obstetrician may have only a diagnostic role in sorting out the

cause of fetal malformations, rather than a therapeutic role in preventing them. The infections of note are syphilis and the 'TORCH' infections (i.e. toxoplasmosis, rubella, CMV, and herpes/varicella-zoster). The fetotoxic infections of note are par-vovirus and listeriosis. HIV infection will also be mentioned as the risk of vertical transmission can be decreased by maternal AZT treatment. Urinary tract infections are mentioned because they are increased in incidence during pregnancy.

Syphilis

Most congenital syphilis can be prevented by treating the maternal infection which is currently identified by screening programmes. Despite the rarity of maternal syphilis in pregnancy, economic analyses have demonstrated the cost-effectiveness of such an approach (Stray-Pederson 1983).

Toxoplasmosis

The prevalence of seronegativity against *Toxoplasma gondii* among women of child-bearing age is 60–80 per cent in Canada, but varies geographically depending on local dietary patterns. However, the incidence of congenital infection is still low, being probably 2–8 per 1000 pregnancies in Canada (Carter and Frank 1986). Routine toxoplasmosis serology at booking is recommended only if the prevalence of toxo-plasmosis is greater than 0.8 per cent (Wang and Smaill 1989); this is not the case in North America or the UK where only education of women about potential sources of toxoplasmosis is recommended.

The primary reservoir for infection is the rodent population and cats which may become chronically infected by eating rodents; transmission to humans occurs via consumption of raw meat and/or faecal contamination.

Maternal infection is usually asymptomatic, but may present with a mononucleosis-like illness. Diagnosis of acute infection is based on finding specific IgM antibodies two weeks after infection. These antibodies reach their peak within one month and become undetectable within six to nine months. IgG-specific antibodies reach their peak concentration one to two months after infection and remain positive indefinitely.

Maternal infection in the first trimester is associated with a low risk of transmission (17 per cent) but severe disease is more common (in 14 per cent of infected infants) and can be associated with fetal loss, malformations, or long term ocular or cerebral involvement which may take months or years to develop (Desmonts and Couvreur 1974). This contrasts with maternal infection in the third trimester which is associ-ated with a high risk of transmission (65 per cent) but no serious sequelae.

The following treatments have been recommended for maternal infection in preg-nancy: sulphadiazine/pyrimethamine and folinic acid (due to their successful treatment of congenitally infected children) or spiramycin therapy (due to efficacy in animal studies). Non-randomized studies in humans have suggested both approaches can decrease the risk of congenital toxoplasmosis after demonstrated seroconversion, but spiramycin has no haematological side-effects (Wang and Smaill 1989). Neither approach has been associated with drug-induced teratogenicity. In seronegative individuals, prophylaxis against acute infection (with spiramycin 1.5 g twice daily) has been recommended in high risk populations, although there are few data about efficacy.

Rubella

Maternal rubella infection may manifest as polyarthritis/arthralgia, but half of infections are subclinical. Screening programmes may pick up women who were vaccinated but who now have 'negative' titres; they are probably protected because viraemia has rarely occurred in such non-pregnant individuals when confronted by virus challenge (O'Shea *et al.* 1983).

Serological diagnosis is problematic. Primary infection is associated with rubella-specific IgM antibody or a four-fold rise in IgG antibody. However, IgM may be negative early after exposure to rubella, and IgG rise may be missed if the first sample is drawn more than one week after the onset of rash. An IgG rise must also be distinguished from that associated with reinfection.

Primary infection is associated with fetal loss, malformations (i.e. deafness, cataracts, congenital heart disease, hepatosplenomegaly and mental retardation), and low birth weight. The risk of severe congenital rubella is high (possibly 100 per cent based on a small number of cases) after maternal infection in the first trimester, but no severe sequelae (e.g. 0/63) have followed infection after 16 weeks, gestation. No teratogenicity has followed reinfection (Fogel *et al.* 1985; Forsgren and Soren 1985; Morgan-Capner *et al.* 1985). Maternal rubella in the first trimester is considered by many to be an indication for therapeutic abortion; post-exposure immune globulin may be tried if termination is not an option. It has been estimated that 33–50 per cent of congenital rubella could be prevented if postpartum vaccination programmes were implemented (Orenstein *et al.* 1984; Smithells *et al.* 1985).

Cytomegalovirus (CMV)

Approximately 20–80 per cent of women of child-bearing age are seronegative against CMV. Maternal infection may be subclinical or present as a seronegative mononucleosis-type illness. Seronegative women may be exposed to asymptomatic CMV excretors at work or in their social and family lives, and they should not be isolated during pregnancy.

Maternal infection is diagnosed by IgM anticytomegalovirus (for primary infection), rising titres of IgG anti-CMV (for secondary infection), and viruria (for both). Congenital infection is confirmed postnatally by neonatal nasopharyngeal and urine cultures.

Both primary and reactivated maternal infection may be transmitted to the fetus, in 40 per cent and 1–2 per cent (Trofattes 1992) of cases, respectively. However, congenital CMV is associated with long term sequelae in a minority of infected fetuses, whether maternal infection is primary (6 per cent) or reactivated (i.e. < 0.01 per cent). Put another way, diagnosis of *in utero* infection does not predict long term prognosis unless no infection is found.

Varicella zoster

Most women have protective antibodies against varicella zoster, even without a history of clinical chickenpox. Varicella infection (presumably in non-immune individuals) in pregnancy is rare (i.e. 0.7/1000 pregnancies).

The issue to be dealt with here is the 'congenital varicella syndrome' which occurs in no more than about 5 per cent of women who have primary exposure to chickenpox in early gestation (Paryani and Arvin 1986). The syndrome is characterized by intrauterine growth restriction, limb hypoplasia, brain atrophy, cicatricial scars, mental retardation, and ocular lesions, all of which may be due to congenital infection and then subsequent in utero shingles; the level of neurological insult has been correlated with the level of skin dermatome involvement (Alkalay *et al.* 1987). If varicella serology can be obtained within 48–72 h of exposure to chickenpox or shingles, then varicella immune globulin (VZIg) may decrease the risk of congenital infection.

Parvovirus

Parvovirus B19 is a small DNA virus transmitted by respiratory secretions. The incubation period is approximately one week after which the patient experiences a mild, self-limited febrile illness associated with a skin rash, symmetric arthralgia and/or arthritis of the hands, wrists, and knees. Only half of adults have evidence of past infection, although serological tests are not widely available to permit determination of who is at risk.

Fetal anomalies resulting from maternal parvovirus infection have not been demonstrated. However, the virus has a predilection for red cell precursors in fetal bone marrow, and can cause fetal anaemia, high output congestive heart failure, and hydrops fetalis. Most reported cases have occurred during the first half of pregnancy, with a fetal loss rate reported to be 3–9 per cent at four to six weeks after infection. Serial fetal ultrasound should be used after the first trimester to screen for hydrops.

Listeriosis

Listeria is ubiquitous, but since the avoidance of high-risk foods (i.e. unpasteurized cheese and pâté) has been advised in pregnancy (*While you are pregnant: safe eating and how to avoid infection from food and animals*, Department of Health and the Central Offfice of Information), the number of reported cases of maternal listeriosis has declined in the UK. Maternal manifestations of infection may be absent, mimic an influenza-like illness, and/or be associated with a urinary tract infection, or be very severe (e.g. meningitis, acute respiratory distress syndrome). This is usually a problem of later pregnancy, but is mentioned here to reinforce dietary recommendations, as fetal infection may be associated with midtrimester abortion or stillbirth. Specific cultures must be requested for *Listeria monocyto*genes which is not easily grown. The organism is susceptible to ampicillin and trimethoprim–sulfamethoxazole.

HIV infection

The incidence of HIV infection in pregnancy varies dramatically depending on geographical location and prevalence of local risk factors, such as intravenous drug abuse and bisexuality. Almost all women found to be HIV positive will develop clinical AIDS over the decade after infection.

There is no evidence that women who are HIV positive but well have a more rapid decline in the their CD4 counts during pregnancy. However, there is some evidence that women with AIDS may deteriorate more rapidly during pregnancy. Therefore, an infectious diseases subspecialist should be involved in the care of all women infected with HIV during their pregnancy.

HIV has been found in fetal tissues (Liebes *et al.* 1990), although the incidence of spontaneous abortion has not been consistently higher in HIV-positive women. There is no association of HIV infection with congenital malformations. Vertical transmission occurs in approximately 25 per cent of cases, usually in the peripartum period and more commonly in association with more severe maternal disease (as indicated by lower CD4 counts, higher viral loads, clinical AIDs) and breast feeding (Newell and Gibb 1995). Antenatal treatment with AZT (100 mg orally every 6 h, started at 14–34 weeks' gestation until delivery) has been shown to decrease the risk of vertical transmission from 25 per cent to 8 per cent (Matheson *et al.* 1995) and is not teratogenic. Caesarean section may further decrease the risk of fetal infection. Other prophylactic therapy the patient may be taking (e.g. aerosolized pentamidine, trimethoprim–sulphamethoxasole) should be continued in pregnancy.

Cancer

Cancer and pregnancy are associated in fewer than 0.1 per cent of pregnancies. The most common malignancies encountered in pregnant women are breast, thyroid, lymphoma, leukaemia, melanoma, colon, cervix, and ovarian. Treatment varies widely. Therefore the reader is referred to more detailed sources about the effects of pregnancy on the disease (Koren *et al.* 1995), and the effects of the disease and/or its treatment (by surgery, cytotoxic drug therapy, and/or radiotherapy) on the pregnancy (Schardein 1985).

DISEASES THAT ARE PREGNANCY INDUCED

Recurrent miscarriage

Recurrent fetal loss is defined as three or more consecutive miscarriages and afflicts approximately 1 per cent of pregnant women. An underlying aetiology can be found in over 50 per cent of cases (Clifford *et al.* 1994) when investigations are aimed at ruling out uterine structural abnormalities, polycystic ovarian syndrome, and performing parental peripheral blood karyotyping. The question addressed by this chapter is which *medical conditions* can result in pregnancy loss, and how such conditions should be diagnosed and treated.

It is common knowledge that many medical conditions (e.g. thyroid disease, collagen vascular disease) have been associated with recurrent miscarriage (Gleicher *et al.* 1993). Although fetal loss has been attributed primarily to poor disease control, many of these disorders have an autoimmune aetiology and their associated organ-specific antibodies (e.g. anti-thyroid antibodies) also have predictive value for recurrent miscarriage (Stagnero-Green *et al.* 1990).

When should autoantibodies be sought?
Autoantibodies occur only infrequently (i.e. in a few per cent of patients) among general (El-Roeiy and Gleicher 1988), general obstetric (in the range of 2–5 per cent), and recurrent miscarriage populations (Pratt *et al.* 1993). The occurrence of these antibodies among women with recurrent miscarriage *and* risk factors for autoimmunity is

probably higher (Gleicher *et al.* 1993) and therefore, the search could be restricted to these patients.

Which antibodies should be measured? Both non-specific and organ-specific (e.g. antithyroid) antibodies should be assayed. With respect to non-organ-specific antibodies, much of the literature focuses on the significance of antiphospholipid antibodies specifically, or on anticardiolipin antibodies even more specifically. However, some experts have argued that what is needed is a more general search for abnormal B-cell function, and, therefore, for a panel of autoantibodies (Gleicher *et al.* 1993) against other histones, nucleotides, and nuclear antigen (i.e. SS-A (anti-Ro), SS-B (anti-La), Sm (anti-Smith)) (Gleicher 1992).

A very important point to emphasize is the interlaboratory variation that exists in the measurement of these antibodies. Antibody titres must be compared with the normal ranges for the lab. In addition, there is also substantial intraindividual variation, and anecdotal experience suggests that many patients with recurrent fetal loss (e.g. 20 per cent Gleicher *et al.* 1993) do not manifest abnormalities until after conception. Therefore, antibody titres should be repeated after conception, even when negative results were obtained pre-pregnancy. A final point is that there are cross-reactivities and cross-specificities between phospholipid–phospholipid—antibody reactions, so detection of an antibody does not necessarily imply a causative role, particularly in the patient involved.

Treatment of recurrent miscarriage has focused either on suppression of antibody production, or on antithrombotic therapy. The former approach is based on the assumption that the antibodies themselves are pathogenic (e.g. by affecting signal transduction because many second messengers are phospholipids); however, this approach has not been successful (Laskin *et al.* 1995). The latter approach has been based on pathological findings of thrombotic/ischaemic placental changes in some (but not all) patients with autoimmune pregnancy loss; aspirin, or heparin and aspirin have been used with some success, but heparin can have serious adverse effects (as discussed previously under 'Thromboembolism'). Therefore, with antibodies other than antiphospholipid antibodies, the best treatment approach has not been established. When the antibodies detected are directed against phospholipids, the association of these antibodies with thrombosis and the safety of low-dose aspirin therapy in pregnancy makes prophylactic low-dose aspirin the recommended treatment at present; if such patients fail to improve with aspirin, then consideration should be given to the addition of low-dose heparin (Cowchuck *et al.* 1992). Other potential therapies include gamma globulin which has had some success in anecdotal reports (Orvietto *et al.* 1991) (but is very expensive), and immunotherapy which has shown some success in small trials (Prendiville 1994).

Finally, the long term prognosis of patients with detectable autoantibodies and recurrent fetal loss is apparently good as they are unlikely to develop classical autoimmune disease (Gleicher *et al.* 1993).

Nausea and vomiting of pregnancy (NVP)

Population based cohort studies (Vellacott *et al.* 1988; Gadsby *et al.* 1993) have found that as many as 80 per cent of women experience nausea and/or vomiting of pregnancy (NVP).

The pathogenesis of NVP is unclear, and has been attributed to physiological (i.e. delayed gastric emptying; high levels of oestrogen, HCGβ, or β_1 glycoprotein; HCGβ induced sensitivity of the chemoreceptor trigger zone to endorphins) and psychological factors. Obviously a broad differential diagnosis must be considered, especially when NVP continues into the mid-second trimester, and any women on glucocorticoids should be given extra coverage during this stressful period.

Most NVP is mild in severity and limited to 7–12 weeks' gestation. However, severe disease may occur in 1 per cent of women (de la Ronde 1994) and result in reversible liver enzyme abnormalities (with an AST four times above the upper limit of normal but unassociated with a prolonged PT), Mallory–Weiss oesophageal tears, vitamin deficiency, maternal malnutrition, and the need for hospitalization and intravenous rehydration. Spontaneous fetal loss may be decreased, but fetal complications may include intrauterine growth restriction which has been associated with poor maternal nutrition. Concerns about teratogenicity figure prominently among patients and their care-givers.

Although NVP may be considered part of normal pregnancy physiology given its prevalence, it is undeniable that women tolerate symptoms to varying degrees, and symptoms may have an impact on quality of life (O'Brien and Naber 1992). Therefore, although reassurance about the self-limited nature of NVP and dietary modifications (i.e. dry, carbohydrate-rich meals and avoidance of large volume drinks in the early morning) usually suffice, some women require drug therapy. It is of great importance to recognize that all such women should be considered candidates for vitamin supplements, specifically thiamine, as deficiency may develop over as little as two weeks and Wernicke's encephalopathy has been well documented in association with NVP. Total parental nutrition has also been used and met with success, although optimal daily nutritional needs are not known, and despite supplementation, deficiencies of thiamine have occurred.

NVP may be associated with a slight decrease in the incidence of spontaneous fetal loss, and therapeutic abortion if symptoms are intolerable. However, the concern that figures more prominently in the minds of patients and physicians is that of drug-induced malformations in this post-thalidomide era.

Teratogenicity has not been attributed to modern-day agents, although available data on some agents are limited in quantity and quality. Evidence from small randomized placebo-controlled trials suggests that the following medications are effective for treatment of varying degrees of pregnancy nausea and vomiting: phenothiazines, benzylamine/dramamine, Bendectin® (dicyclomine, doxylamine, pyridoxine), pyridoxine, P6 acupressure, and ginger. The use of metoclopramide (central and peripheral dopamine D_2 receptor antagonist) or ondansetron (a selective 5-HT$_3$ antagonist) have been described in case series/reports; although no teratogenicity has been reported, the limited data do not support first-line use of these agents. For true hyperemesis gravidarum, a number of case reports and case series have also described successful (Nelson-Piercy and de Swiet 1995a,b) and unsuccessful (Magee and Redman 1996) use of corticosteroids for their action on the chemoreceptor trigger zone. No agent has been recognized to be superior as no direct comparisons have been made. Therefore, no firm treatment recommendations can be made.

Patients who present with severe hyperemesis gravidarum need very careful management of their fluid and electrolytes. Rapid correction of hyponatraemia can cause central pontine myelinosis which may be fatal or associated with permanent neurological sequelae.

Most (i.e. 80 per cent) of women who suffered NVP in the past will do so again in their next pregnancy. However, this must be put into perspective; 55 per cent of women with no history of NVP will also have NVP in their next pregnancy (Klebanoff *et al.* 1985).

Anaemia

Iron deficiency anaemia

A normal diet contains 1–2 mg of iron per day, but requirements during pregnancy average 4 mg/day. Therefore, pregnant women routinely mobilize their iron stores. Although this may be detected during the first trimester in a woman with a history of menorrhagia, it is more likely to be a progressive problem over the nine months of pregnancy. The diagnosis is straightforward based on a microcytosis, low serum ferritin (to < 15 μg/l), serum iron (to < 12 μM), and increased total iron-binding capacity (TIBC) (to > 72 μM).

The primary issue to be addressed early in pregnancy is whether iron supplementation is necessary and/or desirable. Controlled trials comparing routine iron supplementation before 24 weeks' gestation with iron treatment for manifest anaemia have been reviewed (Mahomed 1993) and were found to be of good methodological quality. Not surprisingly, routine supplementation resulted in a lower incidence of low serum ferritin (< 10 μg/l) and anaemia (< 100–106 g/l), as well as lower rates of both Caesarean section (total and elective) and maternal blood transfusion. Pregnancy outcome was otherwise no different between groups. Advocates of supplementation (with 60–80 mg/day elemental iron) base their argument on the aforementioned findings, and also on the fact that supplementation may prevent the theoretically detrimental effect of iron deficiency on exercise tolerance, and maternal and/or fetal cognitive function. However, advocates of treatment only for manifest anaemia argue that the decrease in red cell mass is physiological and increasing it artificially could result in adverse perinatal outcomes, although there is no evidence that this occurs. No cost–benefit analysis has been done to determine the relative merits of the two approaches. Therefore, either seems reasonable, as long as patients have haemoglobin monitored during pregnancy and the puerperium.

Folic acid deficiency

Folic acid deficiency is responsible for almost all megaloblastic anaemia, which occurs in 0.2–5.0 per cent of pregnancies; B_{12} deficiency is rare and will not be reviewed. In contrast to iron, folate needs during pregnancy may be met from the diet, except in the case of multiple pregnancy.

Once again, the issue is not so much one of diagnosis, which is likely to develop later in pregnancy, but rather whether or not supplementation is necessary. This is separate from the issue of periconceptional folic acid which has been shown, by an as yet unknown mechanism, to decrease the incidence of neural tube defects. It should be noted that neural tube closure is either complete by 28 days post-conception (i.e. 6

weeks post-LMP) or will remain incomplete, and to be effective, folic acid must be taken before this time.

Akin to the argument for iron, folate needs are increased during pregnancy (by about 100 μg/day), and store depletion has been documented by showing megaloblastic changes in the marrow, and both serum and red blood cell folate decreases during pregnancy. Not surprisingly, trials have shown that supplementation reduced the prevalence of megaloblastic haematopoiesis, low serum and red cell folate levels, and anaemia at term, as well as a possible decrease in prematurity and low birth weight. However, the methodological quality of the trials was poor and all effects occurred in groups receiving concomitant iron supplementation.

Therefore, no recommendations can be made on whether or not all pregnant women should be supplemented with folic acid. What can be agreed upon is that women with multiple gestations, haemolytic anaemias (whether intra- or extravascular), anticonvulsant therapy, or other reasons for folate deficiency (e.g. malaria) should receive 5 mg/day folic acid periconceptionally and throughout pregnancy.

Gestational diabetes mellitus (GDM)

GDM is defined as glucose intolerance discovered during pregnancy. Although GDM may therefore be diagnosed within the first trimester, insulin resistance, increased insulin production, and postprandial hyperglycaemia are progressive changes, and are usually seen after 20 weeks' gestation. Finding an elevated glucose during the first trimester probably reflects pre-existent diabetes mellitus (DM) and raises the issue of an increased risk of pregnancy loss and congenital malformations (as discussed under 'Pre-existent diabetes mellitus').

Pre-eclampsia

The incidence of pre-eclampsia is up to 5 per cent of obstetric populations, depending on geography and possibly also the proportion of primigravidas. It is a syndrome of the second half of pregnancy, recognized by a constellation of easily observable clinical signs (i.e. hypertension, proteinuria, and/or oedema). Such a definition does not define the underlying pathophysiology, which is yet to be elucidated. Although pre-eclampsia is almost invariably a disease of the second half of pregnancy, it is mentioned here for three reasons: (i) pre-eclampsia is regarded as a primary placental disorder with detectable haematological, biochemical, and/or physiological abnormalities in the first half of pregnancy; (ii) pre-eclampsia may present much earlier in the setting of gestational trophoblastic disease; and (iii) women with previous pre-eclampsia need to be assessed early in subsequent pregnancies for identifiable risk factors and considered for closer antenatal care, especially during 20–28 weeks' gestation.

Risk factors for first occurrence or recurrence of pre-eclampsia include the following: previous proteinuric preeclampsia (especially that of early onset), primary or secondary forms of hypertension (especially that associated with renal disease), renal parenchymal disease, family history, possibly obesity, and conditions associated with large placental mass (e.g. multiple pregnancy, hydrops fetalis). Most of these can be ruled out by history, physical examination, and basic laboratory testing. The recurrence rate of approximately 10–25 per cent depends on the gestational age at onset, severity of pre-eclampsia (including HELLP syndrome, see Sullivan *et al.* 1994), and the presence of underlying risk factors.

Baseline bloodwork during the current pregnancy should also be drawn. However, it should be noted that plasma urate concentrations decrease by over 25 per cent before the end of the first trimester, reaching pre-pregnancy levels by the second trimester and rising by about another 50 μmol/l in the third trimester; a relative rise is normal, reflecting decreased tubular secretion, and must not be interpreted as invariably reflecting pre-eclampsia, especially when levels are below 350 μmol/l. There is no evidence that aspirin can prevent pre-eclampsia, as discussed earlier under 'Hypertension'.

Peripartum cardiomyopathy

Peripartum cardiomyopathy is rare. It usually occurs within two months of delivery, but onset can be from two months before to six months after delivery. Full recovery is associated with a good prognosis in the absence of future pregnancies, but peripartum cardiomyopathy is likely to recur in at least one third of future pregnancies, especially if full recovery after the first pregnancy has not occurred (Elkayam *et al.* 1992). Women with a history of this condition should be advised against conceiving again.

Skin rashes

Most skin rashes in pregnancy occur in the third trimester or puerperium, and are benign. Herpes (pemphigoid) gestationis is rare but deserving of specific mention because (i) it may occur in association with trophoblastic disease, (ii) it may cause substantial maternal (and possibly fetal) morbidity, and (iii) it usually recurs in future pregnancies which many experts would advise against.

CONCLUDING REMARKS

This chapter has highlighted the many issues that must be addressed when faced with the most common medical disorders in early pregnancy. There is now no question that pregnancy begins in the first trimester for both the fetus and the mother. Perhaps it is time to reassess the obstetric practice of booking for obstetric care only after spontaneous abortion is unlikely; rather, booking should begin with the recognition of pregnancy and its attendant risks for both mother and fetus.

ACKNOWLEDGEMENT

L.A.M. would like to thank P.V.D. for his patience and professional advice.

REFERENCES

Alkalay, A.L., Pomerance, J.J., and Rimoin, D.L. (1987). Fetal varicella syndrome. *Journal of Pediatrics*, **111**, 320–3.

Andrews, E.B., Yankaskas, B.C., Cordero, J.F., Schoeffler, K., and Hampp, S. (1992). Acyclovir in pregnancy registry: six years' experience. *Obstetrics and Gynecology*, **79**, 7–13.

ATC (Antiplatelet Trialists' Collaboration) (1994). Collaborative overview of randomised trials of antiplatelet therapy—III: Reduction in venous thrombosis and pulmonary embolism by antiplatelet prophylaxis among surgical and medical patients. *British Medical Journal*, **308**, 235–46.

Badaracco, M.A. and Vessey, M. (1974). Recurrence of venous thrombolembolism disease and use of oral contraceptives. *British Medical Journal*, **1**, 215–17.

Barbour, L.A. and Pickard, J. (1995). Controversies in thromboembolic disease during pregnancy: a critical review. *Obstetrics and Gynecology*, **86**, 621–33.

Becker, R.M. (1983). Intracardiac surgery in pregnant women. *Annals of Thoracic Surgery*, **36**, 453–8.

Berkovitch, M., Pastuszak, A., Gazarian, M., Lewis, M., and Koren, G. (1994). Safety of the new quinolones in pregnancy. *Obstetrics and Gynecology*, **84**, 535–8.

Bjerkedal, T. (1982). Outcome of pregnancy in women with epilepsy, Norway, 1967–1978: congenital malformations. In *Epilepsy, pregnancy and the child*, (ed. D. Janz, M. Dam, and A. Richens), pp. 289–95. Raven Press, New York.

Bonnar, J. (1987). Haemostasis and coagulation disorders in pregnancy. In *Haemostasis and thrombosis*, (2nd edn) (ed. A.L. Bloom, and D.P. Thomas), pp. 570–84. Churchill Livingstone, Edinburgh.

Briggs, G.G., Freeman, R.K., and Yaffe, S.J. (1994). *Drugs in pregnancy and lactation*, (4th edn), pp. 65–73. Williams and Wilkins, Baltimore.

Burr, W.A., Evans, S.F., Lee, J., Prince, H.P., and Ramsden, D.B. (1979). The ratio of thyroxine to thyroxine-binding globulin in the assessment of thyroid function. *Clinical Endocrinology*, **11**, 333–42.

Burrow, G.N., Klatskin, E.H., and Genel, M. (1978). Intellectual development in children whose mothers received propylthiouracil during pregnancy. *Yale Journal of Biology and Medicine*, **51**, 151–6.

Burrows, R.F. and Kelton, J.G. (1992). Thrombocytopenia during pregnancy. In *Haemostatisis and Thrombosis in Obstetrics and Gynaecology*, (ed. I.A. Greer, A.G. Turpie, and C.D. Forges), pp. 407–29 Chapman and Hall, London.

Burtin, P., Taddio, A., Ariburnu, O., Einarson, T.R., and Koren, G. (1995). Safety of metronidazole in pregnancy: a metal-analysis. *American Journal of Obstetrics and Gynecology*, **172**, 525–9.

Butler, N.R. and Bonham, D.G. (1963). *Perinatal mortality*, pp. 87–100. E & S Livingstone, Edinburgh.

Buyon, J.P., Winchester, R.J., Slade, S.G., Arnett, F., Copel, J., Fridman, D., *et al.* (1993). Identification of mothers at risk for congenital heart block and other neonatal lupus syndromes in their children. Comparison of enzyme-linked immunosorbent assay and immunoblot for measurement of anti-SSa-A/Ro and anti-SSOB/La antibodies. *Arthritis and Rheumatism*, **36**, 1263–73.

Buyon, J.P., Cronstein, B.N., Morris, M., Tanner, M., Weissmen, G. (1986). Serum complement values (C_3 and C_4 to to differentiate between systemic lupus activity and pre-eclampsia. *American Journal of Medicine*, **81**, 194–200.

Caldwell, D.C., Williamson, R.A., and Goldsmith, J.C. (1985). Hereditary coagulopathies in pregnancy. *Clinical Obstetrics and Gynecology*, **28**, 53–72.

Canadian hydroxychloroquine study group (1991). A randomized study of the effect of withdrawing hydroxychloroquine sulfate in systemic lupus erythematosus. *New England Journal of Medicine*, **324**, 150–4.

Carter, A.O., and Frank, J.W. (1986). Congenital toxoplasmosis; epidemiologic features and control. *Canadian Medical Association Journal*, **135**, 618–23.

CLASP (Collaborative low-dose aspirin study in pregnancy) Collaborative Group (1994). CLASP: a randomised trial of low-dose aspirin for the prevention and treatment of pre-eclampsia among 9364 pregnant women. *Lancet*, **343**, 619–29.

CLASP Collaborative Group (1995). Low dose aspirin in pregnancy and early childhood development: follow-up of the collaborative low dose aspirin study in pregnancy. *British Journal of Obstetrics and Gynaecology*, **102**, 861–8.

Clifford, K., Rai, R., Watson, H., and Regan, L. (1994). An informative protocol for investigation of recurrent miscarriage: preliminary experience of 500 consecutive cases. *Human Reproduction*, **9**, 1328–32.

Colvin, B.T. and Barrowcliff, T.W. (1993). The British Society for Haematology guidelines on the use and monitoring of heparin 1992: second revision. *Journal of Clinical Pathology*, **46**, 97–103.

Conard, J., Horellou, M.H., Van Dredan, P., Lecompte, T., and Samama, M. (1990). Thrombosis and pregnancy in congenital deficiencies in anti-thrombin III, protein C or protein S: study of 78 women. *Thrombosis and Haemostasis*, **63**, 319–20.

Connolly, H.M., Ammsh, N.M., and Warnes, C.A. (1996). Pregnancy in women with coarctation of the aorta. *Journal of American College of Cardiology*, **27**, 43A (abstract).

Cowchuck, F.S., Rece, E.A., Balaban, D., Branch, D.W., and Plouffe, L. (1992). Repeated fetal losses associated with antiphospholipid antibodies: a collaborative randomized trial comparing prednisolone with low-dose heparin treatment. *American Journal of Obstetrics and Gynecology*, **166**, 1318–23.

D'Alauro, F., Lee, R.V., Pao-in, K., and Khairollah, M. (1985). Intestinal parasites and pregnancy. *Obstetrics and Gynecology*, **66**, 639–43.

Dahlman, T.C. (1993). Osteporotic fractures and the recurrence of thromboembolism during pregnancy and the puerpium in 184 women undergoing thromboprophylaxis with heparin. *American Journal of Obstetrics and Gynecology*, **168**, 1265–70.

Davis, L.E., Lucas, M.J., Hankins, G.D.V., Roark, M.L., and Cunningham, F.G. (1989). Thyrotoxicosis complicating pregnancy. *American Journal of Obstetrics and Gynecology*, **160**, 63–70.

Davison, J.M., Dunlop, W., and Ezimokhai, M. (1980). Twenty-four hour creatinine clearance during the third trimester of normal pregnancy. *British Journal of Obstetrics and Gynaecology*, **87**, 106–9.

de la Ronde, S. (1994). Nausea and vomiting in pregnancy. *Journal of the Society of Obstetric and Gynaecology*, **16**, 2035–41.

de Leeuw NKM., Lowenstein, L., and Hsieh, Y.S. (1966). Iron deficiency and hydremia in normal pregnancy. *Medicine, Baltimore*, **45**, 291–315.

Department of Health and the Central Office of Information (1992). *While you are pregnant: safe eating and how to avoid infection from food and animals*.

De Santis, M., Noia, G., Caruso, A., and Mancuso, S. (1995). Guidelines for the use of zidovudine in pregnant women with HIV infection. *Drugs*, **50**, 43–7.

Desmonts, G. and Couvreur, J. (1974). Congenital toxoplasmosis. A prospective study of 378 pregnancies. *New England Journal of Medicine*, **290**, 1110–16.

Dicker, D., Feldberg, D., Samuel, N., Yeshaya, A., Karp, M., and Goldman, J.A. (1988). Spontaneous abortion in patients with insulin-dependent diabetes mellitus: the effect of preconceptional diabetic control. *American Journal of Obstetrics and Gynecology*, **158**, 1161–4.

Douketis, J.D. and Ginsberg, J.S. (1995). Diagnostic problems with venous thromboembolic disease in pregnancy. *Haemostasis*, **25**, 58–71.

Elkayam, U. and Gleicher, N. (1982). *Cardiac problems in pregnancy. Diagnosis and management of maternal and fetal disease.* Alan R. Liss, New York.

Elkayam, U., Ostrzega, E.L., and Shotan, A. (1992). Periparum cardiomyopathy. In *Principles and practice of medical therapy in pregnancy*, (2nd edn), pp. 812–14. Appleton and Lange, New York.

Elkayam, U., Ostrzega, E., Shotan, A., and Mehra, A. (1995). Cardiovascular problems in pregnant women with Marfan syndrome. *Annals of Internal Medicine*, **123**, 117–22.

El-Roeiy, A. and Gleicher, N. (1988). Definition of normal autoantibody levels in an apparently healthy population. *Obstetrics and Gynecology*, **72**, 596–602.

Eymard, B. and Morel, E. (1989). Myasthenie et grossesse: une étude clinique et immunologique de 42 cas (21 myasthenies n!eonatales). *Revue Neurologique (Paris)*, **45**, 696–70.

Fagan, E.A. (1995). In *Medical disorders in obstetric practice*, (3rd edn), pp. 379–422. Blackwell, Oxford.

Feldkamp, M. and Carey, J.C. (1993). Clinical teratology counseling and consultation case report: low dose methotrexate exposure in the early weeks of pregnancy. *Teratology*, **47**, 533–9.

Fennell, D.F. and Ringel, S.P. (1987). Myasthenia gravis and pregnancy. *Obstetrical and Gynecological Survey*, **41**, 414–21.

Fogel, A., Handsher, R., and Barnea, B. (1985). Subclinical rubella in pregnancy—occurrence and outcome. *Israel Journal of Medical Science*, **21**, 133–8.

Forsgren, M. and Soren, L. (1985). Subclinical rubella reinfection in vaccinated women with rubella-specific IgM response during pregnancy and transmission of virus to the fetus. *Scandinavian Journal of Infectious Disease*, **17**, 337–41.

Fuhrmann, K., Reiher, H., Semmler, K., Fischer, F., Fischer, M., and Flockner, E. (1983). Prevention of congenital malformations in infants of insulin dependent diabetic mothers. *Diabetes Care*, **6**, 219–23.

Gadsby, R., Barnie-Adshead, A.M., and Jagger, C. (1993). A prospective study of nausea and vomiting during pregnancy. *British Journal of General Practice*, **43**, 245–8.

Gaily, E.K., Kantola-Sorsa, E., and Granstrom, M.L. (1990). Specific cognitive dysfunction in children with epileptic mothers. *Developmental Medicine and Child Neurology*, **32**, 403–14.

Galvoa-Teles, A. and Burke, C.W. (1973). Cortisol levels in toxaemic and normal pregnancy. *Lancet*, **i**, 737–40.

Ginsberg, J.S. and Hirsh, J. (1992). Use of antithrombotic agents during pregnancy. *Chest*, **102**, 385–90S.

Gleicher, N. (1992). Autoimmunity. In *Principles and practice of medical therapy in pregnancy*, (2nd edn) (ed. N. Gleicher, S.A., Gall, B.M., Sibai, U. Elkayam, R.M., Galbraith and (G.E., Sarto). Appleton and Lange, New York.

Gleicher, N., Pratt, D., and Dudkiewicz, A. (1993). What do we really know about autoantibody abnormalities and reproductive failure: a critical review. *Autoimmunity*, **16**, 115–40.

Hanson, J.W. and Buehler, B.A. (1982). Fetal hydantoin syndrome. *Journal of Pediatrics*, **101**, 816–18.

Hayslett, J.P. and Lynn, R.I. (1980). Effect of pregnancy in patients with lupus nephropathy. *Kidney International*, **18**, 207.

Heinonen, O.P., Sloan, D., and Shapiro, S. (1977). *Birth defects and drugs in pregnancy*, pp. 358–60. Publishing Sciences Group, Littleton, MA.

Hench, A.B. (1938). The ameliorating effect of pregnancy on chronic atrophic (infectious rheumatoid) arthritis; fibrositis and intermittent hydrothosis. *Proceedings of the Mayo Clinic*, **13**, 161.

Hirsh, J., Cade, J.F., and Gallus, A.S. (1972). Anticoagulation in pregnancy: a review of indications and complications. *American Heart Journal*, **83**, 301–5.

Hirsh, J. and Fuster, V. (1994). Guide to anticoagulant therapy. *Circulation*, **89**, 1449–68.

Hod, M., Sharony, R., Friedman, S., and Ovadia, J. (1989). Pregnancy and thyroid carcinoma: a review of incidence, course and prognosis. *Obstetrics and Gynecological Survey*, **44**, 774–9.

Hollingsworth, D.R. (1989). Endocrine disorders of pregnancy. In *Maternal–fetal medicine: principles and practice*, (2nd edn) (ed. R.K. Creasy and R. Resnik), pp. 989–1031. W.B. Saunders, Philadelphia.

Jacobson, S.L. and Redman, C.W.G. (1989). Basilar migraine with loss of consciousness in pregnancy: case report. *British Journal of Obstetrics and Gynaecology*, **96**, 495.

Jarnerot, G., Into-Maimberg, M.B., and Esbjorner, E. (1981). Placental transfer of sulphasalazine and sulphayridine and some of its metabolites. *Scandinavian Journal of Gastroenterology*, **16**, 693–7.

Jones, K.L., Lacro, R.V., Johnson, K.A., and Adams, J. (1989). Pattern of malformations in the children of women treated with carbamazepine during pregnancy. *New England Journal of Medicine*, **320**, 1661–6.

Kammerer, W.S. (1979). Non-obstetric surgery during pregnancy. *Medical Clinics of North America*, **63**, 1157–64.

Karlen, J.G. and Cook, W.A. (1974). Renal scleroderma and pregnancy. *Obstetrics and Gynecology*, **44**, 349–54.

Khoury, M.J., Becerra, J.E., and d'Almada, P.J. (1989). Maternal thyroid disease and the risk of birth defects in offspring: a population-based case–control study. *Paediatric and Perinatal Epidemiology*, **3**, 402–20.

Klebanoff, M.A., Koslowe, P.A., Kaslow, R., and Rhoads, G.G. (1985). Epidemiology of vomiting in early pregnancy. *Obstetrics and Gynecology*, **66**, 612–16.

Knight, A.H. and Rhind, E.G. (1975). Epilepsy and pregnancy: a study of 153 pregnancies in 59 patients. *Epilepsia*, **16**, 99–110.

Koopman, M.M.W., Prandoni P., Piovella, F., Ockelford, P.A., Brandjes, D.P.M., Van Der Meer, J., *et al.* (1996). Treatment of venous thrombosis with intravenous unfractionated heparin administered in the hospital as compared with subcutaneous low-moleclar-weight - weight heparin administered at home. *New England Journal of Medicine*, **334**, 682–7.

Koren, G., Lishner, M., and Farine, D., (ed.) (1995). *Cancer in pregnancy: maternal and fetal risks*. Cambridge University Press, Cambridge.

Koshy, M., Burd, L., Wallace, D., Moawad, A., and Baron, J. (1988). Prophylactic red-cell transfusions in pregnant patients with sickle cell disease. *New England Journal of Medicine*, **319**, 1447–52.

Krogmann, O.N., Kramer, K.H., Rammos, S., Heusch, A., and Bourgeois, M. (1993). Non-invasive evaluation of left ventricular systolic function late after coarctation repair: influence of early vs. late surgery. *European Heart Journal*, **14**, 764–9.

Kupersmith, M.J., Rosenberg, C., and Kleinberg, D. (1994). Visual loss in pregnant women with pituitary adenomas. *Annals of Internal Medicine*, **121**, 73–7.

Laifer, S.A., Darby, M.J., Scantlebury, V.P, Harger, J.H., and Curtis, S.N. (1990). Pregnancy and liver transplantation. *Obstetrics and Gynecology*, **76**, 1083–8.

Laskin, C., Bombardier, C., Mandel, F., Ritchie, K., Hannah, M., Farine, D., *et al.* (1996). A randomized controlled trial of prednisone and ASA in women with autoantibodies and unexplained recurrent fetal loss. Meeting of the Society of Perinatal Obstetricians, Kona Village (abstract).

Letsky, E.A. (1995*a*). Blood volume, haematinics, anaemia. In *Medical disorders in obstetric practice*, (3rd edn), pp. 33–70. Blackwell, Oxford.

Letsky, E.A. (1995*b*). Coagulation defects. In *Medical disorders in obstetric practice*, (3rd edn), pp. 71–115. Blackwell, Oxford.

Levine, M., Gent, M., Hirsh, J., Leclerc, J., Anderson, D., Weitz J., *et al.* (1996). A comparison of low-molecular-weight heparin administered primarily at home with unfractionated heparin administered in the hospital for proximal deep-vein thrombosis. *New England Journal of Medicine*, **334**, 677–81.

Levy, N., Lemberg, E., and Sharf, M. (1971). Bowel habit in pregnancy. *Digestion*, **4**, 216–22.

Liebes, L., Mendoza, S., Wilson, D., and Dancis, J. (1990). Transfer of zidovudine (AZT) by human placenta. *Journal of Infectious Disease*, **161**, 203–7.

Lindheimer, M.D. and Davison, J.M. (ed.) (1994). *Baillière's clinical obstetrics and gynaecology. Renal disease in pregnancy*. Baillière Tindall, London.

Littlejohns, P.I., Ebrahim, S., and Anderson, R. (1989). Prevalence and diagnosis of chronic respiratory symptoms in adults. *British Medical Journal*, **298**, 1556–60.

Lockshin, M.D., Bonfa, E., Elkon, K., and Druzin, M.L. (1988). Neontal lupus risk to newborns of mothers with systemic lupus erythematosus. *Arthritis and Rheumatism*, **31**, 697–701.

Long, T.J., Felice, M.E., and Hollingsworth, D.R. (1985). Goiter in pregnant teenagers. *American Journal of Obstetrics and Gynecology*, **152**, 670–4.

Magee, L.A., Downer, Sermer, M., Boulton, B.C., Cameron, D., Rosengarten, M., et al. (1995). Pregnancy outcome following gestational exposure to amiodarone in Canada. *American Journal of Obstetrics and Gynecology*, **172**, 1307–11.

Magee, L.A. and Redman, C.W.G. (1996). An N-of-1 trial for treatment of hyperemesis gravidarum. *British Journal of Obstetrics and Gynaecology*, **103**, 478–80.

Mahomed, K. (1993). Routine iron supplementation in pregnancy. In *Pregnancy and childbirth module Cochrance database of systematic reviews* (ed. M.W. Enkin, M.J.N.C. Keirse, M.J., Renfrew, and J.P., Neilson), Review No 03157, 28 April 1993. Cochrane, Oxford.

Mandel, S.J., Larsen, P.R., Seely, E.W., and Brent, G.A. (1990). Increased need for thyroxine during pregnancy in women with primary hypothyroidism. *New England Journal of Medicine*, **323**, 91–6.

Matheson, P.B., Abrams, E.J., Thomas P.A., Hernan, M.A., Thea, D.M., Lambert, G., et al. (1995). Efficacy of antenatal zidovudine in reducing perinatal transmission of human immunodeficiency virus type 1. The New York City Perinatal HIV Transmission Collaborative Study Group. *Journal of Infectious Diseases*, **172**, 353–8.

McCaw-Binns, A. and the Jamaica low-dose aspirin study group (1996). Low dose aspirin in pregnancy—are there any benefits? *10th World Congress International Society for the Study of Hypertension in Pregnancy*, August 4–8, Seattle (Abstract).

Miller, J.P. (1986). Inflammatory bowel disease in pregnancy: a review. *Journal of the Royal Society of Medicine*, **79**, 221–5.

Mills, J.L., Knopp, R.H., Simpson, J.L, Jovanovic-Peterson, L., Metzger, B.E., Holmes, L.B., et al. (1988). Lack of relation of increased malformation rates in infants of diabetic mothers to glycemia control during organogenesis. *New England Journal of Medicine*, **318**, 671–6.

Milne, J.A., Howie, A.D., and Pack, A.I. (1978). Dyspnoea during normal pregnancy. *British Journal of Obstetrics and Gynaecology*, **84**, 448.

Milne, J.A., Mills, R.J., Howie, A.D., and Pack, A.L. (1977). Large airways function during normal pregnancy. *British Journal of Obstetrics and Gynaecology*, **84**, 448–51.

MNHWP (Maternal and Neonatal Haemostasis Working Party) of the Haemostasis and Thrombosis Talk (1993). Guidelines on the presentation, investigation, and management of thrombosis associated with pregnancy. *Journal of Clinical Pathology*, **46**, 489–96.

Montoro, M., Collea, J.V., ??? et al. (1981). Successful outcome of pregnancy in women with hypothyroidism. *Annals of Internal Medicine*, **94**, 31–4.

Morgan-Capner, P., Hodgson, J., Hambling, M.H., Dulake, C., Coleman, T.J., Boswell, P.A., et al. (1985). Detection of rubella-specific IgM in subclinical rubella reinfection in pregnancy. *Lancet*, i, 244–6.

Nachman R.L. and Silverstein, R. (1993). Hypercoagulable states. *Annals of Internal Medicine*, **119**, 819–27.

National High Blood Pressure Education Program Working Group (1990). Report on high blood pressure in pregnancy. *American Journal of Obstetrics and Gynecology*, **163**, 1691–712.

Nelson-Piercy, C. and de Swiet, M. (1995*a*). Corticosteroids for the treatment of hyperemesis gravidarum. *British Journal of Obstetrics and Gynaecology*, **101**, 1013–15.

Nelson-Piercy, C. and de Swiet, M. (1995*b*). Complications of the use of corticosteroids for the treatment of hyperemesis gravidarum. *British Journal of Obstetrics and Gynaecology*, **102**, 507–9.

Nelson-Piercy, C. and Moore-Gillon, J. (1995): Treatment of Asthma. In *Prescribing in pregnancy*, (2nd edn), (ed. P Rubin), pp. 46–58. BMJ Publishing Group, London.

Newell, M.L. and Gibb, D.M. (1995). A risk–benefit assessment of zidovudine in the prevention of perinatal HIV transmission. *Drug Safety*, **12**, 274–82.

Niswander, K.R. and Gordon, M. (1972). *Women and their pregnancies*, p. 246. W.B. Saunders, Philadelphia.

Nora, J.J. and Nora, A.H. (1987). Maternal transmission of congenital heart diseases: new recurrent risk figures and the question of cytoplasmic inheritance and vulnerability to teratogens. *American Journal of Cardiology*, **59**, 459–63.

O'Brien, B. and Naber, S. (1992). Nausea and vomiting during pregnancy: effects on the quality of women's lives. *Birth*, **19**, 138–43.

Orenstein, W.A., Bart, K.J., Hinman, A.R., Preblud, S.R., Greaves, W.L., Doster, S.W., *et al.* (1984). The opportunity and obligation to eliminate rubella from the United States. *Journal of the American Medical Association*, **251**, 1988–94.

Orvietto, R., Achiron, A., Ben-Rafael, Z., and Achiron, R. (1991). Intravenous immunoglobulin treatment of recurrent abortion caused by antiphophoslipid antibodies. *Fertility and Sterility*, **56**, 1013–20.

O'Shea, S., Best J.M., and Banatvala, J.E. (1983). Viremia, virus excretion and antibody responses after challenge in volunteers with low levels of antibody to rubella virus. *Journal of Infectious Disease*, **148**, 639–47.

Owen, J. and Hauth, J.C. (1989). Polyarteritis nodosa in pregnancy: a case report and brief literature review. *American Journal of Obstetrics and Gynecology*, **160**, 606–7.

Pabringer, I., Bruckner, S., Kyle, P.A., Schneider, B., Korniger, H.C., Niessner, H, *et al.* (1992). Hereditary deficiencies of antithrombin III, protein C and protein S: prevalence in patients with a history of venous thrombosis and criteria for rational patient screening. *Blood Coagulation and Fibrinolysis*, **3**, 547–53.

Paryani, S.G. and Arvin, A.M. (1986). Intrauterine infection with varicella-zoster virus after maternal varicella. *New England Journal of Medicine*, **314**, 1542–6.

Pratt, D., Novotny, M., Kaberlein G., Dudkiewicz, A., and Gleicher, N. (1993). Antithyroid-antibodies and the association with nonorganspecific antibodies in recurrent pregnancy loss. *American Journal of Obstetrics and Gynecology*, **168**, 837–41.

Prendiville, W.J. (1994). Immunotherapy for recurrent miscarriage. In *Pregnancy and childbirth module Cochrane database of systematic reviews* (ed. M.W., Enkin, M.J.N.C., Keirse, M.L., Renfrew, and J.P., Neilson), Review No 06814, 4 May 1994. Cochrane, Oxford.

Price, H.V., Salaman, J.R., Laurence, K.M., and Langmaid, H. (1976). Immunosuppressive drugs and the fetus. *Transplantation*, **21**, 294–8.

Pumphrey, C.W., Fay, T., and Weir, I. (1986). Aortic dissection during pregnancy. *British Heart Journal*, **55**, 106–8.

RCEMD, (1991). Report on confidential enquiries into maternal deaths in the United Kingdom 1985–87. HMSO, London.

RCEMD, (1994). *Report on Confidential Enquiries into Maternal Deaths in the United Kingdom 1988–1990*. HMSO, London.

Redman, C.W.G. (1995). Hypertension in pregnancy. In *Medical disorders in obstetric practice*, (3rd edn), pp. 182–225. Blackwell, Oxford.

Reimers, T.J. and Sluss, P.M. (1978). 6-mercaptopurine treatment of pregnant mice. Effects on second and third generations. *Science*, **201**, 65–7.

Romero, R., Duffy, T., Berkowitz, R.L., Change, E., and Hobbins, J.C. (1986). Prolongation of a preterm pregnancy complicated by death of a single twin *in utero* and disseminated intravascular coagulation. *New England Journal of Medicine*, **310**, 772–4.

Rosen, I.B. and Walfish, P.G. (1986). Pregnancy as a predisposing factor in thyroid neoplasia. *Archives of Surgery*, **121**, 1287–90.

Rosenblum, N.G., Grossman, A.R., Gabbe, S.G., Mennuti, M.T., and Cohen, A.W. (1983). Failure of serial echocardiographic studies to predict aortic dissection in a pregnant patients with Marfan's syndrome. *American Journal of Obstetrics and Gynecology*, **146**, 470–1.

Rosenn, B.M., Miodovnik, M., Holcberg, G., Khoury, J.C., and Siddiqi, T.A. (1995). Hypoglycemia: the price of intensive insulin therapy for pregnant women with insulin-dependent diabetes mellitus. *Obstetrics and Gynecology*, **85**, 417–22.

Rosman, J. (1992). Pulmonary physiology. In *Principles and practice of medical therapy in pregnancy*, (2nd edn), (ed. N. Gleicher, S.A. Gall, B.M. Sibai, U. Elkayam, R.M. Galbraith, and G.E. Sarto). Appleton and Lange, New York.

Sbarouni, E. and Oakley, C.M. (1994). Outcome of pregnancy in women with valve prostheses. *British Heart Journal*, **71**, 196–201.

Schardein, J.L. (1985). *Chemically induced birth defects*. Marcel Dekker, New York.

Schatz, M., Zieger, R.S., and Hoffman, C.P. (1990). Intrauterine growth is related to gestational pulmonary function in pregnant asthmatic women. *Chest*, **98**, 389–92.

Schwerk, W.B., Wichtrup B, Rothmund, M., and Ruschoff, J. (1989). Ultrasonography in the diagnosis of acute appendicitis: a prospective study. *Gastroenterology*, **97**, 630–9.

Scolnick, D. (1994). *Journal of the American Medical Association*, **271**, 767–70.

Shennan, A., Gupta, M., Halligan, A., Taylor, D.J., and de Swiet, M. (1996). *Lancet*, **347**, 139–42.

Shiraki, K., Yoshihara, Sakurai, M., Eto, T., and Kawana, T. (1980). Acute hepatitis B in infants born to carrier mothers with the antibody to hepatitis B e antigen. *Journal of Pediatrics*, **97**, 768–70.

Shores, J., Berger, K.R., Murphy, E.A., and Pyertiz, R.E. (1994). Progression of aortic dilatation and the benefit of long-term β-adrenergic blockade in Marfan's syndrome. *New England Journal of Medicine*, **330**, 1335–41.

Sibai, B.M., Caritis, S.N., Thom, E., Klebanoff, M., McNellis, D., Rocco, L., *et al.* (1993). Prevention of pre-eclampsia with low-dose aspirin in healthy, nulliparous pregnant women. *New England Journal of Medicine*, **329**, 1213–18.

Siu, S.C., Sermer, M., Harrrison, D.A., Grigoriadis, E., Liu, G., Sorensen, S., *et al.* (1996). Risk and predictors for pregnancy-related complications in women with heart disease. *Journal of American College of Cardiology*, **27**, 543A (abstract).

Soloninka, C.A., Laskin, C.A. Chin W, and Droppo, L. (1989). A noncytotoxic antilymphocyte antibody is highly specific in identifying women with unexplained recurrent fetal loss and subclinical autoimmunity. *Arthritis and Rheumatism*, **32**, S123.

Smithells, R.W., Sheppard, S., Holzel, H., and Dickson, A. (1985). National congenital rubella surveillance programme 1 July 1971–30 June 1984. *British Medical Journal*, **291**, 40–1.

Stagnoro-Green, A., Roman, SH., Cogin, R., El-Harazy, E., Alvarez-Margany, M., and Davies, T.F. (1990). Detection of atrisk pregnancy by means of highly sensitive assays for thyroid autoantibodies. *Journal of the American Medical Association*, **264**, 1422–5.

Steel, J.M., Johnstone, F.D., Hepburn, D.A., and Smith, A.F. (1990). Can prepregnancy care of diabetic women reduce the risk of abnormal babies? *British Medical Journal*, **301**, 1070–4.

Steven, M.M., Buckley, J.B., and Mackay, I.R. (1979). Pregnancy in chronic active hpeatitis. *Quarterly Journal of Medicine*, **48**, 519–33.

Stray-Pederson, B. (1983). Economic evaluation of maternal screening to prevent congenital symphilis. *Sexually Transmitted Diseases*, **10**, 167–72.

Sullivan, C.A., Magann, E.F., Perry, K.G., Roberts, W.E., Blake, P.G., and Martin, J.N. (1994). The recurrence risk of the syndrome of hemolysis, elevated liver enzymes, and low platelets (HELLP) in subsequent gestations. *American Journal of Obstetrics and Gynecology*, **171**, 940–3.

Trofatter, Jr K.F. (1992). Cytomegalovirus. In *Principles and practice of medical therapy in pregnancy*, (2nd edn), (ed. N. Gleicher, S.A., Gall, B.M. Sibai, U. Elkayam, R.M., Galbraith, and G.E., Sarto), pp. 633–7. Appleton and Lange, New York.

Valle, D. (1994). Treatment and prevention of genetic disease. In *Harrison's Principles of Internal Medicine*, (13th edn), pp. 387–91. McGraw-Hill, New York.

Van Allen, M.I. (1994). 'Folate up' for healthy babies. *Canadian Medical Association Journal*, **151**, 151–66.

Van den Hof, M.C., Nicolaides, K.H., Campbell, J., and Campbell, S. (1990). Evaluation of the lemon and banana signs in one hundred thirty fetuses with open spina bifida. *American journal of Obstetric and Gynecology*, **162**, 322–7.

Van Dijke, C.P., Heyendael, R.J., and De Kleine, M.J. (1987). Methimazole, carbimazole and congenital skin defects. *Annals of Internal Medicine*, **106**, 60–1. (1978). *Yale Journal of Biological Medicine*, **51**, 151

Van Thiel, D. (1987). Effects of pregnancy and sex hormones on the liver. *Seminars in Liver Disease*, 7, 1–66.

Veille, J.C., Morton, M.J., and Burry, K.J. (1985). Maternal cardiovascular adaptations to twin pregnancy. *American Journal of Obstetrics and Gynecology*, **153**, 261–3.

Vellacott, I.D., Cooke, E.J.A., and James, C.E. (1988). Nausea and vomiting in early pregnancy. *International Journal of Gynecology*, **27**, 57.

Villar, J., Klebanoff, M., and Kester, E. (1989). The effect on fetal growth of protozoan and helminthic infection during pregnancy. *Obstetrics and Gynecology*, **74**, 915–20.

Vulsma, T., Gons, M.H., and de Vijlder, J.J.M. (1989). Maternal–fetal transfer of thyroxine in congenital hypothyroidism due to a total organifcation defect or thyroid agenesis. *New England Journal of Medicine*, **321**, 13–16.

Wainscott, G., Sullivan, F.M., Volans, G.N., and Wilkinson, M. (1978). The outcome of pregnancy in women suffering from migraine. *Postragraduate Medical Journal*, **54**, 98–102.

Wald, N.J., Cuckle, H., Boreham, J., Stirrat, G.M., and Turnbull, A.C. (1979). Maternal serum alpha-fetoprotein and diabetes mellitus. *British Journal of Obstetrics and Gynaecology*, **86**, 101–5.

Wang, E. and Smaill, F. (1989). Infection in pregnancy. In *Effective care in pregnancy and childbirth*, (ed. I. Chalmers, M. Enkin, and M.J.N.C. Keirse). Oxford University Press, Oxford.

Whittaker, P.G., Wilcox, T., and Lind, T. (1982). The effect of stress upon serum prolactin concentrations in pregnancy and nonpregnant women. *Journal of Obstetrics and Gynaeclogy*, **2**, 149–52.

WHO (World Health Organization) (1972). *Nutritional anaemias*. Technical Report Series No. 503. WHO, Geneva.

Wig, J.D., Bushnurmath, S.R., and Kaushik, S.P. (1984). Complications of amoebiasis in pregnancy and puerperium. *Indian Journal of Gastroenterology*, **3**, 37–8.

Williams, M.A., Lieberman, E., Mittendorf, R., Monson, R.R., and Schoenbaum, S.C. (1991). Risk factors for abruptio placentae. *American Journal of Epidemiology*, **134**, 965–72.

Wright, D.S. and Patel, M.K. (1986). Focal migraine and pregnancy. *British Medical Journal*, **293**, 1557–8.

FURTHER READING

Briggs, G.G., Freeman, R.K., and Yaffe, S.J. (1994). *Drugs in pregnancy and lactation* (4th edn), pp. 65–73. Williams and Wilkins, Baltimore.

Chalmers, I., Enkin, M., and Keirse, M.J.N.C. (eds). *Effective care in pregnancy and childbirth.* Oxford University Press, Oxford.

de Swiet, M. (1995). *Medical disorders in obstetric practice*, (3rd edn). Blackwell, Oxford.

Elkayam, U. and Gleicher, N. (1982). *Cardiac problems in pregnancy. Diagnosis and management of maternal and fetal disease.* Alan R. Liss, New York.

Gleicher, N., Gall, S.A., Sibai, B.M., Elkayam, U., Galbraith, R.M., and Sarto, G.E. (eds) (1992). *Principles and practice of medical therapy in pregnancy*, (2nd edn). Appleton and Lange, New York.

23 | *Regulation of deleterious effects of environmental xenobiotic exposure during early pregnancy*

Mrinal K. Sanyal

INTRODUCTION

Numerous studies have demonstrated that human exposure to various toxic agents is extensive. These agents may arise from various sources, including food (Table 23.1), water (Fig. 23.1), ambient and indoor air, lifestyle patterns, industrial effluents, agricultural pesticides, preservatives, urban life, and countless natural botanical sources (Grasso 1984; Bjorseth and Becher 1986; Lewtas 1989; Loforth 1989; Seinfeld 1989; Appel *et al.* 1990; Sugimura and Wakabayashi 1990; Vartiainen *et al.* 1988; Tuomisto and Vartiainen 1990). Environmental exposure to agents is often completely involuntary and associated with human survival processes. Human exposure to man-made chemicals may also be voluntary, and it is greatly amplified by activities related to industrialization and uncontrolled pollution. Ames *et al.* (1987) ranked a list of hazardous agents in the immediate environment with exposure possibilities for relative toxicity, and showed that overall exposure of agents is a massive and critical factor in assessing risk–benefit ratios. The toxicity of a specific agent is only a small component. Human adaptation to various environmental xenobiotic exposure is considerable, and a highly variable process among different individuals.

Exposure to environmental toxic agents can interfere with all aspects of reproduction including gametogenesis and fertilization, preimplantation development and implantation, and pregnancy and parturition processes (Wen *et al.* 1990; Schoendorf and Kiely 1992; Ekwo *et al.* 1993; Li *et al.* 1993; Lieberman *et al.* 1994; DiFranza and Lew 1995;). The early pregnancy period is a highly sensitive period for a normal embryonic organogenesis and progressive continuation of the pregnancy. Deleterious xenobiotic exposure may cause termination of the pregnancy and/or induce dysmorphogenesis of the embryo (birth defects). The conceptus has the potential to protect itself by a number of metabolic processes (Juchau 1989, 1990). Of interest are the progressive expression of various enzymes for the metabolism of environmental xenobiotics (teratogens) in the developing conceptus and their availability in the maternal system for the protection of the conceptus from the harmful effects of environmental agents.

Table 23.1 Polycyclic aromatic hydrocarbon (PAH) content in some common foodstuffs

Type of food	Benzo[*a*]pyrene (ppb)	Benz[*a*]anthracene (ppb)
Fresh vegetables	2.85–24.5	0.3–43.6
Vegetable oils	0.4–1.4	0.8–1.1
Coconut oil	43.7	98.0
Margarine	0.4–0.5	1.4–3.0
Mayonnaise	0.4	2.2
Coffee	0.3–1.3	1.3–3.0
Tea	3.9	2.9–4.6
Grain	0.19–4.13	0.40–6.85
Oysters and mussels	1.5–9.0	—
Smoked ham	3.2	2.8
Smoked fish	0.83	1.9
Smoked bonito	37	189
Cooked sausage	12.5–18.8	17.5–26.2
Singed meat	35.99	28–79
Grilled meat	0.17–0.63	0.2–0.4
Charcoal-grilled steak	8.0	4.5
Grilled mackerel	0.9	2.9
Barbecued beef	3.3	13.2
Barbecued spareribs	10.5	3.6

Some high figures have also been included to indicate the probable maximum PAH content. From Grasso (1984).

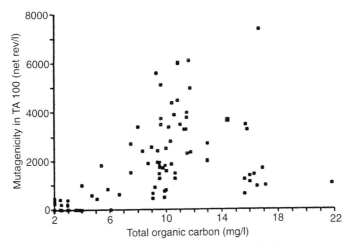

Fig. 23.1 The correlation between total organic carbon levels in raw waters and the mutagenic activities in *Salmonella* test system (TA 100) of drinking waters (from Vartiainen *et al.* 1988). These data reflect genotoxic potential of drinking water indicated by mutation of the bacterial strain (rev = mutation/litre water).

The placenta is the anatomical link between the mother and the embryo/fetus. The well-being of the trophoblast cells of the placenta is critical for the continuation of pregnancy and embryo–fetal development. The strategic location of trophoblast cells as an interface layer between the maternal and embryo/fetal compartments is of functional significance. Metabolism of xenobiotics in the conceptus is presumably supplementary to that of the mother, and it is likely that placental tissues regulate the transfer of metabolized xenobiotics into the fetal compartment. Transfer of toxic agents into the fetal compartment may affect fetal development, and presumably also increases its susceptibility to cancer in postnatal life (Tomatis 1994).

This chapter deals with the metabolic adaptations for xenobiotics which lead to normal embryo–fetal development and the metabolic conditions associated with deleterious effects.

XENOBIOTIC METABOLISM DURING PREGNANCY

Environmental xenobiotics may reach the cells and organs of the mother through the epithelial lining of the external skin or internal organs of the respiratory and digestive systems. Xenobiotic effects on the maternal–fetal compartments could be classified as either direct toxicity such as heavy metals and some alkylating agents or indirect toxicity requiring bioactivation by enzymes such as polycyclic aromatic hydrocarbon, (PAH). Diverse processes of toxicity on cells and organs and the metabolic bioactivation and detoxification for different environmental agents have been described in the literature. PAH type environmental toxic agents, generated by combustion processes, are widely distributed. The regulatory metabolic aspects of PAH will be discussed in detail in this chapter (Fig. 23.2).

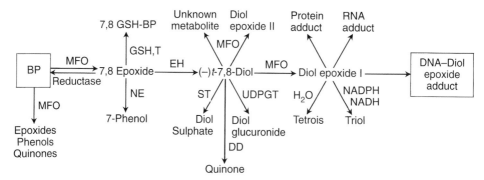

Fig. 23.2 A summary of detoxification and activation pathways from PAH, benzo[a]pyrene (BP). Detoxification by mixed function oxidase (MFO; CYP-cytochrome P450), glutathione S-epoxide transferase (GSH-T), epoxide hydrolase (EH), uridine diphosphoglucuronic acid transferase (UDGAT), dihydrodiol dehydrogenase (DD) and non enzymatic (NE) processes have been outlined. Activation pathway leads to macromolecular binding to reactive diol epoxide metabolite. Determinants in these processes are major regulatory factors for genotoxicity (from Gelboin *et al.* 1984).

The basic enzyme system in this process for PAH and a large variety of xenobiotics is phase I mixed function oxidases (cytochrome P450; CYPs) (Kadlubar and Hammons 1987; Nelson *et al.* 1996). The CYP monooxygenase family of enzymes introduce oxygen into the xenobiotic compound. The CYPs are available in more than 20 different forms and are functional for specific groups of xenobiotics. These enzymes are often induced by various forms of environmental exposure (e.g. smoke). An important regulatory metabolic pathway for further detoxification of hydroxy-lated metabolites is the participation of phase II enzymes. Epoxide hydroxylase can catalyse such substrates into epoxides which are the reactive intermediates for a number of carcinogens and teratogens. There are two forms of epoxide hydrolases in tissues, microsomal and cytosolic, and their differential functions with regard to reactive metabolite formation remain unclear. The phase II enzymes, transferases (glutathione *S*-transferase (GST), glucuronyl transferase, methyltransferase, sulpho-transferase, reductases, and peroxidases also participate actively in detoxification processes. The relative expression and function of these enzymes determine toxic product formation and detoxification of the environmental xenobiotic substrate.

The human tissues metabolize PAH into primary metabolites: dihydrodiols, epox-ides, quinones, and phenols. They are then converted into numerous secondary metabolites, some of which are detoxified and conjugate with ligands; others may be highly reactive products that bind with macromolecules (Gelboin *et al.* 1984; Jerina *et al.* 1986). The hydroxylated reactive metabolites of PAH produced by tissues may bind with DNA, forming PAH-metabolite–DNA adducts as outlined in Fig. 23.2. Adduct generation can be regulated by glutathione and GST enzyme and other detoxification systems (Jernstrom *et al.* 1990).

The human conceptus tissues have resources for metabolism of xenobiotics. They express mixed function oxidase (MFO) and related enzymes associated with reactive metabolite formation and detoxification of xenobiotics. These are aryl hydrocarbon hydroxylase (cytochrome P450; CYP1A1); epoxide hydrolases; glutathione *S*-transferase; quinone reductase, catechol-*O*-methyl transferase, and others which may biotransform PAH into various products (Manchester and Jacoby 1982; Pasanen *et al.* 1988; Wixtrom *et al.* 1988; Pacifici and Rane 1982; Aiso *et al.* 1989; Huel *et al.* 1989; Barnea and Avigdor 1990, 1991; Pasanen and Pelkonen 1990, 1994; Avigdor *et al.* 1992; Barnea *et al.* 1993, 1995; Sanyal *et al.* 1993, 1994). Exposure to xenobi-otic agents (e.g. cigarette smoke) markedly augments the metabolic processes of PAH substrates in human conceptus tissues. The cigarette smoke is a rich source of differ-ent classes of toxins including PAH, and the exposure can be readily quantified by nicotine and cotinine levels in the serum. Recent studies of mothers with exposure to active cigarette smoke showed that such exposure, in general, induced intrauterine growth retardation (IUGR) of fetuses. However, in a small number of conceptuses, IUGR was relatively mild and apparently normal neonates were born in spite of toxic exposure to maternal cigarette smoke (Sanyal *et al.* 1994). These data are indicative of the fact that there are natural processes which can effectively combat and prevent cigarette smoke toxicity (Fig. 23.3).

The toxic effects of xenobiotics on the conceptus compartments depend upon numerous factors. Among these, the important regulatory factors are: rates of absorp-

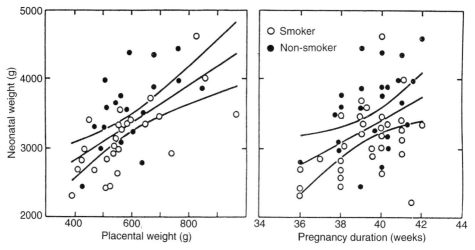

Fig. 23.3   Scatter diagrams of birth weight related to placental weights (left) and to pregnancy duration (right). The regression lines (middle) and 95% confidence intervals on the regression line show that birth weight is correlated with placental weights and with pregnancy duration. An increase in birth weights is associated with an increase in placental weight and prolongation of pregnancy for both smokers and non-smokers (from Sanyal *et al.* 1994). An important feature is that deleterious effects on neonatal/placental growth and development (weight and pregnancy duration) due to maternal cigarette exposure are not apparent in some samples resembling normal.

tion by the maternal lung epithelium; concentration gradients through haemodilution and presence of receptor systems for xenobiotics; excretion capabilities in the maternal and fetal compartments (maternal urine and fetal amniotic fluid); and, finally, metabolic potential of different maternal and fetal tissues. The toxicity on placental and fetal cells varies considerably. The metabolic potential of placental tissues for a PAH substrate (e.g., benzo-[α]-pyrene) is highly variable, but markedly augmented only in some samples in response to environmental cigarette smoke exposure. The increase in overall metabolism correlates with relative potentials for reactive metabolite generation or detoxification of xenobiotics. The specific metabolic conditions favouring these processes, yet remain unknown.

Detailed analyses of toxic bioactivation and detoxification processes in human trophoblast cells in a more defined system of trophoblastic explant and cell cultures have revealed interesting facts, in particular, on detoxification processes (Sanyal *et al.* 1993; Barnea *et al.* 1993). PAH xenobiotics may induce MFO enzyme systems in isolated trophoblast cells. Maternal serum derived from smokers and non-smokers or PAHs added to such cultures also differentially influence metabolic activities related to detoxification. Since placental cells contain enzymes associated with detoxification of a variety of xenobiotics, and environmental exposure, such as, that of cigarette smoke may induce detoxification processes in trophoblast cells, establish the possibility that placental tissues may indeed be an important site of detoxification.

XENOBIOTIC METABOLITE–DNA ADDUCTS IN HUMAN CONCEPTUS TISSUES

The reactive xenobiotics when produced in cells may bind covalently with macromolecules (nucleic acids and proteins) forming adducts (Fig. 23.3). Such adducts are specific markers for toxic xenobiotic exposure and their metabolic conditions in tissues. Various studies now show that human conceptus tissues of early pregnancy and term placentas produce and accumulate such adducts (Everson *et al.* 1986, 1988; Manchester *et al.* 1988, 1990, 1992; Hatch *et al.* 1990; Hansen *et al.* 1993; Randerath and Randerath 1993). Maternal cigarette smoke exposure generates a number of xenobiotic–DNA adducts including PAH–DNA adducts in term human placentas. The relative levels of such adducts in term placental tissues together with other exposure parameters of cigarette smoke have been shown to predict a deleterious fetal outcome (Everson *et al.* 1988). It is known that such binding may inhibit DNA (gene) replication, reduce DNA template activity, break DNA strands, or induce somatic mutations (Mizusawa and Kakefuda 1979; Haseltine *et al.* 1980; Obi *et al.* 1986; Arce *et al.* 1987; Reardon *et al.* 1989). The presence of one single adduct on the gene could profoundly affect that gene's expression (Koch *et al.* 1993). The replicating cells containing DNA adducts of reactive metabolites exhibit various mutations because the DNA polymerase may bypass such molecular lesions, and induce base substitutions in the new DNA that is synthesized (Eisenstadt *et al.* 1982; Vousden *et al.* 1986; Lawley 1987; Basic-Zaninovic *et al.* 1992). The nucleotide sequence modifications GC to AT for aliphatic alkylating agents and GC to TA for epoxide diol derivatives of PAH are the most prevalent.

The rate of spontaneous mutations per gene related to malformations during gestation in humans is approximately 0.7×10^{-5} to 1.4×10^{-5} (Nelson and Holmes 1989; Holland and Sielken 1993). Major congenital malformation due to a single gene mutation is estimated to be 0.07 per cent, and nearly 20 per cent of these are new spontaneous mutations. Mutational changes producing structurally variant human insulin by substitution of the amino acid Phe[B24/25] by Leu, resulting in diabetes mellitus, or changes in growth by alteration of Gly[119] of growth hormone, have been shown (Shoelson *et al.* 1983; Chen *et al.* 1991).

Xenobiotic–DNA adducts are a major source of somatic mutation in tissues. Such lesions of the genome are constantly repaired by base excision-repair mechanisms (Chen *et al.* 1990). Approximately 2.5×10^5 lesions of DNA occur in each cell per day, and reduced efficiency of this process, together with xenobiotic exposure, may increase the probability of such mutations (Swenberg *et al.* 1990). Thus, genotoxicity in conceptus tissues, in part, is presumably due to combined interactions of DNA-adduct generation and functions of repair system.

PHARMACOGENETICS RELATED TO METABOLISM OF XENOBIOTICS

The relative expression of such enzymes, based on hereditary determinants, influences adduct formation and other toxic processes in cells. Genetic polymorphisms of the principal metabolic enzymes related to PAH-metabolism have been shown to alter the capability of DNA–adduct generation in tissues (Seidegard *et al.* 1988; Guengerich 1991; Nebert *et al.* 1991, 1993; Shields *et al.* 1993; Hassett *et al.* 1994). The initial RFLP studies with lymphocytes showed that amplification of CYP1A1 activity is associated with a homozygosity of *Msp1* 1.9 kb DNA fragment with 12 per cent allelic frequency (Kawajiri *et al.* 1990; Peterson *et al.* 1991). Recent studies have demonstrated that polymorphism in the human CYP1A1 gene is due to mutations at two different sites, on exons 7 and 3′ in the non-coding region of the gene, and augmented expression of the CYP1A1 gene (mRNA levels) is related to such mutations (Crofts *et al.* 1994). In addition, since the Ah receptor system for PAH is the controlling element for CYP1A1 gene expression, functions of the Ah receptor and the nuclear translocator protein associated with Ah receptor, may also be important factors in regulating PAH metabolism (Manchester *et al.* 1987; Hankinson 1994).

The interindividual variation in different detoxifying enzyme activities is wide and specific allelic combination characteristics also determine their expression. The possibility of phenotyping and genotyping individuals for GST has been suggested in various recent studies. Deficiencies of GST-1 (μ class) produce an increase in the amount of DNA–adduct by xenobiotic exposure (Ichiba *et al.* 1994). The homozygosity and heterozygosity of genes for such enzymes influence their expression in tissues (Caporaso 1991). Thus, these hereditary metabolic determinants could be major regulatory factors in detoxification and toxic product formation from xenobiotics in both the maternal and fetal compartments.

In summary, it is likely that a combination of exposure to xenobiotics and influences of various hereditary factors associated with the expression of metabolic enzymes for reactive metabolite generation and detoxification processes in tissues may determine the toxicity processes. The rapidly dividing developing conceptus cells of early pregnancy are at a higher risk of genotoxic effects because the DNA adducts can be readily converted into mutations which will be reflected in innumerable cells with the progressing pregnancy. The human placental tissues may be an important site for detoxification of xenobiotics, supplementing maternal metabolic potential, is a developing concept. Since the trophoblast cell layer is the interface between the maternal and fetal compartments and expresses some of the principal enzymes involved in xenobiotic metabolism, these cells may participate in regulating transplacental toxicity of growing and differentiating embryo–fetal tissues.

ACKNOWLEDGEMENTS

Supported by grants from the NIH (ES -05337) and Neuroengineering and Neuroscience Center. The author thanks Dr Eytan R. Barnea for his interest and editorial help in preparation of this manuscript.

REFERENCES

Aiso, S., Yasuda, K., Shiozwa, M., Yamamoto, H., and Sogo, T. (1989). Preparation of monoclonal antibodies to glutathione S-transferase-π and application to immunohistochemical study. *Journal of Histochemistry and Cytochemistry*, 37, 1247–52.

Ames, B.N., Magaw, R., and Gold, L.S. (1987). Ranking possible carcinogenic hazards. *Science* **236**, 271–80.

Appel, B.R., Guirgis, G., Kim, I.S., Garbin, O., Fracchia, M., Flessel, *et al.* (1990). Benzene, benzo[*a*]pyrene and lead in smoke from tobacco products other than cigarettes. *American Journal of Public Health*, 80, 560–4.

Arce, G.T., Allen, J.W., Doerr, C.L., Elmore, E., Hatch, G.C., Moore, M.M., *et al.* (1987). Relationships between benzo[*a*]pyrene DNA adduct levels and genotoxic effects in mammalian cells. *Cancer Research*, 47, 3388–95.

Avigdor, S., Zekheim, D., and Barnea E.R. (1992). Quinone reductase activity in the first trimester placenta: effect of cigarette smoking, and polycyclic aromatic hydrocarbons. *Reproductive Toxicology*, 6, 363–6.

Barnea, E.R. (1993). Modulatory effect of maternal serum on xenobiotic metabolizing activity of placental explants: modification by cigarette smoking. *Human Reproduction*, 9, 1017–21.

Barnea, E.R., and Avigdor, S. (1990). Coordinated induction of estrogen hydroxylase activity and catechol-*O*-methyl transferase by xenobiotics in first trimester human placental explants. *Journal of Steroid Biochemistry*, 35, 327–31.

Barnea, E.R. and Avigdor, S. (1991). Aryl hydrocarbon hydroxylase activity in the first trimester placenta: induction by carcinogens and chemoprotectors. *Gynecological and Obstetrical Investigation*, 32, 4–9.

Barnea, E.R., Avigdor, S., Boady, W.Y., and Check, J.H. (1993). Effect of xenobiotics on quinone reductase activity in first trimester placental explants. *Human Reproduction*, 8, 102–6.

Barnea, E.R., Sorkin, M., and Barnea, J.D. (1995). Peroxidase activity and glutathione content in the first trimester placenta and decidua. *Early Pregnancy Biology and Medicine*, 1, 141–7.

Basic-Zaninovic, T., Palombo, F., Bignami, M., and Dogliotti, E. (1992). Fidelity of replication of the leading and lagging DNA strands opposite N-methyl-N-nitrosourea-induced DNA damage in human cells. *Nucleic Acid Research*, 20, 6543–8.

Bjorseth, A. and Becher, G. (1986). *PAH in work atmospheres: occurrence and determination.* CRC Press, Boca Raton, FL.

Caporaso, N.E. (1991). Genetic polymorphism of drug metabolism and host susceptibility to cancer in humans: current work with debrisoquine. In *Origins of cancer* (ed. J. Brugge, T. Curran, E. Harlow and F. McCormick), pp. 753–73. Cold Spring Harbor Laboratory Press.

Chen, R.H., Maher, V.M., and McCormick, J.J. (1990). Effect of excision repair by diploid human fibroblasts on the kinds and locations of mutation induced by (+/–) –7 beta, 8 alpha dihydroxy-9 alpha, 10 alpha-epoxy-7,8,9,10-tetrahydrobenzo *a*:pyrene in the coding region of the HPRT gene. *Proceedings of the National Academy of Sciences, USA*, 87, 8680–4.

Chen, W.Y., Wright, D.C., Mehta, B., Wagner, T.E., and Kopchick, J.J. (1991). Glycine 119 of bovine growth hormone is critical for growth-promoting activity. *Molecular Endocrinology*, 5, 1845–52.

Crofts, F., Taioli, E., Trachman, J., Cosma, G.N., Currie, D., Toniolo, P., *et al.* (1994). Functional significance of different human CYP1A1 genotypes. *Carcinogenesis*, 15, 2961–3.

DiFranza, J.R. and Lew, R.A. (1995). Effect of maternal cigarette smoking on pregnancy complications and sudden infant death syndrome. *Journal of Family Practice*, 40, 385–94.

Eisenstadt, E., Warren, A.J., Porter, J., Atkins, D., and Miller, J.H. (1982). Carcinogenic epoxides of benzo[*a*]pyrene and cyclopenta (*c,d*) pyrene induce base substitution. *Proceedings of the National Academy of Sciences, USA*, 79, 1945–9.

Ekwo, E.E., Gosselink, C.A., Woolson, R., and Moaward, A. (1993). Risk for premature rupture of amniotic membranes. *International Journal of Epidemiology*, **22**, 495–503.

Everson, R.B., Randerath, E., Santella, R.M., Cefalo, R.C., Avitts, T.A., and Randerath, K. (1986). Detection of smoking-related covalent DNA-adducts in human placenta. *Science*, **231**, 54–7.

Everson, R.B., Randerath, E., Santella, R.M., Avitts, T.A., Weinstein, I.B., and Randerath, K. (1988). Quantitative association between DNA damage in human placenta and maternal smoking and birth weight. *Journal of the National Cancer Institute*, **80**, 567–75.

Gelboin, H.V., Fujino, T., Song, B.J., Park, S.S., Cheng, K.C., West, D., *et al.* (1984). Monoclonal antibody-directed phenotyping of cytochrome P-450 by enzyme inhibition, immunopurification, and radioimmunoassay. In *Genetic variability in response to chemical exposure*, (ed. G.S. Omen and H.V. Gelboin), Branbury Report 16, pp. 65–85. Cold Spring Harbor Laboratory Press, NY.

Grasso, P. (1984). Carcinogens in food. In *Chemical carcinogens*, (ed. C.E. Searle), ACS Monograph, Vol. **182**, pp. 1205–39. American Chemical Society, Washington, DC.

Guengerich, F.P. (1991). Interindividual variation in biotransformation of carcinogens: basis and relevance. In *Molecular dosimetry and human cancer*, (ed. J.D. Groopman and P.L. Skipper), pp. 27–51. CRC Press, Boca Raton, FL.

Hankinson, O. (1994). A genetic analysis of processes regulating cytochrome P4501A1 expression. *Advances in Enzyme Regulation*, **34**, 59–171.

Hansen, C., Asmussen, I., and Autrup, H. (1993). Detection of carcinogen–DNA-adducts in human fetal tissues by ^{32}P-postlabeling procedure. *Environmental Health Perspectives*, **99**, 229–31.

Haseltine, W.A., Lo, K.M., and D'Andrea, A.D. (1980). Preferred sites of strand scission in DNA modified by anti-diol epoxide of benzo[*a*]pyrene. *Science*, **209**, 929–31.

Hassett, C., Aicher, L., Sidhu, J.S., and Omiecinski, C.J. (1994). Human microsomal epoxide hydrolase: genetic polymorphism and functional expression *in vitro* of amino acid variants. *Human Molecular Genetics*, **3**, 421–8.

Hatch, M.C., Warburton, D., and Santella, R.M. (1990). Polycyclic aromatic hydrocarbon–DNA-adducts in spontaneously aborted fetal tissues. *Carcinogenesis*, **11**, 1673–5.

Holland, C.D. and Sielken, R.L. (1993). *Quantitative cancer modeling and risk assessment*. Prentice-Hall, Englewood Cliffs, NJ.

Huel, G., Godin, J., and Moreau, M. (1989). Aryl hydrocarbon hydroxylase activity in human placenta of passive smokers. *Environmental. Research*, **50**, 173–83.

Ichiba, M., Hagmar, L., Rannug, A., Hogstedt, B., Alexandrie, A.K., Carstensen, U., and Hemminki, K. (1994). Aromatic DNA adducts, micronuclei and genetic polymorphism for CYP1A1 and GST1 in chimney sweeps. *Carcinogenesis*, **15**, 1347–52.

Jerina, D.M., Sayer, J.M., Agrawal, S.K., Yogi, H., Levin, W., Wood, A.W., *et al.* (1986). Reactivity and tumorigenicity of bay-region diol epoxide derived from polycyclic aromatic hydrocarbons. In *Biological reactive intermediates III*, (ed. J.J. Kocsis, D.J. Jollow, C.M. Witmer, J.O. Nelson, and R. Snyder), pp. 11–30. Plenum Press, New York.

Jernstrom, B., Martinez, M., and Dock, L. (1990). Glutathione transferase catalysed conjugation of benzo-[α]-pyrene diol-epoxide with glutathione in rat hepatocytes. In *Glutathione S-transferase and drug resistance*, (ed. J.D. Hayes, C.B. Pickett, and T.J. Mantle), pp. 111–20. Taylor and Francis, London.

Juchau, M.R. (1989). Bioactivation in chemical teratogenesis. *Annual Review of Pharmacology and Toxicology*, **29**, 165–87.

Juchau, M.R. (1990). Fetal and neonatal drug biotransformation. In *Drug toxicity and metabolism in pediatrics*, (ed. S. Kacew), pp. 15–34. CRC Press, Boca Raton, FL.

Kadlubar, F.F. and Hammons, G.J. (1987). The role of cytochrome P-450 in the metabolism of chemical carcinogens. In *Mammalian cytochrome P-450*, Vol. II, (ed. F.P. Guengerich), pp. 1–139. CRC Press, Boca Raton, FL.

Kawajiri, K., Nakachi, K., Imai, K., Yoshii, A., Shinoda, N., and Watanabe, J. (1990). Identification of genetically high risk individuals to lung cancer by DNA polymorphism on cytochrome P 450 A1 gene. *FEBS Letters*, 263, 131–3.

Koch, K.S., Fletcher, R.G., Groun, M.P., Inyang, A.I., Lu, X.P., Brenner, D.A., *et al.* (1993). Inactivation of plasmid reporter gene expression by one benzo[*a*]pyrene diol-epoxide DNA adduct in adult rat hepatocytes. *Cancer Research*, 53, 2279–86.

Lawley, P.D. (1987). Concepts of carcinogenesis. In *Biology of carcinogenesis*, (ed. M.J. Waring and B. Ponder), pp. 1–21. MTP Press, Boston.

Lewtas, J. (1989). Toxicology of complex mixture of indoor air pollutants. *Annual Review of Pharmacology and Toxicology*, 29, 415–32.

Li, C.Q., Windsor, R.A., Perkins, L., Goldenberg, and Lowe, J.B. (1993). The impact of infant birth weight and gestational age of cotinine validated smoking reduction during pregnancy. *Journal of the American Medical Association*, 269, 1519–24.

Lieberman, E., Gremy, I., Lang, J.M., and Cohen, A.P. (1994). Low birth weight at term and the timing of fetal exposure to maternal smoking. *American Journal of Public Health*, 84, 1127–31.

Loforth, G. (1989). Environmental tobacco smoke: overview of chemical composition and genotoxic components. *Mutation Research*, 222, 73–80.

Manchester, D.K. and Jacoby, E.H. (1982). Glutathione S-transferase activities from smoking and nonsmoking women. *Xenobiotica*, 12, 543–7.

Manchester, D.K., Gordon, S.K., Golas, C.L., Roberts, E.A., and Okey A.B. (1987). Ah receptor in human placenta: stabilization by molybdate and characterization of binding of 2,3,7,8-tetra chloro-dibenzo-*p*-dioxin, 3-methylcholanthrene and benzo[*a*]pyrene. *Cancer Research*, 47, 4861–8.

Manchester, D.K., Weston, A., Choi, J.S., Trivers, G., Fennessey, P.V., Quintana, E., *et al.* (1988). Detection of benzo[*a*]pyrene diol epoxide–DNA adducts in human placenta. *Proceedings of the National Academy of Sciences, USA*, 85, 9243–7.

Manchester, D.K., Wilson, V.L., Hsu, I.C., Choi, J.S., Parker, N.B., Mann, D.L., *et al.* (1990). Synchronous fluorescence spectroscopic, immunoaffinity chromatographic, and ^{32}P-postlabeling analysis of human placental DNA known to contain benzo[*a*]pyrene diol epoxide adducts. *Carcinogenesis*, 11, 553–9.

Manchester, D.K., Bowman, E.D., Parker, N.B., Caporaso, N.E., and Weston, A. (1992). Determinants of polycyclic aromatic hydrocarbon–DNA-adducts in human placenta. *Cancer Research*, 52, 1499–503.

Mizusawa, H. and Kakefuda, T. (1979). Inhibition of DNA synthesis *in vitro* by binding of benzo[*a*]pyrene metabolite diol-epoxide 1 to DNA. *Nature*, 279, 775–7.

Nebert, D.W. (1991). Role of genetics and drug metabolism in human cancer risk. *Mutation Research*, 247, 267–81.

Nebert, D.W., Puga, A., and Vasiliou, V. (1993). Role of Ah receptor and the dioxin-inducible (Ah) gene battery in toxicity, cancer and signal transduction. *Annals of the New York Academy of Sciences*, 685, 624–40.

Nelson, D.R., Koymans, L., Kamataki, T., Stegeman, J.J., Feyerisen, R., Waxman, D.J., *et al.* (1996). The P450 gene superfamily: update of new sequences, gene mapping accession numbers and nomenclature. *Pharmacogenetics*, 6, 1–42..

Nelson, K. and Holmes, L.B. (1989). Malformations due to presumed spontaneous mutations in newborn infants. *New England Journal of Medicine*, 320, 19–23.

Obi, F.O., Ryan, A.J., and Billett, M.A. (1986). Preferential binding of carcinogen to DNA in active chromatin and nuclear matrix. *Carcinogenesis*, 7, 907–13.

Pacifici, G.M. and Rane, A. (1982). Metabolism of styrene oxide in different human fetal tissues. *Drug Metabolism and Disposition*, 10, 302–5.

Pasanen, M. and Pelkonen, O. (1990). Xenobiotic and steroid-metabolizing monooxygenase catalyzed by cytochrome P-450 and glutathione S-transferase conjugations in the human placenta and their relationships to maternal cigarette smoking. *Placenta*, 11, 75–85.

Pasanen, M. and Pelkonen, O. (1994). The expression and environmental regulation of P450 enzymes in human placenta. *Critical Reviews in Toxicology*, **24**, 211–29.

Pasanen, M., Stenback, F., Park, S.S., Gelboin, H.V., and Pelkonen, O. (1988). Immuno-histochemical detection of human placental cytochrome P-450-associated mono-oxygenase system inducible by maternal cigarette smoking. *Placenta*, **9**, 267–75.

Peterson, D.D., McKinney, C.E., Ikeya, K., Smith, H.H., Bale, A.E., McBride O.W., and Nebert, D.W. (1991). Human CYP1A1 gene: cosegregation of the enzyme inducibility phenotype and an RFLP. *American Journal of Human Genetics*, **48**, 720–5.

Randerath, E. and Randerath, K. (1993). Monitoring tobacco smoke-induced DNA damage by ^{32}P-postlabeling. In *Postlabeling methods for detection of DNA-adducts*, (ed. D.H. Phillips and H. Bartsch), pp. 305–13. IACR, Lyon.

Reardon, D.B., Bigger, C.A.H., Strandberg, J., Yagi, H., Jerina, D.M., and Dipple, A. (1989). Sequence selectivity in reaction of optically active hydrocarbon dihydrodiol epoxides with rat *H-ras* DNA. *Chemimal Research and Toxicology*, **2**, 12–14.

Sanyal, M.K., Li, Y.L., and Belanger, K. (1994). Metabolism of polynuclear aromatic hydrocarbon in human placenta influenced by cigarette smoke exposure. *Reproductive Toxicology*, **8**, 411–18.

Sanyal, M.K., Li, Y.L., Biggers, W.J., Satish, J., and Barnea, E.R. (1993). Augmentation of polynuclear aromatic hydrocarbon metabolism of human placental tissues of first trimester pregnancy by cigarette smoke exposure. *American Journal of Obstetrics and Gynecology*, **168**, 1587–97.

Schoendorf, K.C. and Kiely, J.L. (1992). Relationship of sudden infant death syndrome to maternal smoking during and after pregnancy. *Pediatrics*, **90**, 905–8.

Seidegard, T., Voracheck, W.R., Pero, R.W., and Pearson, W.R. (1988). Hereditary differences in the expression of human glutathione transferase active on trans-stilbene oxide are due to gene deletion. *Proceedings of the National Academy of Sciences, USA*, **85**, 7293–7.

Seinfeld, J.H. (1989). Urban air pollution—state of the science. *Science*, **243**, 745–52.

Shields, P.G., Bowman, E.D., Harrington, A.M., Doan, V.T., and Weston, A. (1993). Polycyclic aromatic hydrocarbon–DNA adducts in human lung and cancer susceptibility genes. *Cancer Research*, **53**, 3486–92.

Shoelson, S., Haneda, M., Blix, P., Nanjo, A., Sanke, T., Inouye, K., et al. (1983). Three mutant insulins in man. *Nature*, **302**, 540–3.

Sugimura, T. and Wakabayashi, K. (1990). In *Mutagens in food*. Mutagens and carcinogens in the diet. (ed. M.W. Pariza, J.S. Felton, H. Aeschbacher, and S. Sato), pp. 1–18. Wiley-Liss, New York.

Swenberg, J.A., Fedtke, N., Fennelll, T.R., and Walker, V.E. (1990). Relationship between carcinogen exposure, DNA adducts and carcinogenesis. In *Progress in predictive toxicology*, (ed. D.B. Clayson, J.C. Munro, P. Shubick, and J.A. Swenberg), pp. 161–84. Elsevier, New York.

Tomatis, L. (1994). Transgeneration carcinogenesis: a review of the experimental and epidemiological evidence. *Japanese Journal of Cancer Research*, **85**, 443–54.

Tuomisto, J. and Vartiainen, T. (1990). In *Genotoxicity of drinking waters*. Complex mixtures and cancer risk. (ed. H. Vainio, M. Sorsa, and A.J. McMichael), pp. 307–13. IARC publication No 104. International Agency for Cancer Research, Lyon.

Vartiainen, T., Liimatainen, A., Kauranen, P., and Hiisvirta, L. (1988). Relation between drinking water mutagenicity and water quality parameters. *Chemosphere*, **17**, 189–202.

Vousden, K.H., Bos, J.L., Marshall, C.J., and Phillips, D.H. (1986). Mutations activating human *c-a-ras1* proto-oncogene (*H-ras 1*) induced by chemical carcinogens and depurination. *Proceedings of the National Academy of Sciences, USA*, **83**, 1222–6.

Wen, S.W., Goldenberg, R.L., Culter, G.R., Hoffman, H.J., Clivers, S.P., Davis, R.O., et al. (1990). Smoking, maternal age, fetal growth, and gestational age at delivery. *American Journal of Obstetrics and Gynecology*, **162**, 53–8.

Wixtrom, R.N., Silva, M.H., and Hammock, B.D. (1988). Cytosolic epoxide hydrolase in human placenta. *Placenta*, **9**, 559–63.

V | *Relevance of the embryo to medicine*

24 | *Transgenesis: molecular manipulation of the genome*

Paul N. Schofield

Transgenesis is the procedure by which a novel piece of DNA is inserted into the genome of a plant or animal *in vivo*; it is now fifteen years since the first transgenic mice were born and more than six years since the first gene was successfully knocked out by homologous recombination. The facility to make specific mutations at will in the mammalian genome has not only revolutionized our ability to analyse the biology of genetic disorders but has also allowed the probing of the molecular mechanisms of development and normal physiology. The genetic approach to such analyses has always been extremely powerful, particularly in organisms with small genomes and short reproductive cycles such as the fruit fly *Drosophila*. However, reliance on naturally occurring mutations in vertebrates carries with it the enormous task of mapping and characterizing the locus, even if appropriate mutations are available. This approach has clearly been of great utility, for example in the study of muscular dystrophy (see Davies *et al.* 1995). However, the approach of reverse genetics, making the mutation first then analysing its effects, has proved to be comparatively rapid and capable of providing enormous amounts of information.

The area of transgenesis has expanded rapidly, and the rate of technological innovation has accelerated in recent years. Consequently this chapter can only scratch the surface of the techniques of manipulating the mammalian genome and the potential applications of this current technology. The reader is referred to recent excellent reviews on specialized areas of transgenesis which are much more detailed that the account given here (Brinster 1993; Camper *et al.* 1995; Ward *et al.* 1995).

INSERTIONAL TRANSGENESIS: TECHNIQUES AND APPLICATIONS

The addition of genetic material to the genome may be achieved in a variety of ways. Most transgenics are produced by the injection of DNA constructs directly into the pronuclei of the fertilized mouse egg. Following replacement into pseudopregnant foster mothers the zygote develops to term and all of the cells in the animal contain copies of the gene. Integration of the gene is effectively a random event due to non-homologous recombination, which gives rise to the source of much variability in expression of transgenes as a result of position effect. Such an effect may either silence or enhance expression from a given transgene or possibly place it in a region subject to other forms of regulation such as genomic imprinting. A transgene may sometimes interrupt an endogenous gene causing an insertional mutagenic event in its own right. Insertional mutagenesis is estimated to occur in 5–10 per cent of all transgenic lines, and has proved to be a useful tool for the discovery of genes involved in embryonic and adult growth (e.g. Xiang *et al.* 1990; Perry *et al.* 1995; see Copp 1995 and Meisler 1992 for extensive reviews).

Insertional transgenesis may also be carried out using replication defective retroviruses expressing the gene under investigation from either the LTR, or from an internal promoter. Direct infection of embryos with packaged retroviral genomes was amongst one of the earliest techniques used and leads to insertion of the viral construct into the genomic DNA of the embryo. As with pronuclear injections this technique also generates insertional mutations as was noted with the inactivation of the $\alpha(1)1$ collagen gene (Barker *et al.* 1991).

More recently, insertion of DNA or retroviral constructs into embryonic stem (ES) cells derived from the inner cell mass of the blastocyst, either by electroporation or retroviral infection, has proved a powerful technique. ES cells are transfected in culture and then reinjected into a host blastocyst to generate a chimera. Chimeras which transmit the transgene through the germ line are then identified and the mutations bred to homozygosity. This technique has several advantages. Firstly it is possible to check that the construct is active in the clone selected for blastocyst injection, and secondly the possibility of working with genetically chimeric animals may obviate the problems associated with an embryonic lethal effect of the transgene.

TRANSGENESIS AS A TOOL IN THE ANALYSIS OF REGULATION OF GENE EXPRESSION

Some of the earliest studies of integrated transgenes demonstrated that there was no simple relationship between the number of transgenes and the level of expression, and that certain regulatory properties were missing, even though all of the gene and its immediate regulatory sequences were present in the construct (see Chada *et al.* 1985). This led investigators to increase the size of DNA injected in an attempt to search for distal *cis*-acting sequences. The β-globin cluster has been most extensively analysed in this way, by the search for position-independent expression and appropriate regulation. This study demonstrated that large stretches of DNA had to be used in the constructs carrying distal regulatory elements (e.g. Strouboulis *et al.* 1992). These contain DNAase I sensitive sites which appear to delineate domains of chromatin probably corresponding to functional domains with respect to regulatory mechanisms together with distal enhancer elements and the LCR sequences (locus control regions) (Grosveld *et al.* 1993). Similar studies have been carried out with the chicken lysozyme gene (Bonifer *et al.* 1994). Whilst DNA fragments of around 70 kb were used in these studies, the use of yeast artificial chromosomes has now opened up the possibility of the insertion of much larger DNA fragments. Interestingly, the use of human genes in a transgenic mouse has lead to a greater understanding of the evolutionary divergence of control of individual members of the β-globin cluster. The analysis of a novel method of gene control, genomic imprinting (see below), is in principle also approachable by this strategy and Efstratiadis and co-workers have demonstrated a parent-of-origin effect for one out of six transgenes containing DNA from the IGF-II locus, implying the presence of *cis*-acting regulatory elements in this domain (Lee *et al.* 1993).

Extensive flanking sequences are not always required to generate position-independent appropriate regulation of gene expression, and for example the sequences required by the insulin gene to target its expression to the pancreatic β cells are substantially smaller (Bucchini *et al.* 1986; Dandoy-Dron *et al.* 1991), although it is as yet unclear which sequences are responsible for the extrapancreatic expression found during development (Dandoy-Dron *et al.* 1995). Similar approaches have been taken with other genes which generally involve the use of a reporter gene such as bacterial β-galactosidase (*LacZ*), chloramphenicol acetyl transferase (CAT), or SV40T antigen attached to the promoter and regulatory sequences. In some cases, species-specific features of the normal gene product allow discrimination between the transgenic and endogenous proteins. The expression of the reporter or generation of tumours (SV40T) then defines the tissue-specific domain of gene expression driven by the promoter sequences. These approaches have defined regulatory elements in renin (Sigmund *et al.* 1990), β-lactoglobulin (Whitelaw *et al.* 1992), the dopamine β-hydroxylase promoter (Mercer *et al.* 1991), and IGF-II (Lee *et al.* 1993) for example.

TRANSGENESIS TO ANALYSE DEVELOPMENTAL AND PHYSIOLOGICAL MECHANISMS

Not only do the above studies give us information on the promoter elements present in the constructs, but they also provide tools for the targeting of proteins of interest to specific lineages or tissues. This is invaluable in the analysis of both physiological and developmental processes. Lineage analysis may be carried out so long as a promoter is available which will drive the expression of a gene in the lineage under investigation. In one strategy a deliberate frame shift mutation is created in the *LacZ* reporter gene which inactivates it (Sanes 1994). Reverting mutations restoring the reading frame occur at a frequency of about 10^{-6}, consequently LacZ-expressing cells are only likely to occur very rarely and if sufficient animals are examined their presence gives information on clonal lineage relationships.

Two complementary approaches have been taken in the analysis of pancreatic islet lineage. In one case the SV40T antigen (TAg) is attached to the rat insulin promoter (RIP), pancreatic tissue is then examined at differing times of development in the preneoplastic phase of tumour formation, and co-expression of the reporter gene and other endogenous lineage markers established (Alpert *et al.* 1988; Teitelman 1993). An alternative approach is to ablate specific lineages with peptide toxins (e.g. diphtheria toxin) expressed from highly lineage-specific promoters. This approach in the pancreas, using regulatory elements for insulin, glucagon, and pancreatic polypeptide, has led to differing conclusions from those of Hanahan and co-workers (Herrera *et al.* 1994). Interestingly this discrepancy may reflect inter-lineage interactions in the formation of the pancreas, and demonstrates the power of the combined approaches to unravelling cell/cell interactions in development.

Targeting of genes to ectopic sites or dyschronic periods of expression is a powerful tool in the analysis of a wide variety of processes. Problems arise when appropriate promoters are not readily available or when continuous expression may be deleterious or even lethal in the embryo. For example, attempts to express IGF-II from the ubiquitous H2k^b promoter failed to generate transgenic mice in one study (C. Ellis, personal communication) and in a second, only lines expressing the gene at relatively low levels proved viable (Van Buul-Offers *et al.* 1995), probably as a result of overexpression having a toxic effect on the embryo. Consequently targeting to particular tissues using heterologous promoters is often the method of choice. This has been carried out with IGF-II driven by a major urinary protein (MUP) promoter directing expression to the liver (Rogler *et al.* 1994), a cytokeratin promoter to the skin (Ward *et al.* 1994a,b), and a β-lactoglobulin (BLG) promoter to the mammary epithelium (Bates *et al.* 1995). In all of these cases expression is of a relatively late onset and although systemic levels of the growth factor are elevated this is sufficiently late so as not to compromise development. Viral promoters have been useful, for example in the MoMulv LTR driven GM-CSF expression (Lang *et al.* 1987) and the relatively ubiquitous metallothionein promoter (Palmiter *et al.* 1983) which has the advantages of inducibility, albeit limited. Recent developments have generated a transactivator system responsive to derivatives of tetracycline, which has very low levels of constitutive activity and will induce expression by two or three orders of magnitude (Gossen *et al.* 1995; Shockett *et al.* 1995). Such a system is very promising for future widespread use, where inducible expression is required to prevent embryonic lethality.

Targeted oncogenesis, usually by the expression of a temperature sensitive (ts) TAg is now a widely used technique for generating conditionally immortalized cells from tissues, and the 'oncomouse', which expresses SV40T antigen from the H2k promoter, provides a rapid route into generation of permanent cell lines (Jat *et al.* 1991). Targeted tumour formation can in addition give useful information on the process of tumourigenesis and has been used in the study of pancreatic tumour formation (Christofori and Hanahan 1994) and in examining the role of cyclin D1 in mammary carcinogenesis (Wang *et al.* 1994).

TRANSGENESIS AND HUMAN DISEASE MODELS

Although gene ablation has now been extensively used to model several specific single gene disorders (see below), insertional transgenesis has proved valuable in assessing the potential for human gene therapy and in examining mechanisms involved in gene action. One of the first successful genome repairs was the correction of the hypogonadal mouse by expression of GnRH (Mason *et al.* 1986). Several groups have corrected the dystrophic phenotype in the naturally occurring dystrophic (*mdx*) mouse (eg. Phelps *et al.* 1995), which suffers from a similar lesion to that found in humans. The dwarf *lit/lit* mouse, which lacks growth hormone, has been corrected by expression of both GH and IGF-I (Hammer *et al.* 1984, Behringer *et al.* 1990), indicating IGF-I as a potential therapeutic agent in GH-dependent disease, and sex reversal has been generated by the insertion of *sry* into the genome (Koopman *et al.* 1991). While there are frequently differences between the human and murine disorders, of greater or lesser significance, the value of the transgenic mouse as a system in which to test potential therapies is invaluable. One such therapy recently excluded by this method is the use of apodystrophin 71 (Dp71) (Hoffmann 1995) to alleviate the *mdx* phenotype, which had been a potentially more tractable approach, involving the insertion of a functional but shorter isoform of dystrophin. A more successful approach has been reported with cystic fibrosis (Hyde *et al.* 1993).

GENE INACTIVATION AND TARGETED MUTAGENESIS

Observations of the apparent randomness of gene insertion in vertebrates suggested that the mechanism of homologous recombination operating in yeast and other organisms either did not operate on exogenously introduced DNA or was extremely rare. In order to select for such potential rare events where homologous DNA inserted into the endogenous gene, elegant selectable constructs were developed by Capecchi and co-workers (Mansour *et al.* 1988). These relied on having a stretch of cellular DNA interrupted by a selectable marker, Neo^r, conferring resistance to G418 selection to select for recombinants. This selection alone is not specific for homologous recombination, and all integrants will confer resistance. In order to select for this small number of homologous recombination events a negative selectable marker, herpes simplex virus thymidine kinase (HSV TK), was introduced. In homologous recombination events this marker is lost, and consequently clones in which the endogenous gene is targeted are insensitive to the lethal effects of gancyclovir (Mansour *et al.* 1988). This positive/negative selection has proved a most reliable method, and coupled with the sensitive PCR technique for positively identifying homologous recombinants, has proved very effective. The frequency of knockouts by this technique was originally reported to be at least 5 per cent of antibiotic resistant clones obtained, depending on the gene targeted, which represents a significant enhancement over vectors without the facility for negative selection. Use of isogenic DNA in the homology regions of the targeting construct in itself can markedly increase the frequency of knockouts in the absence of negative selection (te Riele *et al.* 1992). More recently a technique based on an enhancer trap has been developed by Smith and co-workers (Mountford *et al.* 1994) which increases the efficiency of knockout substantially; up to 80 per cent of colonies screened in the reported knockout of the transcription factor *Oct-4* resulted from homologous recombination. So long as the gene targeted is expressed in ES cells at significant levels, then construction of a targeting vector without a promoter driving the reporter/resistance gene only yields G418-resistant colonies on homologous recombination, transcription of the selectable marker (β-geo) being driven by the endogenous promoter and translation assisted by the presence of an internal ribosome entry site (IRES). The availability of these techniques has now made homologous recombination a relatively routine operation, though very much gene dependent.

Whilst most experiments are aimed at generating functional gene deletions by the insertion of material into the coding sequence of the target gene, the technique is capable of inserting specific mutations constructed *in vitro* into the germ line, and even replacing an endogenous gene with a completely different gene which will then be driven off the endogenous promoter. Such an approach has been successful with the α-lactalbumin gene (Stacey *et al.* 1994). This is potentially a way of expressing the gene of choice in a pattern shown by another gene or introducing subtle function-altering mutations directly into the germ line (Wu *et al.* 1994).

The great advantage of homologous recombination ('gene knockout') is that it provides a method of generating recessive mutations in specific genes which may be bred to homozygosity in the absence of a wild type allele. This obviates the problem with insertional transgenics where usually only dominant mutations will have a potential phenotype, and widens the applicability and power of the technique enormously. In the situation where haploid insufficiency generates a phenotype it may not even be necessary to breed to homozygosity. The power of this technique is amply demonstrated by the number of analyses which have been undertaken. In a recently published survey (Brandon *et al.* 1995) at least 263 knockouts had been reported, with the number increasing year by year.

Gene ablation has been used extensively to examine the role of specific genes during development and adult life. For example the deletion of LIF (Stewart *et al.* 1992) and cadherin (Larue *et al.* 1994) has profound effects on preimplantation development, and deletion of Mash-2 affects placentation (Guillemot *et al.* 1995). Deletion of, for example, particular homeodomain-containing or related genes (Jonsson *et al.* 1994; Subramanian *et al.* 1995) results in anteriorization of vertebrae (amongst other effects) or deletion of the pancreatic rudiment respectively. Severe organism-lethal phenotypes are problematical with knockout experiments, and it is often the case that gene ablation kills the embryo before the time window of interest. Consequently, inducible gene ablation is an attractive system. This has now become possible thanks to the exploitation of the *cre/lox* system in which *loxP* recombinase target sequences are placed on either side of the target gene by homologous recombination. Until the activation of the *cre* recombinase the gene functions perfectly well, then at a predetermined point a recombinase under the control of an inducible or tissue-specific promoter is turned on; this induces recombination between the *lox* sites, generating a tissue- or time-specific gene deletion. Inducible recombination has been demonstrated under the control of an interferon-inducible promoter (Kuhn *et al.* 1995), and it will only be a matter of time now before other inducible systems are available to generate deletion of genes in specific tissues at specific times of development.

GENE ABLATION AND MULTI-GENE PROCESSES

One of the most powerful applications of the gene knockout system is in the analysis of multicomponent systems. The activin/inhibin system has been extensively studied, as have the genes involved in establishing the muscle lineage in development (Rudnicki *et al.* 1992; Hasty *et al.* 1993; Tajbahksh and Buckingham 1994), factors involved in the metabolism of low density lipoprotein (Ishibashi *et al.* 1994), and the insulin-like growth factor system (reviewed by Efstratiadis 1994). In many cases of single gene knockouts the phenotype has either been observed to be much less severe than might have been predicted by other experimental approaches, or in some cases to have profound or unexpected effects. In the deletion of TGFβ, it appears that compensation for gene inactivation may come from transplacental transport of maternal protein (Letterio *et al.* 1994), but in other cases, particularly the IGFs, there is the added complication of redundancy between members of the same growth factor family. Such problems are probably the most profound facing the interpretation of gene ablation. Should functional redundancy be widespread in essential systems, then a lack of apparent effect may well simply reflect that redundancy, although it should be stressed that one might get normal development of an organ or organism through different routes depending on the lesions made. Increasingly, examples where knockout seems to have a minimal effect are being seen to suffer from defects in specific systems when examined in detail, and there are few mutants which can genuinely be claimed to be neutral. The way around problems of this nature is to combine gene ablations made in individual lines by breeding. In this way all of the receptors and ligands, for example in a growth factor family, can be removed in whatever combination is required and the effects noted. This has been achieved for the IGF family of molecules by Efstratiadis and co-workers over the last few years and this work has generated a paradigm for other investigations. The area has recently been exhaustively reviewed by Ward *et al.* (1995) and Efstratiadis (1994), and so will only be discussed in outline here.

The IGFs are part of a family of peptides related to insulin, which interact with at least three receptors. The two highest affinity receptors, the type 1 IGF and the type 2 receptor are profoundly different. The type 1 receptor is an $\alpha_2\beta_2$ transmembrane tyrosine kinase related to the insulin receptor, whilst the type 2 is the cation-independent mannose 6-phosphate receptor and seems to have a bifunctional role in that it is involved in targeting lysosomal enzymes to lysosomes and binds extracellular IGF-II. There has been considerable controversy not only about the role of the IGFs in individual developmental and other growth processes, but also the role of the type 2 receptor, previously suggested to either signal independently or to be simply acting as a sink for extracellular IGF-II. Deletion of the *Igf2* gene itself held a great many surprises, and led to the discovery that the gene was regulated by genomic imprinting. Deletion of IGF-II leads to a greatly reduced birth weight (60 per cent of normal) and placental mass (75 per cent of normal) with effects visible from embryonic day. However, unexpectedly, this effect is seen when the deletion is heterozygous in the animals carrying the deficient chromosome from the father and not from the mother. This gamete-of-origin effect is termed 'genomic imprinting' and was found to reflect the normal expression pattern of IGF-II where the maternal allele is normally expressed at about 5 per cent or less of the paternal allele (de Chiara *et al.* 1991). Consequently, mice inheriting the deficiency from the father are effectively homozygous nulls and have the same phenotype as true homozygous null mice. Type 1 receptor deletion leads to a more severe phenotype than expected from the ligand ablation, but when mutants were combined it led to the unexpected conclusion that whilst

IGF-I only acts through the type 1 receptor, IGF-II seems to act through a combination of a type 1 receptor and a second unknown receptor, not the type 2, which seemed in addition to be the sole mediator of the effects of IGF-II on placental growth (Liu *et al.* 1993). Cells derived from animals lacking type 1 receptors are now proving invaluable for the dissection of IGF-I-dependent processes such as cell growth and transformation (Sell *et al.* 1994). Recent deletion of the type 2 receptor seems to lead to an increase in IGF levels with concomitant hypertrophy, as expected from the postulated role for the type 2 receptor in turnover of extracellular IGF-II (Lau *et al.* 1994).

The implication of genomic imprinting in regulation of the *IGF-II* gene led to a search for the same phenomenon at other loci, and it is now clear that several other genes, often clustered, share the same mode of regulation. A combination of powerful genomic knockout experiments combined with a gene-introduction transgenic approach are beginning to unravel something of the mechanism of genomic imprinting, which may be effected within domains of contiguous genes (Leighton *et al.* 1995*a*, *b*; Viville and Surani 1995). The observation that removal of the DNA methylase enzyme by gene ablation (Li *et al.* 1992, 1993) leads to the loss of imprinting of some genes further supports the hypothesis that CpG methylation may be important in either initiating or maintaining the imprinted status.

GENE ABLATION AND HUMAN DISEASE

In several genes we know from the experience of human genetics that single gene defects may have a catastrophic effect on the individual, specifically in cases such as growth hormone deficiency (Behringer *et al.* 1988), cystic fibrosis (Snouwaert *et al.* 1992), and other disorders such as citrullinaemia (Patejunas *et al.* 1994) or fragile-X syndrome (Bakker *et al.* 1994). In these cases gene ablation has allowed the generation of a mouse model of the human disease, which whilst not always precisely the same as in the human, provides aspects of the disease which can be used as therapeutic targets in experimental procedures, such as gene therapy, aimed at alleviating the disease pathology.

The usefulness of transgenic techniques in looking at disease in model organisms (Clarke 1994) raises the question of whether it would be possible to treat genetic disease in humans by similar techniques. The possibility of human gene replacement may now appear to be a reality, with the advancement of *in vitro* fertilization techniques. However, we must consider very seriously the feasibility and desirability of carrying out transgenic procedures on humans in the same way as we do on mice.

For the most part only recessive disorders may be treated by gene replacement. The requirement for ES cells from each individual makes homologous recombination an impossible route to replace dominant mutations. Diseases which would be amenable to treatment must be those with a familial history or where parental carrier status is known, and those such as Duchenne muscular dystrophy or Huntington's chorea which arise sporadically with a high incidence do not present the possibility of intervention at conception.

The frequency of successful transgenesis in mice is estimated at about 20 per cent of transferred embryos in the most successful laboratories. To reach this figure several hundred eggs have to be injected, and the rate of successful embryo transfer is relatively high. In humans few eggs may be aspirated during any one cycle of IVF, and the rate of establishment of successful pregnancy is relatively low. The logistics clearly show that even if it were considered desirable to correct gene defects at conception, the procedure is highly unlikely to work at an acceptable rate in humans. In addition, about 5 per cent of transgenes in mice interrupt existing genes and cause insertional mutagenesis. Such a frequency suggests that the mutagenic risk in itself might be unacceptable and, by way of comparison, is enormously higher than the risk, for example, of Down syndrome in a 40-year-old woman. An additional unknown is the effect of genetic background on the expression levels of particular genes. This is known to be significant in mice, and we have no indication of how the diverse genetic backgrounds found in human populations may affect the expression of transgenes. On balance the most useful intervention at pre-implantation stages is still the selection of embryos lacking the mutant allele of a disease gene for reimplantation.

The most optimistic approach for human gene therapy still lies in the correction of the defect in a subpopulation of stem cells. In adults this is frequently problematic as, with the exception of the blood, stem cells are often uncharacterized and inaccessible. Inevitably as research progresses some systems will become efficiently targetable. However, to return a gene to all of the stem cells of an affected tissue, such as muscle, is a major technical challenge which so far has not been met. The only success has been in the replacement of the adenosine deaminase (ADA) gene in patients suffering from ADA deficiency where medium term success has recently been reported (Blaese *et al.* 1995). A much more attractive option is to target fetal stem cells in a particular organ. This has the advantage of targeting a population which will contribute extensively to the affected tissue and reduces the potential target number of tissue-specific essential genes whose insertional mutagenesis would cause significant pathology. Such targeting would require the development of novel methods of *in utero* delivery, and carries with it the risk of transformation of the germ line, either deliberately or incidentally, itself a major cause for concern.

There are inevitably ethical and moral problems raised by the possibilities discussed above which are beyond the scope of this review, but the prospects for fetal stem cell therapy are now real and are dealt with in Chapter 26.

ACKNOWLEDGEMENTS

The author wishes to thank Dr Catherine Boulter for helpful comments on the manuscript. Related research in the author's laboratory is funded by the UK Medical Research Council the Wellcome Trust and the National Kidney Research Fund.

REFERENCES

Alpert, S., Hanahan, D., and Teitelman, G. (1988). Hybrid insulin genes reveal a developmental lineage for pancreatic endocrine cells and imply a relationship with neurons. *Cell*, 53, 295.

Bakker, C.E., Verheij, C., Willemsen, R., Van der Helm, R., Oerlemans, F., Vermey, M., *et al.* (1994). Fmr-1 knockout mice: a model to study fragile X mental retardation. *Cell*, **78**, 23–33.

Barker, D.D., Wu, H., Hartung, S., Breindl, M., and Jaenisch, R. (1991). Retrovirus induced insertional mutagenesis; mechanism of collagen mutation in mov13 mice. *Molecular and Cellular Biology*, **11**, 5154–63.

Bates, P., Fisher, R., Ward, A., Richardson, L., Hill, D.J., and Graham, C.F. (1995). Mammary cancer in transgenic mice expressing insulin-like growth factor II (IGF-II). *British Journal of Cancer*, **72**, 1189–93.

Behringer, R.R., Mathews, L.S., Palmiter, R.D., and Brinster, R.L. (1988). Dwarf mice produced by genetic ablation of growth hormone expressing cells, *Genes and Development*, **2**, 453–61.

Behringer, R.R., Lewin, T.M., Quaife, C.J., Palmiter, R.D., Brinster, R.L., and DErcole, A.J. (1990). Expression of insulin-like growth factor I stimulates normal somatic growth in growth hormone-deficient transgenic mice. *Endocrinology*, **127**, 1033–40.

Blaese, R.M., Culver, K.W., Miller, A.D., Carter, C.S., Fleisher, T., Clerici, M., *et al.* (1995). Trophoblast lymphocyte directed gene therapy for ADA-SCID; initial trial results after four years. *Science*, **270**, 475–80.

Bonifer, C., Yannoutsos, N., Kruger, G., Grosveld, F., and Sippel, A.E. (1994). Dissection of the locus control function located on the chicken lysozyme gene domain in transgenic mice. *Nucleic Acids Research*, **22**, 4202–10.

Brandon, E.P., Idzerda, R.L., and McKnight, G.S. (1995). Targeting the mouse genome: a compendium of knockouts. *Current Biology*, **5**, 625–34.

Brinster, R.L. (1993). Stem cells and transgenic mice in the study of development. *International Journal of Developmental Biology*, **37**, 89–99.

Bucchini, D., Ripoche, M.-A., Stinnakre, M.-G., Desbois, P., Lores, P., Monthioux, E., *et al.* (1986). Pancreatic expression of human insulin gene in transgenic mice. *Proceedings of the National Academy of Sciences USA*, **83**, 2511–15.

Camper, S.A., Saunders, T.L., Kendal, S.K., Keri, R.A., Seasholtz, A.F., Gordon, D.F., *et al.* (1995). Implementing transgenic and embryonic stem cell technology to study gene expression cell/cell interactions and gene function. *Biology of Reproduction*, **52**, 246–57.

Chada, K., Magram, J., Raphael, K., Radice, G., Lacy, E., and Constantin, F. (1985). Specific expression of a foreign beta-globin gene in erythroid cells of transgenic mice. *Nature*, **314**, 377–80.

Christofori, G. and Hanahan, D. (1994). Molecular dissection of multi-stage tumorigenesis in transgenic mice. *Seminars in Cancer Biology*, **5**, 3–12.

Clarke, A.R. (1994). Murine genetic models of human disease. *Current Opinion in Genetics and Development*, **4**, 453–60.

Copp, A.J. (1995). Death before birth: clues from gene knockouts and mutations. *Trends in Genetics*, **11**, 87–93.

Dandoy-Dron, F., Monthioux, E., Jami, J., and Bucchini, D. (1991). Regulatory regions of rat insulin 1 gene necessary for expression in transgenic mice. *Nucleic Acids Research*, **19**, 4925–30.

Dandoy-Dron, F., Itler, J.M., Monthioux, E., Bucchini, D., and Jami, J. (1995). Tissue-specific expression of the rat insulin 1 gene *in vivo* requires both the enhancer and promoter regions. *Differentiation*, **58**, 291–5.

Davies, K.E., Tinsley, J.M., and Blake, D.J. (1995). Molecular analysis of Duchenne muscular dystrophy: past, present and future. *Annals of the New York Academy of Sciences*, **758**, 287–96.

de Chiara, T.M., Efstratiadis A., and Robertson, E.J. (1991). Parental imprinting of the mouse insulin-like growth factor gene. *Cell*, **64**, 849–59.

Efstratiadis, A. (1994). IGFs and dwarf mice: genetic and epigenetic control of embryonic growth. In *Developmental endocrinology*, (ed. P.C. Sizonenko, M.L. Aubert, and J.-D. Vassalli), Frontiers in Endocrinology, Vol. 6, pp. 27–42. Ares Serono Publications, Rome.

Gossen, M., Freundlieb, S., Bender, G., Muller, G., Hillen, W., and Bujard, H. (1995). Transcriptional activation by tetracyclines in mammalian cells. *Science*, **268**, 1766–9.

Grosveld, F., Antoniou, M., Berry, M., deBoer, E., Dillon, N., Ellis, J., *et al.* (1993). The regulation of human globin gene switching. In *Transgenic modification of the germline and somatic cells*, (ed. R.B. Flavell and R.B. Heap), pp. 45–53. Chapman and Hall, London.

Guillemot, F., Caspary, T., Tilghman, S.M., Copeland, N.G., Gilbert, D.J., Jenkins, N.A., *et al.* (1995). Genomic imprinting of Mash2, a mouse gene required for trophoblast development. *Nature Genetics*, **9**, 235–42.

Hammer, R.E., Palmiter, R.D., and Brinster, R.L. (1984). Partial correction of murine hereditary growth disorder by germ-line incorporation of a new gene. *Nature*, **311**, 65–7.

Hasty, P., Bradley, A., Morris, J.H., Edmondson, D.G., Venuti, J.M., Olson, E.N., *et al.* (1993). Muscle deficiency and neonatal death in mice with a targeted mutation in the myogenin gene. *Nature*, **364**, 501–6.

Herrera, P.L., Huarte, J., Zuffery, R., Nichols, A., Mermillod, B., Philipe, J., and Vassalli, J.-D. (1994). Ablation of islet endocrine cells by targeted expression of hormone promoter driven toxigenes. *Proceedings of the National Academy of Sciences, USA*, **91**, 12999–3003.

Hoffman, E.P. (1994). Dystrophin associated proteins fail in filling dystrophin's shoes. *Nature Genetics*, **8**, 311–12.

Hyde, S.C., Gill, D.R., Higgins, C.F., Trezise, A.F., MacVinish, L.J., Cuthbert, A.W., *et al.* (1993). Correction of the ion transport defect in cystic fibrosis trangenic mice by gene therapy. *Nature*, **362**, 250–3.

Ishibashi, S., Herz, J., Maeda, N., Goldstein, J.L., and Brown, M.S. (1994). The two-receptor model of lipoprotein clearance: tests of the hypothesis in 'knockout' mice lacking the low density lipoprotein receptor, apolipoprotein E, or both proteins. *Proceedings of the National Academy of Sciences USA*, **91**, 4431–5.

Jat, P.S., Noble, M.S., Ataliotis, P., Tanaka, Y., Yannoutsos, N., Larsen, L., *et al.* (1991). Direct derivation of conditionally immortal cell lines from an H-2K^{b}tsA58 transgenic mouse. *Proceedings of the National Academy of Sciences, USA*, **88**, 5096–100.

Jonsson, J., Carlsson, L., Edlund, T., and Edlund, H. (1994). Insulin-promoter-factor 1 is required for pancreas development in mice. *Nature*, **371**, 606–9.

Koopman, P., Gubbay, J., Vivian, N., Goodfellow, P., and Lovell-Badge, R. (1991). Male development of chromosomally female mice transgenic for Sry. *Nature*, **351**, 117–21.

Kuhn, R., Schwenk, F., Aguet, M., and Rajewsky, K. (1995). Inducible gene targeting in mice. *Science*, **269**, 1427–9.

Lang, R.A., Metcalf, D., Cuthbertson, R.A., Lyons, I., Stanley, E., Kelso, A., *et al.* (1987). Transgenic mice expressing a hemopoietic growth factor gene (GM-CSF) develop accumulations of macrophages, blindness, and a fatal syndrome of tissue damage. *Cell*, **51**, 675–86.

Larue, L., Ohsugi, M., Hirchenhain, J., and Kemler, R. (1994). E-cadherin null mutant embryos fail to form a trophectoderm epithelium. *Proceedings of the National Academy of Science, USA*, **91**, 8263–7.

Lau, M.M.H., Stewart, C.E.H., Liu, Z., Bhatt, H., Rotwein, P., and Stewart, C.L. (1994). Loss of the imprinted IGF2/cation-idependent mannose 6-phosphate receptor results in fetal overgrowth and perinatal lethality. *Genes and Development*, **8**, 2953–63.

Lee, J.E., Tantravahi, U., Boyle, A.L., and Efstratiadis, A. (1993). Parental imprinting of an IGF-2 transgene. *Molecular and Reproductive Development*, **35**, 382–90.

Leighton, P.A., Ingram, R.S., Eggenschwiler, J., Efstratiadis, A., and Tilghman, S.M. (1995a). Disruption of imprinting caused by deletion of the H19 gene region in mice. *Nature*, **375**, 34–9.

Leighton, P.A., Saam, J.R., Ingram, R.S., Stewart, C.L., and Tilghman, S.M. (1995*b*). An enhancer deletion affects both H19 and Igf2 expression. *Genes and Development*, 9, 2079–89.

Letterio, J.J., Geiser, A.G., Kulkarni, A.B., Roche, N.S., Sporn, M.B, *et al.* (1994). Maternal rescue of transforming growth factor b1 null mice. *Science*, 264, 1936–8.

Li, E., Bestor, T.H., and Jaenisch, R. (1992). Targeted mutation of the DNA methyltransferase gene results in embryonic lethality. *Cell*, 69, 915–26.

Li, J.E., Beard, C., and Jaenish, R. (1993). Role for DNA methylation in genomic imprinting. *Nature*, 366, 362–5.

Liu, J., Baker, J., Perkins, A.S., Robertson, L.J., and Efstratiadis, A. (1993). Mice carrying null mutations of the genes encoding insulin like growth factor I and type 1 IGF receptor. *Cell*, 75, 59–72.

Mansour, S.L., Thomas, K.R., and Capecchi, M.R. (1988). *Nature*, 336, 348–52.

Mason, A.J., Pitts, S.L., Nikolics, K., Szonyi, E., Wilcox, J.N., Seeberg, P.H., and Stewart, T.A. (1986). The hypogonadal mouse. Reproductive functions restored by gene therapy. *Science*, 234, 1372–8.

Meisler, M. (1992). Insertional mutations of classical and novel genes in transgenic mice. *Trends in Genetics*, 8, 341–4.

Mercer, E.H., Hoyle, G.W., Kapur, R.P., Brinster, R, L., and Palmiter, R.D. (1991). The dopamine-β-hydroxylase gene promoter directs expression of *E. coli lac z to* sympathetic and other neurones in adult transgenic mice. *Neuron*, 7, 703–16.

Mountford, P., Zevnik, B., Duvel, A., Nichols, J., Li, M., Dani, C., *et al.* (1994). Dicistronic targeting constructs: reporters and modifiers of mammalian gene expression. *Proceedings of the National Academy of Sciences USA*, 91, 4303–7.

Palmiter, R.D., Norstedt, G., Gelinas, R.E., Hammer, R.E., and Brinster, R.L. (1983). Metallothionein-human GH fusion genes stimulate growth of mice. *Science*, 222, 809–14.

Patejunas, G., Bradley, A., Beaudet, A.L., and O'Brien, W.E. (1994). Generation of a mouse model for citrullinemia by targeted disruption of the argininosuccinate synthetase gene. *Somatic Cell and Molecular Genetics*, 20, 55–60.

Perry, W.L. III, Vasicek, T.J., Lee, J.J., Rossi, J.M., Zeng, L., Zhang, T., *et al.* (1995). Phenotypic and molecular analysis of a transgenic insertional allele of the mouse fused locus. *Genetics*, 141, 321–32.

Phelps, S.F., Hauser, M.A., Cole, N.M., Rafael, J.A., Hinkle, R.T., Foulkner, J.A., *et al.* (1995). Expression of full-length and truncated dystrophin mini-genes in transgenic mdx mice. *Human Molecular Genetics*, 4, 1251–8.

Rogler, C.E., Yang, D., Rossetti, L., Donohoe, J., Alt, E., Chang, C.J., *et al.* (1994). Altered body composition and incresed frequency of diverse malignancies in Insulin-like growth factor-II transgenic mice. *Journal of Biological Chemistry*, 269, 13779–84.

Rudnicki, M.A., Braun, T., Hinuma, S., and Jaenisch, R. (1992). Inactivation of *MyoD* in mice leads to up-regulation of the myogenic HLH gene *Myf-5* and results in apparently normal muscle development. *Cell*, 71, 383–90.

Sanes, J.R. (1994). The latest in lineage. *Current Biology*, 4, 1162–4.

Sariola, H., Saarma, M., Saino, K., Arumae, I.J., Polgi, J., and Vaahto Ravi, A., *et al.* (1991). Dependence of kidney morphogenesis on the expression of nerve growth factor receptor. *Science*, 254, 571–3.

Sell, C., Dumenil, G., Deveaud, C., Miura, M., Coppola, D., DeAngelis, T., *et al.* (1994). Effect of a null mutation of the insulin-like growth factor I receptor gene on growth and transformation of mouse embryo fibroblasts. *Molecular and Cellular Biology*, 14, 3604–12.

Shockett, P., Difilippantonio, M., Hellman, N., and Schatz, D.G. (1995). A modified tetracycline-regulated system provides autoregulatory, inducible gene expression in cultured cells and transgenic mice. *Proceedings of the National Academy of Sciences, USA*, 92, 6522–26.

Sigmund, K.D., Jones, C.A., Mullins, J.J., Kim, U., and Goross, K.W. (1990). Expression of murine renin genes in subcutaneous conective tissue. *Proceedings of the National Academy of Sciences, USA*, **87**, 7993–7.

Snouwaert, J.N., Brigman, K.K., Latar, A.M., Malouf, N.N., Barker, R.C., *et al.* (1992). An animal model for cystic fibrosis made by gene targeting. *Science*, **257**, 1046–7.

Stacey, A., Schnieke, A., McWhir, J., Cooper, J., Colman, A., and Melton, D.W. (1994). Use of double-replacement gene targeting to replace the murine alpha-lactalbumin gene with its human counterpart in embryonic stem cells and mice. *Molecular and Cellular Biology*, **14**, 1009–16.

Stewart, C.L., Kaspar, P., Brunet, L.J., Bhatt, H., Gadi, I., Kontgen, F., *et al.* (1992). Blastocyst implantation depends on maternal expression of leukaemia inhibitory factor. *Nature*, **359**, 76–9.

Strouboulis, J., Dillon, N., and Grosveld, F. (1992). Developmental regulation of a complete 70-kb human betaglobin locus. *Genes and Development*, **6**, 1857–64.

Subramanian, V., Meyer, B., and Gruss, P. (1995). Disruption of the murine homoeobox *cdx1* affects axial skeletal identities by altering the mesodermal expression domains of *hox* genes. *Cell*, **83**, 641–54.

Tajbakhsh, S. and Buckingham, M.E. (1994). Mouse limb muscle is determined in the absence of the earliest myogenic factor myf-5. *Proceedings of the National Academy of Sciences, USA*, **91**, 747–51.

te Riele, H., Maandag, E.R., and Berns, M. (1992). Highly efficient gene targetting in embryonic stem cells through homologous recombination. *Proceedings of the National Academy of Sciences, USA*, **89**, 5128–32.

Teitelman, G (1993). On the origin of pancreatic endocrine cells, proliferation and differentiation. *Tumor Biology*, **14**, 167–73.

Van Buul-Offers, S.C., DeHaan, K., Rijnengresnigt, M.R., Meinsma, D., Jansen, M., Oei, S.L., *et al.* (1995). Overexpression of human IGF-II in transgenic mice causes increased growth of the thymus. *Journal of Endocrinology*, **144**, 491–502.

Viville, S. and Surani, A. (1995). Towards unravelling the *Igf2/H19* imprinted domain. *BioEssays*, **17**, 835–8.

Wang, T.C., Cardiff, R.D., Zukerberg, L., Lees, E., and Arnold, A. (1994). Mammary hyperplasia and carcinoma in *mmtv-cyclinD1* transgenic mice. *Nature*, **369**, 669–71.

Ward, A., Bierke, P., Pettersson, E., and Engström, W. (1995). Insulin-like growth factors: growth, transgenes and imprinting. *Zoological Science*, **11**, 167–74.

Ward, A., Bates, P., Fisher, R., Richardson, L., and Graham, C.F. (1994*a*). Disproportionate growth in mice with *Igf-2* transgenes. *Proceedings of the National Academy of Sciences, USA*, **91**, 10365–9.

Whitelaw, C.B.A., Harris, S., McClenaghan, M., Simons, J.P., and Clark, A.J. (1992). Position-independent expression of the ovine β-lactoglobulin gene in transgenic mice. *Journal of Biochemistry*, **286**, 31–9.

Wu, H., Liu, Y., and Jaenisch, R. (1994). Double replacement: strategy for efficient introduction of subtle mutations into the mouse *colla-1* gene by homologous recombination in ES cells. *Proceedings of the National Academy of Sciences, USA*, **91**, 2819–23.

Xiang, X., Benson, K.F., and Chada, K. (1990). Mini-mouse: disruption of the pygmy locus in a trangenic insertional mutant. *Science*, **247**, 967–9.

25 | Transplantation of fetal haematopoietic tissues

Jean-Louis Touraine, Daniel Raudrant, and
Sylvie Laplace

INTRODUCTION

Transplantation of fetal liver stem cells results in haematopoietic and lymphopoietic reconstitution (Uphoff 1958; Touraine 1983; Touraine *et al.* 1987). Due to immaturity of the lymphoid system of the fetal donor (especially characterized by the absence of T lymphocytes) in the early ontogenetic phase, no or mild graft-versus-host reaction (GvHR) develops, provided that donor age is below 13 weeks post-fertilization.

Recently, fetal liver transplantation (FLT) has been applied to the treatment of human fetuses *in utero*, with significant success (Touraine *et al.* 1989; Touraine 1992). The immaturity of both the recipient and the donor has then been responsible for easier engraftment, lack of rejection, and stable chimerism with immunological tolerance to both donor and host antigens (Spits *et al.* 1990; Bacchetta *et al.* 1992). Many years after the pioneering work of Billingham, Brent, and Medawar on neonatal tolerance in mice, similar results have been obtained in humans: tolerance without conditioning of the recipient and even in a patient without immunodeficiency disease. Instead of being induced at birth, the immunological tolerance was obtained by cell injection during early fetal development in the human. The immaturity of T cell immunity in the murine new-born appears to be comparable to that of the human fetus at the border between the first and the second trimesters (Royo *et al.* 1987).

POSTNATAL FLT

Over the past 20 years, 242 fetal tissue transplants (especially FLTs associated with syngeneic fetal thymus) have been performed in our institution to treat 63 patients with severe immunodeficiency diseases (IDD), severe aplastic anaemia, or inborn errors of metabolism (IEM). At present, 73 per cent of all patients with IEM and 50 per cent of all patients with IDD are alive and well, with a follow-up of 1–20 years (Fig. 25.1). They are either completely cured or significantly improved. Despite HLA mismatch between donor and recipient, in these cases, there is no noticeable restriction of T-cell functions *in vivo*, *ex vivo*, and *in vitro*, provided that investigations are carried out several years after the transplant (Touraine 1983; Roncarolo *et al.* 1986).

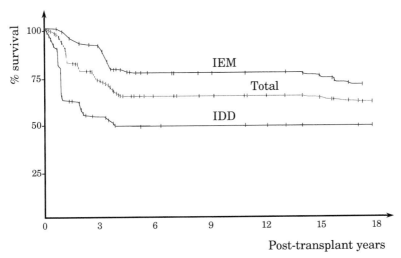

Fig. 25.1 Survival of patients with severe immunodeficiency diseases (IDD) or inborn errors of metabolism (IEM) treated by fetal tissue transplantation. The global survival of all patients from these two groups is shown by the line 'Total'.

PRENATAL FLT

The first patient treated by *in utero* FLT had bare lymphocyte syndrome (BLS), i.e. a genetically transmitted form of combined immunodeficiency disease due to the lack of expression of HLA molecules (Touraine *et al.* 1978). Infections, especially with opportunistic microorganisms, are responsible for the death of these infants, unless they grow up isolated in a fully sterile atmosphere while they are successfully reconstituted with stem cell transplants (SCTs). When carried out postnatally, however, such a SCT—in the form of either a bone marrow transplant or a FLT—is usually associated with graft failure due to the presence of allogeneic reactions in the host (persisting transplant immunity) and to high susceptibility to infections (defective immunity to infectious antigens).

Prenatal diagnosis of BLS in this human fetus was followed by *in utero* FLT (Touraine *et al.* 1989). The transplant was carried out in June 1988. It involved the infusion of 7 ml of culture medium containing a suspension of 16×10^6 fetal liver and thymic epithelial cells, into the fetus umbilical vein, under ultrasound visualization. The child has evidence of engraftment: initially, 10 per cent of lymphocytes had normal expression of class I HLA and these cells expressed the HLA-A9 specificity of donor origin. The number of cells deriving from the *in utero* transplant increased up to 26 per cent among peripheral blood lymphocytes at 14 months and stabilized between 17 and 21 per cent after the sixth year of age. As a result, cell-mediated immunity was reconstituted (Table 25.1), enabling the child to live normally (Touraine 1992). The seven-year-old boy has not experienced any severe infection, his T-lymphocyte functions are presently normal and his clinical condition is excellent.

Table 25.1 Modalities and results of *in utero* transplants into human fetuses

Patients	Diseases	Age of fetal patients[a]	Age of fetal donors[a]	Date of transplant	Route of cell infusion	Date of birth	Evidence for engraftment	Correction of initial disease	Clinical status
D.T.	BLS[b]	28	7 and 7.5	30.06.1988	IV	17.08.1988	HLA markers	Reconstitution of T cells with normal functions	Alive and well
M.H.	SCID[c]	26	7.5	08.06.1989	IV	07.08.1989	HLA markers	Reconstitution of T cells with subnormal functions	Alive and well
M.R.	TM[d]	12	9.5	10.10.1989	IP	25.03.1990	Y chromosome	Presence of HbA coexisting with abnormal Hb	Alive and well
R.M.	TM[d]	17	11.5	30.04.1991	IV	–	–	–	Bradycardia and fetal death
A.V.	CGD[e]	17 21	13.5 14	22.04.1992 22.05.1992	IV IV	–	–	–	Bradycardia and fetal death
C.D.	N–P (A)[f]	14 16	12 13	07.03.1995 21.03.1995	IP IP	22.08.1995	HLA markers	ND	Alive and well

[a] Weeks post-fertilization; [b] bare lymphocyte syndrome; [c] severe combined immunodeficiency disease; [d] β^0 thalassaemia major; [e] chronic granulomatous disease; [f] Niemann–Pick disease (type A). ND, not yet determined; IV, intravenous; IP, intraperitoneal.

A second patient with a complete form of severe combined deficiency was then treated by *in utero* FLT. Engraftment has also been obtained and donor stem cells differentiated into T lymphocytes with adequate immune function (Table 25.1). This young girl is now healthy, with a satisfactory immunological reconstitution (Touraine 1992), and she lives normally despite a viral hepatitis.

These results obtained in immunodeficiency diseases prompted us to attempt *in utero* FLT in fetal patients with severe non-immune haematological disorders. In such conditions, however, graft take may not be facilitated by an abnormally incompetent immunity in the fetal host and we assumed that FLT had to be carried out during the first trimester or at the beginning of the second trimester of pregnancy, when normal fetuses have not yet developed cell-mediated immunity.

A pregnant woman with a family history of thalassaemia solicited precocious prenatal diagnosis. By molecular biology techniques, the fetus was demonstrated to have β^0 thalassaemia major. The mother refused abortion for religious reasons, and she asked for *in utero* FLT. FLT was carried out in the fetal patient whose age was 12 weeks post-fertilization. The transplant consisted of the intraperitoneal injection of 3×10^8 viable cells from a fetus of 9.5 weeks post-fertilization age (Table 25.1). There was no adverse effect in the mother nor in the fetus. Birth occurred in March 1990. The site of puncture could hardly be seen on the abdominal skin of the new-born infant and ultrasound investigations demonstrated no modification of the abdominal wall.

Studies performed after birth showed the presence of thalassaemia. However, there were a few cells of donor origin: PCR gene amplification techniques revealed Y chromosome-specific DNA fragments in the peripheral blood lymphocytes (PBL) of this girl. In addition, haemoglobin A (HbA) was found to account for 0.9 per cent of all haemoglobin at 6 months.

No further transplant was done in this infant who is presently in very good general condition. Investigations have been carried out one year after birth, 3 months after she had received a single blood transfusion; the total haemoglobin level was slightly below normal, and the HbA percentage was 30 per cent. These data suggest that the engraftment of only a few donor cells has been followed by some cell proliferation resulting in improvement and partial correction of this haematologic disorder. The number of donor red cells does not, however, reach a level that would permit avoidance of any blood transfusion.

The fourth fetal patient also had thalassaemia major. Unfortunately, the intravenous infusion into the umbilical vein was followed by bradycardia and fetal death (Table 25.1).

The fifth fetal patient received two FLTs to treat chronic granulomatous disease (Table 25.1). The first transplant was carried out uneventfully by umbilical vein infusion at 17 weeks post-fertilization but the number of cells available for infusion was considered insufficient. A second transplant was therefore attempted at 21 weeks but unfortunately it resulted in fetal bradycardia (possibly due to a relatively rapid infusion of a larger number of cells) and it led to fetal death within one hour.

More recently, in 1995, we have performed two FLTs *in utero* into a fetus with Niemann–Pick disease (type A) (Table 25.1). Birth occurred in August 22, 1995. The new-born infant is now in good condition despite preliminary results on sphingomyelinase activity that appears to be very low and the liver enzymes which are elevated. However, there are a few cells of donor origin: the presence of cells expressing the HLA-A2 specificity of one fetal donor could be demonstrated in the peripheral blood of the new-born by cytofluorimetry analysis. Further investigations have to be performed to determine whether the Niemann–Pick disease will be partially improved in this young girl.

TOLERANCE AND MHC RESTRICTION IN HUMAN CHIMERAS

Both in patients treated by postnatal FLT and in fetuses receiving FLT *in utero*, full reconstitution could develop despite a complete mismatch of HLA class I and class II antigens between donor and host. The separation of T and B lymphocyte populations, and the development of cell lines and clones from PBL of these patients, followed by HLA typing, showed that all T lymphocytes were of donor origin, while most B lymphocytes and monocytes were of host origin in the reconstituted and now chimeric patients, cured of severe immunodeficiency disease.

Tolerance between donor-derived T cells and host-derived B cells/ monocytes was confirmed *in vitro*. Specific unresponsiveness of lymphocytes towards the host cells in a primary mixed leucocyte culture was observed (Bacchetta *et al.* 1992). However, by clonal analysis, CD4+ and CD8+ T-cell clones were isolated and shown to be specifically reactive to the host HLA class II and class I molecules. The frequency of CD8+ host-reactive T cells was high, in the same range as that found for CD8+ alloreactive T cells (Bacchetta *et al.* 1992). By contrast, no donor-reactive CD8+ T cells were observed, indicating that in these patients treated with allogeneic FLT, donor-reactive but not host-reactive cells are deleted from the T-cell repertoire (Bacchetta *et al.* 1992). Similar findings have been obtained very recently in the Severe combined immunodeficiency (SCID)-hu mouse (Vandckerckhove *et al.* 1992), suggesting tolerance to antigens of the stem-cell donor via clonal deletion and tolerance to antigens of the host thymus via clonal anergy.

Tolerance is therefore exerted towards all donor and host antigens, in these patients. In contrast, the HLA restriction of antigen recognition was shown to be imposed upon the patient's T cells by the host determinants only. Antigen-presenting cells of the host could effectively present tetanus toxoid antigens or Epstein–Barr virus antigens to the allogeneic T lymphocytes (Roncarolo *et al.* 1986, 1988*a*; Plotnicky and Touraine 1993). The antigenic peptide was, as usual, presented in the groove of an HLA molecule but, in this case, it was a different HLA molecule from that of the T lymphocyte itself. The study of numerous clones has demonstrated that T cells from these patients recognize antigen in the context of the allogeneic HLA determinants (Roncarolo *et al.* 1986, 1988*a*,*b*).

Similarly, the *in vivo* defence against virus infections of various kinds has been normal and has not been hindered by the HLA mismatch between infected cells and cytotoxic T lymphocytes able to control the infection. Both *in vivo* and *in vitro* data led us to postulate the 'Allo + X' hypothesis (Fig. 25.2), according to which some T lymphocytes can develop a recognition for the X antigen in the context

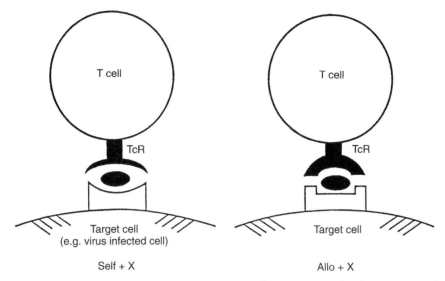

Fig. 25.2 Two distinct varieties of T lymphocytes differentiating in the thymus, one with 'Self + X' recognition structures (left), the other with 'Allo + X' recognition structures (right). TcR is T-cell receptor for antigen.

of allogenic determinants instead of the previously known recognition for 'Self + X' (Touraine and Bétuel 1981; Touraine 1983).

The ontogenetic development of T lymphocytes with such recognition structures takes place primarily in the fetal thymus and might be envisioned schematically to occur as follows. A first degree of diversity develops with a variety of thymocytes which have a primary recognition structure for the histocompatibility antigens (possibly associated with a common peptide) (Fig. 25.3). In normal circumstances, only those T cells with recognition for self-histocompatibility antigens are solicited, since the alloantigens are not encountered in the thymus. These cells are induced to proliferate and to develop the full repertoire of antigen recognition in association with self recognition. In chimeric patients, a given set of other histocompatibility antigens is also presented continuously to the differentiating T cells. Those T cells with recognition for the given alloantigens are then solicited, they expand by proliferation, and they develop the gene rearrangement leading to the expression of the T cell receptor. Antigen recognition is then associated with alloantigen recognition. 'Self + X' and 'Allo + X' recognitions are supported by distinct T cells as shown by the analysis of T-cell clones: each T-cell clone is able to recognize the antigen presented by one histocompatibility determinant only. In chimeric patients, T cells that recognize antigen in the context of allospecificities are positively selected.

CONCLUDING REMARK

In utero transplantation of fetal cell stems is a therapy with remarkable advantages: (a) tolerance induction due to immune immaturity of host, (b) lack of GvHD due to

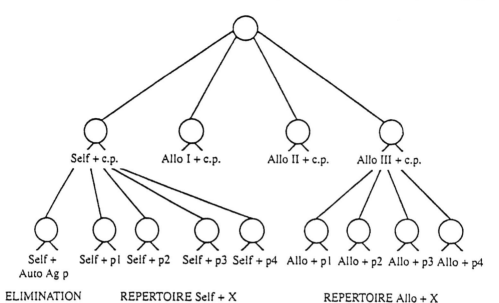

Fig. 25.3 Development and selection of a large variety of T lymphocytes with distinct recognition structures, during the differentiation process from the stem cell after migration to the thymus. In the figure, c.p. is 'common peptide'; Auto Ag is 'autoantigenic peptide'; p1–p4 are 'peptide 1–peptide 4'.

immaturity of donor, (c) ideal isolation of the fetus in the maternal uterus, and (d) optimal environment for donor fetal cell development in the vicinity of host fetal cells and growth factors.

REFERENCES

Bacchetta, R., Vandekerckhove, B.A.E., Bigler, M., and Roncarolo, M.G. (1992). Human and mouse SCID models to study tolerance after HLA-mismatched fetal stem cell transplantation. *Experimental Hematology*, 20, 722.

Plotnicky, H. and Touraine, J.-L. (1993). Cytotoxic T cells from a human chimera induce regression of Epstein–Barr virus-infected allogeneic host cells. *International Immunology*, 5, 1413–20.

Roncarolo, M.G., Touraine, J.-L., and Banchereau, J. (1986). Cooperation between major histocompatibility complex mismatched mononuclear cells from a human chimera in the production of antigen-specific antibody. *Journal of Clinical Investigation*, 77, 673–80.

Roncarolo, M.G., Yssel, H., Touraine, J.-L., Bacchetta, R., Gebuhrer, L., de Vries, J., and Spits, H. (1988*a*). Antigen recognition by MHC-incompatible cells of a human mismatched chimera. *Journal of Experimental Medicine*, 67, 2139–52.

Roncarolo, M.G., Yssel, H., Touraine, J.-L., Bétuel, H., de Vries, J., and Spits, H. (1988*b*). Autoreactive T-cell clones specific for class I and class II HLA antigens isolated from a human chimera. *Journal of Experimental Medicine*, 167, 1523–34.

Royo, C., Touraine, J.-L., and de Bouteiller, O. (1987). Ontogeny of T-lymphocyte differentiation in the human fetus: acquisition of phenotype and functions. *Thymus*, **10**, 57–73.

Spits, H., Touraine, J.-L., Yssel, H., de Vries, J., and Roncarolo, M.G. (1990). Presence of host-reactive and MHC restricted T-cells in a transplanted severe combined immunodeficient (SCID) patient suggest a positive selection and absence of clonal deletion. *Immunology Reviews*, **116**, 101–16.

Touraine, J.-L. (1983). Bone marrow and fetal liver transplantation in immunodeficiencies and inborn errors of metabolism: lack of significant restriction of T-cell function in long-term chimeras despite HLA-mismatch. *Immunology Reviews*, **71**, 103–21.

Touraine, J.-L. (1992). Rationale and results of *in utero* transplants of stem cells in humans. *Bone Marrow Transplantation*, **10**, (Suppl. 1), 121–6.

Touraine, J.-L. and Bétuel, H. (1981). Immunodeficiency diseases and expression of HLA antigens. *Human Immunology*, **2**, 147–53.

Touraine, J.-L., Bétuel, H., Souillet, G., and Jeune, M. (1978). Combined immunodeficiency disease associated with absence of cell-surface HLA A and B antigens. *Journal of Pediatrics*, **93**, 47–51.

Touraine, J.-L., Roncarolo, M.G., Royo, C., and Touraine, F. (1987). Fetal tissue transplantation, bone marrow transplantation and prospective gene therapy in severe immunodeficiencies and enzyme deficiencies. *Thymus*, **10**, 75–87.

Touraine, J.-L., Raudrant, D., Royo, C., Rebaud, A., Roncarolo, M.G., Souillet, G., et al. (1989). *In utero* transplantation of stem cells in the bare lymphocyte syndrome. *Lancet*, **i**, 1382.

Uphoff, D.E. (1958). Preclusion of secondary phase of irradiation syndrome by inoculation of fetal hematopoietic tissue following total-body X-irradiation. *Journal of the National Cancer Institute*, **20**, 625–32.

Vandekerckhove, B.A.E., Namikawa, R., Bacchetta, R., and Roncarolo, M.G. (1992). Human hematopoietic cells and thymic epithelial cells induce tolerance via different mechanisms in the SCID-hu mouse thymus. *Journal of Experimental Medicine*, **175**, 1033–43.

26 | Fetal stem cell therapy

Jack Goldberg

The development of biologic assays to study haematopoietic precursor cells significantly contributed to our current understanding of haematopoiesis. These assays, termed 'colony forming units, spleen' (CFU-S) and 'colony forming units, culture' (CFU-C) were developed in the 1970s. Prior to that time, our understanding of haematopoiesis was dependent on detailed histologic descriptions of haemato-poietic organs and by radiosotopic studies of bone marrow kinetics. The existence of a population of haematopoietic stem cells had always been speculated but never identified. Diseases such as chronic myelogenous leukaemia (CML) also supported the presence of a population of lineage-specific haematopoietic precursor cells. CML is a proliferative disorder characterized by the presence of an abnormal chromosome known as the Philadelphia chromosome in red blood cells, white blood cells, and platelets but not in somatic tissues. Thus, CML appears to arise from a haemato-poietic precursor cell. There is now a growing list of diseases such as chronic myelo-proliferative, myelodysplastic, and acute myeloid leukaemia that arise from a disordered haematopoietic precursor cell. These pathological conditions further stim-ulated interest and research in the study of haematopoietic stem cells.

The first assay of haematopoietic precursor cells was known as the 'colony forming unit, spleen' (CFU-S) (Till and McCulloch 1961). This assay is an *in vivo* system in which marrow is removed from a healthy mouse donor and injected systemically into lethally irradiated mouse recipients. The infusion of bone marrow into these lethally irradiated mice resulted in the formation of cellular aggregates on the surface of the spleens of the recipient animal. These cellular aggregates arose from a single cell. This assay was the first to reproducibly quantitate haematopoietic precursor cells but required an *in vivo* system. Obviously this was not applicable to humans and thus investigators continued to search for an *in vitro* assay system. Such a system was identified in the 70s and was termed 'colony forming units in culture' (CFU-C) (Pluznik and Sachs 1965; Bradley and Metcalf 1966; Pike and Robinson 1970). The CFU-C assays were semi-solid culture systems in which agar, methyl cellulose, or plasma clots provided a matrix on which cells could grow, nutrient medium, includ-ing fetal calf serum, was an absolute requirement, as well as the addition of a source of stimulating factor (Parker and Metcalf 1974; McLeod *et al.* 1974). Target haematopoietic cells were suspended in the semi-solid culture system and after 10–14 days of incubation, cellular aggregates of greater than 40 cells were identified and these growths were termed colonies. Culture systems were modified to assay different types of haematopoietic precursor cells based on the semi-solid matrix, nutient medium, and most importantly, the type of stimulating factors used. Researchers were now able to quantitate and study haematopoietic progenitor cells committed to granulocyte macrophage (CFU-GM), erythroid (BFU-E and CFU-E), or megakaryocytic (CFU-meg) lineages or combinations of all three. The *in vitro* assay systems noted above, however, only detect a group of precursor cells that are capable of proliferation and differentiation but are unable to self-replicate. These cells are called progenitor cells. The CFU-S cells are capable of multi-lineage proliferation, differentiation, and also self-replication. Until recently, the haematopoietic stem cell (capable of self-replication), has not been assayable in *in vitro* systems. Several investigators have developed assays for these haematopoietic stem cells *in vitro* but these assays are still not consistently available or reliable.

The haematopoietic progenitor cells are a small fraction of the bone marrow cells. For example, 50–100 granulopoietic progenitor cells are present in cultures of 5×10^5 bone marrow mononuclear cells. Peripheral blood also contains haematopoietic progenitor cells but their frequency is lower than that of bone marrow, with approximately 1–10 granulopoietic progenitor cells for every 5×10^5 cells plated in culture (Kirshner *et al.* 1980). Our laboratory attempted to increase the plating efficiency of these cellular sources. We obtained enriched populations of haematopoietic progenitor cells (Goldberg *et al.* 1979; Goldberg *et al.* 1980*a*; Kirshner *et al.* 1980). Ten years later, investigators reported nearly 100 per cent yields of haematopoietic precursor cells. These purified precursor cells appear morphologically as normal lymphocytes and contain the CD34 surface marker. These isolated haematopoietic precursor cells are non-adherent and do not contain any T-cell or B-cell markers.

The stimulating factors which are absolute requirements for cellular proliferation and differentiation in the *in vitro* assay systems have been defined and isolated. Erythropoietin was successfully purified from human urine. The other growth factors were much more difficult to isolate and it took advances in the field of molecular biology to provide tools for the isolation and subsequent production of these factors. Colony stimulating factor(s), interleukins, stem cell factor, and TPO are groups of substances that have been isolated and produced by recombinant technology. These factors have a variety of stimulatory effects on haematopoietic precursor cells. The advances in our understanding and isolation of the haematopoietic progenitor cells and stimulating factors resulted in direct clinical benefits to patients and provided an important resource for supporting cancer chemotherapy and bone marrow transplantation.

With the CFU assay systems in hand, investigators began to evaluate pathological states with these assays and to use the assay for prognosis and diagnosis of a variety of haematological disorders, both benign and malignant (Goldberg *et al.* 1978, 1980*b*, 1983; Kirshner *et al.* 1980, 1982). A variety of tissue sources of haematopoietic progenitor/stem cells and stimulating factors were also examined, including liver, spleen, and placenta. Liver and spleen tissue contained progenitor cell numbers equivalent to those observed in normal peripheral blood (Kirshner *et al.* 1980). Approximately 50–100 granulopoietic progenitor cells can be found in cultures of 5×10^5 umbilical cord blood mononuclear cells (similar to bone marrow yields). Three sources of human haematopoietic progenitor cells (peripheral blood, bone marrow, and umbilical cord blood) have been identified since the development of the CFU-C assay.

Advances in the field of *in vitro* haematopoiesis were paralleled by advances in the clinic, namely bone marrow transplantation. As the efficacy and safety of bone marrow transplantation improved over the years, investigators began to look toward expanding the use of this treatment, including finding donors outside of identical sibling HLA matches. As a result, there has been a great deal of interest and excitement in the use of umbilical cord blood as a source of transplantable haematopoietic tissue. The first successful cord blood transplant was performed in 1965 (Ende 1966; Ende and Ende 1972). In the past few years, several other successful cord blood transplants have been performed (Gluckman *et al.* 1989, 1992).

Cord blood from a single birth contains sufficient numbers of stem/progenitor cells for HLA-compatible allogeneic transplantation of a child based on the number of cells per kg of body weight and provides comparable numbers of precursor cells, as measured *in vitro* for long-term culture initiating cells (LTC-IC) or high proliferative potential colony-forming cells (HPP-CFC), to that found in bone marrow tissue (Broxmeyer *et al.* 1990). Cord blood appears to be a novel and unique source of transplantable haematopoietic precursors. Cord blood, which is normally discarded, can be readily collected without discomfort or danger to mother or infant. The technical feasibility of using cord blood for transplantation and the optimal conditions for cryopreservation to maintain cell viability have been established (Broxmeyer *et al.* 1990, 1992; Gluckman *et al.* 1992; Wagner *et al.* 1992). Further, cord blood now has been used successfully, albeit in a limited number of cases, in the clinic to reconstitute HLA-identical siblings (Gluckman *et al.* 1989). However, the use of cord blood for the transplantation of HLA-identical, non-related children or adults remains to be established. Cord blood has been demonstrated to have a stem/progenitor cell precursor frequency significantly greater than adult peripheral blood and equal to that of adult bone marrow (Kirshner and Goldberg 1980). This high progenitor cell frequency is thought to result from stem cell expansion during the last months of fetal life and probably represents the final phases of bone marrow colonization from other sites. Cord blood LTC-ICs can be maintained in long-term culture and this greater proliferative capacity may reflect their production by more primitive stem cells (Broxmeyer *et al.* 1989). This experimental observation suggests the presence of qualitatively distinct fetal, as opposed to adult, precursor cells in cord blood.

T-cell depletion of bone marrow is commonly used to decrease the incidence of graft-versus-host disease (GvHD), which frequently occurs after allogeneic transplants, even in patients with HLA-matched sibling donors. Unfortunately, T-cell depletion is associated with an increased failure to engraft. Interestingly, GvHD does not seem to be as serious a problem when using cord blood for haematopoietic transplantation. This clinical observation was made in a recent case in which a child with CML was treated with an HLA-matched cord blood transplant from his sister and engrafted without any GvHD. When this patient relapsed, GvHD occurred upon subsequent re-transplantation with bone marrow from the same donor. Mouse cord blood also does not induce GvHD under experimental conditions. Thus, cord blood haematopoietic precursors may be less immunogenic than other transplantable haematopoietic tissues.

A successful bone marrow transplantation requires the transfer to the host of multi-potential cells (capable of self-renewal). In humans these cells are identified by the lack of mature haematopoietic lineage markers in combination with expression of the CD34 antigen (Vilmer *et al.* 1992). Successful engraftment of bone marrow has been correlated to the number of CFU-GM transferred to the recipient. However, there exists considerable controversy as to the predictive value of this parameter for tissue such as cord blood. Broxmeyer (1995) has indicated that the average cord blood collection consists of 75–150 ml and contains sufficient numbers of CFU-GM for allogeneic transplantation of both children and adults. However, this question is still open. The primitive nature of cord blood precursors has been supported by the finding that 100 per cent of primary cord blood colonies give rise to secondary colonies upon replating, indicative of a more primitive stem cell subset than that found in peripheral blood or bone marrow.

Cord blood has the potential to be the graft of choice for transplantation in the future and currently complements conventional bone marrow needs. The establishment of a cord blood bank could open new avenues in the procurement of donors for both autologous and allogeneic transplantation. A bank of cryopreserved cord blood could overcome some of the present limitations of the bone marrow registry. Storing cord blood from the large number of potential donors available would ensure that an ethnic balance of the donor pool was maintained. Cord blood also contains a substantially lower incidence of age-dependent infectious agents than adult tissue (e.g. Epstein–Barr virus; cytomegalovirus). This aspect is particularly important as primary infection as well as viral reactivation can be a contributing factor to post-transplant mortality. Significantly, cord blood does not appear as capable of causing GvHD, which is frequently a problem when using unrelated bone marrow for transplantation. GvHD, when it occurs in cord blood transplants, has been observed to be mild in degree and readily eliminated by short-term drug therapy. Chronic GvHD is seen in approximately 50 per cent of all HLA-matched, unrelated grafts. In view of the serious problems associated with both GvHD and immunosuppressive therapy (including organ/tissue failure, bacterial and viral infections, reactivation of EBV, leukaemia, and lymphoma, and severe growth and developmental defects in children), cord blood could have a significant advantage over bone marrow tissue.

In summary, umbilical cord blood contains sufficient numbers of haematopoietic precursor cells to routinely allow long-term haematopoietic reconstitution in children requiring an allogeneic bone marrow transplant. As noted in Dr Broxmeyer's review in 1995, there are a significant number of questions that need to be answered regarding the use of this tissue in bone marrow transplantation. There are sufficient numbers of repopulating cells in umbilical cord blood to support a child, but will this number of cells be sufficient for adult allogeneic transplants? There are significant data accruing demonstrating that umbilical cord blood contains more primitive haematopoietic elements including stem cells and progenitor cells. There appears to be qualitative differences between haematopoietic repopulating cells in cord blood as compared to peripheral blood and bone marrow tissue. If there are not sufficient numbers of repopulating cells in cord blood for adult transplantation, it is very conceivable that this obstacle may be solved through *ex vivo* expansion of haematopoietic stem cells and progenitor cells. There are currently a number of new *in vitro* culture systems and 'cocktails' of growth factors which can reproducibly expand various haematopoietic progenitor cell subgroups. Thus, this approach may be of use in the future to support a variety of different therapeutic needs. Another important characteristic of cord blood appears to be that this tissue is less immunologically reactive and thus has the potential to provide better engraftment in HLA-mismatched settings and less GvHD than other mismatched haematopoietic tissues such as peripheral blood and bone marrow. This characteristic feature would make cord blood a much more attractive source for unrelated HLA transplants and would supplement the 'National Marrow Donor Program' in identifying persons with appropriate HLA type for transplant. Finally, cord blood cell banks have been established as an allogeneic cell repository for unrelated, HLA-matched transplant needs. In addition, banks can be used for autologous donation or related matched or mismatched allogeneic transplants. Thus family members can provide directed donations in families at high risk for certain lethal immunodeficiency or haematological congenital disorders. Cord blood banks would also provide individuals with their own sources of haematopoietic stem cells to be used at a later date in the event that these patients develop a cancer or bone marrow disorder that requires marrow ablative therapy followed by haematopoietic reconstitution.

There are a significant number of severe congenital disorders of the haematopoietic and immune system. One of these disorders, X-linked severe combined immunodeficiency disorder (SCID), generally results in the death of these children by the age of 10. Current curative treatment for this condition in the postnatal period is either HLA-matched or T-cell depleted haplo-identical bone marrow transplantation. This procedure is usually successful in restoring the immune system in 75–90 per cent of patients; but significant problems occur including graft failure, GvHD, and delayed immunological reconstitution. Recently Dr A.W. Flake and colleagues reported at the American Society of Hematology's 37th Annual Meeting, December 1995 (Flake *et al.* 1995), successful treatment of an X-linked recessive severe combined immunodeficient fetus with *in utero* transplantation of CD34-enriched paternal bone marrow cells. In their report, the investigators identified in the first trimester of pregnancy a fetus that carried genetic abnormalities for X-linked SCID. A previous male sibling in this family died at seven months of age. Thus, the family wished for a successful outcome to the pregnancy and consented to *in utero* transplantation. The fetus is immunotolerant during the first trimester of pregnancy and there are a number of reports in the literature of chimerism among twins *in utero*, including haematopoietic chimerism due to exchange of haematopoietic cells during the first trimester of gestation. Thus, the investigators attempted to establish chimerism in the fetus by collecting CD4-enriched paternal bone marrow cells and infusing them intraperitoneally at 16, 17.5, and 18.5 weeks of gestation. The fetus was delivered by Caesarean section at 36 weeks gestation because of fetal compromise by a double nuchal cord. At delivery, the infant had only mild macular rash consistent with grade 1 GvHD. Cord blood revealed a normal absolute lymphocyte count and molecular HLA analysis revealed a strong donor band of equal intensity to the host antigens. HLA analysis by flow cytometry confirmed the presence of mixed chimerism with 100 per cent of the patient's Trophoblast lymphocytes being of donor origin. The patient's rash completely resolved with a short course of steroids and the infant has remained healthy and had normal growth with no evidence of GvHD. Thus, this was a very successful *in utero* transplant of paternal haematopoietic cells which resulted in reconstitution of T and B lymphocytes, allowing the infant to have a fully competent immune system at birth. This technique avoids the need of allogeneic bone marrow transplantation in the postnatal period which, as noted above, is often complicated by graft failure, GvHD, and the need for an appropriate donor. This case illustrates the important potential of this type of procedure for infants who are identified as having severe congenital haematologic and immunologic disorders that require bone marrow transplantation. Genetic counselling is obviously critical in establishing the diagnosis in the first trimester of pregnancy. Once diagnosis is made, it appears that chimerism can be established by *in utero* transplantation of paternal haematopoietic tissue without graft failure or inducing significant GvHD.

REFERENCES

Bradley, T.R. and Metcalf, D. (1966). The growth of mouse bone marrow cells *in vitro*. *Australian Journal of Experimental Biological and Medical Science*, **44**, 287–300.

Broxmeyer, H.E., Douglas, G.W., Hangoc, G., Cooper, S., Bard, J., English, D. *et al.* (1989). Human umbilical cord blood as a potential source of transplnatable hematopoietic stem/progenitor cells. *Proceedings of the National Academy of Sciences, USA*, **86**, 3828–32.

Broxmeyer, H.E., Gluckman, E., Auerbach, A., Douglas, G.W., Friedman, H., Cooper, S., *et al.* (1990). Human umbilical cord blood: A clinically useful source of transplantable hematopoietic stem/progenitor cells. *International journal of Cell Clonning*, **8**, (Suppl. 1), 76–91.

Broxmeyer, H.E., Hangoc, G., Cooper, S., Ribeiro, R.C., Graves, V., Yoder, M., *et al.* (1993). Growth charcteristics and expansion of human umbilical cord blood and estimation of its potential for transplantation in adults. *Proceedings of the National Academy of Sciences, USA*, **89**, 4109–13.

Broxmeyer, H.E. (1995). Questions to be answered regarding umbilical cord blood hematopoietic stem and progenitor cells and their use in transplantation. *Transfusion*, **35**, 694–702.

Broxmeyer, H.E., Douglas, G.W., Hangoc, G., *et al.* (1989). Human umbilical cord blood as a potential source of transplantable hematopoietic stem/progenitor cells. *Proceedings of the National Academy of Sciences, USA*, **86**, 3828–32.

Broxmeyer, H.E., Gluckman, E., Auerbach, A., *et al.* (1990). Human umbilical cord blood: a clinically useful source of transplantable hematopoietic stem/progenitor cells. *International Journal of Cell Cloning* **8**, (Suppl. 1), 76–91.

Broxmeyer, H.E., Hangoc, G., Cooper, S., *et al.* (1993). Growth characteristics and expansion of human umbilical cord blood and estimation of its potential for transplantation in adults. *Proceedings of the National Academy of Sciences, USA*, **89**, 4109–13.

Ende, M. (1966). Lymphangiosarcoma. Report of a case. *Pacific Medical Surgery*, **74**, 80–2.

Ende, M. and Ende, N. (1972). Hematopoietic transplantation by means of fetal (cord) blood. A new method. *Vancouver Medical Monthly*, **99**, 276.

Flake, A.W., Puck, J.M., Almeida-Porada, G., Evans, N.I., Johnson, M.P., Roncarolo, M.G., and Zanjani, E.D. (1995). Successful treatment of X-linked recessive severe combined immunodeficiency (X-scid) by the *in utero* transplantation of CD34 in rich paternal bone marrow cells. *Blood*, **86**, (Suppl. 1), 125a.

Gluckman, E., Broxmeyer, H.E., Auerbach, A.D., Friedman, H.S., Douglas, G.W., Devergie, A., *et al.* (1989). Hematopoeitic reconstitution in a patient with Fanconi's anemia by means of umbilical cord blood from an HLA identical sibling. *New England Journal of Medicine*, **321**, 1174–8.

Gluckman, E., Broxmeyer, H.E., Auerbach, A.D., *et al.* (1989). Hematopoietic reconstitution in a patient with Fanconi's anemia by means of umbilical cord blood from an HLA identical sibling. *New England Journal of Medicine*, **321**, 1174–8.

Gluckman, E., Devergie, A., Thierry, D., *et al.* (1992). Clinical applications of stem cell transfusion form cord blood and rationale for cord blood banking. *Bone Marrow Transplantation*, **9**, (Suppl.) 114–17.

Goldberg, J. (1990). Systems used to study the nature of the leukemic cell and predict treatment outcome in patients with myeloproliferative disorders. *Clinics in Laboratory Medicine*, **10**, 809–24.

Goldberg, J., Tice, D., Nelson, D.A., and Gottlieb, A.J. (1978). Predictive value of *in vitro* colony and cluster formation in acute non-lymphocytic leukemia. *Medical Science*, **277**, 81–4.

Goldberg, J., Williams, W.J., and Nelson, D.A. (1979). Platelet pheresis residues: enrichment of committed stem cells (CFU-C) from human peripheral blood. *Proceedings of the Society for Experimental Biology and Medicine*, **161**, 378–81.

Goldberg, J., McGuire, L.A., Dock, N.L., Williams, W.J., and Davey, F.R. (1980). Purification of human peripheral blood colony forming cells (CFU-C). *Experimental Hematology*, **8**, 1086–93.

Goldberg, J., Zamkoff, K.A., Nelson, D.A., Davey, F.R., and Gottlieb, A.J. (1983). The *in vitro* effects of vincristine on peripheral blood leukocyte progenitor cells (CFU-C) in patients with blast crisis of chronic granulocytic leukemia: correlation with clinical response. *Hematology*, **14**, 149–57.

Kirshner, J.J. and Goldberg, J. (1980). Types of colonies formed by normal human bone marrow, peripheral blood and umbilical cord blood CFU-C. *Experimental Hematology*, **8**, 1202–7.

Kirshner, J.J., Goldberg, J., and Landaw, S.A. (1980). The spleen as a site of colony forming cell (CFU-C) production in myelofibrosis. *Proceedings of the Society for Experimental Biology and Medicine*, **165**, 279–82.

Kirshner, J.J., Goldberg, J., Nelson, D.A., and Gottlieb, A.J. (1982). Predictive value of the CFU-C assay in acute nonlymphocytic leukemia. *Medicine*, **72**, 615–19.

McLeod, D.L., Shreeve, M.M., and Axelrad, A.A. (1974). Improved plasma culture system for production of erythrocytic colonies *in vitro*: quantitative assay method for CFU-E. *Blood*, **44**, 517–34.

Parker, J.W. and Metcalf, D. (1974). Production of colony-stimulating factors in mitogen-stimulated lymphocyte cultures. *Journal of Immunology*, **112**, 502–10.

Pike, B.L. and Robinson, W.A. (1970). Human bone marrow colony growth in agar gel. *Journal of Cellular Physiology*, **76**, 77–84.

Pluznik, D.H. and Sachs, L. (1965). The cloning of normal 'mast' cells in tissue culture. *Journal of Cellular and Comparative Physiology*, **66**, 319–24.

Till, J.E. and McCulloch, E.A. (1961). A direct measurement of the radiation sensitivity of normal mouse bone marrow cells. *Radiation Research*, **14**, 213–18.

Vilmer, E., Sterkers, G. Rahimy, C., Elion, J., Broyart, A., Lescoeur, B., *et al.* (1992). HLA-mismatched cord blood transplantation in a patient with advanced leukemia. *Transplantation*, **53**, 1155–7.

Vilmer, E., Sterkers, G., Rahimy, C., *et al.* (1992). HLA-mismatched cord blood transplantation in a patient with advanced leukemia. *Transplantation*, **53**, 1155–7.

Wagner, J.E., Broxmeyer, H.E., and Cooper, S. (1992). Umbilical cord and placental blood hematopoietic stem cells: collection, cryopreservation, and storage. *Journal of Hematotherapy*, **1**, 167–73.

27 | *Practical teratology*

J.M. Friedman

INTRODUCTION

Every infant has at least a 5 per cent risk of being born with a serious congenital anomaly or mental retardation that is apparent within the first year of life (Baird *et al.* 1988). The cause of most congenital anomalies is unknown. Purely genetic factors, i.e. chromosomal aberrations and abnormalities of a single gene or gene pair, account for about a quarter of all congenital anomalies; environmental factors by themselves probably account for no more than one-tenth (Brent and Beckman 1990). Nevertheless, congenital anomalies caused by environmental and drug exposures are especially important because such birth defects are potentially preventable.

A teratogen is often defined as an agent that can produce a permanent abnormality of structure or function in an organism exposed during embryonic or fetal life. Definitions such as this, despite their wide use, are potentially misleading because they suggest that teratogenicity is an inherent property of some agents but not of others. In fact, it is much more useful to think of teratogenic *exposures* than of teratogenic *agents* because teratogenicity actually depends on the dosage, route, and gestational timing of the exposure as well as on the chemical and physical nature of the agent itself. Most agents can damage the embryo or fetus if given to a pregnant animal or woman in a manner and dose that produces severe maternal toxicity. It is differences in conditions of exposure that explain the fact that there are so many 'animal teratogens' and so few 'human teratogens' recognized.

HOW TERATOGENS WORK

Physical agents, drugs, and other chemicals can cause various kinds of reproductive toxicity. The observation that a certain exposure produces one kind of reproductive toxicity does not necessarily mean that similar exposures cause other kinds of reproductive toxicity as well. One cannot predict whether an exposure will be teratogenic in women on the basis of studies that show increased mutation rates in bacteria or reduced sperm counts in men. In fact, the mechanisms involved in teratogenesis often differ greatly from those involved with other kinds of toxicity, and understanding these differences is useful in interpreting potential teratogenic risks in patients.

Embryonic development is controlled by the genome. The zygote contains all of the information necessary to produce an entire organism, but the molecular processes involved in development are only beginning to be understood. This complex and coordinated system of developmental control offers many potential targets for teratogenic action. Damage caused by teratogenic exposures often is repaired at least partially, and some of the effects observed at birth may result from unsuccessful attempts at repair of the initial damage.

In mammals, embryonic development does not proceed clonally. Thus, there is a fundamental difference between teratogenesis and the process of tumour development, which occurs by the accumulation of mutations within the progeny of a single cell (Brent 1986*a*). Although many mutagens can be shown to have teratogenic activity in experimental animals under appropriate conditions of exposure, some teratogenic exposures do not have any measurable effect on the genome itself.

Teratogens may affect developmental processes by inducing or preventing programmed cell death, by distorting or disrupting morphogen gradients, or by inhibiting, delaying, advancing, or altering regulatory cascades. Some teratogenic effects are simply manifestations of the same pharmacological action an agent exhibits in adults or children. For example, the virilization of female genitalia that may occur in fetuses of women who take danazol during pregnancy (Brunskill 1992) is simply a manifestation of the androgenic properties of this agent. More often, however, teratogenic effects differ from the pharmacological effects of an agent in children and adults. Thalidomide provides a striking example of this. It is not surprising that pharmacological activity often does not predict teratogenic action: the biological processes involved in forming a structure in an embryo do not necessarily have anything to do with the processes that are necessary for function and maintenance of the structure once it has developed. These differences between pharmacological action and teratogenic activity make it difficult to predict which exposures are likely to be teratogenic in humans.

Exposures that are teratogenic characteristically perturb certain aspects of embryogenesis but not others. As a result, teratogenic exposures usually result in characteristic patterns of congenital anomalies in affected infants. Familiar examples include the fetal alcohol syndrome and rubella embryopathy (South and Sever 1985; Preblud and Alford 1990; Ginsburg *et al.* 1991; Coles 1992).

Because of the complexity of embryogenesis and the many genetic factors that underlie it, it is not surprising that individual differences in susceptibility to teratogenic effects exist. In experimental mammals, such effects can sometimes be partitioned into those that depend on the fetal genotype and others that depend on the maternal genotype. In humans, these interactions are more difficult to study, but clear evidence of differences in individual susceptibility to a few teratogenic exposures has been found. For example, infants with malformations characteristic of the fetal hydantoin syndrome often exhibit a pharmacogenetic variant of epoxide hydrolase with decreased activity (Buehler *et al.* 1990). It seems likely that such variations in susceptibility are widespread because even strong teratogenic exposures such as those to therapeutic doses of thalidomide or isotretinoin during early embryogenesis produce characteristic malformations in less than half of all cases (Lenz and Knapp 1962; Lenz 1966; Rosa *et al.* 1986; Chen *et al.* 1990).

Teratogens act at vulnerable periods of embryonic or fetal development. For most teratogenic exposures, the period of organogenesis, i.e. approximately 2–10 weeks after conception or 4–12 weeks after the last normal menstrual period, is the time of greatest susceptibility. In some teratogenic exposures, such as those to therapeutic doses of thalidomide, more precise localization of the specific time in embryonic development that is associated with greatest susceptibility to particular congenital anomalies has been possible (Lenz and Knapp 1962; Lenz 1966).

It is important to realize that many potentially teratogenic exposures occur before a woman has recognized that she is pregnant. This has clear implications with respect to the prevention of congenital anomalies that result from teratogenic exposures. It means that physicians should consider the teratogenic potential of any drug prescribed for a woman of child-bearing age and discuss this with her at the time the prescription is written. Similarly, attempts to reduce the teratogenic effects of maternal diseases such as diabetes by improved control should be implemented prior to conception.

Although embryogenesis is usually the period of greatest susceptibility to teratogenic effects, some exposures act later in development and some may act earlier. Susceptibility to fetal renal dysfunction, oligohydramnios, and death is greatest when exposure to captopril or another angiotensin-converting enzyme inhibitor occurs during the second or third trimester of pregnancy (Brent and Beckman 1991; Hanssens et al. 1991; Shotan et al. 1994). There is no evidence that similar exposures during the first trimester of gestation pose a substantial risk to the embryo. Similarly, the dental staining that may occur in children of women who take tetracycline during pregnancy is only seen with treatment in the second or third trimester of gestation (Cohlan 1977).

The first two weeks after conception have been considered an 'all-or-none' period with respect to adverse effects of teratogenic exposures. Many exposures that are teratogenic during a later period of embryogenesis do not produce malformations before implantation because any damage that occurs either causes death of the conceptus or is repaired without apparent effect on the infant at birth (Austin 1973; Kimmel et al. 1993). However, some exposures have been shown to cause malformations in mammalian offspring after maternal treatment prior to implantation (Generoso et al. 1991; Kimmel et al. 1993).

One difficulty in determining the risks related to potentially teratogenic exposures in humans is that such exposures usually do not occur in isolation. Many women who have had one potentially teratogenic exposure have concomitant exposure to other agents as well. In addition, women who have teratogenic exposures often differ greatly from those who do not. Exposed women may have medical illnesses, lifestyles, or occupations that are quite different from those in unexposed populations.

HOW WE RECOGNIZE POTENTIALLY TERATOGENIC EXPOSURES

Identification of human teratogenic exposures requires careful interpretation of data obtained from several different kinds of studies (Cordero and Oakley 1983; Brent 1986b; Shepard 1994).

The first evidence that an exposure is teratogenic in humans often comes from clinical case reports. Case reports are most useful if they reveal a recurrent pattern of anomalies in babies who experienced similar well-defined exposures at similar points during embryonic development. While case reports are important in raising suspicion that a particular exposure may produce a given congenital anomaly or pattern of anomalies, most such associations are merely coincidental. Coincidental occurrence of an environmental or drug exposure in a pregnant woman and congenital anomalies in her child is common, especially if the exposure or the defects or both are relatively frequent.

Clinical series are an effective means of recognizing the patterns of congenital anomalies that characterize most human teratogenic exposures. For example, the fetal alcohol syndrome and thalidomide embryopathy were first recognized in clinical series (McBride 1961; Lenz 1962; Jones *et al.* 1973). Such studies may involve the children of a group of women who all experienced a similar exposure during pregnancy or a group of children who all have a similar congenital anomaly or pattern of anomalies.

Epidemiologic studies provide the only means of obtaining quantitative estimates of the strength and statistical significance of associations between teratogenic exposures in pregnant women and abnormalities in their offspring. Epidemiologic investigations used in teratology are mostly of two types: cohort studies and case–control studies. In cohort studies, the frequencies of certain anomalies are compared in the children of women with and without a given exposure. In case–control studies, the frequency of prenatal exposure is compared among children with and without a given congenital anomaly.

If a teratogenic exposure increases the risk of anomalies in the offspring only slightly, very large epidemiological studies may be necessary to demonstrate the increase. In interpreting epidemiological studies, one must remember that the maternal disease or situation which occasioned the exposure rather than the agent itself may be responsible for an observed association. Biases of ascertainment and recall may also produce spurious associations. Spurious associations regularly occur in investigations involving large numbers of comparisons between exposed and unexposed or affected and unaffected subjects. Moreover, the usefulness of most published epidemiological studies is limited by failure to consider the aetiological heterogeneity of human congenital abnormalities or the subtle patterns of anomalies characteristic of many human teratogens.

Although human investigations are necessary to demonstrate that an exposure is teratogenic in humans, such studies are not informative until the exposure has already damaged many children. Experimental animal studies provide a means of identifying exposures with teratogenic potential before any children have been harmed. Unfortunately, it is usually difficult to extrapolate findings in animals to a clinical situation involving a pregnant woman. Species differences in placentation, pharmacodynamics, embryonic development, and innate predisposition to various fetal anomalies are well recognized. Moreover, teratology experiments in animals often employ doses or methods of exposure that are much greater than those likely to occur in humans. Maternal toxic effects may confound interpretation of fetal outcome in such experiments.

One can never conclude that an association found in a single study between a maternal exposure and congenital anomalies in the offspring indicates causality without adducing other evidence to support such a conclusion. Establishing that a particular exposure is potentially teratogenic in humans requires the demonstration of a reproducible, consistent, and biologically plausible effect (Brent 1986*b*; Shepard 1994).

Reproducibility means that similar findings have been obtained in independent studies. Concordance is considered particularly important if the studies are of different design and if the types of anomalies observed in various studies are consistent. Effects seen in animal investigations should be weighed more heavily if the exposure is similar in dosage and route to that encountered in pregnant women and if the species tested are closely related to humans phylogenetically.

Of critical importance is that the observed association make biological sense. Exposures that produce malformations in the embryo or fetus are expected to do so only during particular periods of development. In most cases, exposure to a greater quantity of the agent should increase the likelihood of abnormalities. Systemic absorption of the agent by the mother and its presence at susceptible sites in the embryo or placenta should be demonstrable. Finally, a causal inference is supported if a reasonable pathogenic mechanism can be established for the observed effect. Experimental animal and *in vitro* studies are very useful in elucidating pathogenic mechanisms.

There are three ways that diverse data available on a particular exposure can be synthesized. The first and most commonly used is the *ad hoc* approach in which a clinician reviews the relevant scientific literature and interprets it for the patient. This approach is time-consuming and the quality of the interpretation depends greatly on the clinician's training and experience and on the rigor and thoroughness of the review.

A second approach is meta-analysis (Einarson *et al.* 1988). This is a formal method of combining the results of similar epidemiological studies and testing for consistency and overall trends. Although powerful when used appropriately, meta-analysis cannot be applied unless a sufficient number of epidemiological studies of sufficiently high quality has been performed regarding a particular exposure. Relatively few teratogenic exposures have been subjected to such extensive epidemiological study. In addition, meta-analysis ignores mechanistic information and suffers from the same limitations as its component studies in dealing with aetiological heterogeneity and subtle patterns of anomalies.

A third approach to integrating the results of various studies to arrive at an overall interpretation is the use of expert consensus. Expert consensus has been used to estimate the teratogenic risk associated with many common exposures (Friedman and Polifka 1994).

HUMAN TERATOGENIC EXPOSURES

Exposures that are known to cause congenital anomalies in humans include some kinds of maternal metabolic imbalance, infectious agents, environmental toxins, physical agents, drugs of abuse, and medications. Information regarding the teratogenic effects of these exposures is summarized below and in Tables 27.1–27.3.

Maternal metabolic imbalance (Table 27.1)

Alterations of the maternal internal milieu, although intrinsic to the mother, affect the external environment of the embryo or fetus. Diabetes mellitus is the most common teratogenic maternal condition. Children of women with insulin-dependent diabetes mellitus have a risk of congenital anomalies that is two to three times greater than that of the general population (Reece and Hobbins 1986, Rosenn and Tsang 1991). The most common malformations among infants of diabetic mothers are congenital heart disease (occurring in 2–3 per cent) and neural tube defects (occurring in 1–2 per cent). Some other congenital anomalies, such as caudal dysplasia and proximal femoral hypoplasia, are rare but occur much more often in the infants of diabetic mothers than in other infants.

Malformations develop early in gestation. Improved control of maternal diabetes later in pregnancy cannot influence the frequency of malformations in infants of diabetic mothers. Thus, pregnancies in women with insulin-dependent diabetes should be planned so that excellent control can be maintained from the moment of conception.

Many of the congenital anomalies associated with maternal diabetes can be detected prenatally by high-resolution ultrasound examination, fetal echocardiography, or measurement of the α-fetoprotein concentration in maternal blood or amniotic fluid. Prenatal diagnosis should be offered to all pregnant women with insulin-dependent diabetes mellitus.

The children of women with phenylketonuria (PKU) that is untreated during pregnancy are almost certain to be born with mental retardation, microcephaly, and other anomalies (Lenke and Levy 1980; Rohr *et al.* 1987). Such children usually do not have PKU themselves but are damaged by developing in a hyperphenylalaninaemic intrauterine environment.

Infectious agents (Table 27.2)

Infection of the embryo or fetus may occur transplacentally. Congenital rubella is the best known teratogenic infection in humans. Rubella embryopathy is preventable by immunization of children with rubella vaccine. Parvovirus infection of the fetus may produce severe anaemia, hydrops, and death (Shmoys and Kaplan 1990; Berry *et al.* 1992). Spontaneous recovery of the fetus may also occur.

Ionizing radiation

Radiation causes DNA damage and can injure the developing embryo. *In utero* exposure to large doses of X-rays, such as those used for cancer radiotherapy, can produce microcephaly and mental retardation (Schull *et al.* 1990; Mole 1993). Although unnecessary diagnostic radiographs should be avoided and necessary exposures minimized during pregnancy, diagnostic radiography is rarely associated with radiation doses that pose a substantial risk to the embryo or fetus.

Radioactive iodine is concentrated in the fetal thyroid gland after the twelfth week of pregnancy and may produce cretinism (Stoffer and Hamburger 1976).

Table 27.1. Human teratogenic exposures: Maternal metabolic imbalance.

Agent	Most susceptible period	Nature	Risk Comments	References
Maternal insulin-dependent diabetes mellitus	Organogenesis	Malformations, especially congenital heart disease and spina bifida	1) Risk may be decreased if diabetes is well controlled from the time of conception and throughout the first trimester. 2) Diabetic pregnancies are also at increased risk for various obstetrical and neonatal complications including abnormal fetal growth and neonatal hypoglycaemia. 3) Prenatal diagnosis of severe cardiac malformations and neural tube defects is available.	Garner 1995 Miller 1994
Maternal phenylketonuria	Organogenesis	Microcephaly, mental retardation, congenital heart disease	1) Risk is almost 100% in the children of untreated women with PKU. 2) The risk is substantially reduced in pregnancies of women with PKU who are treated beginning before conception.	Lenke & Levy 1980 Rohr et al. 1987
Excess maternal androgen secretion	Cliteromegaly: any time; labioscrotal fusion: first trimester	Cliteromegaly, labioscrotal fusion in female fetus	1) Similar genital virilization in female fetuses may occur when the mother takes exogenous androgens during pregnancy.	Bilowus et al. 1986
Maternal systemic lupus erythematosus	Unknown	Heart block; fetal death		Petri 1994, 1995

Table 27.2. Human teratogenic exposures: Infectious agents.

Exposure		Risk		References
Agent	Most susceptible period	Nature	Comments	
Rubella virus	First trimester	Rubella embryopathy: growth retardation, cardiovascular anomalies, cataracts, retinopathy, glaucoma, deafness	1) Rubella immunization of children and susceptible women prior to conception can prevent rubella embryopathy. 2) Fetal infection to often persistent and deterioration may occur later in life. 3) Prenatal diagnosis can be performed by fetal blood sampling or chorionic villus sampling.	Preblud & Alford 1990 South & Sever 1985
Treponema pallidum	Unknown	Intrauterine or perinatal death; Congenital syphilis: jaundice, anemia, rhinitis, arthritis, osteochondritis	1) Most liveborn infants of women with untreated syphilis during pregnancy have congenital infection. 2) Treatment is indicated when maternal syphilis is diagnosed during pregnancy.	Mascola et al. 1985
Toxoplasma gondii	Risk of fetal infection increases with gestational age, but risk of symptomatic congenital infection is greatest between 10 and 24 weeks gestation.	Congenital toxoplasmosis: encephalitis, hydrocephalus, chioretinitis, anaemia, jaundice, hepatosplenomegaly, glomerulitis, myocarditis, myositis	1) Most infants of women infected during pregnancy are clinically normal, even if intrauterine infection has occurred. 2) Treatment of primary maternal infection during pregnancy is recommended.	Remington & Desmonts 1990 Dubey & Beattie 1988

Table 27.2. Human teratogenic exposures: Infectious agents. (continued)

Agent	Exposure — Most susceptible period	Risk — Nature	Comments	References
Cytomegalovirus (CMV)	First half of pregnancy	Congenital CMV infection: growth retardation, microcephaly, petechiae, hepatosplenomegaly, jaundice, chorioretinitis, migration defects of brain	1) Most infants of women infected during pregnancy are clinically normal, even if intrauterine infection has occurred. 2) Prenatal diagnosis of fetal anomalies by ultrasound examination is sometimes possible.	Adler 1992 Stagno 1990
Human immunodeficiency virus (HIV)	Unknown	Congenital AIDS: failure to thrive, interstitial pneumonia, recurrent bacterial and other infections, chronic diarrhea, generalized lymphadenopathy, death in infancy or early childhood	1) The risk of maternal-fetal HIV transmission can be reduced by treatment of the mother with zidovudine.	Abrams & Rogers 1991 Sicklick & Rubinstein 1992
Parvovirus B19	Unknown	Anaemia, hydrops fetalis, death	1) Spontaneous resolution of hydrops may occur. 2) Survival of infected hydropic fetus after intrauterine transfusion has been reported. 3) Most infants of women infected during pregnancy are clinically normal, even if intrauterine infection has occurred. 4) Fetal hydrops can be diagnosed prenatally by ultrasound examination.	Berry *et al.* 1992 Shmoys & Kaplan 1990

Environmental agents and occupational chemicals

'Chemicals' are often of concern to pregnant women, but exposure to only two such agents has been shown to be teratogenic in humans. Maternal poisoning during pregnancy by food contaminated with methyl mercury can cause damage to the fetal central nervous system (Burbacher *et al.* 1990). Ataxia, weakness, and features of cerebral palsy may result. Maternal ingestion of large amounts of polychlorinated biphenyls (PCBs) during pregnancy produces fetal growth retardation, diffuse hyper-pigmentation, and natal teeth (Lione 1988; Tilson *et al.* 1990).

Hyperthermia that produces sustained elevation of maternal body temperature to levels substantially above normal causes central nervous system anomalies in laboratory animals (Warkany 1986). A similar effect may occur in humans, but this has not been clearly established. Hyperthermia in pregnant women is usually caused by fever but may occur with extreme use of saunas or hot tubs or because of excessive exercise in hot conditions.

Maternal exposure to large amounts of lead during pregnancy has been associated with central nervous system damage in the offspring, but available studies do not permit clear separation of the effects of prenatal and postnatal exposures (Davis *et al.* 1990; Ernhart 1992).

Drugs of abuse

Drug abuse may not only damage the health of the mother but also interfere with the development of the embryo or fetus. Maternal alcohol abuse is a particularly important cause of congenital anomalies.

Classic fetal alcohol syndrome occurs among the children of women with chronic, severe alcoholism during pregnancy (Ginsburg *et al.* 1991; Coles 1992). Mothers of infants with fetal alcohol syndrome usually drink more, and often much more, than 90 ml of absolute alcohol daily—the equivalent of about six 12 ounce 4% beers, six glasses of wine, or cocktails.

Features of fetal alcohol syndrome include growth deficiency, mental retardation, behavioural disturbances, and typical facial appearance characterized by short palpebral fissures, hypoplastic midface, long flat philtrum, and narrow upper lip vermilion. Congenital heart disease and structural brain anomalies are common.

The risks of maternal binge drinking during pregnancy have not been clearly defined but may be substantial. Smaller amounts of maternal drinking during pregnancy have been associated with less severe disturbances of growth, intellectual performance, and behaviour among offspring. No safe level of maternal drinking during pregnancy has been established.

Maternal use of cocaine during pregnancy has been associated with placental abruption and the occurrence of encephaloclastic lesions and other vascular disruptions in the fetus (Behnke and Eyler 1993; Frank *et al.* 1993; Singer *et al.* 1993). Other teratogenic effects of cocaine have been suggested but are controversial.

Although usual occupational exposures to toluene are unlikely to produce fetal damage, chronic maternal abuse of toluene by inhalation during pregnancy has been associated with central nervous system dysfunction and characteristic physical abnormalities in the offspring (Arnold *et al.* 1994; Pearson *et al.* 1994). Features of this 'toluene embryopathy' include developmental delay, attention deficit disorder, microcephaly, short palpebral fissures, deep-set eyes, micrognathia, abnormal auricles, small fingernails, and growth deficiency.

Heavy maternal cigarette smoking during pregnancy is associated with increased rates of fetal growth retardation and miscarriage (Rosenberg 1987; Fredricsson and Gilljam 1992). Most epidemiological studies show no association between the frequency of major congenital anomalies and maternal smoking during pregnancy. Weak associations have been observed in some studies between smoking in pregnant women and various congenital anomalies in their children, but these associations have not been consistently reproducible.

Medications (Table 27.3)

Maternal treatment with some medications in usual therapeutic doses early in pregnancy can cause congenital anomalies in infants.

Isotretinoin and etretinate are vitamin A congeners that can produce craniofacial, brain, cardiac, and other serious fetal malformations (Rosa *et al.* 1986; Chen *et al.* 1990; Mitchell 1992; Adams and Lammer 1993). Maternal use early in pregnancy of very high doses of vitamin A taken as retinol or retinyl esters has also been associated with fetal anomalies (Rosa *et al.* 1986; Rothman *et al.* 1995; Oakley and Erickson 1995). The dose at which this occurs has not been determined but is clearly much greater than the recommended dietary allowance (RDA). Maternal use of β-carotene, which is converted to vitamin A in the body, does not appear to be associated with any teratogenic risk (Fonda Allen and Rosenbaum 1992).

An increased rate of congenital anomalies occurs among the children of epileptic women treated with anticonvulsant medications during pregnancy. It is uncertain whether this increased risk is a consequence of the mother's epilepsy, a teratogenic effect of the medications, or some combination thereof. In general, however, therapy with multiple anticonvulsant drugs is associated with a higher risk than therapy with a single anticonvulsant. Drugs that have been implicated as having teratogenic effects when used as anticonvulsants include phenytoin (Hanson 1986; Delgado-Escueta and Janz 1992; Lindhout and Omtzigt 1992), trimethadione (Goldman and Yaffe 1978; Dansky and Finnell 1991), valproic acid (Dansky and Finnell 1991; Lindhout and Omtzigt 1994; Yerby and Devinsky 1994), carbamazepine (Lindhout and Omtzigt 1992; Yerby and Devinsky 1994), primidone (Dansky and Finnell 1991), and phenobarbital (Dansky and Finnell 1991).

Maternal treatment with valproic acid during pregnancy has also been associated with about a 2 per cent risk of spina bifida among the offspring. The risk of spina bifida may also be somewhat increased among the children of women treated with carbamazepine during pregnancy. Epileptic women who take valproic acid or carbamazepine can reduce their risk of having a child with a neural tube defect if they also take folic acid supplements before conception and through the first two months of pregnancy. Prenatal diagnosis of neural tube defects should be offered to women who have been treated with valproic acid or carbamazepine during early pregnancy.

Table 27.3. Human teratogenic exposures: Medications

Agent	Exposure Dose	Most susceptible period	Nature	Risk Comments	References
Thalidomide	Usual therapeutic	Gestational days 27–40	Phocomelia, malformed ears, tetralogy of Fallot, oesophageal or duodenal atresia, renal agenesis, cranial nerve anomalies, facial haemangioma.	1) Malformations occur in about 20% of infants whose mothers took this medication during the sensitive period of pregnancy.	Lenz & Knapp 1962 Lenz, 1966
Aminopterin	1–3 mg/d or more	Organogenesis	Short stature, delayed calvarial ossification, craniosynostosis, hydrocephalus, abnormal auricles, ocular hypertelorism, micrognathia, cleft palate		Warkany 1978, 1981
Methotrexate	12.5 mg/week or more	Organogenesis	Large fontanelles, abnormal head shape, craniosynostosis, ocular hypertelorism, skeletal defects	1) The frequency of malformations among the children of women treated with methotrexate during early pregnancy appears to be dose related. Most infants of women treated with low-dose methotrexate for arthritis during pregnancy are normal. 2) The rate of miscarriage is high in women treated with methotrexate early in pregnancy.	Warkany 1978 Wiebe & Sipila 1994

Table 27.3. Human teratogenic exposures: Medications (continued)

Agent	Exposure			Risk		References
	Dose	Most susceptible period	Nature	Comments		
Cyclophos-phamide	Usual therapeutic (for cancer)	Organogenesis	Skeletal defects, cleft palate, eye malformations			Kirshon et al. 1988
						Mutchinick et al. 1992
Phenytoin	Usual therapeutic	Organogenesis	Fetal hydantoin syndrome: ocular hypertelorism, flat nasal bridge, distal digital hypoplasia, nail hypoplasia, developmental delay	1) Typical fetal hydantoin syndrome occurs in about 10% of infants born to epileptic women treated with phenytoin during pregnancy. 2) Cleft palate, congenital heart disease, and growth deficiency may be less common manifestations of fetal hydantoin syndrome 3) The risk is greater if the treatment involves multiple anticonvulsants.		Hanson 1986 Delgado-Escueta & Janz 1992. Lindhout & Omtzigt 1992.
Valproic acid	Usual therapeutic	Organogenesis	Fetal valproate syndrome: growth retardation, microcephaly, unusualfacial features; spina bifida	1) The risk of major congenital anomalies among the children of epileptic women treated with valproic acid during pregnancy is 2–3 times greater than expected. 2) The risk of neural tube defects among the children of epileptic women treated with valproic acid during pregnancy is about 2%. 3) The risk is greater if the treatment involves multiple anticonvulsants.		Dansky & Finnell 1991 Lindhout & Omtzigt 1994 Yerby & Devinsky 1994

494

Table 27.3. Human teratogenic exposures: Medications (continued)

Agent	Exposure		Risk		References
	Dose	Most Susceptible Period	Nature	Comments	
				4) Folate supplementation is recommended for women who are taking valproic acid and who are or may become pregnant to reduce the risk of neural tube defects in the offspring. 5) Prenatal diagnosis of fetal neural tube defects is available by means of ultrasound examination and measurement of the alpha-fetoprotein concentration in maternal blood or amniotic fluid.	Lindhout & Omtzigt 1994 Yerby & Devinsky 1994
Carbamaze-pine	Usual therapeutic	Organogenesis	Fetal carbamazepine syndrome with unusual facial features and other anomalies similar to those seen among the children of women treated with other anticonvulsants during pregnancy, spina bifida	1) The risk of major congenital anomalies among the children of epileptic women treated with carbamazepine during pregnancy is 2–3 times greater than expected. 2) The risk of neural tube defects among the children of epileptic women treated with carbamazepine during pregnancy is 1–2%. 3) The risk is greater if the treatment involves multiple anticonvulsants. 4) Folate supplementation is recommended for women who are taking carbamazepine and who are or may become pregnant to reduce the risk of neural tube defects in the offspring.	

Table 27.3. Human teratogenic exposures: Medications (continued)

Agent	Exposure		Risk		References
	Dose	Most susceptible period	Nature	Comments	
				5) Prenatal diagnosis of fetal neural tube defects is available by means of ultrasound examination and measurement of the alpha-fetoprotein concentration in maternal blood or amniotic fluid.	Goldman & Yaffe 1978
Trimethadione	Usual therapeutic	Organogenesis	Fetal trimethadione syndrome: growth retardation, microcephaly, cleft lip and/or palate, unusual facial features, cardiovascular malformations, mental retardation	1) Malformations are observed in about 30% of children born to epileptic women treated with trimethadione during pregnancy. 2) The rates of miscarriage and stillbirth appear to be increased in women treated with trimethadione during pregnancy 3) The risk is greater if the treatment involves multiple anticonvulsants.	Dansky & Finnell 1991
Primidone	Usual therapeutic	Organogenesis	Facial clefts, congenital heart disease; facial features similar to those seen in other 'fetal anticonvulsant syndromes'		Dansky & Finnell 1991
Phenobarbital	Usual therapeutic (chronic)	Organogenesis	Facial clefts, congenital heart disease, facial features similar to those seen in other 'fetal anticonvulsant syndromes'	1) The risk is unlikely to be increased in an infant whose mother has taken a single or occasional therapeutic dose of phenobarbital during pregnancy. 2) The risk may be greater with a toxic overdose of phenobarbital during pregnancy.	Dansky & Finnell 1991

Table 27.3. Human teratogenic exposures: Medications (continued)

Agent	Exposure		Risk		References
	Dose	Most Susceptible Period	Nature	Comments	
				3) The risk is greater if the treatment involves multiple anticonvulsants.	
Danazol	200 mg/d or greater		Virilization of external genitalia in female		Brunskill 1992
Norethindrone	Large therapeutic	First trimester	Virilization of external genitalia in female	1) Virilization has been observed in a few percent of female infants born to women who took norethindrone during pregnancy in doses greater than those used for oral contraception.	Schardein 1980 Wilson & Brent 1981
Ethisterone	Usual therapeutic	First trimester	Virilization of external genitalia in female	1) Virilization has been observed in about 15% of female infants born to women who took ethisterone during pregnancy.	Schardein 1980 Wilson & Brent 1981
Penicillamine	Usual therapeutic		Connective tissue abnormalities resembling cutis laxa with loose skin, hernias, loose joints, flat face, small jaw	1) The risk of this syndrome occurring in the child of a woman treated with penicillamine during pregnancy appears to be no more than a few percent. 2) Death in infancy is frequent in affected individuals. Appearance of the skin improves markedly with age in children who survive.	Roubenoff et al. 1988
Lithium	Usual therapeutic	Organogenesis	Cardiovascular malformations, especially Ebstein's anomaly of the	1) The risk of congenital heart disease in the child of a woman treated with lithium during pregnancy appears to be no more than a few percent.	Cohen et al. 1994

Table 27.3. Human teratogenic exposures: Medications (continued)

Agent	Exposure		Nature	Risk	References
	Dose	Most susceptible period		Comments	
			tricuspid valve	2) Prenatal diagnosis by fetal echocardiography is available for major cardiac malformations.	
Isotretinoin	Usual therapeutic (oral)	Organogenesis	Retinoid embryopathy: central nervous system malformations, ear malformations, cleft palate, micrognathia, cardiovascular anomalies, thymic abnormalities, eye defects, developmental delay	1) About half of children born to women treated with isotretinoin during the first trimester of pregnancy exhibit developmental delay and/or major malformations. 2) Many, but not all, serious manifestations of retinoid embryopathy can be visualized prenatally by ultrasonography.	Rosa *et al.* 1986 Chen *et al.* 1990 Adams & Lammer 1993
Etretinate	Usual therapeutic	Organogenesis	Central nervous system malformations, craniofacial anomalies, skeletal defects	1) Etretinate persists in the body for an extremely long time after administration. The length of time that teratogenic effects may occur after discontinuation of therapy is unknown. 2) Many, but not all, serious manifestations or retinoid embryopathy can be visualized prenatally by ultrasonography.	Rosa *et al.* 1986 Mitchell 1992
Vitamin A (retinoid)	> 25 000 IU per day	Organogenesis	'Retinoid embryopathy' with malformations similar to those seen in children of women treated with isotretinoin early in pregnancy	1) The risk of congenital anomalies appears to be small, even in children of women who take very large doses (> 25 000 IU per day) during early pregnancy.	Rothman *et al.* 1995 Oakley & Erickson 1995

498

Table 27.3. Human teratogenic exposures: Medications (continued)

Agent	Exposure		Risk		References
	Dose	Most susceptible period	Nature	Comments	
				2) There is no evidence of an increased risk of congenital anomalies among children of women who take less than 10 000 IU of vitamin A (retinoid) per day. 3) Maternal use during pregnancy of beta-carotene, which is contained in some supplements as a source of vitamin A, has not been associated with an increased risk of congenital anomalies in the offspring.	Rosa et al. 1986
Warfarin	Usual therapeutic	Second half of first trimester	Warfarin embryopathy: nasal hypoplasia, stippled epiphyses on radiographs, growth retardation, central nervous system malformations, eye anomalies	1) 8–10% of infants born to women who take conventional doses of warfarin during early pregnancy have features of this syndrome. The frequency appears to be lower with low-dose treatment.	Wong et al. 1993
Captopril	Usual therapeutic doses	Second or third trimester	Oligohydramnios, fetal growth retardation, neonatal renal failure, hypotension, pulmonary hypoplasia, hypocalvaria, joint contractures, death	1) There is no evidence that maternal treatment with captopril early in pregnancy increases the risk of malformations in the offspring.	Brent & Beckman 1991 Hanssens et al. 1991 Shotan et al. 1994

Table 27.3. Human teratogenic exposures: Medications (continued)

Agent	Exposure		Risk		References
	Dose	Most susceptible period	Nature	Comments	
Enalapril	Usual therapeutic doses	Second or third trimester	Oligohydramnios, fetal growth retardation neonatal renal failure, hypotension, pulmonary hypoplasia, hypocalvaria, joint contractures, death	1) There is no evidence that maternal treatment with enalapril early in pregnancy increases the risk of malformations in the offspring.	Brent & Beckman 1991 Hanssens et al. 1991 Shotan et al. 1994
Tetracycline	Usual therapeutic	Second or third trimester	Staining of primary teeth	1) Maternal treatment with tetracycline early in pregnancy does not appear to increase the risk of malformations in the offspring substantially.	Cohlan 1977
Methylene blue	Intra-amniotic administration	Second trimester	Jejunal atresia	1) The risk of jejunal atresia in an infant after second trimester intra-amniotic administration of methylene blue is about 20%. 2) It is unlikely that topical administration of methylene blue to a pregnant woman poses any teratogenic risk. 3) Haemolytic anaemia and jaundice may occur in infants born after intra-amniotic injection of methylene blue late in pregnancy.	Nicolini & Monni 1990 van der Pol et al. 1992
Indomethacin	Usual therapeutic premature	Third trimester	Olighydramnios, anuria, closure of the ductus arteriosus, necrotizing enterocolitis		Van den Veyver & Moise 1993

Maternal treatment later in pregnancy with some medications can have serious adverse effects on the offspring. For example, oligohydramnios, fetal renal failure, and fetal or neonatal death occur with greatly increased frequency among women treated with angiotensin-converting enzyme (ACE) inhibitors such as captopril and enaiapril late in pregnancy (Brent and Beckman 1991; Hanssens *et al.* 1991; Shotan *et al.* 1994). ACE inhibitors are not known to pose a substantial teratogenic risk in early pregnancy.

TERATOGEN RISK ASSESSMENT AND COUNSELLING

Pregnant women should avoid unnecessary exposure to any potentially harmful agent whenever possible. Unfortunately, avoiding exposure is sometimes impossible. Inadvertant exposure occurs when a woman is exposed after conception but before she recognizes that she is pregnant. Intended exposure occurs when a woman knowingly takes a drug or is otherwise exposed to an agent after she knows that she is pregnant. It is widely recognized that a pregnant woman should not be given any medication unless its benefit is clearly greater than the risk to both her and her fetus, but it is often difficult to determine whether the risk exceeds the benefit in practice.

The purpose of teratogen risk assessment is to determine whether the risk of congenital anomalies is increased in the child of a woman who has been exposed to a particular agent (or combination of agents) during pregnancy and, if so, to define the nature and magnitude of the extra risk. Teratogen risk counselling seeks to provide a patient with accurate information about her risk in a manner that enables her to participate more effectively in decisions regarding further management of the pregnancy.

Teratogen risk assessment requires knowledge of an individual patient's state of health, previous and current pregnancy history, and family history. Sometimes other factors increase the risk in a pregnancy as much as, or more than, the exposures. This must be considered when providing counselling and discussing options for management.

It is always necessary to determine as accurately as possible what the route and dose of an exposure was and whether there were concurrent exposures to other agents. Most agents that exhibit teratogenic effects do so only when the dose exceeds a certain threshold value. A woman who has had an exposure in an amount or by a route that produces an absorbed dose below this critical threshold is usually *not* at increased risk of having a child with congenital anomalies. On the other hand, almost any agent may produce fetal damage in a pregnant woman whose exposure is great enough to cause systemic toxicity in her. This is a clinically important consideration when a pregnant woman has taken a drug overdose or has had a massive exposure to a toxic industrial chemical.

Simultaneous exposure to more than one agent may modify the associated fetal risk. Studies in experimental mammals demonstrate that the teratogenic effects of two or more concomitant exposures may not be predictable from the effects of the exposures individually. Sometimes concomitant exposures result in effects that are simply additive. In other cases one exposure may substantially potentiate the effect of another or provide protection against the adverse effect of another exposure. In humans, the effect of a combination of agents is usually unknown. In such circumstances one must use the risks associated with the individual agents to estimate the overall risk but decrease the certainty of the assessment because of the combined exposure.

A clinician must consider all of the information available on the agent(s), dose, route of exposure, gestational timing, and other medical factors together in order to determine whether the risk of congenital anomalies in a particular pregnancy is similar to, greater than, or less than that usually associated with exposure to the agent under consideration. In other words, one must determine if the teratogenic risk estimate given in standard references applies to the patient under consideration. *The most frequent mistake made in teratogen risk counselling is failure to recognize that the circumstances in a particular pregnancy differ from those for which a risk has been established.*

Counselling provided as the result of this comprehensive risk assessment should be tailored to each patient's intellectual, educational, psychosocial, and cultural background. The risk associated with an exposure should be presented with reference to the background risk of congenital anomalies or mental retardation that attends every pregnancy. Any additional risk must be explained in qualitative as well as quantitative terms. A pregnant woman may be much more comfortable with a high risk for dental staining, for example, than a small risk of severe mental handicap in her child. Decisions regarding prenatal diagnosis and continuation or termination of pregnancy should be made by the patient in consultation with her physician, family, and other appropriate individuals.

Counselling a pregnant woman about possible effects of an environmental or drug exposure on her developing embryo or fetus is an important component of her medical care. Such counselling should be provided by physicians and other health professionals with competence in clinical teratology. Difficult or complex cases should be referred to appropriate specialists.

PREVENTION OF CONGENITAL ANOMALIES

The ultimate goal of clinical teratology is the prevention of congenital anomalies. There are a few examples of interventions that have been successful in this regard. Probably the best known is widespread rubella immunization of children (Preblud and Alford 1990), but passive immunization of rhesus-negative women to prevent hydrops fetalis provides another important instance (Bowman 1991).

The knowledge of health professionals about potential teratogenic risks is very important in avoiding dangerous exposures. Public education is crucial to avoiding self-inflicted exposures such as the use of 'recreational' drugs. Scientists and physicians have a social responsibility to ensure that the information provided to the public about teratogenic risks is as accurate and balanced as possible.

Regulation and legislation are important means of protecting pregnant women from harmful exposures. Regulatory restriction of thalidomide, for example, has certainly prevented many birth defects. Regulation is often a crude tool, however, and official labelling of drugs sometimes does more harm than good by causing unnecessary alarm among patients and their physicians (Friedman 1993).

The most spectacular current opportunity for prevention of congenital anomalies lies in dietary supplementation with folic acid. Folic acid supplementation before and during pregnancy reduces the risk of spina bifida and certain other birth defects substantially (Czeizel and Dudas 1992). The typical Western diet is deficient in folic acid, at least in terms of preventing birth defects. Fortification of staple foods with folic acid has been recommended, but until this is implemented women who are pregnant or are capable of becoming pregnant should take folic acid supplements (*Morbidity and Mortality Weekly Reports* 1993).

REFERENCES

Abrams, E.J. and Rogers, M.F. (1991). Pediatric HIV infection. *Baillière's Clinical Haematology*, 4, 333–59.

Adams, J. and Lammer, E.J. (1993). Neurobehavioral teratology of isotretinoin. *Reproductive Toxicology*, 7, 175–7.

Adler, S.P. (1992). Cytomegalovirus and pregnancy. *Current Opinion in Obstetrics and Gynecology*, 4, 670–5.

Arnold, G.L., Kirby, R.S., Langendoerfer, S., and Wilkins-Haug, L. (1994). Toluene embryopathy: clinical delineation and developmental follow-up. *Pediatrics*, 93, 216–20.

Austin, C.R. (1973). Embryo transfer and sensitivity to teratogenesis. *Nature*, 224, 333–4.

Baird, P.A., Anderson, T.W., Newcombe, H.B., and Lowry, R.B. (1988). Genetic disorders in children and young adults: a population study. *American Journal of Human Genetics*, 42, 677–93.

Behnke, M. and Eyler, F.D. (1993). The consequences of prenatal substance use for the developing fetus, newborn, and young child. *International Journal of Addiction*, 28, 1341–91.

Berry, P.J., Gray, E.S., Portar, J.H., and Burton, P.A. (1992). Parvovirus infection of the human fetus and newborn. *Seminars in Diagnostic Pathology*, 9, 4–12.

Bilowus, M., Abbassi, V., and Givvons, M.D. (1986). Female pseudohermaphroditism in a neonate born to a mother with polycystic ovarian disease. *Journal of Urology*, 136, 1098–100.

Bowman, J.M. (1991). Antenatal suppression of Rh alloimmunization. *Clinical Obstetrics and Gynecology*, 34, 296–303.

Brent, R.L. (1986*a*). Editorial comment: definition of a teratogen and the relationship of teratogenicity to carcinogenicity. *Teratology*, 34, 359–60.

Brent, R.L. (1986*b*). Evaluating the alleged teratogenicity of environmental agents. *Clinical Perinatology*, 13, 609–14.

Brent, R.L. and Beckman, D.A. (1990). Environmental teratogens. *Bulletin of the New York Academy of Medicine*, 66, 123–63.

Brent, R.L. and Beckman, D.A. (1991). Angiotensin-converting enzyme inhibitors, an embryopathic class of drugs with unique properties: information for clinical teratology counselors. *Teratology*, 43, 543–6.

Brunskill, P.J. (1992). The effects of fetal exposure to danazol. *British Journal of Obstetrics and Gynaecology*, 99, 212–15.

Buehler, B.A., Delimont, D., van Waes, M., and Finnell, R.H. (1990). Prenatal prediction of risk of the fetal hydantoin syndrome. *New England Journal of Medicine*, 322, 1567–72.

Burbacher, T.M., Rodier, P.M., and Weiss, B. (1990). Methylmercury developmental neurotoxicity: a comparison of effects in humans and animals. *Neurotoxicology and Teratology*, 12, 191–202.

Chen, D.T., Jacobson, M.M., and Kuntzman, R.G. (1990). Experience with the retinoids in human pregnancy. In *Basic science in toxicology*, (ed. G.N. Volans), pp. 473–82. Francis Taylor, London.

Cohen, L.S., Friedman, J.M., Jefferson, J.W., *et al.* (1994). A reevaluation of risk of *in utero* exposure to lithium. *Journal of the American Medical Association*, 271, 146–50.

Cohlan, S.Q. (1977). Tetracycline staining of teeth. *Teratology*, 15, 127–30.

Coles, D.C. (1992). Prenatal alcohol exposure and human development. In *Development of the central nervous system: effects of alcohol and opiates*, (ed. M.W. Miller), pp. 9–36. Wiley-Liss, New York.

Cordero, J.F. and Oakley, G.P. (1983). Drug exposure during pregnancy: some epidemiological considerations. *Clinical Obstetrics and Gynecology*, 26, 418–28.

Czeizel, A.E. and Dudas, I. (1992). Prevention of the first occurrence of neural tube defects by periconceptional vitamin supplementation. *New England Journal of Medicine*, 327, 1832–5.

Dansky, L.V. and Finnell, R.H. (1991). Parental epilepsy, anticonvulsant drugs, and reproductive outcome: epidemiologic and experimental findings spanning three decades. 2. Human studies. *Reproductive Toxicology*, 5, 301–35.

Davis, J.M., Otto, D.A., Weil, D.E., and Grant, L.D. (1990). The comparative developmental neurotoxicity of lead in humans and animals. *Neurotoxicology and Teratology*, 12, 215–29.

Delgado-Escueta, A.V. and Janz, D. (1992). Consensus guidelines: preconception counselling, management, and care of the pregnant woman with epilepsy. *Neurology*, 42, (Suppl. 5), 149–60.

Dubey, J.P. and Beattie, C.P. (1988). *Toxoplasmosis of animals and man*. CRC Press, Boca Raton.

Einarson, T.R., Leeder, J.S., and Koren, G. (1988). A method for meta-analysis of epidemiological studies. *Drug Intelligence and Clinical Pharmacy*, 22, 813–24.

Ernhart, C.B. (1992). A critical review of low-level prenatal lead exposure in the human: 1. effects on the fetus and newborn. *Reproductive Toxicology*, 6, 9–19.

Fonda Allen, J.F. and Rosenbaum, K.N. (1992). Counselling after exposure to excessive amounts of beta-carotene in the first trimester: a case report. *Teratology*, 45, 459–60.

Frank, D.A., Bresnahan, K., and Zuckerman, B.S. (1993). Maternal cocaine use: impact on child health and development. *Advances in Pediatrics*, 40, 65–99.

Fredricsson, B. and Gilljam, H. (1992). Smoking and reproductions: short and long term effects and benefits of smoking cessation. *Acta Obstetrica et Gynecologica Scandinavica*, 71, 580–92.

Friedman, J.M. (1993). Report of the Teratology Society public affairs committee symposium on FDA classification of drugs. *Teratology*, 48, 5–6.

Friedman, J.M. and Polifka, J.E. (1994). *Teratogenic effects of drugs: a resource for clinicians* (TERIS). The Johns Hopkins University Press, Baltimore.

Garner, P. (1995). Type I diabetes mellitus and pregnancy. *Lancet*, 346, 157–61.

Generoso, W.M., Shourbaji, A.G., Piegorsch, W.W., and Bishop, J.B. (1991). Developmental response of zygotes exposed to similar mutagens. *Mutation Research*, 250, 439–46.

Ginsburg, K.A., Blacker, C.M., Abel, E.L., and Sokol, R.J. (1991). Fetal alcohol exposure and adverse pregnancy outcomes. *Contributions to Gynecology and Obstetrics*, 18, 115–29.

Goldman, A.S. and Yaffe, S.J. (1978). Fetal trimethadione syndrome. *Teratology*, 17, 103–6.

Hanson, J.W. (1986). Teratogen update: fetal hydantoin effects. *Teratology*, 33, 349–53.

Hanssens, M., Keirsc, M.J.N.C., Vankelecom, F., and Van, Assche, F.A. (1991). Fetal and neonatal effect of treatment with angiotensin-converting enzyme inhibitors in pregnancy. *Obstetrics and Gynecology*, 78, 128–35.

Jones, K.L., Smith, D.W., Ulleland, C.N., and Streissguth, A.P. (1973). Pattern of malformation in offspring of chronic alcoholic mothers. *Lancet*, i, 1267–71.

Kimmel, C.A., Generoso, W.M., Thomas, R.D., and Bakshi, K.S. (1973). A new frontier in understanding the mechanisms of developmental abnormalities. *Toxicology and Applied Pharmacology*, 119, 159–65.

Kirshon, B., Wasserstrum, N., Wlllis, R., Hermn, G.E., and McCabe, E.R.B. (1988). Teratogenic effects of first trimester cyclophosphamide therapy. *Obstetrics and Gynecology*, 72, 462.

Lenke, R.R. and Levy, H.L. (1980). Maternal phenylketonuria and hyperphenylalaninemia. *New England Journal of Medicine*, 303, 1202–8.

Lenz, W. (1962). Thalidomide and congenital abnormalities. *Lancet*, i, 271–2.

Lenz, W. (1966). Malformations caused by drugs in pregnancy. *American Journal of Diseases of Children*, 112, 99–106.

Lenz, W. and Knapp, K. (1962). Thalidomide embryopathy. *Archives of Environmental Health*, 5, 100–5.

Lindhout, D. and Omtzigt, J.G.C. (1992). Pregnancy and the risk of teratogenicity. *Epilepsia*, 33, (Suppl. 4), S41–8.

Lindhout, D. and Omtzigt, J.G.C. (1994). Teratogenic effects of antiepileptic drugs: implications for the management of epilepsy in women of childbearing age. *Epilepsia*, 35, (Suppl. 4), S19–28.

Lione, A. (1988). Polychlorinated biphenyls and reproduction. *Reproductive Toxicology*, 2, 83–90.

McBride, W.G. (1961). Thalidomide and congenital abnormalities. *Lancet*, ii, 1358.

Mascola, L., Pelosi, R., Blont, J.H., Alexander, C.E., and Cates, W. (1985). Congenital syphilis revisited. *American Journal of Diseases of Children*, 139, 575–80.

Miller, E.H. (1994). Metabolic management of diabetes in pregnancy. *Seminars in Perinatology*, 18, 414–31.

Mitchell, A.A. (1992). Oral retinoids. What should the prescriber know about their teratogenic hazards among women of child-bearing potential? *Drug Safety*, 7, 79–85.

Morbidity and Mortality Weekly Report (1993). Recommendations for use of folic acid to reduce number of spina bifida cases and other neural tube defects. *Journal of the American Medical Association*, 269, 1233–8.

Mole, R.H. (1993). The biology and radiobiology of *in utero* development in relation to radiological protection. *British Journal of Radiology*, 66, 1095–102.

Mutchinick, O., Aizpuru, E., and Grether, P. (1992). The human teratogenic effect of cyclophosphamide. *Teratology*, 45, 329.

Nicolini, U. and Monni, G. (1990). Intestinal obstruction in babies exposed *in utero* to methylene blue. *Lancet*, 336, 1258–9.

Oakley, G.P. and Erickson, J.D. (1995). Vitamin A and birth defects: continuing caution is needed. *New England Journal Medicine*, 333, 1414–15.

Pearson, M.A., Hoyme, H.E., Seaver, I.J., and Rimsza, M.E. (1994). Toluene embryopathy: delineation of phenotype and comparison with fetal alcohol syndrome. *Pediatrics*, 93, 211–15.

Preblud, S.R. and Alford, C.A. (1990). Rubella. In *Infectious diseases of the fetus and newborn infant*, (ed. pp. 196–240 J.S. Remington and J.O. Klein), W.B. Saunders, Philadelphia.

Reece, E.A. and Hobbins, J.C. (1986). Diabetic embryopathy: pathogenesis, prenatal diagnosis, and prevention. *Obstetric and Gynecological Surveys*, 41, 325–35.

Remington, J.S. and Desmonts, G. (1990). Toxoplasmosis. In *Infectious diseases of the fetus and newborn infant*, (ed. J.S. Remington and J.O. Klein), pp. 89–95. W.B. Saunders, Philadelphia.

Rohr, F.J., Doherty, L.B., Waisbren, S.E., Bailey, I.V., Ampola, M.G., Benacerraf, B., and Lavy, H. (1987). New England maternal PKU project: prospective study of untreated and treated pregnancies and their outcomes. *Journal of Pediatrics*, 110, 391–8.

Rosa, F.W., Wilk, A.L., and Kelsey, F.O. (1986). Teratogen update: vitamin A congeners. *Teratology*, 33, 355–64.

Rosenberg, M.J. (ed.) (1987). *Smoking and reproductive health*. PSG publishing Company, Littleton, Massachusetts.

Rosenn, B. and Tsang, R.C. (1991). The effects of maternal diabetes on the fetus and neonate. Annals of *Clinical Laboratory Science*, **21**, 153–70.

Rothman, K.J., Moore, L.L., Singer, M.R., Nguyen, U-S., Mannino, S., and Milunsky, A. (1995). Teratogenicity of high vitamin A intake. *New England Journal of Medicine*, **333**, 12369–73.

Roubenoff, R., Hoyt, J., Petri, M., Horchberg, M.C., and Hellnann, D.B. (1988). Effects of antiinflamatory and immunosuppressive drugs on pregnancy and fertility. *Seminars on Arthritis and Rheumatism*, **18**, 88–110.

Schardein, J.L. (1980). Congenital abnormalities and hormones during pregnancy: a clinical review. *Teratology*, **22**, 251–70.

Schull, W.H., Norton, S., and Jensch, R.P. (1990). Ionizing radiation and the developing brain. *Neurotoxicology and Teratology*, **12**, 249–60.

Shepard, T.H. (1994). 'Proof' of human teratogenicity. *Teratology*, **50**, 97–8.

Shmoys, S. and Kaplan, C. (1990). Parvovirus and pregnancy. *Clinical Obstetrics and Gynecology*, **33**, 268–75.

Shotan, A., Widerhorn, J., Hurst, A., and Elkayam, U. (1994). Risk of angiotensin-converting enzyme inhibition during pregnancy: experimental and clinical evidence, potential mechanisms, and recommendations for use. *American Journal of Medicine*, **96**, 451–6.

Sicklick, M.J. and Rubinstein, A. (1992). Types of HIV infection and the course of the disease. In *HIV infection and developmental disabilities: a resource for service providers*, (ed. A.C. Crocker, H.J. Cohen and T.A. Kastner), pp. 15–23. Paul H. Brookes, Baltimore.

Singer, L., Arendt, R., and Minnes, S. (1993). Neurodevelopmental effects of cocaine. *Clinical Perinatology*, **20**, 245–62.

South, M.A. and Sever, J.L. (1985). Teratogen update: the congenital rubella syndrome. *Teratology*, **31**, 297–307.

Stagno, S. (1990). Cytomegalovirus. In *Infectious diseases of the fetus and newborn infant*, (ed. J.S. Remington and J.O. Klein), pp. 241–81. W.B. Suanders, Philadelphia.

Stoffer, S.S. and Hamburger, J.I. (1976). Inadvertent I^{131} therapy for hyperthyroidism in the first trimester of pregnancy. *Journal of Nuclear Medicine*, **17**, 146–9.

Tilson, H.A., Jacobson, J.L., and Rogan, W.J. (1990). Polychlorinated biphenyls and the developing nervous system: cross-species comparisons. *Neurotoxicology and Teratology*, **12**, 239–48.

Van den Veyver, I.B. and Moise, K.J. (1993). Prostaglandin synthetase inhibitors in pregnancy. *Obstetric and Gynecologyical Surveys*, **48**, 493–502.

van der Pol, J.G., Wolf, H., Boer, K., Treffers, P.E., Leschot, N.J., Hey, H.A., *et al.* (1992). Jejunal atresia related to the use of methylene blue in genetic amniocentesis in twins. *British Journal Obstetrics and Gynaecology*, **99**, 141–3.

Warkany, J. (1978). Aminopterin and methotrexate: folic acid deficiency. *Teratology*, **17**, 353–8.

Warkany, J. (1981). Teratogenicity of folic acid antagonists. *Cancer Bulletrin*, **33**, 76–7.

Warkany, J. (1986). Teratogen update: hyperthermia. *Teratology*, **33**, 365–71.

Wiebe, V.J. and Sipila, P.E.H. (1994). Pharmacology of anitneoplastic agents in pregnancy. *Critical Reviews in Oncology and Hematology*, **16**, 75–112.

Wilson, J.G. and Brent, R.L. (1981). Are female sex hormones teratogenic? *American Journal of Obstetrics and Gynecology*, **141**, 567–80.

Wong, V., Cheng, C.H., and Chan, K.C. (1993). Fetal and neonatal outcome of exposure to anticoagulants during pregnancy. *American Journal of Medical Genetics*, **45**, 17–21.

Yerby, M.S. and Devinsky, O. (1994). Epilepsy and pregnancy. *Advances in Neurology*, **64**, 45–63.

28 | *Ethics of embryo research: What status the embryo, which duties to future generations?*

Francoise Shenfield and Claude Sureau

INTRODUCTION

What is included in any title may enlighten us as to what is discussed beneath. We attempt here an analysis of what and why it may be, between description and prescription, ethically or morally (Quere 1992) right or wrong to perform research on the human embryo. We are particularly concerned with the embryo *in vitro*, especially since the scientific and clinical landmark of the first human *in vitro* fertilization (IVF), resulting in a live pregnancy (Steptoe and Edwards 1978), has made the embryo available to the scrutiny of scientists outside the maternal environment. The subtitle of this chapter reflects two fundamental points, based on the important philosophical theories of deontology and consequentialism: can and should the respect firmly articulated by Kant in his categorical imperative (Raphael 1981) as owed to the person, be shown to the human embryo? And, how do we place research on this entity in the context of its consequence, the child to be, necessarily a symbol of future generations towards whom we should be acting responsibly (Fagot-Largeault 1995)?

The term embryo, however, needs to be further defined, as it covers several stages, starting at the fertilization of gametes and up to 10–12 weeks of pregnancy, before it becomes a fetus. This entity has already given rise to a famous semantic debate: the use of the term pre-embryo, or 'the stage of the conceptus for the interval from the completion of the process of fertilization until the establishment of biologic individuation' (Jones and Schrader 1989), led to controversy and suspicion that its human essence was deliberately being ignored or diminished by this prefix, when it was branded as 'circumstantial ontology' (Seve 1994).

In order to allay this concern, the explanatory subtitle places the subject firmly into the context of research on an entity, the embryo, whose status must be defined. If academic lawyers have written essays on how this may fit with only two categories known by the law, a '*res*' (a 'thing') which could then become property; or a person, which cannot be treated as such (Kennedy 1988; Grubb 1992), a consensus seems to have emerged. Indeed, this consensus encompassed societies as culturally different as the French and the American, when the embryo was called practically simultaneously a 'potential person' by the *Comité Consultatif National d'Ethique pour les Sciences de la Vie et de la Santé* (CCNE 1995) and in the Supreme Court of Tennessee at the occasion of a famous case concerning the battle of divorced parents (Davis v. Davis) for their cryopreserved embryos (Reid *et al.* 1992). Thus, the human embryo deserves respect because of its human 'potential' and kinship. Furthermore, this very notion of respect is enshrined in both the French legislation of 1994 (*Loi 94–653*, concerning 'respect of the human body and its products') and the British '*Human Fertilisation and Embryology Act*' (*HUFE Act* 1990). The British Act set up the Human Fertilization and Embryology Authority (HFEA), whose *Code of practice* (HFEA 1990) spells out that the respect of the embryo is 'fundamental to the Act' and delineates the duties and responsibilities of scientists and practitioners to their patients and the potential offspring this embryo may represent.

The practice of research on human beings, whether therapeutic or non-therapeutic, has been subjected to strict regulations in order to assure protection against abuse, many of which, established since the ten 'basic principles ... [of] moral, ethical and legal concepts' enunciated at the judgment of the Nuremberg trials, became known as the Nuremberg Code (Kennedy and Grubb 1989). The purpose of research must withstand scientific analysis and be of a nature which is impossible to achieve in animal research. Consent to the research is the key to the respect for the autonomy of the subject concerned and in the case of the embryos, may only be given by proxies, i.e. the male and female persons providing the gametes at its origins. Most of our analysis will concentrate on the research performed on the embryo *in vitro*. It is important to note, however, that if performed on the embryo *in vivo*, or embryonic or fetal material expulsed or evacuated from the uterus, the question of consent becomes complicated by the analogy with the necessary legal consent to termination of pregnancy, where the putative father of the pregnancy has no legal say (European Court of Human Rights 1980).

The notion of the fetus as a patient is relatively recent, because of its increased accessibility and visibility, particularly with modern ultrasound. The ethical implications have been well described, particularly in the rare instances of 'feto-maternal conflict' (McCullough and Chervenak 1994). It is thus not surprising that this concept of an embryo as a potential patient followed closely afterwards.

Society in general has added its scrutiny to that of the microscope, from lay attention concerning the quintessential human endeavour of reproduction, to the specialist and focused attention of philosophers, stating that the real question is 'when does life begin to matter morally?', rather than 'what is a person?' (Harris 1985); or that an 'abstract philosophical question (the moral status of the embryo) may be turned into a practical question, moral action concerning the embryo' (Dunstan 1989). Many debates on the subject have concentrated on the care and precautions to be taken, often dictated by legal limits (*HUFE Act* 1990, *Loi 94–654*) and duty towards the future generation, symbolized by the embryo and its human potential.

We will first outline the ethical dilemmas raised by embryo research *per se* and argue for the inevitability of discussing, if not determining, the status of the embryo, and the necessity of research, then analyse its implications with regards to the applications of the research accomplished to diagnosis and therapy. In conclusion, we will examine the possibility of consensus in Europe, and our duty to future generations by ensuring the safety of the applications of research.

EMBRYO RESEARCH: THE NECESSITY

Animal embryo research, when performed on species which reproduce rapidly, allows us to forecast possible problems resulting from assisted reproduction techniques which might affect future generations. But it may not answer all the questions relative to the human embryo and its eventual ability to fulfil its potential. Not only does pathology often differ between species (for instance ectopic pregnancy or repeated miscarriage specific to the human species), but the goals are often dissimilar, concentrating on 'quality' and commercial value in animals. The 'tools and strategies' gained, however, may be applied to human medicine, 'if they contribute to ethically acceptable goals in human medicine' (Baird 1995). Of these goals, one is the improvement of success rates in IVF: if IVF is morally acceptable, so is embryo research, the latter being necessary to the improvement of the former. The position of the Catholic Church, which forbids both, is just as logical. In this context, the end does not justify the means.

The consequentialist argument has been thrashed out in debates like this, organized under the aegis of the Ciba Foundation (1984), or the different '*avis*' published by the CCNE during its first 10 years of existence (CCNE 1995).

Advice and reflection are essential, but may only serve as guidelines at most. When society feels strongly enough about the matter concerned, legislation is enacted. The time interval between the Warnock report (Warnock 1984) and legislation (*HUFE Act* 1990), and the rapport Lenoir (Lenoir 1991) and the July 1994 *Loi* (*Loi* 94–653, *Loi* 94–654) reflect, respectively in the UK and France, the intensity and breadth of public concern in matters of reproduction. Both avoid qualifying the status of the embryo as such, within the only two categories known in law: '*res*' (or thing, property) or person. The HFEA *Code of practice* (HFEA 1990) stresses 'that the special status of the embryo is fundamental to the provisions of the Act' without defining this special quality, and French law underlines the respect due to the human body 'as soon as life begins' without defining this precise moment (*Loi* 94–653, *Relative au respect du corps humain*).

National differences in legislation reflect cultural as well as historical influences: for instance, German legislation forbids embryo 'consumptive' research (Beier and Beckman 1991). It is interesting to compare, however, the British and French legislation, where some research is allowed to rather different degrees, within specific boundaries and circumstances. The framework of the British legislation is dual: each research project has to be approved and granted a three year licence by the HFEA, as long as it falls within any one of five categories allowed in the Act (promoting advances in the treatment of infertility, increasing knowledge about the causes of congenital disease and causes of miscarriages, developing more effective techniques of contraception, or methods for detecting the presence of gene or chromosome abnormalities in embryos before implantation). Section 3 of the Act details the activities prohibited, amongst which are cloning, the creation of chimeras, trans-species transfer, or the alteration of the embryonic genome. Finally there is a time limit for *in vitro* research of 14 days, or the apparition of the neural plate, for which the consensus is internationally far-reaching (FIGO 1994). This does not so much reflect the principle of graduation and potentiality as a compromise between varied interests, as in fact a 14 day embryo *in vitro* loses its potential to become human, and thus could arguably be experimented on more easily than a younger one (Baird 1995).

The French legislation passed in July 1994 symbolizes the difficulty in finding a compromise which makes sense: it leaves a void of interpretation, stipulating that embryo 'experimentation' is forbidden, as is the conception *in vitro* of human embryos specifically for studies, research, or experimentation. 'Studies' are allowed with a couple's consent 'in exceptional (undefined) circumstances', as long as they do not threaten the integrity of the embryo (*Loi 94–659*), and with approval of the *Commission nationale de medecine et de biologie de la reproduction et du diagnostic prénatal*. As the terms 'study', 'experimentation', and 'research' are not defined, it is not surprising that the '*décrets d'application*' are eagerly awaited.

If one accepts that embryo research is permissible, two further problems arise: the source of embryos, and their fate. In most cases embryos used for research will be destroyed, as safety of the potential child who might ensue could not be assured, and it can actually be argued that it would be unethical to replace such embryos *in utero*. Since the possibility of cryopreservation of embryos (Downing *et al.* 1985) has enabled couples to have further attempts at embryo transfer from one stimulatory IVF cycle, the creation of embryos purely for research purposes has been even more topical. French legislation makes this a criminal offence (*Loi 94–654*), and the HUFE Act leaves to the HFEA the control of every single research project in the UK, for which a three-year license is granted. A draft convention on bioethics issued by the steering committee on bioethics set up by the Council of Europe states that embryos may not be created with the intention of conducting research on them (Council of Europe 1994).

The same issue has given rise to a complex debate in the US, after the report of the National Institute of Health (NIH) embryo research panel had endorsed pre-implantation embryo research on the grounds that it offers potential benefits to infertile couples, and because the pre-embryo 'does not have the same moral status as infants or children' (Fletcher 1995). In the case of fertilization of embryos for research alone, the panel outlined two special categories according to the nature of the research and its 'outstanding scientific and therapeutic value', including, for instance, research on freezing of oocytes followed by fertilization, or the comparison of embryos from couples 'at risk' of congenital defects and 'controls'. Within a few hours, a presidential statement directed the NIH not to support such research.

This dilemma about the source of embryos can go one step further, with the theoretical possibility of using fetal material from animal research or ovarian grafts as a source of oocytes (Gosden 1990). In the UK, a public consultation by the HFEA on the matter of fetal sources, relating to both therapeutic use (when it would be technologically feasible) and research, was undertaken in 1994. Mostly for psychological reasons of unease, fetal material was deemed suitable for research, but not therapeutic use (HFEA 1994). This consultation went into depth on the problem of who gives consent for the use of fetal material, outlined the specificity of the gift of gametes and reproducible cells (as compared to other cells), and challenged the separation principle. This had been recommended in the Polkinghorne report, in order to enable the woman contemplating a termination of pregnancy to consider, without undue pressure, the donation of the ensuing material (Polkinghorne 1989).

Finally, the proposals from the HFEA to lengthen the statutory limit for cryo-preservation of embryos from five years (by the application of the 1990 statute) to ten years (DoH 1995) have been accepted. This may reflect, in part, the difficulty encountered when trying to come to terms with the consequences of the technique and, particularly, contemplating the destruction of embryos, although the *Code of practice* recommends it should be done 'in a sensitive manner' (Shenfield *et al.* 1993). Another question may be raised though: is destruction, howeve, sensitive, better than allocation to research which might prove of benefit to future generations, if the couple donating their gametes have not jointly decided to offer their supernumary embryos to another couple in need?

EMBRYO RESEARCH: THE CONSEQUENCES OF ITS ACCEPTANCE

Once pre-implantation embryo research is accepted, it follows that its status as a non-person is implicitly recognized: this is not because its consent cannot be obtained, as there are several instances in law where proxy consent is accepted (of children, or adults unable to give proper consent for reasons of 'incapacity'); but rather that its destruction is necessarily planned, distancing the embryo more remotely from full human status. By definition, when the technique researched has proven to be safe and useful, it may become therapeutic or diagnostic. Then the embryo concerned may be allowed to fulfil its potential to become a person, which, in British law, it is not until it is born alive (Kennedy and Grubb 1989).

New techniques applied to the pre-implantation embryo have also raised new dilemmas: pre-implantation diagnosis is a good example of a technique which has only recently left the field of research to become a diagnostic tool (Handyside *et al.* 1990). Its practice is submitted to stringent controls, both in the UK via the HFEA licensing system, and in France. The '*Loi*' allows the practice in 'exceptional circumstances', if a 'couple has a strong probability to give birth to a child suffering from a particularly grave and incurable genetic disease' (*Loi* 94–654). Such safeguards should allay lay fears and fantasies concerning the selection of future children according to particular non-pathological characteristic, like the colour of their eyes (Robertson 1992). Similarly, the choice of the sex of a child for social reasons (i.e. other than sex-linked congenital abnormality), was deemed to be unethical (Shenfield 1994) and rejected in the UK after public consultation by the HFEA. This applies to pre-conceptual selection (when efficient and reliable) as well as pre-implantation, whilst its falls within legislation for termination of pregnancy when we consider prenatal selection.

Nevertheless, there remain other matters of reproduction linked to research on pre-implantation embryos which have given rise to public concern, and cloning is one of them. All of the different types of cloning, namely nuclear transplantation, blastomere separation, or bisection (Jones and Edwards 1994) elicit discomfort. Indeed, blastomere separation gave rise to debate and strong statements ('if the aim of research is morally objectionable, all other ethical preconditions for research become irrelevant') in the pages of *Fertility and Sterility* (Nisker and Baylis 1994). The main objection to cloning, however, stems from the threat of trivializing the individual by replicating the entity that is the embryo, with the consequence of creating identical potential persons: it would 'violate the inherent uniqueness and dignity of individuals' by deliberate twinning, if used to 'increase the number of embryos transferred, avoid subsequent egg retrieval, become a form of life insurance, or, enable the selection of a desirable genome' (Robertson 1994). The latter, especially, raises the spectre of attempts, forcibly conducted in Nazi Germany, to enhance the 'Aryan race' by marriage legislation (Arendt 1972). This type of imposition from a State without consent individuals is akin to the 'eugenism' expressly forbidden in the French legislation, where it is described as 'an organised selection of persons' (*Loi* 94–653). Indeed, consent is one of the safeguards recognized internationally as an essential protection against the possible abuses stemming from embryo research (American Fertility Society Ethics Committee 1994).

GUIDELINES FOR THE FUTURE

Thus, in Europe and North America, consent represents one of the keys to consensus on the acceptability of pre-implantation embryo research. Consent of the gamete donors is the subject of the whole of Schedule 3 of the *HUFE Act* (1990), and is also enshrined in the French *Loi*. The subject of research on the embryo *in vivo* is not covered here. This more mature embryo has, by virtue of its successful implantation, greater potential to become a person and hence, even firmer claims to protection, and certainly to non-destruction, or protection from harm resulting from research.

The other common principle, that of '*res extra commercio*', is also enshrined in the *HUFE Act* (1990), with the exception of 'a sum as directed by the *Code of practice*' for gamete donation. Its phasing out, considered in the HFEA *Annual report* (HFEA 1996) would certainly increase the consistency of the principle stated (i.e. no money or benefit (to be exchanged) in respect of gametes and embryos) and strengthen the spirit of donation (Shenfield and Steele 1995).

Amongst other safeguards, as in all research, openness is necessary, in order to enhance public participation in a debate which involves not only the professionals involved, but all members of society. As pointed out by a recent *Avis* of the CCNE, the role of those purveying scientific infomation is particularly sensitive and responsible (CCNE 1995). This also means that all results should be published; that advice is sought from scientific and representative authorities on the French or British model; and that periodic reviews are planned to ensure updating of the legal constraints, if necessary. This is the case for the French *loi*, which will be reviewed within five years.

Indeed there has been a recent call in the US for 'independant regulations of assisted reproductive technologies' (Jones 1996).

Finally, the child which might ensue from an embryo replaced *in utero*, when the research can be safely applied, has interests which must be considered (Fagot-Largeault 1995). In order to behave responsibly towards future generations, there is a need to follow up those embryos who have achieved their potential to become persons, thanks to what was only research yesterday. The mother, recipient and carrier, hopefully to term, of the potential person, may also be watched, in order to ensure that no harm comes to her, but this is unlikely to cause legal problems as she was, as an adult, able to give consent, or refuse to participate.

As far as the children are concerned, several problems arise: the length of time the follow-up may be necessary entails an invasion of the privacy of the family concerned. Furthermore, the more mature the child, the more inappropriate it becomes to perform any test or observation with the consent of the parents rather than the child itself. This is reflected in British law by the notion of the 'Gillick competent child', after a case concerning the legality of prescribing contraception to an under-age child (Kennedy and Grubb 1989). The *HUFE Act* (1990) also underlines the respect for privacy, with great concern for confidentiality. Thus, there is no obligation for parents to inform their child that 'they may be the product of an assisted method' of fertility treatment. If informed, however, the child will subsequently have rights to anonymous information in the case of gamete donation at 18, for instance.

The psychological aspects are intricate and demand sensitive handling, which legislation may not necessarily portray, although the provision of counselling is mandatory in British law (*HUFE Act* 1990).

In order to promote public understanding and tolerance of the advances of science, it is essential to inform patients better of the rapid advances seen regularly in the field of reproduction, and their full implications. It is just as essential for the professional to listen to the concerns of potential patients and society in general, as we do not function in a vacuum. But it is very rare indeed that our aims should not coincide: that is, to fulfil our duty to the present and future generations.

REFERENCES

American Fertility Society Ethics Committee (1994). Ethical considerations of assisted reproductive technologies. *Fertility and Sterility*, **62**, Suppl. 1, Chapter 10, 355–75.

Arendt, H. (1972). Le systeme totalitaire. *Points Politique*, Po53 (transl. J.L. Bourget, R. Davreu, and P. Lévy), p. 115. Editions du Seuil, Paris.

Baird, P. (1995). Research on pre-embryos (zygotes). In *Ethical aspects of human reproduction Ethique et Sciences*, (ed. Claude Sureau and Francoise Shenfield), p. 327–40. John Libbey Eurotext, Paris.

Beier, H.M. and Beckman, J.O. (1991). Implications and consequences of the German embryo protection Act, 1991. *Human Reproduction*, **6**, 607–8.

CCNE (Comité Consultatif National d'Ethique pour les Sciences de la vie et de la Santé) (1995). Avis concernant l'embryon, 1986, 1990; Avis relatif aux recherches sur les embryons humains *in vitro*, et sur les recherches soumises à un moratoire depuis 1986. Centre de documentation et d'information d'ethique, 101 rue de Tolbiac, 75–654 Paris, Cedex 13. Avis no 45 sur les questions éthiques posées par la transmission de l'information scientifique relative à la recherche biologique et médicale. In *Les cahiers du CCNE*, No 5, Octobre 1995, pp. 3–8. Biomedition, Levallois-Perret.

Ciba Foundation (1984). *Human embryo research: Yes or No?* Tavistock, London.

Council of Europe (1994). Draft convention for the protection of human rights and dignity of the human being with regard to the application of biology and medicine: bioethics convention and explanatory report, Strasbourg, July 1994. *Dir/Jur*, 94, 2.

DoH (Department of Health) (1995). Press release, 19 December 1995. HFEA recommends extension to five-year storage period for human embryos. Richmond House, 79 Whitehall, London SW1A 2NS.

Downing, B.J., Mohr, L.R., Tronson, A., Freeman, L.E., and Wood, C. (1985). Pregnancy after transfer of frozen thawed embryo. *Medical Journal of Australia*, 142, 489–91.

Dunstan, G. (1989). The moral status of the embryo. In *Philosophical ethics in reproductive medicine*, (ed. D.R. Bronham, M.E. Dalton, and J.C. Jackson). Manchester University Press.

European Court of Human Rights (1980). Paton v. United Kingdom, 3 EHRR 408.

Fagot-Largeault, A. (1995). Procréation responsable. In *Ethical aspects of Reproduction Ethique et Sciences*, (ed. C. Sureau and F. Shenfield), pp. 3–18. John Libbey Eurotext, Paris.

FIGO, (1994). The FIGO Committee for the study of ethical aspects of human reproduction. FIGO Secretariat, 27 Sussex Place, Regents Park, London NW1 4RG.

Fletcher, J.C. (1995). US public policy on embryo research: two steps forward, one large step back. *Human Reproduction*, 10, 875–8.

Gosden, R.G. (1990). Restitution of fertility in sterilised mice by transferring primordial ovarian follicles. *Human Reproduction*, 5, 117–22.

Grubb, A. (1992). The legal status of the frozen human embryo. In *Challenges in Medical care*, pp. 69–87. Wiley, London.

Handyside, A.H., Kontogianni, E.H., Hardy, K., and Winston, R.L.M. (1990). Pregnancies from biopsied human pre-implanation embryos sexed by Y-specific DNA amplification. *Nature*, 244, 768–70.

Harris, J. (1985). Beings, human beings and persons. In *The value of life*, p. 10–18. Routledge, London and New York.

HFEA (Human Fertilisation and Embryology Authority) (1990). *Code of practice*. HMSO, London.

HFEA (Human Fertilisation and Embryology Authority) (1993). *Annual report*. HMSO, London.

HFEA (Human Fertilisation and Embryology Authority) (1994). *Donated ovarian tissue in embryo research and assisted conception*. HMSO, London.

HFEA (Human Fertilisation and Embryology Authority) (1995). *Annual report*. HMSO, London.

HUFA Act (Human Fertilisation and Embryology Act) (1990). HMSO, London.

Jones, H.W. (1996). The time has come. *Fertility and Sterility*, 65(6), 1090–2.

Jones, H.W. and Edwards R.G. (1994). On attempts at cloning in the human. *Fertility and Sterility*, 61, 423–7.

Jones, H.W. and Schrader, C. (1989). And just what is a pre-embryo? *Fertility and Sterility*, 52, 189–91.

Kennedy, I. (1988). The moral status of the embryo. In *Treat me right*, Ch. 6. Clarendon Press, Oxford.

Kennedy, I. and Grubb, A. (1989). A case study in medical law and ethics, Ch. 1, p. 17; Research, Ch. 11, p. 860; Facilitating conception, Ch. 8, p. 655. In *Medical law, text and material*. Butterworth, London.

Lenoir, N. (1991). Rapport au Premier Ministre. *Aux frontie*res de la vie. La documentation francaise, Paris.

Loi 94–653 du 29 Juillet 1994. *Relative au respect du corps humain.*

Loi 94–654 du 29 Juillet 1994. *Relative au don, assistance medicale à la procréation et diagnostic prénatal.*

McCullough, A.B. and Chervenak, F.A. (1994). *Ethics in obstetrics and gynaecology*, p. 117. Oxford University Press, New York and Oxford.

Nisker, J.A. and Baylis, F. (1994). The best of us (Letter to the editor). *Fertility and Sterility*, **62**, 893–4.

Polkinghorne, J. (1989). Review of the guidance on the research use of fetuses and fetal material. HMSO, London.

Quere, F. (1992). *L'éthique et la vie.* Editions Odile Jacob, Paris.

Raphael, D.D. (1981). *Kanthian ethics, moral philosophy.* Oxford University Press.

Reid, C.J., Anderson, Daughtrey, Drowota, and O'Brien J.J. (1992). Frozen embryos: legal status, disposition and control, Davis v. Davis. In *Medical law review*, (ed. I. Kennedy and A. Grubby), Vol. 1, No 2, pp. 273–8.

Robertson, J.A. (1992). Legal and ethical issues arising with preimplantation human embryos. *Archives of Pathology and Laboratory Medicine*, **116**, 430–6.

Robertson, J.A. (1994). The question of human cloning. *Hastings Center Report*, **24**, 6–14.

Séve, L. (1994). *Pour une critique de la raison bioéthique.* Editions Odile Jacob, Paris.

Shenfield, F. (1994). Sex selection: a matter for fancy or for ethical debate?. *Debates in Human Reproduction*, **9**, 569.

Shenfield, F. and Steele, S.J. (1995). A gift is a gift is a Gift, or why gametes donors should not be paid. *Human Reproduction* , **10**, 253–5.

Shenfield, F., Matson, P.L., Hamer, F., Lieberman, B.A., and Steele, S.J.S. (1993). The statutory limit for embryo storage in the UK: a potential problem for 1996. In *Dispatches*, Vol. 4, No 1, pp. 8–9. Centre of Medical Law and Ethics, King's College, The Strand, London.

Steptoe, P.C. and Edwards, R.G. (1978). Birth after the replacement of a human embryo. *Lancet*, ii, 366.

Warnock, M. (1984). *Report of the committee of inquiry into human fertilisation and embryology.* HMSO, London.

Index